MW00846660

Hospital Management and Emergency Medicine:

Breakthroughs in Research and Practice

Information Resources Management Association
USA

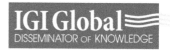

Published in the United States of America by
IGI Global
Medical Information Science Reference (an imprint of IGI Global)
701 E. Chocolate Avenue
Hershey PA, USA 17033
Tel: 717-533-8845
Fax: 717-533-8661
E-mail: cust@igi-global.com
Web site: http://www.igi-global.com

Copyright © 2020 by IGI Global. All rights reserved. No part of this publication may be reproduced, stored or distributed in any form or by any means, electronic or mechanical, including photocopying, without written permission from the publisher. Product or company names used in this set are for identification purposes only. Inclusion of the names of the products or companies does not indicate a claim of ownership by IGI Global of the trademark or registered trademark.

Library of Congress Cataloging-in-Publication Data

Names: Information Resources Management Association, editor.
Title: Hospital Management and emergency medicine : breakthroughs in research and
    practice / Information Resources Management Association, editor.
Description: Hershey, PA : Medical Information Science Reference, [2020] |
    Includes bibliographical references and index. | Summary: "This book
    examines the latest scholarly material on emerging strategies and
    methods for delivering optimal emergency medical care and examines the
    latest techniques and methods of critical care. It also shows how
    revolutionary technologies and methods are vastly improving how
    healthcare is implemented globally"-- Provided by publisher.
Identifiers: LCCN 2019040954 (print) | LCCN 2019040955 (ebook) | ISBN
    9781799824510 (hardcover) | ISBN 9781799824527 (ebook)
Subjects: MESH: Emergency Medical Services | Critical Care | Telemedicine |
    Models, Organizational | Cell Phone Use
Classification: LCC RC86.8 (print) | LCC RC86.8 (ebook) | NLM WX 215 |
    DDC 616.02/8--dc23
LC record available at https://lccn.loc.gov/2019040954
LC ebook record available at https://lccn.loc.gov/2019040955

British Cataloguing in Publication Data
A Cataloguing in Publication record for this book is available from the British Library.

The views expressed in this book are those of the authors, but not necessarily of the publisher.

For electronic access to this publication, please contact: eresources@igi-global.com.

Editor-in-Chief

Mehdi Khosrow-Pour, DBA
Information Resources Management Association, USA

Associate Editors

Steve Clarke, *University of Hull, UK*
Murray E. Jennex, *San Diego State University, USA*
Ari-Veikko Anttiroiko, *University of Tampere, Finland*

Editorial Advisory Board

Sherif Kamel, *American University in Cairo, Egypt*
In Lee, *Western Illinois University, USA*
Jerzy Kisielnicki, *Warsaw University, Poland*
Amar Gupta, *Arizona University, USA*
Craig van Slyke, *University of Central Florida, USA*
John Wang, *Montclair State University, USA*
Vishanth Weerakkody, *Brunel University, UK*

List of Contributors

Table of Contents

Section 2
Information Systems

Section 3
Management and Operations

Section 4
Quality and Performance

Preface

During times of medical emergencies, patients turn to hospitals for treatment, expecting emergency personnel to be well-trained and for the center to be well-equipped to effectively and efficiently meet their needs. Poorly managed emergency departments yield frustrating wait times and unnecessary charges and jeopardize patient health and can lead to death through the mismanagement of patient records, data, and resources. Hospitals can easily become chaotic, between high-pressure emergency medical events, unfamiliarity with the environment, and the strain of financial burdens and resource allocation. It is of the utmost importance, then, that hospitals continuously strive to become efficient, informative environments that provide excellent care.

It falls to researchers to analyze and, when needed, redesign hospital tools and management practices to make them as easy to use as possible. To ensure hospitals and emergency services are at an excellent level of quality, a multi-pronged approach is required, and by studying every element of hospitals from the ground up, issues within the day-to-day procedures are revealed.

Many researchers have answered the call and set out to improve hospital practices and facilities by studying its operations at every level, from data collection and organization to management policies. This is why IGI Global is pleased to offer this comprehensive reference that will support hospital directors, hospital staff, emergency medical services, paramedics, doctors, nurses, medical administrators, healthcare records specialists, medical data scientists, healthcare system operators, IT consultants, managers, and medical students.

This compilation is designed to act as a single reference source on conceptual, methodological, and technical aspects and will provide insight into emerging topics including but not limited to information management, patient monitoring, artificial intelligence, and performance improvement. The chapters within this publication are sure to provide readers the tools necessary for further research and discovery in their respective industries and/or fields.

Hospital Management and Emergency Medicine: Breakthroughs in Research and Practice is divided into four distinct sections that provide detailed, all-encompassing coverage of vital topics. These sections are:

1. Data Management;
2. Information Systems;
3. Management and Operations; and
4. Quality and Performance.

Section 1, "Data Management," explores methods and models of gathering and managing patient data. The first chapter in this section is "A New Approach to Generate Hospital Data Warehouse Schema" by Profs. José Machado and António Abelha from the University of Minho, Portugal. It proposes a method of collecting data from across hospitals in order to make them available for decision-making needs. The second chapter is "A Multi-Agent Based Modeling and Simulation Data Management and Analysis System for the Hospital Emergency Department" by Profs. Manel Saad Saoud, Abdelhak Boubetra, and Safa Attia from the University of Bordj Bou Arreridj, Algeria. It uses computer simulations of emergency departments to develop a robust decision support system. The third chapter, "A Case Study Perspective for Balanced Perioperative Workflow Achievement Through Data-Driven Process Improvement," by Prof. Jim Ryan from Auburn University, USA; Prof. Barbara Doster of the University of Alabama Birmingham Hospital, USA; Prof. Sandra Daily from Cullman Regional Medical Center, USA; and Prof. Carmen Lewis from Troy University, USA, illustrates how dynamic technological activities of analysis, evaluation, and synthesis applied to internal and external organizational data can highlight complex relationships within integrated processes to identify process limitations and potential process capabilities, ultimately yielding balanced patient workflow through data-driven perioperative process improvement. The following chapter, "A Soft Computing Approach for Data Routing in Hospital Area Networks (HAN)," by Profs. Rakhee and M. B. Srinivas from Birla Institute of Technology and Science Pilani, India, suggests an alternative model to delivering vital signs of patients within environments with rapidly changing traffic. The next chapter, "Categorize Readmitted Patients in Intensive Medicine by Means of Clustering Data Mining," by Profs. Rui Veloso, Filipe Portela, Manuel Filipe Santos, José Machado, and António da Silva Abelha of the University of Minho, Portugal and Profs. Fernando Rua and Álvaro Silva from the Intensive Care Unit, Centro Hospitalar do Porto, Porto, Portugal, examines methods of collecting data on readmitted patients. In the next chapter, "The Evolution of Comorbidities in Hospital Administrative Databases," by Profs. Alberto Freitas, Isabel Garcia Lema, and Altamiro Costa-Pereira from the University of Porto, Portugal & CINTESIS - Center for Health Technology and Services Research, Portugal, the comparison of comorbidities by administrative databases is discussed. In the following chapter, "Data Quality and Critical Events in Ventilation," by Profs. Filipe Portela and Manuel Filipe Santos from Universidade do Minho, Portugal; Profs. António Abelha and José Machado of Centro de Ciências e Tecnologias de Computação and Universidade do Minho, Portugal; and Prof. Fernando Rua from the Intensive Care Unit, Centro Hospitalar do Porto, Porto, Portugal, the critical events concept was applied to the ventilation system and a quality assessment of the collected data was performed when a new value arrived. Section 1 concludes with the chapter "An Online Neonatal Intensive-Care Unit Monitoring System for Hospitals in Nigeria" by Profs. Peter Adebayo Idowu, Franklin Oladiipo Asahiah, and Jeremiah Ademola Balogun from Obafemi Awolowo University, Nigeria and Prof. Olayinka Olufunmilayo Olusanya of Tai Solarin University of Education, Nigeria. This chapter presents an online monitoring system for the storage and retrieval of physiological data from neonates admitted into the Neonatal Intensive Care Units (NICU) of Obafemi Awolowo University Teaching Hospital.

Section 2, "Information Systems," covers improvements and updates to information systems within hospitals. Opening this section is "Effect of Information Service Competence and Contextual Factors on the Effectiveness of Strategic Information Systems Planning in Hospitals" by Profs. Shin-Yuan Hung and Wei-Min Huang from National Chung Cheng University, Taiwan; Prof. David C. Yen from SUNY at Oneonta, USA; and Profs. She-I Chang and Chien-Cheng Lu from National Chung Cheng University, Taiwan. It examines the effect of contextual factors and information service systems on strategic information systems planning (SISP) in order to lend Taiwanese hospitals a competitive edge. The second chapter, "Lessons Learned From the Implementation of an Emergency Department Information System," by Profs. Paraskevas Vezyridis, Stephen Timmons, and Heather Wharrad from the University of Nottingham, UK, examines social and technical factors for implementing an emergency department information system. In the following chapter, "A Simulation Knowledge Extraction-Based Decision Support System for the Healthcare Emergency Department," by Profs. Manel Saad Saoud, Abdelhak Boubetra, and Safa Attia from the University of Bordj Bou Arreridj, Algeria, a decision support system is outlined that is designed to shorten patient wait times and length of stay in emergency departments. The next chapter, "Step Towards Pervasive Technology Assessment in Intensive Medicine," by Profs. Filipe Portela, Manuel Filipe Santos, José Machado, António Abelha of Universidade do Minho, Braga, Portugal and Prof. Fernando Rua from the Intensive Care Unit, Centro Hospitalar do Porto, Porto, Portugal, evaluates a pervasive intelligent decision support system in intensive medicine making use of Technology Acceptance Model 3 (TAM3). In the following chapter, "Wireless Heartrate Monitoring Along Prioritized Alert Notification Using Mobile Techniques," by Prof. Rajasekaran Rajkumar of the Vellore Institute of Technology, Vellore, India, diverse methods that improve the cost, demands of hospital information systems (HIS), and provide techniques to function efficiently using wireless networks are discussed and a new system is proposed by combining the wireless healthcare system along prioritized alert notification. The next chapter, "Integrated Hospital Information System Architecture Design in Indonesia," by Profs. Putu Wuri Handayani, Puspa Indahati Sandhyaduhita, Achmad Nizar Hidayanto, Ave Adriana Pinem, Haya Rizqi Fajrina, Kasiyah M. Junus, Indra Budi, and Dumilah Ayuningtyas of Universitas Indonesia, Indonesia, designs an information system architecture as part of the enterprise architecture based on The Open Group Architecture Framework in order to support the hospital information system implementation in Indonesia. The section concludes with "Design of a Hospital Interactive Wayfinding System," written by Profs. Ashok Sivaji, Hizbullah Kampo Radjo, Mohd-Faizal Amin, and Mohd Azrin Hafizie Abu Hashim from MIMOS Berhad, Malaysia, which analyzes improvements to hospital wayfinding in Malaysia that incorporate ease of use for a multilingual, multicultural population.

Section 3, "Management and Operations," focuses on managerial practices, resource management, and hospital operations that include prioritizing patients, disaster management, managing incoming patients and schedules, and reducing wait time. This section is introduced by "Managing Emergency Units Applying Queueing Theory," by Profs. Salvador Hernández-González, Manuel Dario Hernández-Ripalda, Anakaren González-Pérez, Moises Tapia-Esquivias, and Alicia Luna-González from Instituto Tecnologico de Celaya, Mexico. The chapter applies queueing theory, the study of waiting in queues, to decision making systems in hospitals in order to help hospitals distribute their resources and tend to patients more effectively. The second chapter is "A Simulation Model for Resource Balancing in Healthcare Systems" by Profs. Arzu Eren Şenaras and Hayrettin Kemal Sezen from Uludag University, Turkey. It analyzes resource effectiveness through a model developed by the Arena package program. The next chapter, "Surgery Operations Modeling and Scheduling in Healthcare Systems," by Profs. Fatah Chetouane and Eman Ibraheem from Université de Moncton, Canada, describes a nonlinear mathematical model for surgery scheduling. In the following chapter, "Application of Fuzzy Soft Set in Patients' Prioritization," by Prof. Samira Abbagholizadeh Rahimi from Université Laval, Canada, using fuzzy logic to prioritize patients' safety and quality of life is discussed. The next chapter, "Evaluation of the Length of Hospital Stay Through Artificial Neural Networks Based Systems," by Profs. Vasco Abelha and Fernando Marins of the University of Minho, Portugal and Prof. Henrique Vicente from the University of Evora, Portugal, uses logic programming to evaluate and predict how long a patient should remain in the hospital without overly burdening them with medical costs. The sixth chapter, "Radio Frequency Identification

Technology in an Australian Regional Hospital," by Profs. Chandana Unnithan and Arthur Tatnall from Victoria University, Australia, explores the case study of radio frequency identification applied to the first large hospital in which its implementation was successful. The following chapter, "Community Hospital Disaster Preparedness in the United States," by Prof. Dan J. Vick from St. Vincent, USA; Prof. Asa B. Wilson of Methodist University, USA; Prof. Michael Fisher of Regis University, USA; and Prof. Carrie Roseamelia from SUNY Upstate Medical University, USA, conducts a comprehensive literature review that focuses on studies and other articles pertaining to disaster preparedness in U.S. community hospitals to determine the current state of disaster preparedness among community hospitals. In the next chapter, "E-Commerce and IT Projects," written by Profs. Wenqi Jacintha Hee and Geoffrey Jalleh from Curtin University, Australia; Prof. Hung-Chih Lai of National Chi Nan University, Taiwan; and Prof. Chad Lin of Curtin University, Australia, the outsourcing of Australian and Taiwanese hospitals' e-commerce and IT systems is discussed. This section concludes with "Operations Project and Management in Trauma Centers: The Case of Brazilian Units" by Profs. Thais Spiegel and Daniel Bouzon Nagem Assad from Rio de Janeiro State University, Brazil. It covers the care of poly-trauma patients and the design and management of their operations.

Section 4 is "Quality and Performance," which discusses ways to elevate quality of healthcare with regard to patient service, information delivery, and more. Section 4 opens with "Quality Evaluation of Health Care Establishment Utilizing Fuzzy AHP" by Prof. Mohammad Azam from the Career Institute of Medical Sciences & Hospital, India; Prof. Mohamed Rafik Noor Mohamed Qureshi of King Khalid University, Saudi Arabia; and Prof. Faisal Talib from Aligarh Muslim University, India. This chapter constructs a system of quality evaluation by analyzing three well-constructed healthcare establishments in northern India. The next chapter, "TQM Practices in Public Sector," by Prof. Mian M. Ajmal of Abu Dhabi University, UAE; Profs. Ville Tuomi and. Petri T. Helo from the University of Vaasa, Finland; and Prof. Maqsood Ahmad Sandhu of UAE University, UAE, discusses the evolution, principles, and stages of totally quality management (TQM) in public health care organizations. The third chapter, "Hospital Service Quality from Patients Perspective," by Profs. Puspa Sandhyaduhita, Haya Rizqi Fajrina, Ave Adriana Pinem, Achmad Nizar Hidayanto, Putu Handayani, and Kasiyah Junus from Universitas Indonesia, Indonesia, identifies and analyzes strategic service quality from patients' perspective. The next chapter, "Applied Pervasive Patient Timeline in Intensive Care Units," by Profs. André Braga, Filipe Portela, Manuel Filipe Santos, António Abelha, José Machado from Universidade do Minho, Portugal, and Profs. Álvaro Silva and Fernando Rua from Centro Hospitalar do Porto, Portugal, introduces an innovative way of presenting and representing information concerning patients in intensive care units. In the following chapter, "Estimating Key Performance Indicators of a New Emergency Department Model," by Prof. Soraia Oueida of the American University of Middle East, Kuwait; Prof. Seifedine Kadry of Beirut Arab University, Lebanon; and Prof. Sorin Ionescu from Politehnica University of Bucharest, Romania, the findings of a study on a real-life emergency department are presented to propose improvements on its operations and patient flow. Finally, this section is closed by "A Review on the Contribution of Emergency Department Simulation Studies in Reducing Wait Time" by Prof. Basmah Almoaber of the University of Ottawa, Ottawa, Canada & King Khalid University, Saudi Arabia and Prof. Daniel Amyot from the University of Ottawa, Canada. In analyzing the existing research conducted on emergency room wait times, it found a discrepancy between the conclusions of the research and the implementation of those systems.

Although the primary organization of the contents in this work is based on its seven sections, offering a progression of coverage of the important concepts, methodologies, applications, technologies, and emerging trends, the reader can also identify specific contents by using the extensive indexing system at the end.

Section 1
Data Management

Chapter 1
A New Approach to Generate Hospital Data Warehouse Schema

Nouha Arfaoui

Institut Supérieur de Gestion de Tunis, Tunisia

Jalel Akaichi

Institut Supérieur de Gestion de Tunis, Tunisia

ABSTRACT

The healthcare industry generates huge amount of data underused for decision making needs because of the absence of specific design mastered by healthcare actors and the lack of collaboration and information exchange between the institutions. In this work, a new approach is proposed to design the schema of a Hospital Data Warehouse (HDW). It starts by generating the schemas of the Hospital Data Mart (HDM) one for each department taking into consideration the requirements of the healthcare staffs and the existing data sources. Then, it merges them to build the schema of HDW. The bottom-up approach is suitable because the healthcare departments are separately. To merge the schemas, a new schema integration methodology is used. It starts by extracting the similar elements of the schemas and the conflicts and presents them as mapping rules. Then, it transforms the rules into queries and applies them to merge the schemas.

INTRODUCTION

The healthcare industry is considered as one of the world's largest, fastest-developing and most information-rich industries (Foundation, 2006). It generates huge amount of data related to patients, drugs, doctors, etc. The collected data plays a crucial role to ensure complex statistical analysis. It is used to calculate the measurement and key performance indicators that are vital for the organization to be more agile, flexible and fluent (Mike, 2014).

DOI: 10.4018/978-1-7998-2451-0.ch001

Copyright © 2020, IGI Global. Copying or distributing in print or electronic forms without written permission of IGI Global is prohibited.

The continuous development, the difficulties related to the collection of the data in the healthcare organization for the analysis, the reduction of the computing cost and the explosion of the healthcare data make the use of Hospital Data Warehouse (HDW) an efficient solution to well exploit the collected data to make good decisions.

The DW is defined as *a subject-oriented, integrated, non-volatile and time-variant collection of data in support of management's decisions* (Inmon, 2005). It allows the end-users to self-service their needs (Inmon, 2005). It may provide information to users in areas ranging from research to management (Sen and Jacob, 1998). It facilitates the storage, enhances timely analysis and increases the quality of area time decision making processes (Sahama and Croll, 2007). It offers one space to store the global truth to enable healthcare analysis such as identifying quickly the causal relationship of diseases. It aggregates, then, the data from clinical and financial systems into one repository.

The top-down starts from the description of the needs of all the users to construct the schema corresponding to the entire DW (Malinowski and Zimanyi, 2008). The bottom-up constructs the global schema of DW starting from the different schemas of Data Mart (DM) (Malinowski and Zimanyi, 2008). The hybrid approach takes advantages of the two previous approaches (Malinowski and Zimanyi, 2008). It has the speed and the user-orientation of the top-down and the integration enforced by a DW of the bottom-up.

The healthcare centers are composed by different departments such as accident and emergency, anesthetics, cardiology, diagnostic imaging, general surgery, maternity departments, neurology, Pharmacy, etc. The departments record their own data, they are still stand along, they do not communicate with other health care centers and they do not share their documents with others (Dutta, 2013). Starting by designing the schemas of the Hospital Data Mart (HDM) one for each healthcare department, then, generating the HDW schema using the bottom-up approach is very suitable and profitable in such case.

The DM is defined *as a flexible set of data, ideally based on the most atomic (granular) data possible to extract from an operational source, and presented in a symmetric (dimensional) model that is most resilient when faced with unexpected user queries* (Kimball and Ross, 2002). It is accessed directly by end users, and its data is structured in a way that is easy for users to understand and use (Moody and Kortink, 2000).

In this work, we mix two approaches: hybrid and bottom-up. The first one is used to generate the HDM taking into consideration the healthcare staffs' requirements and the existing data sources. An assistant system is introduced, at this level, to facilitate to the users the specification of their needs. The second approach is applied to build the HDW from HDM schemas. In the two steps, we use a new schema integration methodology to ensure the automatic generation of the schemas.

Starting by generating HDM helps to resolve the different problems that arise within each department because of the various care practices, data types and definitions, the perceived incompleteness of clinical information systems, the type of information that the medicine and healthcare need (Mul et al., 2012) which make the creation of the HDW in one step a very hard task.

As working hypothesis, it is proposed to present the schemas as star or snowflake because they are the most used models and they are easy to understand (Lee and Ling, 1997), (Levene and Loizou, 2003). Concerning the data sources, it is proposed to deal with Entity-Relationship (ER) database because it adopts the more natural view that the real world consists of entities and relationships; it incorporates some of the important semantic information and it can achieve a high degree of data independence (Chen, 1976).

BACKGROUND

In this section, we start by presenting some DW design methodologies to move next to summarize some work proposing the use of DW in healthcare domain.

Data Warehouse Design Methodologies

Several methodologies, in literature, have been proposed to design the DW. The following table (Table 1) presents some of them.

Table 1. Example of DW methodologies

	Step	Input	Output
[Golfarelli and Rizzi, 2009]	Requirement analysis	Requirements collected from users	Glossaries or Goal-oriented diagrams
	Analysis and reconciliation	Data sources	Reconciled schema
	Conceptual design	User requirements and data extracted from the reconciled schema.	Conceptual schema (the form of a set of fact schemata)
	Workload refinement	Preliminary workload	UML use case diagrams
	Logical design	Conceptual schema	Logical schema
	Data staging design	Source schemata, reconciled schema and the DM logical schema.	ETL procedures
	Physical design	Workload and user profiles, logical schema	Physical schema
	Implement	Workload and user profiles, physical schema, logical schema, and ETL procedures	Implementation
[Peralta et al., 2003]	Conceptual level	Non-functional user requirements	multidimensional conceptual schema
	Logical level	multidimensional conceptual schema, mappings, guideline	Logical relational schema
	Physical level	Logical relational schema	The implementation
[Bizarro and Madeira, 2002]	Logical level	Business view, operational data, design rules, predicated usage profile, meta-data	Optimized star scheme
	Physical level	Optimized star scheme	Optimized physical star scheme
	Preliminary administrative tasks	Optimized physical star scheme	Final star scheme
[Hüsemann et al., 2000]	Requirement analysis and specifications	Operational database schema	Semiformal business concept
	Conceptual design	Semiformal business concept	Formal conceptual schema
	Logical design	Formal conceptual schema	Formal logical schema
	Physical design	Formal logical schema	Physical database schema
[Malinowski and Zimanyi, 2008]	Requirements specification	Source systems, users	Document requirements specification
	Conceptual design	Initial schema	Final schema and mapping
	Logical design	Developed schema	Definition of ETL processes
	Physical des	Developed schema	Implementation of ETL processes and staging area

Data Warehouse and Healthcare

According to our knowledge, few works propose the use of the DW in the medical field. In the following, some of them are described. In (Bennett et al., 2009), the authors propose the implementation of the DW because it offers opportunities when it is used in the healthcare domain. It aggregates the data from clinical and financial systems into one repository. It identifies quickly the causal relationship of diseases. It allows the end-users to self-service their needs.

In (Sheta and Eldeen, 2012), the authors develop and implement a prototype healthcare DW specific for cancer diseases. They employ the DW to incorporate large quantity of analysis information needed for healthcare decision-making.

The author introduces, in (Dutta, 2013), DW architecture for the Influenza (Flu) diseases. The developed DW is used by database administrator or executive manager, doctors, nurses, other staff members of the health care. It helps to store all information about the patients to facilitate making decisions. The authors, in (Banek et al., 2006), suggest a multidimensional conceptual model of a federated DW. The conceptual model of the component warehouses offers a traditional view on financial measures, yet it does not enable the processing of time-segmented medicine administration data, whose grain level is even lower than the basic grain level of the model.

In (Berndt et al., 2003), the authors construct a comprehensive healthcare DW that provides automated support for CATCH (Comprehensive Assessment for Tracking Community Health). The innovation is about combining the extensive field experience with CATCH and the application of the DW technology. According to the authors the implementation of this type of DW and its use in monitoring, as well as improving health status, will become a primary role of public health agencies in the future. Darmont in (Darmont, 2008) introduce a DW model of complex DW for the health of elite athletes. This tool allows the storage of complex medical data from various fields of medicine and biology. It allows two types of analysis; the first one supports the personalized medicine of anticipation for well-identified patients. The second one is related the statistical analysis of patients.

In (Berndt et al., 2001), the authors implement the DW to support health assessments of communities throughout the state. It is used to explore the relationship between surgical volume and successful outcomes. The healthcare DW includes fine-grained data, such as hospital discharges, births, deaths, and specific disease registries. It includes also demographic, economic, and marketing data to derive many health status indicators. A large collection of stored procedures calculates the health status indicators, propagating the data from fine-grained structures to higher-level reporting components. In (Einbinder et al., 2001), the authors create clinical data repository CDR. The purpose is to support the research and education functions of the academic medical center, also to provide the data for the managers and administrators.

Discussion

Compared to the previous works, we suggest focusing on each department separately because of the lack of communication and documents exchange. We propose, also, the use of an assistant system to help the healthcare staffs to specify their requirements.

Our approach is composed by the following steps:

- It starts by collecting the requirements of the different healthcare staffs. It uses an assistant system HDwADS (Hospital Data warehouse Assistant Design System) to facilitate the specification of the multidimensional components (fact, measures, dimensions and attributes) basing on the stored traces of the previous users. The collected requirements are represented as star schemas.
- Next, it generates the global schema corresponding to HDM conceptual schema from uses' requirements. It uses the schema integration methodology that extracts the semantically closest elements as well as the conflicts and presents them as mapping rules. Then, it merges the different schemas to get at the end the global schema by generating the queries from the mapping rules and executing them.
- Then, the conceptual schemas are mapped to logical ones. This is done in two steps. In the first one, it extracts all possible multidimensional schemas from the databases. In the second step, it generates the logical schemas. Indeed, it updates the conceptual schemas by adding the necessary information extracted from the multidimensional schemas using the mapping rules.
- Finally, using the schema integration technique, the set of logical schemas of HDM are merged to build the final schema of the HDW.

MAIN FOCUS OF THE CHAPTER

This chapter proposes four contributions:

- A new approach to generate the schema of the HDW by mixing the bottom-up approach and the hybrid approach. The different proposed solutions use one approach bottom-up, top-down or hybrid. Because of the specificity of our case (generating HDM for each healthcare center and then merging them to build the DW), we need to mix two approaches the hybrid and the bottom-up. Indeed, each department has its own database and its own requirements, so we apply the mixed approach to generate HDM i.e. taking into consideration both the needs and the available data sources. Then, using the bottom-up approach the HDW is constructed from the set of HDM schemas.
- An assistant system to facilitate the collect of healthcare staffs' requirements. The healthcare staffs are not experienced with the DW technologies and they can find difficulties to express their requirements. To facilitate this task, we use a system that assists the user during this task by proposing the possible next elements to use basing on the previous experiences that are already stored.
- A new schema integration methodology to ensure the automatic merging of the schemas. Different schema integration (SI) methodologies have been proposed to construct the global schema from a set of local schemas. They are applied mainly with the databases. In this work, we propose its use to automate the bottom-up approach. The new methodology is composed by few steps to deal with specificities structure of DW/DM schemas that they are different compared to the databases schemas.
- Appling the new approach to build HDW. The proposed approach facilitates the construction of HDW faster by taking into account the needs of each department and its available information. The share of information between different departments/centers becomes easier and the communication between them becomes possible. Having a global view of the existing information facilitates the process of making decisions.

COLLECTION OF USERS' REQUIREMENTS

In order to ensure a good design of HDM, it is crucial to start by collecting the requirements that specify *what data should be available and how it should be organized as well as what queries are of interest* (Malinowski and Zimanyi, 2008). We extract, then, the important elements related to the multidimensional schema: facts, measures, dimensions, and attributes that reflect the users' needs.

Hospital Data Warehouse Assistant Design System (HDwADS)

The healthcare staffs find difficulties to specify their needs using the SQL queries especially when they apply the GROUP BY and/or HAVING clauses (Annoni et al., 2006) and (Gyssens and Lakshmanan, 1997). Also, they have difficulties to cooperate with the designers since there is not a common language for sufficiently unambiguous communication between them (Börger, 1998).

In order to facilitate this task, we propose the use of an assistant system named Hospital Data warehouse Assistant Design System (HDwADS) (Figure1) that offers helps basing on previous experiences stored as traces (this latter will be explained later). It compares the current manipulation to the stored traces to propose the new possible object(s). It extracts, then, the objects using the use model and the actions using the observation model. The two models build the traces that are stored into "Trace" database. We have then for each user the information related to his manipulation.

Figure 1. The composition of HDwADS

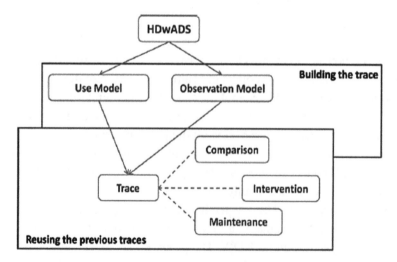

Figure 2. The Use Model schema

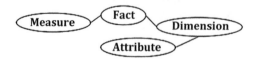

- **Use Model:** It extracts the objects from the current manipulation in order to facilitate their comparison to the objects of the previous experiences. The objects belong to the following categories (C): "C: Fact", "C: Dimension", "C: Attribute", and "C: Measure". These various categories are linked into single schema as presented in Figure 2.
- **Observation Model:** It extracts the actions (∥A: ∥) handled by a single user during his session. It gives a vision on the use and the manipulation of the application and more precisely on how to deal with the existing objects of the use model.
- **Trace:** It is the basis of HDwADS. It is built using the use model and the observation model as consequence it is a secession of objects and actions over the time. It keeps for each user its own trace. Figure 3 presents a portion of a trace where there is a star schema composed by one fact table "Order", three measures "Price, Qty and Cost" and one dimension "PatientDim" with its attributes "Name, LastName and Age".
- **Extraction of Useful Information**: It is about comparing the current manipulation to the previous experiences that are already stored into database. The comparison task helps to locate the user to suggest the possible next objects to manipulate. The detection of similar cases is automatically and in parallel with the use of the system, and the intervention is done in real time i.e. the research of the cases and the proposal of solution are made in parallel with the specification of the requirements.

The comparison: There are two cases of comparison:

- HDwADS takes into consideration the last manipulated object (Figure 4).

Figure 3. Example of trace

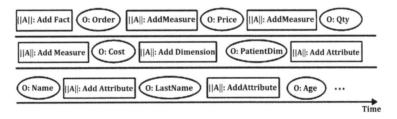

Figure 4. Comparing the last manipulated object

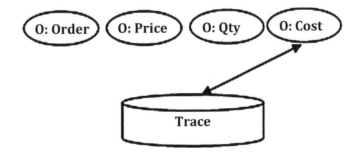

Figure 5. Comparing all the objects of the current manipulation

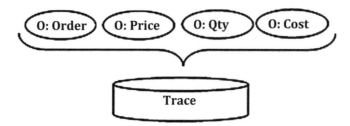

- HDwADS takes into consideration all the manipulation respecting the order of the objects over the time (Figure 5).

In the both cases, if there is the corresponding object(s) in the database "Trace" this implies that there are at least one experience that can be used in the next step, else, the system keeps the new objects until the validation of the final schema, then, it saves them as new trace. In the case of no validation of the final schema, the objects are neglected.

The intervention: It is done in three different ways:

- If the system finds traces from the base that can be used to assist the user in the next step, it intervenes by proposed the next object to manipulate (Figure 6).
- If the system finds traces from the base that can be used to assist the user in the next step, it intervenes by proposed the rest of the trace respecting the order of the existing objects (Figure 7).
- If the system does not find any trace from the base, it proposes the closest objects (by using the degree of similarities and choose the objects with the highest values).

Figure 6. Intervention by proposing the next object extracted from the existing traces

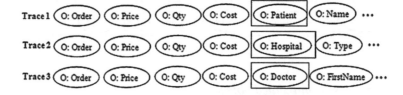

Figure 7. Intervention by proposing the rest of object extracted from the existing traces

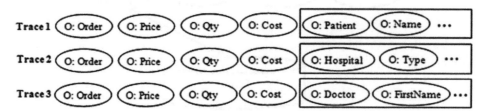

The maintenance: The purpose of the maintenance of the base of the trace is to keep a database running smoothly through saving the most pertinent traces for a reuse. Indeed, we need to keep a reasonable number of trace so that it will not saturate the base, and reduce the response time (to keep real time aspect).

We propose then to assign with each trace its frequency (the number of times that is used i.e. created by the user or exploited in the intervention phase), and we keep the traces with the highest frequency numbers. We give the freedom to the user to specify the threshold.

The Structure of the Generated Schemas

To well exploit the users' requirements, HDwADS presents them as conceptual star schemas having the following structure:

- Fact table corresponds to the subject of analysis. It is defined by: FN and MF{} with:
  - FN: represents the name of the fact.
  - MF {m1, m2, m3, m4, …}: corresponds to the set of measures related to the fact.
- Dimension tables represent the axis of analysis. Each one is composed by: DN, A{} with:
  - DN: corresponds to the name of the dimension.
  - A {a1, a2, a3, a4, …}: presents the set of attributes describing the current dimension.

BUILDING DATA MART CONCEPTUAL SCHEMAS

Semantic Similarity Measure

Let Sch1 and Sch2 be two schemas. Let Cp be the categories of elements existing in the schema with Cp = {fact, dimension, measure, attribute}

$\forall\, e_i \in$ Sch1, $\exists\, e_j \in$ Sch2, so that e_i and e_j belong to the same category Cp.

To calculate the semantic similarity of two elements belonging to the same category, we use the following formula (1):

$$\text{DeSim}(ei, ej) = \text{DeId}(ei, ej) + \text{DeSy}(ei, ej) + \text{SeTy}(ei, ej) + \text{DePost}(ei, ej) + \text{DePre}(ei, ej) + \text{DeAbb}(ei, ej) \tag{1}$$

With:

- DeId $(e_i, e_j) = 1$ if e_i and e_j are identical i.e. they have the same name, and 0 if not.
  Example: Sch1.fact = "Order" and Sch2.fact= "Order".
- DeSy (ei, ej) = 1 if ei and ej are synonymous i.e. they have two different names with the same meaning, and 0 if not.
  Example: Sch1.dimension = "Medication" and Sch2.dimension = "Drug".
- DeTy (ei, ej) =1 if e_i and e_j are the same with the existence of typos.
  Example: Sch1.measure = "Price" and Sch2.measure = "Prace".

- DePost (ei, ej) = 1 if one is the postfix of the other and 0 if not.
  Example: Sch1.attribute = "Name" and Sch2.attribute = "FirstName".
- DePre (ei, ej) = 1 if one is the prefix of the other, and 0 if not.
  Example: Sch1.dimension = "PatientDim" and Sch2.dimension = "Patient".
- DeAbb (ei, ej) = 1 if one is the abbreviation of the other, 0 if not.
  Example: Sch1.measure = "Qty" and Sch2.measure = "Quantity".

The New Schema Integration Methodology

At this level, we have a set of conceptual HDM schemas. We propose their gathering using schema integration technique that starts by generating the necessary rules and then applying those rules to ensure the merging of the schemas. To facilitate this task, we specify a common interface structure, so we are sure that the different schemas have the same data model, and each element of the schema belongs to a specific category (fact, dimension, measure or attribute).

To achieve our task, the new schema integration methodology is composed by the following steps:

- Categorization: It is to specify the category of each element.
- Construction of the similarity matrix: It is to use the similarity matrix as a way to find the closest elements. The cells contain the coefficient of similarity of the different elements belonging to the same category. It is calculated using the formula (1).
- Generation of the mapping rules: The rules visualize the relationships between the instances of the elements belonging to the same category. They are expressed as: "If Similar (X, Y) then Action (X, Y) and Save (X, Y)", with:
  - X and Y: two elements belong to the same category.
  - Similar (): it is a function that specifies if the two inputs are similar or not. It uses the similarity matrix determined in the previous step.
  - Action (): it specifies the action to perform. It can be union, or intersection.
    - Union: R = union (ei, ej) implies that R contains all the components of ei and all components of ej.
    - Intersection: R= intersection (ei, ej) implies that R contains the components that exist in ei and ej.
  - Save (): it saves the two elements.
- Merging the schemas: It is about transforming the previous mapping rules to queries and executing them.

Let us apply the previous steps on Figure 8.

- Categorization:
  - Fact: In Figure 8 (a), the fact is "Order", and in Figure 8 (b) is "Order".
  - Measure: In Figure 8 (a), the measures are "Price, Qty, TotalCost", and in Figure 8 (b), they are "Prace, Quantity, TotalCost".
  - Dimension: In Figure 8 (a), the dimensions are "PatientDim and Medication", and in Figure 8 (b), they are "Patient, Drug and Physician".

Figure 8. (a) (b). Example of schemas corresponding to the users' requirements

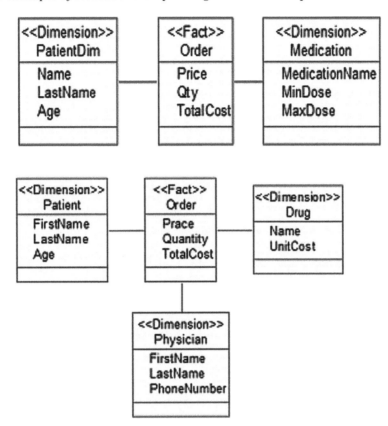

- ◦ Attribute: In Figure 8 (a) the attributes are "Name, LastName, Age, MedicationName MinDose, MaxDose". In Figure 8 (b), they are "FirstName, LastName, Age, Name, UnitCost, FirstName LastName, PhoneNumber".
- • Construction of the similarity matrix: In the following, we give some examples of similarity matrix.

Figure 9 presents the similarity matrix used to compare the two facts. The value of "Max" is 1 so that they are similar.

Figure 10 presents the similarity matrix used to compare the measures. Basing on the values of Max, we have as similar pairs of measures: {{Price, Prace}; {Qty, Quantity}; {TotalCost, TotalCost}}.

Figure 11 presents the similarity matrix used to compare the dimensions. The similar ones are: {PatientDim, Patient} and {Medication, Drug}

Figure 12 presents the similarity matrix used to compare the attributes of the two dimension tables "PatientDim/Patient" existing in the two schemas. According to the matrix, we have the following similar pairs of attributes {Name, FirstName}, {LastName, LastName} and {Age, Age}.

Figure 13 presents the similarity matrix used to compare the attributes of the two dimension tables "Medication/Drug" existing in the two schemas. According to the matrix, we have the following similar pair of attributes {MedicationName, Name}.

Figure 9. Similarity matrix to compare the facts

Fact	Order	Max
Order	1	1

Figure 10. Similarity matrix to compare the measures

Measure	Prace	Quantity	TotalCost	Max
Price	1	0	0	1
Qty	0	1	0	1
TotalCost	0	0	1	1

Figure 11. Similarity matrix to compare the dimensions

Dimension	Patient	Drug	Physician	Max
PatientDim	1	0	0	1
Medication	0	1	0	1

Figure 12. Similarity matrix to compare the attributes of the dimension tables "PatientDim/Patient"

Attributes of the dimensions "PatientDim/Patient"	FirstName	LastName	Age	Max
Name	1	0	0	1
LastName	0	1	0	1
Age	0	0	1	1

Figure 13. Similarity matrix to compare the attributes of the dimension tables "Medication/Drug"

Attributes of the dimensions "Medication/Drug"	Name	UnitCost	Max
MedicationName	1	0	1
MinDose	0	0	0
MaxDose	0	0	0

- Generation of the mapping rules: As example of mapping rules, we can present:
  - If Similar (Order, Order) then Union (Order, Order) and Save (Order, Order)
  - If Similar (Drug, Medication) then Intersection (Drug, Medication) and Save (Drug, Medication)
  - If Similar (PatientDim, Patient) then Intersection (PatientDim, Patient) and Save (PatientDim, Patient)
- Merging the schemas: As example of queries, we can present:
  - Query1 = "Insert into Fact (FactName, idSchema) values ('Order',"+ schemaId +")" ;
  - Query2 = "Insert into Measure (MeasureName, idFact) values (Price',"+ factId +")" ;

- ◦ Query3 = "Insert into Dimension (DimensionName, idSchema) values ('Patient'," +schemaId + ") ";
- ◦ Query4 = "Insert into Attribute (AttributeName, idDimension) values ('FirstName'," +dimensionId +")";

With:

- schemaId: is the identifier of the new schema.
- factId: is the identifier of the new fact table.
- dimensionId: is the identifier of the new dimension table.

The result of executing the queries is stored into specific database composed by the following tables:

- The table "Schema" contains the set of schemas to be merged. Each schema is identified through a unique numeric identifier automatically incremented. At the end of the integration process, "Schema" contains only one element corresponding to the identifier of the final schema.
- The table "Fact" stores the names of the facts. It has one primary key and a foreign key connected to the table "Schema".
- The table "Measure" contains the set of measures. It is defined by a primary key and a foreign key connected to the table "Fact".
- The table "Dimension" contains the set of dimensions for each schema. It is described by a primary key, and a foreign key connected to the table "Schema".
- The table "Attribute" is used to store the attributes of each dimension. This table is defined by one primary key, the name of the attributes, their types, and a foreign key connected to the table "Dimension".

At the end of this step, we obtain the following schema (Figure 14) corresponding to the merging of the two previous schemas (Figure 8). It has one fact "Order" with three measures "Price, Quantity and TotalCost", surrounded by three dimensions "Patient, Drug and Physician". Each dimension contains a set of attributes.

GENERATING MULTIDIMENSIONAL SCHEMAS

In this part, we propose the generation of multidimensional schemas from Entity-Relationship (ER) databases. This choice is because ER adopts the more natural view that the real world consists of entities and relationships, it incorporates some of the important semantic information about the real world; it can achieve a high degree of data independence (Chen, 1976). The generated schemas can be star or snowflake.

To achieve this task, we propose the following algorithm that is composed by three steps:

Step 1: *Normalize the ER model.* Apply the 1NF, 2NF and 3NF to construct the ER normalized:
- ◦ **First Normal Form (1NF):** It should be no nesting or repeating groups in a table.
- ◦ **Second Normal Form (2NF):** The key attributes determine all non-key attributes.

Figure 14. The HDM Conceptual schema

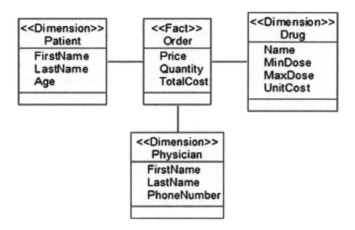

Figure 15. Example of multidimensional schema

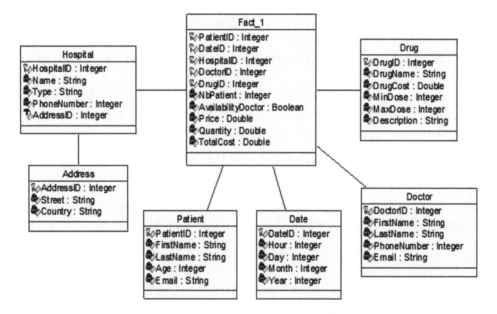

- ◦ **Third Normal Form (3NF):** The non-key attributes should be independent.

Step 2: *Build the tree from ER model.* From the ER model, we extract the entities (Ef) having n-ary relationships with other entities and those having numerical attributes. They represent the potential facts. Every Ef becomes the root of the tree. The number of trees corresponds to the number of Ef entities. From the ER we extract the entities (E) that are directly linked to Ef corresponding to the potential dimensions.

Step 3: *Transform the tree to multidimensional model.*

- ◦ The fact is created having as name "Fact_N" with N is an incremental number.
- ◦ The existing numeric attributes become the potential measures.

- The nodes that are directly linked to the roots are transformed to dimensions keeping their attributes and their identifiers.
- The primary keys of the children nodes become foreign keys in the parents' nodes.

Figure 15 corresponds to a multidimensional schema presented as snowflake with one fact table "Fact_1" having as primary key the set of primary keys of the dimensions. The measures are "NbPatient", "AvailabilityDoctor", "Price", "Quantity" and "TotalCost". Concerning the dimensions, we have "Patient", "Drug", "Doctor", "Date" and "Hospital" that is connected to the parameter "Address". Each table has its primary key and its attributes. The keys and the type of attributes are specified.

GENERATING HOSPITAL DATA MART LOGICAL SCHEMAS

The Structure of the Logical Schemas

The logical HDM schemas can be star or snowflake.
  The star schema has the following structure:

- The fact table is defined by FN, FP and MF{} with:
  - FN represents the name of the fact.
  - FP represents the primary key of the fact table.
  - MF {m1(Tym1), m2 (Tym2), m3 (Tym3), m4 (Tym4), ...} corresponds to the set of measures related to the fact. Each measure has its type.
- Each dimension table is composed by DN, DK and A{}, with:
  - DN corresponds to the dimension name.
  - DK corresponds to the primary key of the dimension table.
  - A {a1 (Tya1), a2 (Tya2), a3 (Tya3), a4 (Tya4), ...} presents the set of attributes describing the current dimension. Each attribute has a type.

The structure of a snowflake schema is as following:

- The fact table is defined by FN, FP, and MF{} with:
  - FN represents the name of the fact.
  - FP represents the primary key of the fact table.
  - MF {m1(Tym1), m2 (Tym2), m3 (Tym3), m4 (Tym4), ...} corresponds to the set of measures related to the fact. Each measure has its type.
- Each dimension table is composed by: DN, DK, A{}, HD{} with
  - DN corresponds to the dimension name.
  - DK corresponds to the primary key of the dimension table.
  - A {a1 (Tya1), a2 (Tya2), a3 (Tya3), a4 (Tya4), ...} presents the set of attributes describing the current dimension. Each attribute has its type.
  - HD {h_{1D}, h_{2D}, h_{3D}, h_{4D}, ...} is a set of ordered hierarchies. Each hierarchy has HN and P { } with
    - HN is the name of the current hierarchy
    - P{p1, p2, p3, p4, ...} is a set of ordered parameters.

From Conceptual Schema to Logical One

The purpose of this step is to move from the conceptual schemas to the logical ones. At this level, we have two types of schemas. The first ones were generated from the requirements. They present the Hospital Data Mart Conceptual Schemas (HDMCS)s and they are modeled as star. The second ones were generated from the different databases. They present Hospital Data Mart Multidimensional Schemas (HDMMS)s and they correspond to star or snowflake schemas. The generated schemas correspond to Hospital Data Mart Logical Schemas (HDMLS) and they can be presented as star or snowflake.

The validation of HDMLS is about adjusting the needs with databases so that we have the source from which we can extract data later.

In order to achieve this task:

- We compare the HDMCSs with HDMMSs to extract the closest ones: we classify the elements of the two schemas into the following categories: fact, measure, dimension, attribute or/and parameter and using the similarity matrix, we extract the closest schemas.
- We generate HDMLS by adding the necessary information from HDMMS to HDMCS. The mapping from the conceptual level to logical one is done by applying the following rules.

Rule 1: *Dimension table.*

Let Dc be the conceptual dimension table, Dl be the logical dimension table, and Dm be the multidimensional dimension table similar to Dc.

The mapping of Dc to Dl is done by keeping the name of Dm.

Example: if Dc is "PatientDim" and Dm is "Patient", the Dl in this case is "Patient".

Rule 2: *Attribute and Primary key.*

Let Ac be the attribute belonging to the conceptual dimension table, Am be the attribute belonging to the multidimensional table similar to Ac and Al be the attribute belonging to the logical dimension table.

The mapping of Ac to Al is done by keeping the name of Am and adding its corresponding type.

Example: if Ac is "FirstName" and Am is "Name" with "String" type, then Al is "Name" with "String" as type. Concerning the primary key, it is extracted from the multidimensional schema.

Rule 3: *Hierarchy.*

The conceptual schema is presented as star schema.

Let Hm be the hierarchy exiting in the multidimensional schema (if it is a snowflake schema), and Hl be the hierarchy of the logical schema having similar dimension tables.

In such case, the mapping is about copying the Hm with its parameters to the corresponding dimension to construct the Hl.

Rule 4: *Fact table.*

Let Fc be the conceptual fact table, Fm be the multidimensional fact table similar to Fc and Fl be the logical fact table. The mapping of Fc to Fl is done by respecting the name of Fm.

Example: Fc is "PharmacyOrderFact", Fm is "PharmacyOrder" the Fl is "PharmacyOrder".
Rule 5: *Measure and Primary key.*

Let Mc be the measure belonging to a specific Fc, Mm be the numeric attributes belonging to the Fm similar to Fc, and Ml be the measure that belong to Fl.

The specification of the measure requires human intervention to specify the numeric attributes and the corresponding function (SUM, MAX, AVG, etc) that should exist in the Fl.

Example: Mc is "TotalCost", Mm is "TotalCost", the Ml is SUM (Quantiy * Cost).

The primary key of the Fl is composed by the primary keys of the surrounded Dl.

Figure 16 presents the logical schema of the HDM after the mapping process. It contains the different measures and attributes with their types, and the fact name as defined by the user. The dimensions are adjusted according to databases.

GENERATING HOSPITAL DATA WAREHOUSE SCHEMA

In order to generate the schema of the HDW, we apply the schema integration technique. Compared to that of the section "The New Schema Integration Methodology", two points are changed. The first one is related to the comparison of the elements. Indeed, we should compare, also, the types of measures and attributes. The second point is about the storage of the elements during the mapping. We need another database that takes into consideration the primary keys, the types, the hierarchies, etc.

Figure 16. Logical HDM schema

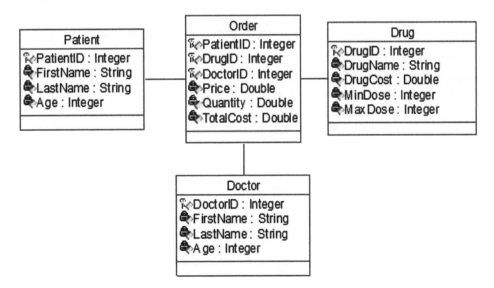

Figure 17. Logical DM schema

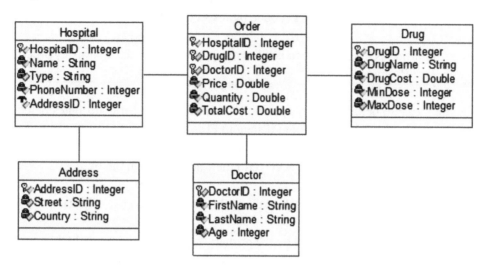

This step is iterative. It takes two HDM logical schemas every time. At the end, it gives HDW schema. To explain this point, let us take sch1 (Figure 16) and sch2 (Figure 17) corresponding to HDM logical schemas. We apply the same steps as defined previously.

- Categorization:
  - Fact {sch1{Order}, sch2 {Order}}
  - FactKey {sch1{PatientID, DrugID, DoctorID}, sch2 {HospitalID, DrugID, DoctorID}}
  - Measure {sch1{Price, Quantity, TotalCost}, sch2{ Price, Quantity, TotalCost }}
  - Dimension {sch1 {Patient, Drug, Doctor}, sch2 {Hospital, Drug, Doctor}}
  - Attribute {sch1 {PatientID, FirstName, LastName, Age, DrugID, DrugName, DrugCost, MinDose, MaxDose, DoctorID, FirstName, LastName, Age}, sch2 { HospitalID, Name, Type, PhoneNumber, AddressID, DrugID, DrugName, DrugCost, MinDose, MaxDose, DoctorID, FirstName, LastName, Age}}
- Construction of the similarity matrix:

Figure 18 presents the similarity matrix used to compare the two fact tables. In this case, they are similar since the value of 'Max'=1.

Figure 19 presents the similarity matrix used to compare the primary keys of the fact tables. In this case, we have the following similar pairs {DrugID, DrugID}, {DoctorID, DoctorID}.

Figure 20 presents the similarity matrix used to compare the measures. In this case, we have the following similar pairs {Price, Price}, {Quantity, Quantity} and {TotalCost, TotalCost} that they have the same type "Double". In the case of different types, we need human intervention.

Figure 21 presents the similarity matrix used to compare the dimension tables. In this case, we have the following similar pairs {Drug, Drug}, {Doctor, Doctor}.

Figure 18. Similarity matrix to compare the fact tables

Fact	Order	Max
Order	1	1

Figure 19. Similarity matrix to compare the fact keys

FactKey	HospitalID	DrugID	DoctorID	Max
PatientID	0	0	0	0
DrugID	0	1	0	1
DoctorID	0	0	1	1

Figure 20. Similarity matrix to compare the measures

Measure	Price (Double)	Quantity (Double)	TotalCost (Double)	Max
Price (Double)	1	0	0	1
Quantity (Double)	0	1	0	1
TotalCost (Double)	0	0	1	1

Figure 21. Similarity matrix to compare the dimension tables

Dimension	Hospital	Drug	Doctor	Max
Patient	0	0	0	0
Drug	0	1	0	1
Doctor	0	0	1	1

Figure 22. Similarity matrix to compare the attributes of the dimension tables 'Drug/Drug

Attribute of the dimension tables: Drug/Drug	DrugID (Integer)	DrugName (String)	DrugCost (Double)	MinDose (Double)	MaxDose (Double)	Max
DrugID (Integer)	1	0	0	0	0	1
DrugName (String)	0	1	0	0	0	1
DrugCost (Double)	0	0	1	0	0	1
MinDose (Double)	0	0	0	1	0	1
MaxDose (Double)	0	0	0	0	1	1

Figure 22 presents the similarity matrix used to compare the attributes of the dimension tables "Drug/Drug". In this case, {DrugID, DrugID} with "Integer" type, {DrugName, DrugName} with "String" type, {DrugCost, DrugCost} with "Double" type, {MinDose, MinDose} with "Double" type and {MaxDose, MaxDose} with "Double" type are the pairs of similar attributes. In the case of different types for two similar attributes, we need human intervention.

Figure 23. Similarity matrix to compare the attributes of the dimension tables 'Doctor/Doctor'

Attribute of the dimension tables: Doctor/Doctor	DoctorID (Integer)	FirstName (String)	LastName (String)	Age (Integer)	Max
DoctorID (Integer)	1	0	0	0	1
FirstName (String)	0	1	0	0	1
LastName (String)	0	0	1	0	1
Age (Integer)	0	0	0	1	1

Figure 23 presents the similarity matrix used to compare the attributes of the dimension tables "Doctor/Doctor". In this case, {DoctorID, DoctorID} with "Integer" type, {FirstName, FirstName} with "String" type, {LastName, LasName} with "String" type, and {Age, Age} with "Integer" type are the pairs of similar attributes related to the dimension "Doctor". In the case of different types, we need human intervention.

- Generation of the mapping rules: in the following, we present some of mapping rules.
  ◦ If Similar (Order, Order) then Intersection (Order, Order) and Save (Order, Order)
  ◦ If Similar (Price (Double), Price (Double)) then Intersection (Price (Double), Price (Double)) and Save (Price (Double), Price (Double))
  ◦ If Similar (PatientID, PatientID) then Intersection (PatientID, PatientID) and Save (PatientID, PatientID)
  ◦ If Similar (Doctor, Doctor) then Intersection (Doctor, Doctor) and Save (Doctor, Doctor)
  ◦ If Similar (FirstName, FirstName) then Intersection (FirstName, FirstName) and Save (FirstName, FirstName)
- Merging the schemas: As explained previously, it transforms the mapping rules into queries, and executes them to generate at the end the final schema of the HDW.

Compared to the previous database, we need, at this level, more details about the tables. We add a new table "FactPrimaryKey" contains the primary key of each fact table and their types. It has a primary key and a foreign key connected to the table "Fact". Concerning the table "Measure", we add the attribute "type" to specify the type of each measure. The table "Dimension" contains a new set of attributes "DimensionPrimaryKey" to specify the primary key of the dimension, "type" corresponding to the type of the primary key. This table specifies also for each dimension its level for a given hierarchy. It is described by a primary key, and a foreign key connected to the table "Schema". Finally, for the table "Attribute" gives information about the type of each attributes.

As example of queries, we can present:

- Query1 = "Insert into Fact (FactName, idSchema) values ('Order',"+ schemaId +")" ;
- Query2 = "Insert into Measure (MeasureName, MeasureType, idFact) values ('TotalCost',"+" 'Double '"+ factId +")" ;
- Query3 = "Insert into Dimension (DimensionName, Hierarchy, Level, DimensionPKName, DimensionPKType, idSchema) values ('Drug'," + null + ", '0', 'DrugID', 'Integer'" +schemaId + ") ";
- Query4 = "Insert into Attribute (AttributeName, AttributeType, idDimension) values ('DrugCost ',"+ ' Integer ' "+dimensionId +")";

With:

- schemaId: is the identifier of the new schema.
- factId: is the identifier of the new fact table.
- dimensionId: is the identifier of the new dimension table.

Once we apply the generated queries, we get the following schema (Figure 24) corresponding to the final HDW schema.

IMPLEMENTATION

To automate the schema integration, we propose the following algorithms.

Figure 25 corresponds to the main algorithm. It takes as input two schemas to give as output one schema. It is iterative. It stops when there is only one schema in the database. This algorithm starts by creating a new schema that will contain all the integrated elements. Next, it extracts the different category (fact, measure, dimension, attribute and parameter) using "Categorization" algorithm. Then, using "SchemaIntegrationFact" algorithm, it ensures the integration of the two fact tables. For each fact, it extracts the set of its corresponding measures that are integrated using "SchemaIntegrationMeasure" algorithm.

In the next step, it extracts the set of dimension tables from the two schemas, and stores them into two different lists. Using "SchemaIntegrationDimension_and_Attribute", it integrates the dimensions and their attributes. It treats also the hierarchies in the case of snowflake schemas. Finally, it deletes the two schemas that were used by applying "Delete_Schema" function that deletes the elements of each schema.

Since each fact table can have many measures, we use lists that contain the measures of the fact tables. "SchemaIntegrationMeasure" algorithm (Figure 26) starts by verifying the existence of a rule corresponding to the two measures in the input. If there is one, then it applies it. If not, it calculates the degree of similarity of two measures using the formula (1). If they are similar, and have the same type,

Figure 24. Hospital Data Warehouse schema

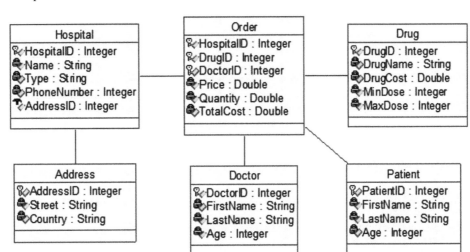

Figure 25. "SchemaIntegration" algorithm

```
1    Begin
2      Repeat
3        Categorization (sch1)
4        Categorization (sch2)
5        Create_NewSchema ( )
6        Fact1 = sch1.Fact
7        Fact2 = sch2.Fact
8        FactF = SchemaIntegrationFact (Fact2, sch1)
9        ListMeasure1 [ ] = sch1.ListMeasure (Fact1)
10       ListMeasure2 [ ] = sch2.ListMeasure (Fact2)
11       SchemaIntegrationMeasure (ListMeasure1, ListMeasure2)
12       ListDimension1 [ ] = sch1.ListDimension ( )
13       ListDimension2 [ ] = sch2.ListDimension ( )
14       SchemaIntegrationDimension_and_Attribute (ListDimension1, ListDimension2)
15       Delete_Schema ( )
16     Until (SchemaNumber = = 1)
17   End
```

Figure 26. "SchemaIntegrationMeasure" Algorithm

```
1    Begin
2      While (i <  ListMeasure1.lenght)
3        While (j < ListMeasure2.lenght)
4          exist = Exist_Rule (ListMeasure1 [i], ListMeasure2[j])
5
6          If (exist) then
7            Rule = Extract_Rule (ListMeasure1[i], ListMeasure2[j])
8            Apply_Rule (Rule, FactF)
9          Else
10             sim = DegSim (ListMeasure1[i], ListMeasure2[j])
11             If (ListMeasure1[i].type.equals (ListMeasure2[j].type)
12               simType = 1
13             Else
14               simType= 0
15             Fin if
16
17             If  (sim = = 1 && simType = = 1)
18                Rule = Generate_Rule (ListMeasure1[i], ListMeasure2[j])
19                Apply_Rule (Rule)
20                 Save_Rule (Rule, meas1, meas2)
21             ElseIf (sim = = 1 && simType = = 0)
22                 Rule = Human_Generate_Rule (ListMeasure1[i], ListMeasure2[j])
23                 Apply_Rule (Rule)
24                 Save_Rule (Rule, meas1, meas2)
25               End If
26           End if
27         j++
28         i++
29       End While
30     End While
31   ListMeasNotSim [ ] = insertRest(ListMeasure1, ListMeasure2)
32   Insert (ListMeasNotSim, FactF)
33
34   End
```

then it generates their corresponding rule, applies it and saves it. If they have different types, then we need human intervention thanks to the function Human_Generate_Rule ().

It is possible to get a set of no similar measures which are added to the chosen fact table in the previous algorithm. Concerning the rest of elements, the same steps are applied.

In the following, we give the implementation of "Extract_Rule", "Generate_Rule" and "Apply_Rule" that are implemented using eclipse as JAVA editor.

The algorithm "Extract-Rule" verifies the existence of a specific rule into the database "ruledatabase". The research is done using the names of the elements.

```
public String Extract_Rule (String elem) {
String rule = "";
try {
        String pilote = "com.mysql.jdbc.Driver";
        String login = "root";
        String mdp = "root";
        String url = new String
        ("jdbc:mysql://localhost:3307/ruledatabase");
        Class.forName(pilote);
        Connection conn = DriverManager.getConnection(url, login, mdp);
        String requete2 = "Select * from integrationrule where Elements =
'"+elem+"';";
        Statement requete = conn.createStatement();
        ResultSet resultat = requete.executeQuery(requete2);
        while (resultat.next())
         rule = resultat.getString("Rule");}
}catch(Exception e){e.getMessage();}
return rule;}
Concerning the following algorithm, it generates the rule for each element.
Here, we present the case for "Measure". The same thing is done with the rest
of elements.
public String Generate_Rule (String type, String elem, int IdParent) {
String rule = "";
        if (Type.equals ("Measure"))
        rule = "Insert into Measure (MeasureName, MeasureType, idFact) values
('"+ elem + "', '"+ type  "','"+IdParent+")";
return rule;}
The following algorithm executes the queries.
public void Apply_Rule (String rule) {
try{
        String pilote = "com.mysql.jdbc.Driver";
        String login = "root";
        String mdp = "root";
        String url = new String("jdbc:mysql://localhost:3307/hsidatabase");
        Class.forName (pilote);
```

```
        Connection conn = DriverManager.getConnection(url, login, mdp);
        java.sql.Statement stm = conn.createStatement();
        int resultats = stm.executeUpdate(rule);
}catch (Exception e){e.getMessage ();}}
```

CONCLUSION

The healthcare industries generate huge amount of data which makes their exploitation and their mastering a hard task. For this reason, the use of DW is considered as the best solution to store the historical data for the analysis purpose.

In this work, we proposed a new approach to generate HDW. It combines the bottom-up and hybrid. The bottom-up is necessary since the different healthcare departments do not communicate and they do not share their information and their documents. We generate, then, for each one its HDM schema then we merge them to get at the end the final HDW schema.

Concerning the HDM, they are constructed using the hybrid approach taking into consideration the users' requirements and the databases.

Concerning the collect of the needs, we proposed an assistant system (HDwADS) that facilitates the task by exploiting the previous experiences stored as traces.

As perspective, we propose extending this work by exploiting other types of data sources such as the UML databases and the XML files.

REFERENCES

Annoni, E., Ravat, F., Teste, O., & Zurfluh, G. (2006). Towards Multidimensional Requirement Design. *Proceedings of the 8th International Conference Data Warehousing and Knowledge Discovery (DaWaK)* (pp. 75-84). 10.1007/11823728_8

Banek, M., Tjoa, A. M., & Stolba, N. (2006). Integrating Different Grain Levels in a Medical Data Warehouse Federation. In A. M. Tjoa & J. Trujillo (Eds.), *DaWak, LNCS* (Vol. 4081, pp. 185–194). Heidelberg: Springer. doi:10.1007/11823728_18

Bennett, W., Boone, E., Parker, D., Thorpe, A., Wang, M., & White, P. T. (2009). *Data Warehousing a New Focus in Healthcare Data Management.* Retrieved from http://www.himss.org/files/HIMSSorg/content/files/EHR/DataWarehousing.pdf

Berndt, D. J., Fisher, J. W., Hevner, A. R., & Studnicki, J. (2001). Healthcare Data Warehousing and Quality Assurance. *IEEE Computer, 34*(12), 56–65. doi:10.1109/2.970578

Berndt, D. J., Hevner, A. R., & Studnicki, J. (2003). The Catch Data Warehouse: Support for Community Health Care Decision-Making. *Decision Support Systems, 35*(3), 367–384. doi:10.1016/S0167-9236(02)00114-8

Bizarro, P., & Madeira, H. (2002). Adding a Performance-Oriented Perspective to Data Warehouse Design. *Proceedings of 4th International Conference Data Warehousing and Knowledge Discovery* (pp. 232-244). 10.1007/3-540-46145-0_23

Börger, E. (1998). High Level System Design and Analysis using Abstract State Machines. In D. Hutter, W. Stephan, P. Traverso, & M. Ullmann (Eds.), Current Trends in Applied Formal Methods FM-Trends '98, LNCS (Vol. 1641, pp. 1-43). Springer-Verlag.

Chen, P. P. S. (1976). The Entity-Relationship Model-Toward a Unified View of Data. *ACM Transactions on Database Systems*, *1*(1), 9–36. doi:10.1145/320434.320440

Darmont, J. (2008). Entreposage de Données Complexes pour la Medicine d'Anticipation Personalisée. *Proceedings of the 9th International Conference on System Science in Health Care* (p. 75).

Dutta, R. (2013). Health care data warehouse system architecture for influenza (flu) diseases. Proceedings of ACER (pp. 77–89).

Einbinder, J. S., Pates, R. D., & Reynolds, R. E. (2001). Case Study: A Data Warehouse for an Academic Medical Center. *Journal of Healthcare Information Management*, *15*(2), 165–175. PMID:11452578

Foundation, K. F. (2006). *Comparing Projected Growth in Health Care Expenditures and the Economy, Snapshots: Health Care Costs*. Retrieved from http://www.kff.org/insurance/snapshot/chcm050206oth2.cfm

Golfarelli, M., & Rizzi, S. (2009). *Data Warehouse Design: Modern Principles and Methodologies*. McGraw-Hill Osborne Media.

Golfarelli, M., & Rizzi, S. (2010). WAND: A CASE Tool for Data Warehouse Design. *Proceedings of 17th International Conference on Data Engineering (ICDE)* (pp. 7-9).

Gyssens, M., & Lakshmanan, L. V. S. (1997). A Foundation for Multi-dimensional Databases. *Proceedings of 23rd International Conference on Very Large Data Bases (VLDB)* (pp. 106-111).

Hüsemann, B., Lechtenbörger, J., & Vossen, G. (2000). Conceptual data warehouse design. *Proceedings International Workshop on Design and Management of Data Warehouses, Stockholm*, (pp. 3-9).

Inmon, W. H. (2005). *Building the Data Warehouse*. John Wiley & Sons Inc.

Kimball, R., & Ross, M. (2002). *The Data Warehouse Toolkit*. John Wiley & Sons.

Lee, M. L., & Ling, T. W. (1997). Resolving Constraint Conflicts in the Integration of Entity-Relationship Schemas. *Proceedings of the 16th International Conference on Conceptual Modeling,* Los Angeles, California, USA (pp. 394-407). 10.1007/3-540-63699-4_32

Levene, M., & Loizou, G. (2003). Why is the Snowflake Schema a Good Data Warehouse Design? *Information Systems Journal*, *28*(3), 225–240. doi:10.1016/S0306-4379(02)00021-2

Malinowski, E., & Zimanyi, E. (2008). *Advanced Data Warehouse Design, From Conventional to Spatial and Temporal Applications*. Springer Verlag Berlin Heidelberg.

Mike, D. (2014). *Clinical Data Warehouse: Why You Really Need One*. Retrieved from http://www.healthcatalyst.com/clinical-data-warehouse-why-you-need-one

Moody, D. L., & Kortink, M. A. R. (2000). From Enterprise Models to Dimensional Models: a Methodology for Data Warehouse and Data Mart Design. *Proceedings of the Second International Workshop on Design and Management of Data Warehouses (DMDW)* (pp.1-12).

Mul, M. D., Alons, P., Velde, P. V. D., Konings, I., Bakker, J., & Hazelzet, J. (2012). Development of a Clinical Data Warehouse from an Intensive Care Clinical Information System. *Computer Methods and Programs in Biomedicine*, *105*(1), 22–30. doi:10.1016/j.cmpb.2010.07.002 PMID:20728956

Peralta, V., Illarze, A., & Ruggia, R. (2003). On the Applicability of Rules to Automate Data Warehouse Logical Design. *Proceedings of the 15th Conference on Advanced Information Systems Engineering* (pp. 329-340).

Sahama, T. R., & Croll, P. R. (2007). A Data Warehouse Architecture for Clinical Data Warehousing. *Proceedings of the fifth Australasian symposium on ACSW frontiers* (vol. 68, pp. 227-232).

Sen, A., & Jacob, V. S. (1998). Industrial Strength Data Warehousing. *Communications of the ACM*, *41*(9), 28–31. doi:10.1145/285070.285076

Sheta, O. E., & Eldeen, A. N. (2012). Building a Health Care Data Warehouse for Cancer Diseases. *International Journal of Database Management Systems*, *4*(5), 39–46. doi:10.5121/ijdms.2012.4503

This research was previously published in Applying Business Intelligence to Clinical and Healthcare Organizations edited by José Machado and António Abelha; pages 84-115, copyright year 2016 by Medical Information Science Reference (an imprint of IGI Global).

Chapter 2
A Multi-Agent Based Modeling and Simulation Data Management and Analysis System for the Hospital Emergency Department

Manel Saad Saoud
University of Bordj Bou Arreridj, Algeria

Abdelhak Boubetra
University of Bordj Bou Arreridj, Algeria

Safa Attia
University of Bordj Bou Arreridj, Algeria

ABSTRACT

In the last decades, multi-agent based modeling and simulation systems have become more increasingly used to model the dynamic and the complex healthcare systems which contain many variabilities and uncertainties such as the hospital emergency departments (ED). Modeling and creating virtual societies almost identical and similar to the reality are considered as the strongest advantages of these agents systems. However, during the dynamic development of the artificial societies, a massive volume of data, which generally contains non-express and shrouded information and even knowledge, is involved. Therefore, dealing with this data, to study and to analyze the unclear relationships and the emerging phenomena, is a well-known weakness and bottleneck that the multi-agent systems is suffering from. In conjunction, data mining techniques are the most powerful tools that can help simulation experts to tackle this issue. This paper presents an ongoing research that combines the multi-agent based modeling and simulation systems and data mining techniques to develop a decision support system to improve the operation of the emergency department.

DOI: 10.4018/978-1-7998-2451-0.ch002

Copyright © 2020, IGI Global. Copying or distributing in print or electronic forms without written permission of IGI Global is prohibited.

INTRODUCTION

Nowadays, the multi-agent based modeling and simulation systems have generously demonstrated their efficiency in many scientific fields, in particular with the open problems of the dynamic and the complex systems, such as the healthcare systems. Adopting simulation systems offers, in one hand, the possibility to model and to create virtual systems almost identical and similar to the real ones, where the individuals and even the organizations are directly represented with their interactions. On the other hand, using these artificial societies facilities the test and the evaluation of the possible policies and the different "what-if" scenarios, which avoid the costly and uncertain changes in the real system.

Complex systems are composed of many individuals and entities, each one of them is mainly characterized by its architecture, its behavior, and its degree of reasoning (Ferber, 1999). Based on these characteristics (Wooldridge, 2009) divided the agents into three main types: cognitive agents, reactive agents, and hybrid agents.

The cognitive agent is an intelligent agent owns a necessary knowledge base to perform its tasks and manage its interactions with the other agents and its environment. It has a symbolic representation of its environment and the agents and explicit goals and plans to decide his actions. Unlike the cognitive agent, the reactive agent has a straightforward and predefined behavior and responds only to a simple environmental stimulus. The hybrid agent represents the combination of the two previous types.

Multi-agent based modeling and simulation system of complex systems and phenomena is to model virtual societies with various individuals or agents via a computer, to observe their behaviors and to understand the relation between them.

According to (Wooldridge & R. Jennings, 1995) an agent is a software-based computer system characterized by four properties; Autonomy (Agent has the possibility to operate without a direct intervention of humans or other agents, and it has some control over his activities and inside his state), Social ability (agent connects with different agents via an agent communication language), Reactivity (Agent can perceive his environment and respond to changes that occur in it), Pro-activity (the possibility to exhibit a behavior controlled by its objectives rather than a reaction according to its environment only).

During the dynamic evolution of the virtual agents' systems, an enormous amount of data is involved, especially, since simulation massively consume and generate the data. The data delivered generally encase underlying and covered information and even knowledge. Thus, the search in these data is of immense utility to better study and understand the operation of the system. Accordingly, a well-known weakness or bottleneck that the MAMSS is suffering from is the analysis of the unclear relationships and the phenomena that may emerge in these artificial systems. As a solution to this problem, Data Mining techniques are considered as the most powerful tools that can help simulation specialists to tackle these issues.

In conjunction, Knowledge Discovery in Database (Data Mining) (Pujari, 2001; Fayyad, Piatetsky-Shapiro, & Smyth, 1996; Hegland, 2001; Han, Kamber, & Pei, 2011) represents the process of discovering and extracting knowledge from large volumes of data. Data Mining process is divided mainly into three principal phases (Fayyad, Piatetsky-Shapiro, & Smyth, 1996): Data pre-processing, Data Mining, and Data post-processing.

Our methodology presented in this paper points out how can the multi-agent based modeling and simulation systems benefit from Data Mining techniques to solve simulation bottlenecks and to improve the study's quality. The combination approach is demonstrated through a case study on the operation of the emergency department in the public hospital Lakhdar Bouzidi in Bordj Bou Arreridj (Algeria).

The hospital emergency department is a critical and a complex system that involves many variabilities and uncertainties. The Hospital emergency departments are often plagued with the overcrowding, the high variety of patients' illnesses, the different resources with different skills, the uncertain patients' arrival and the need for the same resources simultaneously. These problems contribute to long waiting time and sojourn, low quality of care, and stress situations for both patients and EDs staff.

The objective of this research is to develop a decision support system based on the incorporation of the agent-based modeling and simulation systems and the knowledge extraction methods (Data Mining techniques), to design a robust tool that can help ED managers to improve the quality and the effectiveness of the care provided in the hospital emergency department Lakhdar Bouzidi (LB-ED)in Bordj Bou Arreridj (Algeria).

In this paper, in addition to, the implementation of a multi-agent simulation model using the programmable modeling environment NetLogo (Wilensky, 1999), to improve the operation performance of the studied emergency department and to enhance the quality of care provided. We shed light on the influence of the quality of the simulation inputs on the study results' quality. In order to ensure the credibility and the validation of our simulation model, to improve the quality of its contributions and to increase and the accuracy of its results, Data Mining preprocessing methods (Kantardzic, 2011; Maimon & Rokach, 2005; Fayyad, Piatetsky-Shapiro, & Smyth, 1996; Cios, Pedrycz, & Swiniarski, 1998) are applied to the collected data set (the simulation inputs). The results showed that the contribution of the preprocessing methods to treat the simulation data had a significant and notable impact on the reliability and thoroughness of the outputs of our system proposed. Consequently, the results of the proposed scenarios regarding the average waiting time of patients and their average length of stay in the LB-ED, have been remarkably enhanced.

The remainder of this paper is organized as follows; A literature review focuses on one hand on the existing background that investigates the combination of the multi-agent based modeling and simulation systems and the Data Mining techniques, on the other hand, the simulation studies within the healthcare are presented in section two. The case of study and the operation of the hospital emergency department Lakhdar Bouzidi Bordj Bou Arreridj (Algeria) is described in section three. In section four, the proposed system results and discussion are presented. Finally, we conclude this paper with the conclusion and prospects.

LITERATURE REVIEW

In recent years, a growing body of literature has addressed the ways in which simulation studies can be improved using the knowledge discovery techniques. (Morbitzer, Strachan, & Simpson, 2004) Portrayed how clustering analysis technique can be utilized to build simulation studies performance. The methodology proposed in (Brady & Yellig, 2005) provided knowledge concerning the interrelationship between input variables used in the simulation model, to select the optimization ones. The study exhibited in (Wu, Olson, & Dong, 2006) showed a methodology that uses the Monte Carlo simulation and fuzzy decision-making using the gray related analysis method. (Remondino & Correndo, 2006) The authors investigated the paths in which Data Mining strategies could be effectively connected to Agent-Based Modeling and Simulation, so as to endeavor concealed relations and emergent behavior. To create and keep up the parameters of the evaluated costs, an innovative methodology that combines simulation, Data

Mining, and knowledge-based techniques for the life cycle cost was produced in (Painter, Erraguntla, Gary, & Beachkofski, 2006).

A simulation optimization approach that depends on a dynamic knowledge extraction model that recognizes the significant inputs of the simulation and finds the effect of their relationship on the Framework execution was proposed in (Better, Glover, & Laguna, 2007). In (Alnoukari, El Sheikh, & Alzoabi, 2009) the authors proposed a decision support system in light of the combination of Data Mining and simulation systems. (Dudas, Amos, & Boström, 2009) This work examines the methods for extracting knowledge from simulation based multi-objective optimization, with a specific goal to get data can bolster decision makers to take the right choices so as to upgrade the manufacturing process. In (Baqueiro, Wang, McBurney, & Coenen, 2009) a bi-directional integration study which combines Data Mining (DM) and Agent-Based Modeling and Simulation (ABMS) was introduced. (Arroyo, Hassan, Gutiérrez, & Pavón, 2010) showed and Illustrated with a case study the application of Data Mining techniques for the improvement and development of agent-based models. Understanding of the relationship between the inputs and the outputs parameters of the simulation system using Data Mining techniques has been proposed in (Ghasemi, Ghasemi, & Ghasemi, 2011). In (Saffar, Doniec, Boonaert, & Lecoeuche, 2011) an approach based on clustering techniques using the observation of real word agents to model simulated agents was proposed. (Lytton, 2006) In this study, the authors have built up a neural inquiry framework (NQS) in the NEURON simulator, a system of a relational database, a research function, and Data Mining tools were provided.

In conjunction, Simulation has profusely used to solve healthcare systems bottlenecks. This review focus on the use of agent-based modeling and simulation to improve the care quality in the emergency department (Cabrera, Taboada, Iglesias, Epelde, & Luque, 2012) (Cabrera, Taboada, Iglesias, Epelde, & Luque, 2011) (Liu, et al., 2015) offered a decision support system using an agent-based modeling simulation to enhance the operation of EDs. To discover the ideal ED staff configuration (Jones & Evans, 2008) designed an agent-based simulation tool using NetLogo software, the paper assessed the effect of different doctor staffing arrangements on patient waiting times. Agent-based models (ABM) and queuing model (QM) techniques were applied to research patient access and course through the ED. IN (Kaushal, et al., 2015) an agent-based simulation tool is proposed to evaluate fast track treatment (FTT) in an ED. A comprehensive review study is presented in (Gul & Guneri, 2015) to reveal the importance of simulation for disaster preparedness of EDs and the innovative aspects of recent ED simulation applications.

Simulation Data Management

LB-ED System Description

Due to the high demographic development and the strategic location of the region of Bordj Bou Arreridj(Algeria), the public hospital of Bordj Bou Arreridj (Lakhdar Bouzidi) has turned into the first destination for many patients. Lakhdar Bouzidi emergency department is open 24 hours a day and receives more than 170 000 patients a year on average. Three shifts are alternating to cover the high demand for services over the entire day. The LB-ED is mainly composed of; Consultation area (the consultation-physician evaluation), Laboratory (medical analysis), X-ray area, nursing room, observation unit (equipped and devoted to patients whose need a treatment and monitoring), resuscitation area (for seriously and critically ill patients), and administration zone to register admitted patients to the hospital.

Figure 1. LB-ED patient flow diagram

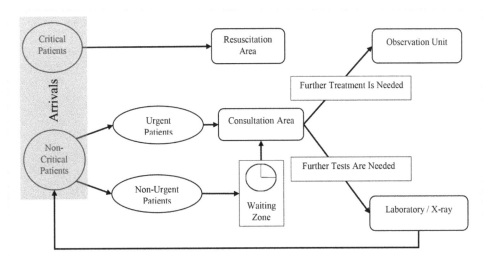

Critically ill patients are immediately rushed and treated in the resuscitation area. Less critical patients get carried directly into the consultation room to be promptly seen by the consultation-physician. Otherwise, the patients wait for the consultation-physician examination. Patients needed further tests, to get the consultation-physician assessment, are sent to the laboratory or the X-ray area. Patients required a continued monitoring or a diagnostic evaluation are sent to the observation unit. The LB-ED patient flow diagram is shown in Figure 1.

LB-ED Simulation Model Design

Data Collection

To build and develop an agent-based modeling and simulation system for the operation of LB-ED, a data collection methodology was carried out. The data collected was mostly derived from LB-ED patients' registries (our database is extracted from the LB-ED patients' registries from January 2013 to December 2013), the remnant of data needed was gotten through the interviews with the ED staff and the system observation.

Simulation Inputs Analysis

To evaluate the impact of the quality of the simulation inputs on the quality of the outputs and the study in general, the inputs data set is separated into two subsets: The preprocessing methods are applied to the first subset before using it in our simulation model. Where the second subset represents the raw data set as illustrates in Figure 2.

Figure 2. Simulation data preparation

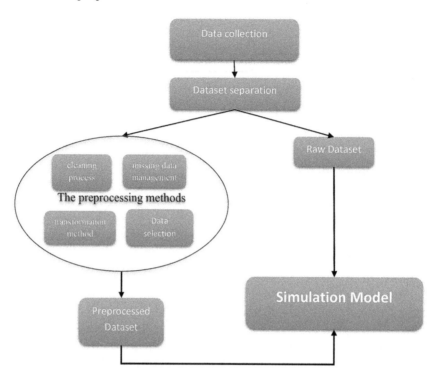

Data Preprocessing

Emergency Department data are often very vulnerable to be inaccurate, corrupted, incomplete, inconsistent, and noisy. To enhance the quality of our inputs and, consequently, of our simulation results the preprocessing phase of the Data Mining is applied on the first subset. First data cleaning process is applied to remove errors, outliers, and anomalies and eliminates duplicated data. Then a missing data management that guarantees the treatment of missing information without losing the force of our original data is created. After that, a transformation method is performed to get the appropriate information form. Finally, before run the simulation model non-useful data as the personal information of patients are eliminated, where target data sets and pertinent information are selected.

Simulation Model Built

A multi-agent based modeling and simulation system for the operation of LB-ED is implemented using the multi-agent programmable modeling environment NetLogo (Wilensky, 1999) Figure 3; an appropriate platform for creating complex Frameworks made out of a vast number of agents all working and acting in parallel and freely. Consequently, it can be conceivable to investigate the association between the micro-level conduct of individuals and the macro-level examples that rise out of their collaboration.

Based on the physical layout and the functioning of the LB-ED our simulation model is built. Contingent upon the patient's state and indications, three patient acuity levels are introduced in our system; low-acuity (non-urgent patients), medium-acuity (urgent patients) and high-acuity (emergency and critical patients). Three kinds of physicians depending on their behaviors and activities in the LB-ED

Figure 3. LB-ED system overview

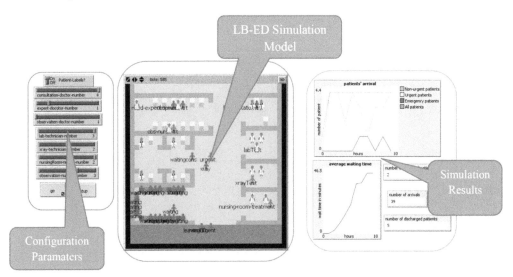

are developed; consultation-physicians are installed in the consultation area to ensure the first examination of patients. Observation-physicians are installed in the observation unit to guarantee the continued monitoring, and diagnostic evaluation of patients needed further treatment. Specialist physicians are requested if the patient's state needs expert assessment.

SIMULATION RESULTS AND DISCUSSION

Under similar setup parameters of the real system, our simulation model has been performed several times using different inputs' data sets. Each execution represents 24 hours of LB-ED activities. To evaluate the performance of our system, simulation results are compared with the real system data. Three key performance indicators have been used:

- **Resources Utilization (%):** The objective is to utilize resources efficiently so as to maximize patients' satisfaction;
- **Average Waiting Time:** Time that the patient spends in the ED waiting to receive treatment;
- **Average Length of Stay:** Of discharged and admitted patients: the total period that the patient pays in ED from his arrival until his discharge or admission.

Simulation Results' Validation

Raw Inputs Results

Intending to assessing the effect of simulation preprocessed inputs on the quality of simulation results, two inputs' data sets have been used in our system. In the first part of our methodology simulation has been executed with the raw data set (non-preprocessed data). After that, a comparison between simulation

Figure 4. Physicians' utilization - simulated results

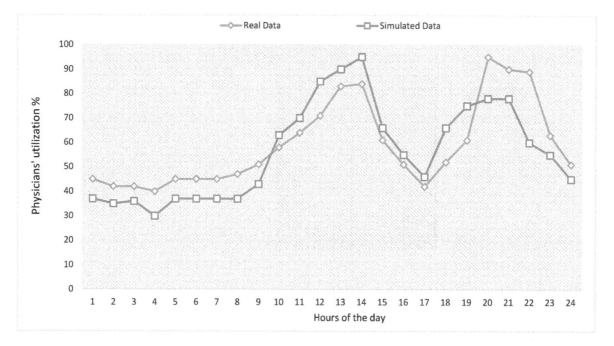

results and the outputs of the real system regarding the key performance indicators mentioned above is carried out. The comparison results are shown in Figure 4, Figure 5, and Figure 6 respectively.

Figure 4 shows the simulated results of the doctors' utilization over the 24 hours of the day compared with the real doctors' utilization data. It can be easily noticed that the simulated results are differe ntiated between good results (Converge to the actual data) and bad results (widely divergent with the real ones).

Reducing the average waiting time is one of the biggest challenges that EDs managers must cope with to improve the ED performances and increase the quality of care and the patients' satisfaction. Figure 5 illustrates our simulation results of the average waiting time for patients depending on their acuity levels (low acuity – medium acuity – high acuity).

According to Figure 5, it is clearly observed that the simulation using the non-preprocessed data provided us better average waiting time for the medium acuity patients, though the quality of simulation results for the high acuity patients and especially for the low acuity patients was not acceptable.

The last key performance indicator that has been identified in our methodology is the average length of stay in the ED (sojourn). Depending on patients' acuity levels, two varieties of sojourn in the ED are distinguished; short sojourn period for the discharged patients (patients who leave the ED as they didn't need a hospitalization) and long sojourn time for the admitted patients who need a hospitalization (in-patients who stay in the ED in order to get available beds in the hospital). Figure 6 shows the simulated results of the average length of stay in the ED for discharged and admitted patients represented with their acuity levels. It is undoubtedly observed that the simulation results are not what we looked forward to since they are not credible and relatively distant from the real outputs.

Figure 5. Average waiting time - simulated results

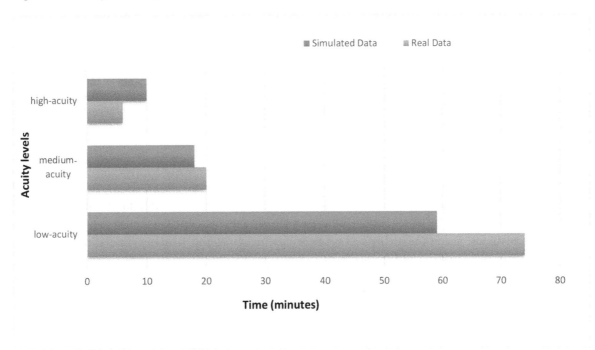

Figure 6. Average length of stay in the ED - simulated results

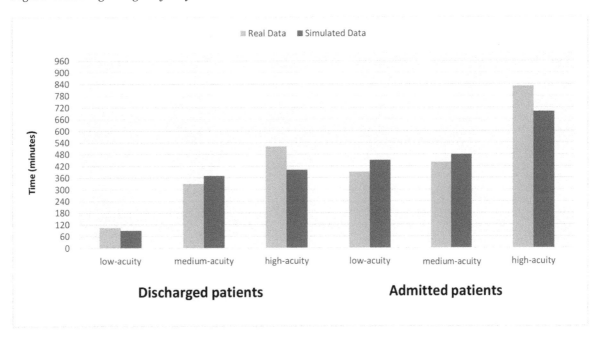

Preprocessed Inputs Results

In this stage, our preprocessed data set is used as an input to the simulation model, to test the performance of our system objectively and to demonstrate the impact of the preprocessed data on the simulation results. A comparison of the achieved results (physicians' utilization, the average waiting time and the average length of stay) using the preprocessed data set with real outputs and obtained results using the raw data setis carried out. The comparison results are shown in Figure 7, Figure 8 and Figure 9 respectively.

Figure 7 summarizes the simulation results (using the raw data set as well as the preprocessed data set) of the physicians' utilization over 24 hours of activity, compared with the results of the physicians' utilization of the real system in the same hours of activity. It is unmistakably remarked that there was a wide variation among physicians' utilization results when we started the simulation model with the non-preprocessed data and the real outputs. While the initialization of our simulation model with the preprocessed data set gave us better results almost identical to the real ones.

Figure 8 illustrates, in addition to the average waiting time of patients with the simulation results that used the raw data set as inputs and the average waiting time results when the preprocessed data set is used, the real average waiting times as a benchmark for comparison. The average waiting time simulation result of the law acuity patients is improved from 59 min when simulation model started with the raw data set to 70 min if the preprocessed data set is used. Consequently, it is more approached to the target which is 74 min in the real system. In the same context, the simulation results for patients with the medium acuity level are as follows; the actual system output is 20 min, 18 min for the raw data set simulation result and 21 min for the simulation result of the preprocessed data set. Where the simulation results for the high acuity patients are 7,2 min for the preprocessed data set, 6 min the real average wait-

Figure 7. Physicians' utilization - simulation results' comparison

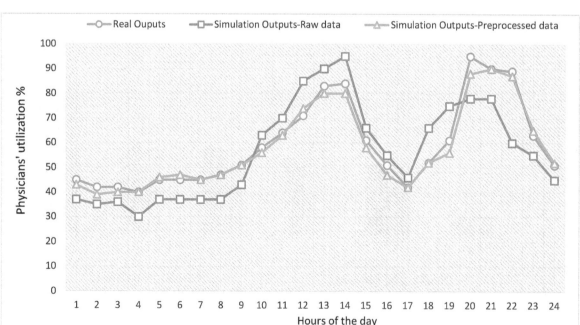

Figure 8. Average waiting time - simulation results' comparison

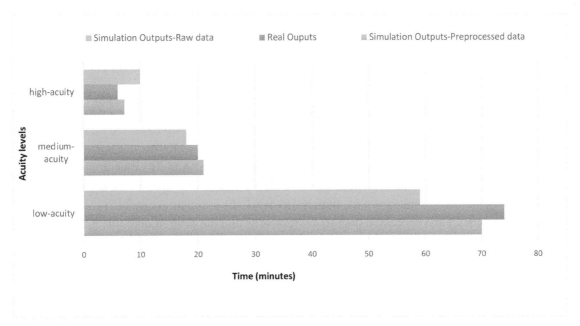

Figure 9. Average length of stay in the ED - simulation results' comparison

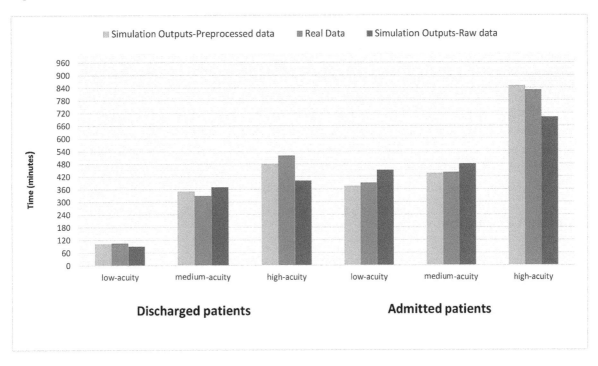

ing time and 10 min for the raw data set. In observing the illustrated results, it can be seen that, the use of the preprocessed data has a significant impact on the quality of our simulation results, where of the average waiting times of patients with their different acuity levels (low acuity – medium acuity – high acuity) have been considerably improved and approached to the real system outputs unlike the obtained results with the raw data set.

Figure 9 shows the simulation results of the average length of stay in the emergency department for both discharged and admitted patient. As described above, our simulation is performed using the preprocessed data as well as the raw data. Hence, the obtained results in the two cases are compared with the real data. The simulation results of the average length of stay in the ED for the discharged patients with low acuity level are as follows; 105 min represents the real and desired data, 102 min the simulation result using the preprocessed data, where the simulation result with the non-preprocessed data set gave us 90 min. For the discharged patients with a medium acuity level, the simulation results are 370 min and 350 min for the raw data set and processed data set respectively, and the desired output is 330 min. Patients with a high acuity level, generally stay in the emergency department more time comparing with medium acuity and low acuity patients. For that category of patients, the simulation results of the discharged patients are 400 min with the use of the raw data set and 480 min with the preprocessed data set which is more approached to the real output 520 min. As well the average length of stay for the discharged patients, simulation performances for the admitted patients demonstrated the significant influence of the contribution of the Data Mining preprocessing methods on the quality of its results. Where the results for the high acuity level patients is enhanced from 700 min when we have initialized the simulation model with the raw data to 830 min and more approached to the real output 850 min. For the medium acuity patients, the actual average length of stay is 440 min, simulation with preprocessed data is 435 min, and with raw data, the simulation result is 480 min. The simulation results for the admitted patients with a low acuity level are 450 min and 375 min when the raw data set and the preprocessed data set are used respectively, and the real system average length of stay, in this case, is 390 min.

In summary, our simulation model has been initialized with two different input data sets; the first one is the raw data set (collected data without any changes or processing). Data Mining preprocessing methods have been applied to the second data set to handle it. Three key performance indicators (the physicians' utilization, the average waiting time of patients (low acuity patients – medium acuity patients – high acuity patients) and their length of stay in the emergency department) have been used to measure and evaluate the performance of our simulation outputs. Our results reveal that the application of the Data Mining preprocessing methods on the simulation inputs has been accordingly, influenced noticeably the quality of its outputs measured with the three key performance indicators selected.

Proposed Scenarios

After guaranteeing the credibility and the reliability of our simulation results using the preprocessed data set, various scenarios are proposed and executed to improve the performance of the LB-EB operation and to enhance the quality of care provided. Due to the limited budget, adding more physicians in each shift to decrease the long waiting time and the length of stay of patients is not the optimal strategy that can be adopted by the LB-ED managers. Therefore, our proposed scenarios are based on adding one more doctor in a particular shift to find out the optimal configuration:

Scenario 1 (S1): A physician is added in the consultation zone between 8.00 am to 2.00 pm (in the first shift).

Scenario 2 (S2): A physician is added in the consultation zone between 2.00 pm to 8.00 pm (in the second shift).

Scenario (S3): A physician is added in the consultation area between 8.00 pm to 8.00 am (in the third shift).

Scenario (S4): A physician is added in the observation unit between 8.00 am to 2.00 pm (in the first shift).

Scenario (S5): A physician is added in the observation unit between 2.00 pm to 8.00 pm (in the second shift).

Scenario (S6): A physician is added in the observation unit between 8.00 pm to 8.00 am (in the third shift).

Scenario S1, S2, and S3 are proposed to reduce the average waiting time of patients before the first assessment of the consultation doctor. To decrease the long length of stay in the emergency department, that is generally caused by the long waiting for the treatment in the observation unit, the scenario S4, S5 and S6 are proposed.

The Simulation Results of the Proposed Scenarios

The simulation results of the proposed scenarios are shown in Figure 10 and Figure 11 respectively.

Figure 10 summarizes the average waiting time results of the low-acuity, medium-acuity, and high-acuity patient for the tree first scenarios proposed. The waiting time of the low-acuity patients is decreased from 74 min in the real system to 55 min, 63 min, and 60 min for scenarios S1, S2, and S3 respectively. For the medium acuity patients, the results were as follows; 20 min for the real data, 12 min, 15 min,

Figure 10. The average waiting time results of the proposed scenarios

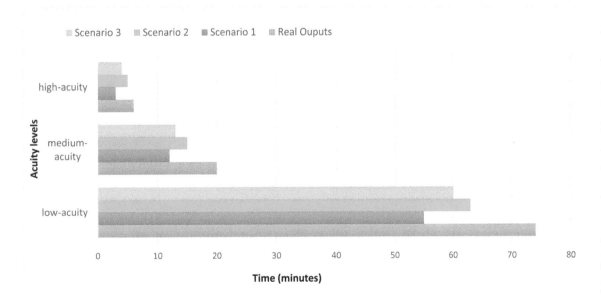

Figure 11. The average length of stay results of the proposed scenarios

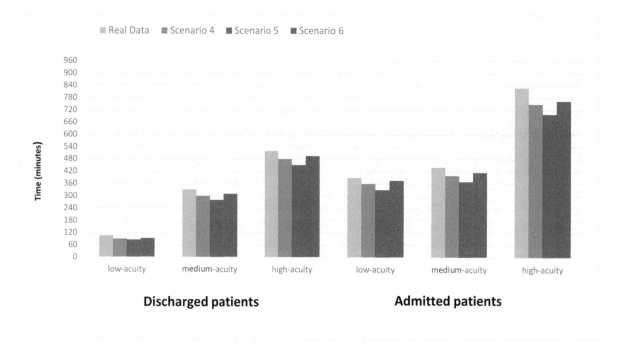

and 13 min for scenarios S1, S2, and S3 respectively. The waiting time of the high-acuity patients is reduced from 6 min the real output to 3 min, 5 min, and 4 min for scenarios S1, S2, and S3 respectively.

Figure 11 illustrates the average length of stay results of the proposed scenarios for both discharged and admitted patient presented with the three acuity levels (low, medium and high). The simulation results for the discharged patients with low acuity level are as follows; 105 min for the real data, 90 min, 85 min, and 92 min for scenarios S4, S5, and S6 respectively. For the discharged patients with medium acuity level the average length of stay is reduced from 330 min for the real data to 300 min, 280 min, and 3s10 min for scenarios S4, S5, and S6 respectively. For the discharged patients with high acuity level the average length of stay is reduced from 520 min for the real data to 480 min, 450 min, and 495 min for scenarios S4, S5, and S6 respectively. The results of the admitted patients are as follows; the average length of stay of patients with low acuity level is decreased from 390 min for the real data to 360 min, 330 min, and 375 min for scenarios S4, S5, and S6 respectively. For patients with medium acuity level the results are as follows; 440 min for the real data, 400 min, 370 min, and 415 min for scenarios S4, S5, and S6 respectively. Finally, for the admitted patients with the high acuity level, the average length of stay is reduced from 830 min in the real system to 750 min, 700 min, and 765 min for scenarios S4, S5, and S6 respectively.

In summary, our simulation model has been initialized with two different input data sets; the first one is the raw data set (collected data without any changes or processing). Data Mining preprocessing methods have been applied to the second data set to handle it. Three key performance indicators (the physicians' utilization, the average waiting time of patients (low acuity patients – medium acuity patients – high acuity patients) and their length of stay in the emergency department) have been used to measure and evaluate the performance of our simulation outputs. Our results reveal that the application of the Data

Mining preprocessing methods on the simulation inputs has been accordingly, influenced noticeably the quality of its outputs measured with the three key performance indicators selected.

The implementation of the proposed scenarios (1,2,3), to reduce the average waiting time of patients before the assessment of the consultation physicians gave us good results comparing to the real output of the system. While the best results obtained of the three proposed scenarios are the results of the second scenario (Adding a physician in the consultation zone between 2.00 pm to 8.00 pm). The results of the average length of stay of the proposed scenarios (4,5,6) have been considerably improved comparing the real output of the system. However, the results of the fifth scenario (Adding a physician in the observation unit between 2.00 pm to 8.00 pm) outperformed the results of the other scenarios (S4 and S6).

CONCLUSION

In this paper, a decision support system based on the integration of the multi-agent based modeling and simulation systems and the Data Mining techniques, for the functioning of the emergency department of the public hospital Lakhdar Bouzidi in Bordj Bou Arreridj (Algeria) has been implemented.

The main contributions of the proposed methodology are, on the one hand, the investigation of the different ways that can be used to advantage from the Data Mining techniques to solve the open problems of the multi-agent based modeling and simulation systems and to improve the exactitude of their results. On the other hand, the present research develops a robust system that can deal with the dynamic nature of the ED, and help the ED managers to check and test various scenarios and strategies, to enhance the operation of the emergency department and improve the quality and the effectiveness of care provided.

To design a reliable system similar and identical to the studied emergency department, an agent-based simulation model using the multi-agent programmable modeling environment NetLogo has been developed. Besides, to explore the influence of the pretreatment of the simulation inputs on the quality of its results and the model credibility, before performing our simulation system, the collected database has been divided into two data sets. Then, the preprocessing methods of the Data Mining techniques have been applied to the first data set, where the second one has been used without any treatment. After that, our simulation model has been initialized and performed using the raw data set, then, the preprocessed data set was used. Thereafter, to evaluate the performance of the simulation model and to measure the exactitude of its outputs, the physicians' utilization, the average waiting time of patients of the low acuity patients, the medium acuity patients and high acuity patients and their length of stay have been used as the key performance indicators of the emergency department. Finally, the simulation results of the three key performances indicators, using the tow datasets have been compared with the outputs of the real system. The comparative study done, showed that the initialization of our simulation model with the pretreated inputs using the preprocessing methods had given better and reliable results comparing to the other ones without the contribution the Data Mining.

To help the ED managers to improve the performance of the LB-EB operation and to enhance the quality of care provided, various scenarios are proposed and performed. Consequently, the results of the proposed scenarios regarding the average waiting time of patients and their average length of stay in the ED, have been remarkably enhanced. To verify and review the performance of our system, the clinical experts have been widely involved throughout all its conceptualization and its development phases. The ED managers test the proposed scenarios, and the results are hugely met their requests. Also, our system provides them the possibility to perform other scenarios and strategies.

Further improvement of our research will be carried out. We plan to go deeply into new issues of the integration of the multi-agent based modeling and simulation systems and the Data Mining techniques. Extracting hidden information and useful knowledge by applying more Data Mining techniques on the simulation outputs to provide a reliable, crucial and decisive system that can help the managers of the emergency department to improve the performance of the system, to decrease the average waiting time and the average length of stay in the ED and to increase the patients' satisfaction will be the primary objectives of our future works.

REFERENCES

Alnoukari, M., El Sheikh, A., & Alzoabi, Z. (2009). An integrated Data Mining and simulation solution. In Handbook of Research on Discrete Event Simulation Environments: Technologies and Applications: Technologies and Applications (p. 359).

Arroyo, J., Hassan, S., Gutiérrez, C., & Pavón, J. (2010). Re-thinking simulation: A methodological approach for the application of Data Mining in agent-based modelling. *Computational & Mathematical Organization Theory*, *16*(4), 416–435. doi:10.100710588-010-9078-y

Baqueiro, O., Wang, Y., McBurney, P., & Coenen, F. (2009). Integrating Data Mining and agent based modeling and simulation. In Advances in Data Mining. Applications and Theoretical Aspects (pp. 220-231). Springer Berlin Heidelberg. doi:10.1007/978-3-642-03067-3_18

Better, M., Glover, F., & Laguna, M. (2007). Advances in analytics: Integrating dynamic Data Mining with simulation optimization. *IBM journal of research and development*, *51*(3.4), 477-487.

Brady, T. F., & Yellig, E. (2005). Simulation Data Mining: a new form of computer simulation output. *Proceedings of the 37th conference on Winter simulation WSC '05* (pp. 285-289). 10.1109/WSC.2005.1574262

Cabrera, E., Taboada, M., Iglesias, M. L., Epelde, F., & Luque, E. (2011). Optimization of healthcare emergency departments by agent-based simulation. *Procedia computer science*, *4*, 1880-1889.

Cabrera, E., Taboada, M., Iglesias, M. L., Epelde, F., & Luque, E. (2012). Simulation optimization for healthcare emergency departments. *Procedia Computer Science*, *9*, 1464–1473. doi:10.1016/j.procs.2012.04.161

Cios, K., Pedrycz, W., & Swiniarski, R. (1998). *Data Mining and Knowledge Discovery*. Springer, US. doi:10.1007/978-1-4615-5589-6_1

Dudas, C., Amos, N., & Boström, H. (2009). Information Extraction from Solution Set of Simulation-based Multi-objective Optimisation using Data Mining. *Proceedings of Industrial Simulation Conference*.

Fayyad, U., Piatetsky-Shapiro, G., & Smyth, P. (1996). From Data Mining to knowledge discovery in databases. *AI Magazine*, *17*(3), 37.

Ferber, J. (1999). *Multi-Agent System: An Introduction to Distributed Artificial Intelligence*. Reading: Addison-Wesley.

Ghasemi, S., Ghasemi, M., & Ghasemi, M. (2011). Knowledge discovery in discrete event simulation output analysis. In *Innovative Computing Technology* (pp. 108–120). Springer Berlin Heidelberg. doi:10.1007/978-3-642-27337-7_11

Gul, M., & Guneri, A. F. (2015). A comprehensive review of emergency department simulation applications for normal and disaster conditions. *Computers & Industrial Engineering*, *83*, 327–344. doi:10.1016/j.cie.2015.02.018

Han, J., Kamber, M., & Pei, J. (2011). *Data Mining: concepts and techniques*. Elsevier.

Hegland, M. (2001). Data Mining techniques. *Acta Numerica*, *10*, 313–355. doi:10.1017/S0962492901000058

Jones, S. S., & Evans, R. S. (2008). An agent based simulation tool for scheduling emergency department physicians. *AMIA ... Annual Symposium Proceedings / AMIA Symposium. AMIA Symposium*, *2008*, 338. PMID:18998871

Kantardzic, M. (2011). *Data Mining: concepts, models, methods, and algorithms*. John Wiley & Sons. doi:10.1002/9781118029145

Kaushal, A., Zhao, Y., Peng, Q., Strome, T., Weldon, E., Zhang, M., & Chochinov, A. (2015). Evaluation of fast track strategies using agent-based simulation modeling to reduce waiting time in a hospital emergency department. *Socio-Economic Planning Sciences*, *50*, 18–31. doi:10.1016/j.seps.2015.02.002

Liu, Z., Cabrera, E., Taboada, M., Epelde, F., Rexachs, D., & Luque, E. (2015). Quantitative Evaluation of Decision Effects in the Management of Emergency Department Problems. *Procedia Computer Science*, *51*, 433–442. doi:10.1016/j.procs.2015.05.265

Lytton, W. (2006). Neural Query System: Data-mining from within the NEURON simulator. *Neuroinformatics*, *4*(2), 163–176. doi:10.1385/NI:4:2:163 PMID:16845167

Maimon, O., & Rokach, L. (2005). *Data Mining and knowledge discovery handbook*. New York: Springer. doi:10.1007/b107408

Morbitzer, C., Strachan, P., & Simpson, C. (2004). Data Mining analysis of building simulation performance data. *Building Services Engineering Research and Technology*, *25*(3), 253–267. doi:10.1191/0143624404bt098oa

Painter, M., Erraguntla, M., Gary, L., & Beachkofski, B. (2006). Using simulation, Data Mining, and knowledge discovery techniques for optimized aircraft engine fleet management. *Proceedings of the 38th conference on Winter simulation* (pp. 1253-1260). 10.1109/WSC.2006.323221

Pujari, A. K. (2001). *Data Mining techniques*. Universities press.

Remondino, M., & Correndo, G. (2006). Mabs validation through repeated execution and Data Mining analisys. International Journal of Simulation: Systems. *Science & Technology*, *7*(6), 10–21.

Saffar, I., Doniec, A., Boonaert, J., & Lecoeuche, S. (2011). Multi-Agent simulation design driven by real observations and clustering techniques. *Proceedings of the 2011 23rd IEEE International Conference Tools with Artificial Intelligence (ICTAI)* (pp. 555-560). IEEE. 10.1109/ICTAI.2011.89

Wilensky, U. (1999). *NetLogo*. Evanston, IL: Center for Connected Learning and Computer Based Modeling, Northwestern University. Retrieved from http://ccl.northwestern.edu/netlogo/

Wooldridge, M. (2009). *An introduction to multiagent systems*. John Wiley & Sons.

Wooldridge, M., & Jennings, R. (1995). Intelligent agents: Theory and practice. *The Knowledge Engineering Review*, *10*(2), 115–152. doi:10.1017/S0269888900008122

Wu, D., Olson, D. L., & Dong, Z. Y. (2006). Data Mining and simulation: A grey relationship demonstration. *International Journal of Systems Science*, *37*(13), 981–986. doi:10.1080/00207720600891521

This research was previously published in the International Journal of Healthcare Information Systems and Informatics (IJHISI), 12(3); edited by Joseph Tan and Qiang (Shawn) Cheng; pages 21-36, copyright year 2017 by IGI Publishing (an imprint of IGI Global).

Chapter 3

A Case Study Perspective for Balanced Perioperative Workflow Achievement through Data–Driven Process Improvement

Jim Ryan
Auburn University at Montgomery, USA

Barbara Doster
University of Alabama Birmingham Hospital, USA

Sandra Daily
Cullman Regional Medical Center, USA

Carmen Lewis
Troy University, USA

ABSTRACT

Based on a 143-month longitudinal study of an academic medical center, this paper examines operations management practices of continuous improvement, workflow balancing, benchmarking, and process reengineering within a hospital's perioperative operations. Specifically, this paper highlights data-driven efforts within perioperative sub-processes to balance overall patient workflow by eliminating bottlenecks, delays, and inefficiencies. This paper illustrates how dynamic technological activities of analysis, evaluation, and synthesis applied to internal and external organizational data can highlight complex relationships within integrated processes to identify process limitations and potential process capabilities, ultimately yielding balanced patient workflow through data-driven perioperative process improvement. Study implications and/or limitations are also included.

DOI: 10.4018/978-1-7998-2451-0.ch003

Copyright © 2020, IGI Global. Copying or distributing in print or electronic forms without written permission of IGI Global is prohibited.

INTRODUCTION

The perioperative process yields patient end-state goals: (1) a patient undergoes a surgical procedure; (2) minimal exacerbation of existing disorders; (3) avoidance of new morbidities; and (4) subsequent prompt procedure recovery (Silverman & Rosenbaum, 2009). To these end-state goals, a hospital's perioperative process provides surgical care for inpatients and outpatients during pre-operative, intra-operative, and immediate post-operative periods. Accordingly, the perioperative sub-processes (e.g. pre-operative, intra-operative, and post-operative) are sequential where each activity sequence paces the efficiency and effectiveness of subsequent activities. Furthermore, perioperative sub-processes require continuous parallel replenishment of sterile supplies and removal of soiled materials. Given the multiple sub-processes and associated dynamics, Fowler et al. (2008) views a hospital's perioperative process as complex and workflow complexity as a barrier to change and improvement. Nonetheless, integrated hospital information systems (IS) and information technology (IT) provide measurement and subsequent accountability for healthcare quality and cost, creating a dichotomy (e.g. quality versus cost) that represents the foundation for healthcare improvement (Dougherty & Conway, 2008).

The challenge of delivering quality, efficient, and cost-effective services affects all hospital stake-holders. Perioperative workflow tightly couples patient flow, patient safety, patient quality of care, and hospital stakeholders' satisfaction (i.e. patient, physician/surgeon, nurse, perioperative staff, and hospital administration). Consequently, implementing improvements that will result in timely patient flow through the perioperative process is both a challenge and an opportunity for hospital stakeholders, who often have a variety of opinions and perceptions as to where improvement efforts should focus. Furthermore, perioperative improvements ultimately affect not only patient quality of care, but also the operational and financial performance of the hospital. From an operational perspective, a hospital's perioperative process requires multidisciplinary, cross-functional teams to maneuver within complex, fast-paced, and critical situations—the hospital environment (McClusker et al., 2005). Similarly, from a hospital's financial perspective, the perioperative process is typically the primary source of hospital admissions, averaging between 55 to 65 percent of overall hospital margins (Peters & Blasco, 2004). Macario et al. (1995) identified 49 percent of total hospital costs as variable with the largest cost category being the perioperative process (e.g. 33 percent). Managing and optimizing a quality, efficient, flexible, and cost-effective perioperative process are critical success factors (CSFs), both operationally and financially, for any hospital. Moreover, increased government and industry regulations require performance and clinical outcome reporting as evidence of organizational quality, efficiency, and effectiveness (PwC, 2012).

This 143-month longitudinal case study covers a clinical scheduling IS (CSIS) implementation, integration, and use within an academic medical center's perioperative process. Empowered individuals driven by integrated internal and external organizational data facilitate the case results. The resulting systematic analysis and subsequent contextual understanding of the perioperative process identified opportunity for improvement. Specifically, the extension of data mining into the analysis and evaluation process of CSIS' data feedback from particular perioperative sub-processes provides the framework for the discovery and synthesis of redesign and reengineering within perioperative workflow to yield continuous process improvement. This paper investigates the research question of how data-driven continuous improvements can balance perioperative sub-process workflow to improve overall patient flow. Furthermore, investigation of the research question in this paper explains how analysis of perioperative performance metrics (e.g., key performance indicators), evaluation of perioperative sub-process constraints and capabilities, and synthesis of perioperative sub-process redesign implemented to balance perioperative workflow can attain: (1) improved workflow, efficiency, and utilization; (2) tighter process to hospital IS coupling; and (3) patient care accountability and documentation. This study highlights operations management practices of continuous improvement, workflow balancing, best practices, process reengineering, and business process management within a hospital's perioperative process. Measured improvements across intra-operative, pre-operative, post-operative, and central sterile supply also distinguish complex dynamics within the perioperative sub-processes nested in the hospital environment.

The following sections review previous literature on data design and data mining, process redesign, business process management, and perioperative performance metrics. By identifying a holistic model for evaluation, analysis, and synthesis between data and process design, this paper prescribes an a priori environment to support continuous process improvement. Following the literature review, we present our methodology, case study background, as well as the observed effects and analysis discussion of the continuous improvement and workflow balancing efforts. The conclusion addresses study implications and limitations.

LITERATURE REVIEW

First mover advantage on innovations, adaptation of better management practices, industry competition, and/or government regulations are examples of the many factors that drive process improvement. Traditionally, the hospital environment lacked similar industrial pressures beyond government regulations. However, hospital administration currently faces increasing pressure to provide objective evidence of patient outcomes in respect to organizational quality, efficiency, and effectiveness (CMS, 2005; CMS, 2010; PwC, 2012), all while preserving clinical quality standards. Likewise, hospitals in the United States must report and improve clinical outcomes more now due to the American Recovery and Reinvestment Act of 2009, the Joint Commission on Accreditation of Healthcare Organizations (TJC), and the Centers for Medicare & Medicaid Services (CMS). These performances and reporting challenges require leveraging information systems (IS) and technologies (IT) to meet these demands.

Hospital administrators and medical professionals must focus on both the patient quality of care as well as management practices that yield efficiency and cost effectiveness (PwC, 2012). To this end, operations management practices of continuous improvement, best practices, process reengineering, workflow balancing, and business process management (BPM) provide improvement approaches (Jeston & Nelis, 2008; Kaplan & Norton 1996; Tenner & DeToro, 1997). However, such approaches yield significant variations in implementation success.

Data, IS Design, and Data Mining

Data is a prerequisite for information, where simple isolated facts give structure through IS design to become information. Early in the IT literature, embedded feedback as a control to avoid management misinformation was proposed in IS design (Ackoff, 1967). Likewise proposed was the selection and supervision of defined data as key performance indicators (KPIs) to assist management in qualifying data needs to monitor CSFs that subsequently manage organizational action (i.e. business processes) through IS feedback (Munroe & Wheeler, 1980; Rockart, 1979; Zani, 1970). Similarly, the perioperative process is becoming increasingly information intensive and doubt exists as to whether perioperative process management is fully understood to meet the increasing hospital environmental demands for value and cost management (Catalano & Fickenscher, 2007). Understanding how IS design and particularly how CSIS design embeds processes into data input and information output is a first step toward understanding data as a resource for heuristic development (Berrisford & Wetherbe, 1979).

Given that people perform organizational action, people develop IS, people use IS, and people are a component within IS (Silver et al., 1995); understanding the human mind is a requisite in understanding how organizational action via CSIS occur. Ackoff (1988) proposed a hierarchy of the human mind, where each category is an aggregate of the categories below it. Wisdom descends to understanding, knowledge, information, and then data. Achieving wisdom requires successively upward movement through the other four human mind categories, with each level drawing content from prior levels. Data, information, knowledge, and understanding relate to past events and wisdom deals with the future as it incorporates vision and design. Other authors of knowledge management literature share similar hierarchical views of human mind content (Earl, 1994; Davenport & Prusak, 1998; Tuomi, 2000).

The IT literature contains volumes of studies to offer opinions on system design. For this study, the intent is to provide a basic understanding of system design activities and substantiate the need for iterative improvement through heuristic development. Blanchard and Fabrycky (2010) recognize system design as a requisite within the systems life cycle where technological activities of analysis, evaluation, and synthesis integrate within iterative applications to minimize systems' risk from entropy, obsolescence, and environmental change.

Under ideal terms, an individual's wisdom recognizes that an IS solution can meet an organizational need. Subsequently, individual understanding and knowledge create the IS design, develop the IS, and implement it to meet the organizational need. This ideal situation is hypothetical, yet it does illustrate that during the design, development, and implementation stages of an IS (i.e. the systems life cycle), understanding, knowledge, and information are decontextualized into detached data and semantic data structures that are accessible by IS' processes. Tuomi (2000) called this set of human mind sequences a reversed hierarchy from the traditional model (e.g. data leads to information, on to knowledge, understanding, and wisdom).

Ackoff (1988) concluded that wisdom might well differentiate the human mind from the IS. Consequently, it is understanding and knowledge of the business process that system stakeholders use to develop information requirements and subsequent data requirements for IS design. Furthermore, in reverse logic, it is data within the deployed IS that knowledge workers can use to assist in the organizational action of discovery to develop the knowledge and understanding of how to redesign business processes. Udell (2004) compared data to Play-doh—a tangible substance that can be squeezed, stretched, and explored directly. Witten and Frank (2005) define data mining as the process (i.e. automatic or semiautomatic) of discovering patterns (i.e. structure) within data, where the data already exists within the IS' databases in substantial quantities and the discovered patterns have organizational importance.

Holistic Model for IS Design and Discovery

Data mining can explore raw data to find organizational and environmental connections (bottom up), or search data to test hypothesis (top down) producing data, information, and insights that add to the organization's knowledge (Chung, 1999). Figure 1 depicts data mining as discovery to use the traditional model of the human mind to churn data, existing within the IS, into information that leads on to

Figure 1. Holistic IS design and IS discovery model. Adapted from R. L. Ackoff's (1989, p. 3) hierarchy of the human mind

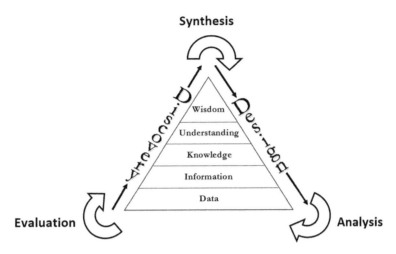

knowledge, understanding, and possibly wisdom. Unfortunately, the healthcare industry has not fully embraced data as a resource and utilized data mining as a knowledge discovery tool (Wickramasinghe & Schaffer, 2006; Catalano & Fickenscher, 2007; Delen et al., 2009; Liu & Chen, 2009; Ranjan, 2009).

Figure 1 also depicts a proposed holistic model for IS design and discovery, which demonstrates the logic for mining perioperative data for business process analysis and redesign. The model incorporates the IT literature we have discussed over data as a resource, system design, and data mining. As stakeholders design a new IS, the system designers draw upon the hierarchy (Tuomi, 2000) to embed and encapsulate organizational actions into the new application. Collected data within an implemented IS represents organizational action (i.e. business processes). Captured and stored CSIS data reflects current and past perioperative actions (i.e. perioperative sub-processes and patient workflow) that is available for heuristic development.

Process Redesign

Specifically, this study examines process redesign approaches over continuous improvement, best practices, and reengineering (Tenner & DeToro, 1997) to balance perioperative patient workflow. Continuous process improvement (CPI) is a systematic approach toward understanding the process capability, the customer's needs, and the source of the observed variation. The incremental realization of improvement gains occurs through an iterative cycle of analysis, evaluation, and synthesis or plan-do-study-act (Walton, 1986) that minimize the observed variation. CPI encourages bottom-up communication at the day-to-day operations level and requires process data comparisons to control metrics. Tenner & DeToro (1997) views CPI as an organizational response to an acute crisis, a chronic problem, and/or an internal driver. CPI rewards are low (i.e. between 3 to 10 percent) with low risk and cost, easy implementation, and short durations. Within a CPI effort, doubt can exist as to: whether the incremental improvement addresses symptoms versus causes; whether the improvement effort is sustainable year after year; and/or whether management is in control of the process (Jensen & Nelis, 2008).

An alternative to CPI is best practices, which offers higher rewards (i.e. between 20 to 50 percent) with similar low risk, longer duration, as well as moderate costs and implementation difficulty (Tenner & DeToro, 1979). Camp (1995) differentiates best practices from benchmarking as finding and implementing industry standard practices that lead to superior performance as opposed to benchmarks that are metric standards or key performance indicators (KPIs). Best practice encourages the imitation or adaptation of external industry standards coupled with internal expertise. However, best practices require more resource allocations versus CPI and a higher degree of understanding about the targeted process, which can lead management to under-estimate the resource requirements necessary for best practice success.

Hammer (1990) summarizes process reengineering in his article, "Reengineering Work: Don't automate, obliterate." Reengineering offers more radical redesign when compared to CPI or best practices (Tenner & DeToro, 1979), assuming more risk with greater reward potential. Hammer & Champy (1993, p.32) defined process reengineering as the fundamental rethinking and radical redesign to achieve dramatic improvements in critical measures of performance (e.g. cost, quality, service, and speed). Three key terms in the definition differentiates reengineering from CPI or best practices—fundamental, radical, and dramatic. Reengineering is a project-oriented effort that utilizes top-down improvement, managed by external and internal expertise, to achieve breakthrough improvement. Reengineering a process offers the highest reward potential, with upwards of 1,000 percent. However, the high potential rewards have very high risk, longer durations, as well as very high costs and the highest implementation difficulty (Tenner & DeToro, 1979). A reengineering project requires extensive resource allocations as opposed to CPI or best practices, as well as seeking an order of magnitude improvement by questioning the relevance of every activity and reinventing new ways to accomplish necessary work.

Business Process Management (BPM)

This study demonstrates business process management (BPM) techniques to monitor process KPIs and measure process improvement within perioperative sub-processes. This study uses the BPM definition provided by Jensen and Nelis (2008, p. 10) as "the achievement of an organization's objectives through the improvement, management, and control of essential business processes." The authors further elaborate that process management and analysis is integral to BPM, where there is no finish line for improvement. Hence, this study views BPM as an organizational commitment to consistent and iterative process performance improvement that meets organizational objectives. To this end, BPM embraces the concept of CPI aligned to organizational strategy.

As BPM requires alignment to strategic objectives, a balanced scorecard (BSC) approach (Kaplan & Norton, 1996) embraces the ability to quantify organizational control metrics aligned with strategy across perspectives of: (1) financial; (2) customer; (3) process; and (4) learning/growth. Furthermore, business analytics is the body of knowledge identified with the deployment and use of technology solutions that incorporate BSCs, dashboards, performance management, definition and delivery of business metrics, as well as data visualization and data mining. Business analytics within BPM focus on the effective use of organizational data and information to drive positive business action (Turban et al., 2008). The effective use of business analytics demands knowledge and skills from subject matter experts and knowledge workers. Similarly, Wears and Berg (2005) concur that IS/IT only yield high-quality healthcare when the use patterns are tailored to knowledge workers and their environment. Therefore, BPM success through BSCs and dashboards has a strong dependence on contextual understanding of end-to-end core business processes (Jensen & Nelis, 2008).

Key Performance Indicators (KPIs)

An integral part of CPI is process information before and after intervention. Hence, performance measurement is essential for purposeful BPM. As we previously mentioned, control feedback in IS avoids management misinformation (Ackoff, 1967) and IS feedback as KPIs (Munroe & Wheeler, 1980; Rockart, 1979; Zani, 1970) assists management in monitoring critical success factors (CSFs) for organizational action (e.g. business processes). However, increasing perioperative process complexity and information intensity (Fowler et al., 2008) challenges perioperative management capabilities to meet performance objectives (Catalano & Fickenscher, 2007).

The following scenario illustrates the complexity, dynamic nature, and nested operational, tactical, and strategic relationships among perioperative KPIs. Operating room (OR) schedules are tightly coupled to an individual OR suite, patient, and surgeon. When preoperative tasks are incomplete or surgical supplies are not readily available at time of surgery, the scheduled case is delayed as well as the subsequent scheduled cases in the particular OR suite or for the particular surgeon. Operational and tactical KPIs in managing and optimizing a hospital's perioperative process include: (1) monitoring the percentage of surgical cases that start on-time (OTS), (2) OR turn-around time (TAT) between cases, (3) OR suite utilization (UTIL), and (4) labor hours per patient care hours or units-of-service (UOS) expended in surgical care (Herzer et al., 2008; Kanich & Byrd, 1996; Peters & Blasco, 2004; Tarantino, 2003; Wright et al., 2010). Tarantino (2003) noted how OR TAT and a flexible work environment are CSFs for physician satisfaction, which in turn is a CSF for hospital margin. Poor KPIs on operational and tactical metrics (i.e., OTS, TAT, UOS, or UTIL) affect strategic CSFs of patient safety, patient quality of care, surgeon/staff/patient satisfaction, and hospital margin (Marjamaa et al., 2008; Peters & Blasco, 2004).

RESEARCH METHOD

The objective of this study is to investigate how data-driven continuous improvements can balance perioperative sub-process workflow to improve overall patient flow through the analysis of perioperative performance metrics (e.g., key performance indicators), evaluation of perioperative sub-process constraints and capabilities, and synthesis of perioperative sub-process redesign. Furthermore, the continuous improvements to yield balance perioperative workflow can attain: (1) improved workflow, efficiency, and utilization; (2) tighter process to hospital IS coupling; and (3) patient care accountability and documentation. To this end, case research is particularly appropriate (Eisenhardt, 1989; Yin, 2003). An advantage of the positivist approach (Weber, 2004) to case research allows concentrating on specific hospital processes in a natural setting to analyze the associated qualitative problems and environmental complexity. Hence, our study took an in-depth case research approach.

Our research site (e.g. University Hospital) is an academic medical center, licensed for 1,046 beds and located in the southeastern United States. University Hospital is a Level 1 Trauma Center, having a robotics program encompassing over eight surgical specialties, as well as a Women's/Infant facility. University Hospital's recognition includes Magnet since 2002 and a Top 100 Hospital by U.S. News and World Report since 2005. Concentrating on one research site facilitated the research investigation and allowed collection of longitudinal data. During the 143-month study, we conducted field research and collected data via multiple sources including interviews, field surveys, site observations, field notes, archival records, and document reviews.

This research spans activities from August 2003 through June 2015, with particular historical data since 1993. Perioperative Services (UHPS) is the University Hospital department that coordinates the perioperative process. Initially, the perspective of this research focused on University Hospital's perioperative process for its 32 general operating room (OR) suites in the main OR campus with Admissions; Surgical Preparations (PRE-OP) having 42 beds; OR Surgery, Endoscopy, and Cystoscopy; Post Anesthesia Care Unit (PACU) having 45 beds, and Central Sterile Supply (CSS). University Hospital administration consolidated all OR management and scheduling within the University Hospital Health System (UHHS) under UHPS in 2008, including cardio-vascular and off-site surgical clinics. In 2011, hospital administration added the Pre-admissions and the preoperative assessment consultation and test (PACT) clinic (Ryan et al., 2012) to UHPS' scope. Currently, UHPS manages 35 general OR suites (GENOR), 6 cardio-vascular OR suites (CVOR), 16 OR suites on the Highlands campus (HHOR), 2 OR suites at Women & Children (WaCOR), and 8 OR suites at the CAL Eye Foundation Hospital (CEFOR). In total, UHPS manages 67 OR suites having a combined FY2014 surgical case volume of 42,741.

CASE BACKGROUND

UHPS implemented a new CSIS in 2003, after using its prior CSIS for 10 years. The old CSIS and its vendor were not flexible in adapting to new perioperative data collection needs. The old CSIS did not have an online analytical processing (OLAP) capability and the perioperative data mart was multiple Microsoft Access databases. The new CSIS from vendor C supports OLAP tools, a proprietary structured query language, and both operational and managerial data stores (i.e. operational data and a separate perioperative data mart). The new CSIS has flexible routing templates (i.e. from 4 to 36 segments to capture point of care data), customizable over generic and surgeon specific surgical procedures, documented in the CSIS as surgeon preference cards (SPCs). Since the new CSIS implementation in August 2003, University Hospital has maintained over 7,775+ SPCs across the surgical specialty services (SSS) represented in Table 1.

Table 1. Surgical specialty services (SSS) with surgeon preference cards (SPCs)

Surgical Specialty Service	SPCs	Surgical Specialty Service	SPCs
BURN – Trauma Burns	26	ORTHO – Orthopedics	1,208
CARDIO – Cardiovascular & Thoracic	946	PLAS – Plastic Surgery	681
ENT – Ear, Nose, & Throat	1,030	SURG ONC – Surgical Oncology	329
GI – Gastro-intestinal	460	TX – Transplants (liver & renal)	194
GYN – Obstetrics & Gynecology	611	TRAUMA – Trauma, MASH	203
NEURO – Neurology	763	URO – Urology	533
ORAL – Oral, Maxilla, & Facial	236	VASCULAR – Arteries & Blood Vessels	558

November 2004

University Hospital opened a new surgical facility in November 2004, with ORs located over two floors and CSS located on a third. The move expanded UHPS to cover an additional floor and nine additional ORs (i.e., 33% capacity increase). The new facility housed 40 state-of-the-art OR suites, each having new standardized as well as surgical specialty equipment. Within six weeks of occupying the new facility, a scheduling KPI reflected chaos. Surgical case OTS plunged to 18% during December 2004. Within a highly competitive hospital industry, having only 18% OTS was unacceptable, as 82% of scheduled surgeries experienced delays and risked patient care and safety.

In January 2005, UHPS expressed concerns before a quickly convened meeting of c-level executive officers and top representatives of surgeons and anesthesia. The meeting yielded a hybrid-matrix management structure and governance in the formation of a multidisciplinary executive team, chartered and empowered to evoke change. The executive team consisted of perioperative stakeholders (i.e., surgeons, anesthesiologists, nurses, and UHPS staff). The executive team's charter was to focus on patient care and safety, attack difficult questions, and remove inefficiencies. No issue was off-limits.

University Hospital's executive team launched a process improvement effort in 2005 to address the perioperative crisis through soft innovations (Ryan et al., 2008). As a result, the executive team enlisted numerous task forces to address specific problems and/or opportunities, which was the foundation for their BPM approach. All initiatives were data-driven from the existing integrated hospital IS. Supporting data identified problem areas, strengths to highlight, and direction for improvement. Each identified problem area presented a new goal proposal and strategy for implementation.

OBSERVED EFFECTS OF PERIOPERATIVE CPI

Since 2005, UHPS has focused on data-driven, systematic analysis of perioperative KPIs to gauge process variance and improve end-to-end workflow balance. Perioperative KPI feedback occurs at strategic, tactical, and operational levels via balanced scorecards and dashboards, aligned to hospital strategy (Ryan et al., 2014b). Using this BPM approach, perioperative CPI efforts have documented OR scheduling (Ryan et al., 2011a); hospital-wide electronic medical record (EMR) integration (Ryan et al., 2011b); preoperative patient evaluations (Ryan et al., 2012); radio-frequency identification (Ryan et al., 2013); CSS/OR supply workflow (Ryan et al., 2014a); unit-of-service charge capture via EMRs in the CSIS (Ryan et al., 2015); and instrument/device reprocessing and tracking (Ryan et al., 2015). Table 2 depicts 14 of the UHPS initiated CPI efforts as well as the specific associated sub-process workflow and implementation year from 2003 to 2015.

Due to the perioperative CPI efforts in Table 2, a balanced workflow exists upstream and downstream of the ORs, yielding improved patient flow throughout the perioperative process via Pre-admissions (PACT Clinic); Admissions; Surgical Preparations (PRE-OP); Central Sterile Supply (CSS); OR Surgery, Endoscopy, and Cystoscopy; as well as Post Anesthesia Care Units (PACU and PACU Phase-II). Surgical patients move through the perioperative workflow via events: (1) A clinic visit resulting in surgery scheduling, (2) PACT Clinic evaluation, (3) day of surgery admission, (4) PRE-OP, (5) Intra-operative, Endoscopy, or Cystoscopy procedure, (6) PACU, (7) PACU Phase-II, and (8) discharge or movement to a medical bed. The following sections highlight particular CPI efforts from Table 2 that reduced or eliminated bottlenecks, delays, and inefficiencies within a specific sub-process workflow.

Table 2. Perioperative continuous process improvement timeline

Perioperative CPI Effort	Sub-process Workflow	Year
Clinical Scheduling IS (CSIS)	OR Surgery, ENDO, CYSTO, CSS	2003
Relocated ORs to NP Building	All	2004
Changed governance – started CPI efforts	All	2005
Heuristic/Modified Block Scheduling	OR Surgery, CSS	2006
Hospital-wide EMR Integration	PRE-OP, OR Surgery, PACU. CSS	2007
Perioperative performance dashboards	All	2008
PACU Nursing Record	PACU Phase-II	2010
Preoperative Assessment (PACT) Clinic	Pre-admissions, PRE-OP	2011
RFID Phased Implementation	OR Surgery	2012
Redesigned CSS / OR Supply Workflow	CSS, OR Surgery, ENDO, CYSTO	2013
PRE-OP & PACU Nursing EMRs	PRE-OP, PACU, PACU Phase-II	2014
UOS CSIS charge capture via EMRs	PRE-OP, PACU, PACU Phase-II	2014
Instrument Reprocessing & Tracking	CSS, OR Surgery, ENDO, CYSTO	2015

Heuristic/Modified Block Scheduling (2006)

In November 2004, University Hospital allocated OR suites by SSS (i.e. for SSS listing refer to Table 1)—scheduling blocks of time for an OR suite between 7 a.m. to 4:30 p.m., regardless of the SSS case-load. Scheduling OR suites by SSS assigned blocks did not reflect actual SSS cases occurring within the scheduling blocks (i.e. the scheduling method did not reflect the OR data collected by the CSIS). The inefficient practice of block scheduling OR suites was directly attributable to University Hospital reaching 100 percent of OR capacity in December 2004, even though the new facility had increased existing OR capacity by 33 percent.

The actual OR hours used by SSS cases (i.e. specific SSS caseload) from the data mart were analyzed against OR hours allocated to each SSS block assignment. The resulting data patterns showed the need to re-design the OR scheduling process. Hence, UHPS discontinued straight SSS block scheduling. Given that physician satisfaction is linked to OR block scheduling by SSS (Peters & Blasco, 2004), block assignments were kept for outside-of-two-weeks planning purposes. However, review of SSS block hour assignments for OR suites occur every three months to reflect the actual SSS caseload history and to reflect individual SSS patient population, similar to marketing segmentation among demographic groups. The perioperative scheduling heuristic review process routinely modifies the block scheduling release rules by analyzing actual SSS caseload versus respective SSS block schedule. SSS with wide variability in scheduling are given consideration and a reduction in the number of early release blocks of OR suites.

Current OR heuristic rules release unscheduled hours of any SSS OR suite block time within: (1) 7 days out to any SSS for robotic rooms, (2) 72 hours out to a surgeon within the same SSS, and (3) 48 hours out to any SSS. Furthermore, any SSS averaging more than 6% of unused OR suite hours per day-of-surgery are penalized during the next OR scheduling heuristic review. Table 3 lists the resulting scheduling windows of OR suite time and the corresponding percentage of OR cases scheduled in each window. Overall, 29.6% of the surgical cases performed were scheduled outside a week and only 2.7%

Table 3. Heuristic / modified block release rule—OR scheduling windows

Scheduling Window	OR cases scheduled (%)	Cumulative OR Cases Scheduled
Beyond 14 days	15.4%	100.0%
7 to 14 days	14.2%	84.6%
1 to 7 days	34.6%	70.4%
24 to 72 hours	18.1%	53.9%
Within 24 hours	33.1%	35.8%
Day-of-surgery	2.7%	2.7%

of the cases were scheduled the day-of-surgery (e.g. emergency cases). Over two-thirds of surgical patients were able to schedule their surgical procedure during the week of their surgery, which indicates the success of the heuristic/modified block release rules for scheduling flexibility.

Hospital-Wide EMR Integration via Project IMPACT (2007)

Project IMPACT, encompassed 11 task forces covering surgeon's orders (CPoE), clinical documentation, electronic medical records (EMRs), pharmacy, physician workflow, critical care, knowledge and content, technical metrics, communications, and testing / training / transition. The hospital-wide integration effort extended the CSIS across the perioperative sub-processes into ancillary hospital processes as well as perioperative tracking information on surgical patients (e.g. outpatient and in-patient) from Admissions through PACU discharge, including the in-patient's location after PACU discharge.

Beyond the enterprise application integration and software coding efforts, the most visible interface into the dissemination of perioperative process information across Admissions, PRE-OP, and PACU were electronic patient status boards. The deployed boards were in each functional area and the perioperative patient information adhered to HIPAA (e.g. Health Insurance Portability and Accountability Act of 1996) compliant formats. Figure 2 depicts Clinical IS departmental views of the electronic boards in PACU.

Additional flat panel displays on wall mounted information boards in each OR waiting room also provided patient tracking status for patient's family members or friends. Clinical staff give documentation to all patient family members, which explains the information boards and how to track your patient. Extending the clinical scheduling IS integration across the hospital gives all stakeholders access to the CSIS modules and tracking of surgical patients. The coded patient information boards in each OR waiting room also ensures patient privacy and HIPAA compliance. Figure 3 depicts patient information boards in one of the OR waiting rooms.

Figure 2. CSIS patient status boards in PACU

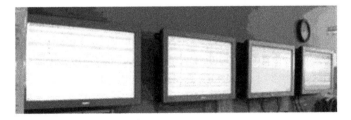

Figure 3. Family link boards in OR waiting rooms

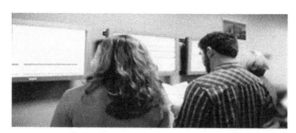

Preoperative Assessment Consultation and Test (PACT) Clinic (2011)

Project IMPACT integrated EMRs from Admissions through PACU in 2007, but omitted parts of the preoperative evaluation documentation such as external medical records (MRs), preoperative assessment consultation (PAC), patient medical history (PMH), surgical history (SH), and former medication history (FMH). Figure 4 represents University Hospital's preoperative patient evaluation flow as of FY2010. Inefficient processes and decision points (see gray areas on Figure 5) delayed scheduled surgical case starts while PRE-OP staff obtained incomplete information. CSIS data reflected incomplete patient information delays for over one out of six surgical cases. As a result, UHPS launched a PACT Clinic task force to reengineer preoperative patient evaluations. Task force members visited four leading academic medical centers in the United States, as well as the two internal University Hospital sites, to gather a transparent and bottom-up view of different perspectives to preoperative evaluation processes. The external sites were located in: (1) Baltimore, MD; (2) Boston, MA; (3) Rochester, MN; and (4) Cleveland, OH.

Essential elements of the preoperative patient flow reengineering required EMR inclusion of all pertinent external records with the initial University Hospital referral as the preoperative evaluation appointment is made simultaneously with the initial surgeon appointment. Patient screening and standardized co-morbidity risk stratification occurs by telephone, the Internet, or by the surgical clinic making the referral. The best practices identified during the site visits afforded University Hospital the opportunity to reengineer their preoperative patient evaluation into a preoperative assessment, consultation, and treatment (PACT) clinic. A "clinic without walls' in that the PACT clinic exists only within the CSIS and evaluations can occur anywhere within University Hospital.

Figure 5 reflects the reengineered PACT Clinic workflow. All surgical patients receive a PACT Clinic evaluation prior to their scheduled procedures. During the same surgeon appointment, a comprehensive preoperative evaluation is performed and recorded via the PACT Clinic ambulatory EMR to include: a complete preoperative history and physical exam (H&P), confirmed informed consent and signed release on surgical procedure (ROS), optimized medications, and patient education. Prompt cardiac/diagnostic testing or cardiac/medical consultations may also occur during the PACT and surgical appointment.

Redesigned CSS / OR Supply Workflow (2013)

Within the perioperative process, CSS pushes supply/instrument inventory to all ORs via three channels: 1) Case carts stocked specifically for a scheduled surgical case according to a specific SPC pick list (i.e. standardized supply/instrument bill of material); 2) standard supplies moved to an OR Core holding area on each OR floor; and/or 3) a specific requisition from OR staff. As early as 2006, UHPS noted multiple

Figure 4. Preoperative patient evaluation FY2010

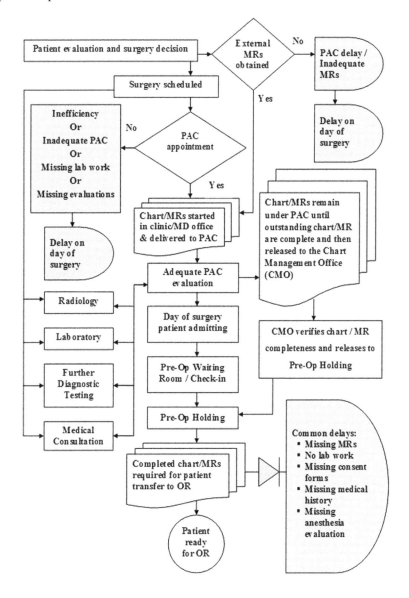

inventory receipts within the perpetual inventory for every inventory usage across particular perioperative supplies. In 2010, the executive team launched an initiative to assess the status of perioperative supply/instrument inventory and workflow due to increasing inventory values and slowing inventory turns metrics. The processes reviewed included: (1) inventory/Par level management, (2) replenishment processes, and (3) technology. The sub-process CSIS data reviewed identified inventory reduction as well as improvement opportunities to sustain reduced perioperative supply/instrument costs. The analysis of the assessment yielded the following themes:

- Scheduling inaccuracy due to lack of SPC maintenance and SPC inaccuracies.
- Work duplication in CSS case cart picking due to lack of trust in case scheduling and SPCs.

Figure 5. Reengineered patient evaluations PACT

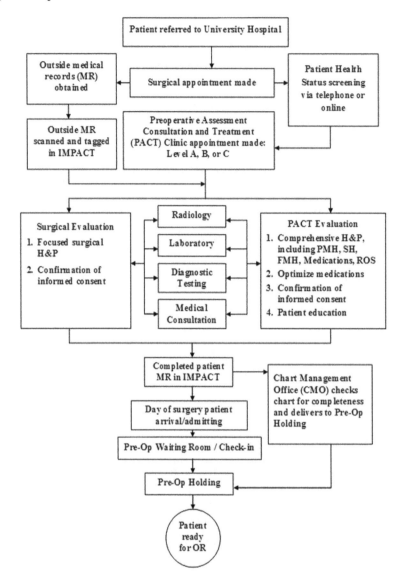

- Charge capture issues where items left off the SPC may not get charged.
- Unused supply/instrument returns to CSS after case completion produce CSS inefficiencies.
- Breakdown in the supply workflow process effects overall inventory management.

Perioperative inventory turns had slowed to 3.7 against an industry average of 9, which represented 3.2 months supply. These KPIs reflected a breakdown in the supply/instrument workflow process. However, responsible actors (e.g. nurses and UHPS staff) interact among the OR case carts, OR Core inventory locations, and CSS. The BPM efforts among CSS and OR perioperative actors yielded a CSS/ OR instruments/supplies workflow redesign to ensure effective instrument/supply inventory management. Likewise, a major task force recommendation was for scheduled surgical cases to have specific and required inventory information that includes accurate location, procedure, specific equipment, and supply needs from consistently updated SPCs.

A review of each of the SPCs yielded the removal of 1,937 SPCs, which reduced the SPC total by 20 percent (e.g. down to 7,778 from 9,315 SPCs) and scrubbed the SPC routings to ensure accuracy. Table 1 lists the frequency counts of current SPCs by SSS. The perpetual maintenance of SPCs, redesigning the perioperative supply workflow, decreasing closing suture and hand-held instrument inventories to industry standards, and managing perioperative inventory turns to 10 turns per 18 months targeted opportunities and evoked changes to the perioperative instruments/supplies inventory in excess of $6.6M over two years.

Unit-of-Service (UOS) CSIS Charge Capture via EMRs (2014)

UHPS developed and configured unique CSIS nursing records as EMRs to manage patient care documentation across the perioperative workflow. UOS standards reflect perioperative staff labor hours associated with particular patient care activity units—one hour of patient care time, an Endoscopy procedure, or a sterilized instrument load. UOS metrics reflect patient care hours in each workflow segment. Table 4 lists the current CSIS nursing record documentation via EMR, the fiscal year of the UOS charge capture implementation, UOS standard labor hours, and UOS unit.

Prior to the implementation of each real-time UOS charge capture via EMR documentation, perioperative staff manually batch-keyed UOS charges. As of March 2014, all CSIS nursing documentation via EMRs capture UOS charge data (e.g., UOS standard multiplied by UOS units) using the appropriate UOS standards and units. UHPS use the granularity in the aggregated UOS charge data for perioperative subprocess OLAP to offer contextual understanding to analyze sub-process variances, target improvement

Table 4. CSIS nursing record documentation via EMR with UOS standards

CSIS Documentation via EMR	FY Start	UOS Standard	UOS Unit
Ancillary Services Record - Family	2007	--	--
PRE-OP Nursing Record	2012	1.93	Time
ENDO PRE-OP Nursing Record	2014	--	Procedure
ENDO Sedation Nursing Record	2014	2.10	Time
Regional Block Nursing Record	2014	2.21	Time
CSS	2003	3.52	Sterilized Loads
OR Nursing Record – CVOR	2007	9.04	Time
OR Nursing Record – Cardiac Perfusion	2012	4.22	Time
OR Nursing Record – GENOR	2003	7.45	Time
OR Nursing Record – ENDO	2014	6.92	Procedure
Ancillary Services Record – Clean-up	2005	--	Time
PACU Nursing Record	2010	2.71	Time
ICU/After Hours PACU Overflow Record	2014	2.71	Time
PACU Phase-II Nursing Record	2014	1.93	Time

areas, and justify resource allocations. CSIS nursing records with UOS standards differentiate staffing labor hours for different levels of patient care (e.g. acute versus ambulatory).

Within PACU, the Phase-II and ICU nursing records also facilitate PACU workflow balancing and bed/resource utilization. Within PRE-OP and PACU, a finite number of acute care beds are valued resources, when compared to ambulatory care beds. The PACU Phase II Nursing Record allows ambulatory nursing documentation via the CSIS in any University Hospital ambulatory bed. Hence, PACU Phase II patients are transferable to PRE-OP or floor beds when PACU beds are in critical supply. Moreover, the ICU Overflow record identifies ICU bed capacity issues to avoid unplanned ICU discharges (Utzolino et al., 2010).

CSIS nursing records without UOS standards facilitate information and data collection on patient family/advocate, Endoscopy (e.g., ENDO) patient status, or surgical case OR suite TAT. All OR Nursing Record EMRs also provide documentation for OR suite OTS and UTIL measures.

DISCUSSION OF BALANCED PATIENT WORKFLOW THROUGH CPI

Figures 6 and 7 depict the resulting patient flow and integrated IS across University Hospital Health System (UHHS) per the CPI efforts described in Table 2 of the observed effects section. As depicted in Figure 6, patient admissions are either medical or surgical. Surgical patient admissions occur via three venues: 1) diagnostic office visits to physicians within the TK Clinic, 2) non-UHHS physician referrals to the PACT clinic, or 3) patients seeking treatment through the Emergency Department. All surgical patients receive a PACT Clinic evaluation prior to their scheduled procedures. The PACT Clinic exists virtually in the CSIS, so the TK Clinic allocated physical space to facilitate PACT evaluations.

All IS depicted in Figure 7 are integrated with either bi-directional data exchange or uni-directional for limited exchange. The seven IS clustered around the CSIS are modules that directly support and extend the CSIS suite, where the Clinical Charting IS houses CPOE and EMRs. The HIPAA compliant Web services and biomedical device interface bus (BDIB) integrate ancillary IS, clinical data sensors, and bio-medical equipment. The institutional intranet serves as a single entry secured portal to extend each IS according to particular user-IS rights and privileges negotiated via user authentication.

Balanced Perioperative Workflow Achievement

Figure 8 depicts CPI efforts to achieve perioperative workflow balancing across sub-processes of preoperative, intra-operative, post-operative, and CSS. The five CPI efforts described in the observed effects section removed inefficiencies and delays in particular perioperative sub-processes to support balanced patient flow through the perioperative process as well as information flow as depicted in Figure 7. The following discussion explains the holistic impact of the workflow balancing efforts.

UHPS is the primary source of admissions to University Hospital and the state of UHPS in early 2005 prohibited streamlining hospital-wide patient flow without first streamlining patient flow through the ORs (e.g. intra-operative). Likewise, the modified block scheduling via heuristic release rules improved the perioperative process planning where OR scheduling yielded a tighter coupling between projected versus actual surgical cases. The structural, process, procedural, and cultural changes achieved in UHPS intra-operative sub-processes over FY2005 and FY2006 allowed the executive committee to move forward in early 2007 to extend the CSIS across University Hospital and address hospital-wide patient flow.

Figure 6. UHHS patient flow

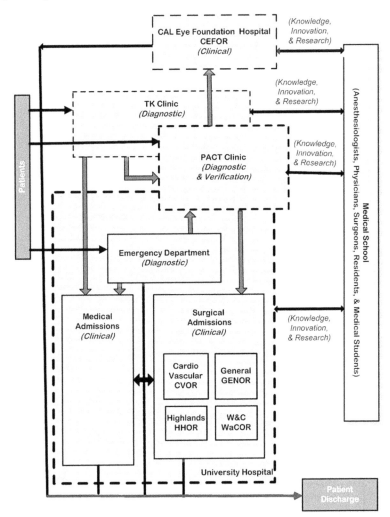

Extending the CSIS across the entire perioperative process in FY2007 through Project Impact provided the basis for perioperative data collection and subsequent CPI efforts. However, Project IMPACT omitted many of the preoperative evaluation activities. The FCOTS KPI for FY2010 was 55.8 percent versus a target of 70 percent. Upon closer analysis of the surgical case delays, 17.5 percent of surgical delays (e.g. more than one out of six cases) were preventable through improved preoperative patient evaluation and improved electronic integration of preoperative documentation and communication. Hence, UHPS identified the need to address the chronic problems in preoperative patient evaluations through a process reengineering effort to yield the Preoperative Assessment, Consultation, and Test (PACT) Clinic to evaluate all surgical patients prior to day-of-surgery.

In May 2011, UHPS identified perioperative supply inventory levels of $15.5M, where inventory turns had slowed to 3.7 versus an industry average of 9, yielding 3.2 months supply. These KPIs reflected a breakdown in the CSS/OR workflow sub-processes. However, responsible actors (e.g. nurses and UHPS

Figure 7. UHHS integrated IS

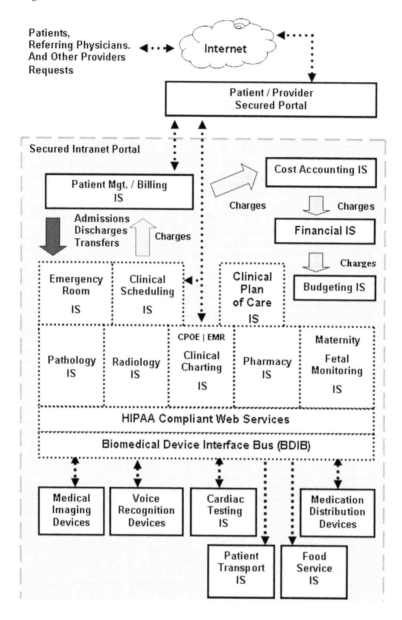

Figure 8. Particular CPI efforts to balance patient flow through perioperative sub-processes

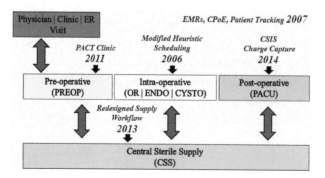

staff) interacting within and among the CSS and intra-operative sub-processes yielded a process redesign effort for an effective solution to improved instrument/supply inventory management and workflow.

Nursing documentation as EMRs with UOS standards differentiate staffing labor hours for different levels of patient care in PRE-OP and PACU. Within PACU, the Phase-II and ICU nursing records facilitate PACU workflow and bed/resource utilization, allowing more critical patients additional surgical recovery time. Moreover, the ICU Overflow record identifies ICU capacity issues to avoid unplanned ICU discharges, while allowing critical patients time to recover in both PACU and ICU. Also Nursing EMRs without UOS standards facilitate information collection on patient family/advocate, Endoscopy patient status, or surgical case OR suite TAT. Similarly, all OR Nursing Record EMRs provide documentation for OR suite OTS and UTIL measures (e.g. KPIs).

Data Visualization of Balanced Perioperative Patient Workflow

Figures 9, 10, and 11 depict aggregated surgical case (e.g. patient) data for perioperative process performance on OTS, UTIL/OTS/TAT, and UOS, respectively. Figure 10 depicts the yearly OTS averages for GENOR, CVOR, and HHOR surgical cases since FY2006 (i.e. UHHS fiscal year begins in October). The chart helps visualization of aggregate workflow performance improvement in providing efficient perioperative patient care while limiting unnecessary patient safety risk. From a BPM approach, these charts also help visualize where perioperative teams and task forces should target CPI efforts. Since the full implementation of the PACT Clinic during FY2012, over 70% of surgical cases in GENOR, CVOR, and HHOR started on time. Prior to FY2013, the OTS 70% target was elusive, in part to incomplete PREOP documentation, which PACT Clinic evaluations eliminated (Ryan et al., 2012).

Figure 9. Surgical OTS FY 2006 to FY 2015

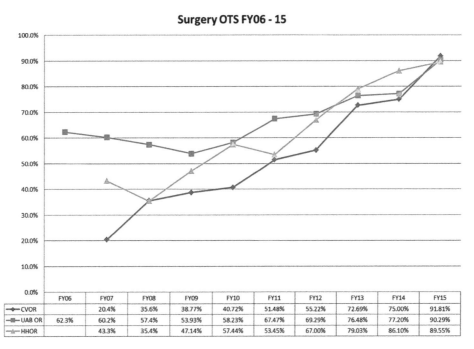

	FY06	FY07	FY08	FY09	FY10	FY11	FY12	FY13	FY14	FY15
CVOR		20.4%	35.6%	38.77%	40.72%	51.48%	55.22%	72.69%	75.00%	91.81%
UAB OR	62.3%	60.2%	57.4%	53.93%	58.23%	67.47%	69.29%	76.48%	77.20%	90.29%
HHOR		43.3%	35.4%	47.14%	57.44%	53.45%	67.00%	79.03%	86.10%	89.55%

Figure 10. OTS/UTIL/TAT by SSS (June 2015)

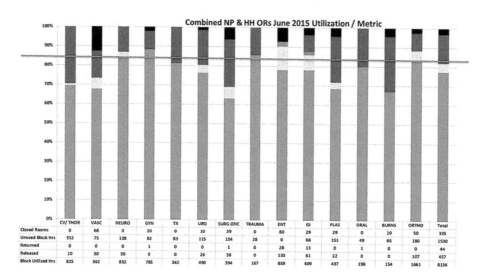

Figure 11. Perioperative UOS FY2006 to FY 2014

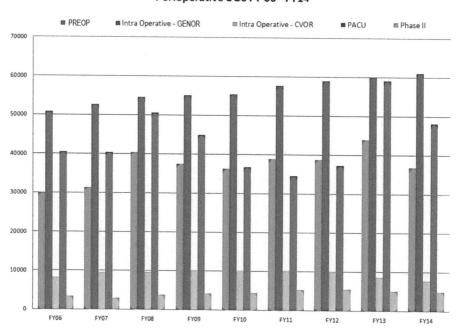

Figure 10 details UTIL, OTS, TAT, and modified- block released time (Ryan et al., 2011a; Peters & Blasco, 2004) by SSS for June 2015. The chart demonstrates granularity and dimensionality of aggregated patient data used in the systematic analysis of process performance. UHPS uses the detailed dimensionality of KPI data to identify specific performance results as well as target specific improvement opportunity.

Aggregated UOS data offers similar analysis capabilities for contextual understanding of patient care workflow dynamics and complexity. Figure 11 reports the UOS patient hours for GENOR and

CVOR workflow since FY2006. In Figure 11, the FY2013 spike in PACU hours, up 12K hours (i.e., 32% increase) from FY2012, is attributable to ICU overflow patient care in PACU (i.e., extended-stay PACU patients waiting for an ICU bed or ICU patients over-nighting in PACU). UHPS use PACU beds to relieve Trauma-ICU and Surgical-ICU patient workflow congestion, moving PACU Phase-II patient care to PREOP beds. In December 2013 (e.g., FY2014), UHPS implemented Phase-II and ICU Overflow nursing records in PACU via the CSIS to document the workflow flexibility and capture UOS charges. As a result, FY2014 hours reflect the virtual PACU flexibility and tightened the CSIS-to-PACU workflow coupling.

Goal Setting and Process Improvement Aligned to Strategy

UHHS "Reach for Excellence" (RFE) goals coordinate and align individual department and employee actions to the UHHS strategic mission and vision of becoming the preferred academic medical center of the 21st century (e.g., AMC21). RFE goals are revised each year as quantitative targets, designed to measure objective outcomes. RFE goals must be aggressive and realistic, where fewer, rather than more, is better. Furthermore, RFE goals change focus as AMC21 progress advances. To this end, UHHS administration annually reviews opportunities for improvement and identifies the most important outcomes needed. Hence, many perioperative KPIs and CPI efforts become RFE goals. As such, UHPS stakeholders focus on RFE process outcomes aligned to AMC21 strategy yielding aligned stakeholder action across departments and employees alike—a very powerful process management tool.

CONCLUSION

Empowered individuals (e.g. nurses, surgeons, anesthesiologists, and perioperative staff), integrated IS, and a holistic model for evaluation, analysis, and synthesis of process data allows UHPS to take control and continuously improve the perioperative sub-processes to balance patient workflow. The perioperative KPIs provide feedback control loops to reflect the perioperative workflow balance as well as identify inefficiencies, delays, and areas for improvement. The RFE goal layer affords UHPS opportunities for process improvement aligned to AMC21 vision. The balanced perioperative workflow improved efficiency, effectiveness, and utilization of perioperative sub-process dynamics within pre-operative, intra-operative, post-operative, and central sterile supply (CSS) activities. Through the CPI efforts, the balanced workflow reflects tighter sub-process to hospital IS coupling as well as patient care accountability and documentation.

Enlisting CPI efforts at strategic, tactical, and day-to-day operations levels further educates hospital stakeholders on the benefits of integrated IS for process measurement, control, and improvement. The cycle of analysis, evaluation, and synthesis reinforces communication and stimulates individual as well as collective organizational learning.

Our case study contributes to the healthcare IT literature by examining how data mining, business analytics, process redesign, and process management are applicable to the hospital environment. This study prescribes an a priori framework to foster their occurrence. This paper also fills a gap in the literature by describing how hospital process data is both a performance measure and a management tool. Furthermore, this study highlighted the complexity and dynamics with the perioperative process.

This study was limited to a single case, where future research should broaden the focus to address this issue along with others that the authors may have inadvertently overlooked. The case examples presented in this study can serve as momentum for healthcare CPI and balanced workflow methodology, comprehension, and extension. The study's results should be viewed as exploratory and in need of further confirmation. Researchers may choose to further or expand the investigation; while practitioners may apply the findings to create their own version of CPI for balanced perioperative workflow.

REFERENCES

Ackoff, R. L. (1967). Management misinformation systems. *Management Science, 14*(4), 147–156. doi:10.1287/mnsc.14.4.B147

Ackoff, R. L. (1989). From data to wisdom: Presidential address to ISGRS. *Journal of Applied Systems Analysis, 16*(1), 3–9.

Berrisford, T., & Wetherbe, J. (1979). Heuristic development: A redesign of systems design. *Management Information Systems Quarterly, 3*(1), 11–19. doi:10.2307/249144

Bird, L. (1997). Computerization in the OR. *AORN Journal, 66*(2), 312–317. doi:10.1016/S0001-2092(06)62800-7 PMID:9513701

Blanchard, B. S., & Fabrycky, W. J. (2010). *Systems Engineering and Analysis* (5th ed.). Upper Saddle River, NJ: Pearson Prentice-Hall.

Caccia-Bava, M., Guimaraes, C., & Guimaraes, T. (2005). Empirically testing determinants of hospital BPR success. *International Journal of Health Care Quality Assurance, 18*(7), 552–563. doi:10.1108/09526860510627238 PMID:16335620

Camp, R. C. (1995). *Business Process Benchmarking: Finding and Implementing Best Practices.* Milwaukee, WI: Quality Press.

Cardoen, B., Demeulemeester, E., & Belien, J. (2010). Operating room planning and scheduling: A literature review. *European Journal of Operational Research, 201*(4), 921–932. doi:10.1016/j.ejor.2009.04.011

Catalano, K., & Fickenscher, K. (2007). Emerging technologies in the OR and their effect on perioperative professionals. *AORN Journal, 86*(6), 958–969. doi:10.1016/j.aorn.2007.07.007 PMID:18068401

Chung, H., & Gray, P. (1999). Data mining. *Journal of Management Information Systems, 16*(1), 11–16. doi:10.1080/07421222.1999.11518231

Davenport, T., & Prusak, L. (1998). *Working Knowledge: How organizations manage what they know.* Boston: Harvard Business School Publishing.

Delen, D., Fuller, C., McCann, C., & Ray, D. (2009). Analysis of healthcare coverage: A data mining approach. *Expert Systems with Applications, 36*(2), 995–1003. doi:10.1016/j.eswa.2007.10.041

Earl, M. J. (1994). Knowledge as strategy: reflections on Skandia International and Shorko Films. In C. Ciborra & T. Jelassi (Eds.), *Strategic Information Systems: A European Perspective* (pp. 53–69). Chichester, UK: John Wiley & Sons.

Eisenhardt, K. (1989). Building theories from case study research. *Academy of Management Review*, *14*(4), 532–550.

Fowler, P., Craig, J., Fredendall, L., & Damali, U. (2008). Perioperative workflow: Barriers to efficiency, risks, and satisfaction. *AORN Journal*, *87*(1), 187–208. doi:10.1016/j.aorn.2007.07.001 PMID:18184599

Hammer, M. (1990). Reengineering work: Don't automate, obliterate. *Harvard Business Review*, *68*(4), 104–112.

Hammer, M., & Champy, J. (1993). *Reengineering the Corporation: A Manifesto for Business Revolution*. New York: Harper Business.

Herzer, K. R., Mark, L. J., Michelson, J. D., Saletnik, L. A., & Lundquist, C. A., (2008). Designing and implementing a comprehensive quality and patient safety management model: A paradigm for perioperative improvement, *Journal of Patient Safety*, 4(2), 84–92.

Jeston, J., & Nelis, J. (2008). *Business Process Management: Practical Guidelines to Successful Implementations* (2nd ed.). Burlington, MA: Elsevier, Ltd.

Kanich, D. G. & Byrd, J. R., (1996). How to increase efficiency in the operating room, *Surgical Clinics of North America*, 76(1), 161–173.

Liu, S., & Chen, J. (2009). Using data mining to segment healthcare markets from patients' preference perspectives. *International Journal of Health Care Quality Assurance*, *22*(2), 117–134. doi:10.1108/09526860910944610 PMID:19536963

Macario, A., Vitez, T., Dunn, B., & McDonald, T. (1995). Analysis of hospital costs and charges for inpatient surgical care. *Anesthesiology*, *83*(6), 1138–1144. doi:10.1097/00000542-199512000-00002 PMID:8533904

Marjamaa, R., Vakkuri, A., & Kirvela, O. (2008). Operating room management: Why, how and by whom? *Acta Anaesthesiologica Scandinavica*, *52*(5), 596–600. doi:10.1111/j.1399-6576.2008.01618.x PMID:18419711

McClusker, J., Dendukuri, N., Cardinal, L., Katofsky, L., & Riccardi, M. (2005). Assessment of the work environment of multidisciplinary hospital staff. *International Journal of Health Care Quality Assurance*, *18*(7), 543–551. doi:10.1108/09526860510627229 PMID:16335619

Meyer, M., & Driscoll, E. (2004). Perioperative surgery in the twenty-first century: Two case studies. *AORN Journal*, *80*(4), 725–733. doi:10.1016/S0001-2092(06)61327-6 PMID:15526705

Munro, M., & Wheeler, B. (1980). Planning, critical success factors, and management's information requirements. *Management Information Systems Quarterly*, *4*(4), 27–37. doi:10.2307/248958

Peters, J., & Blasco, T. (2004). Enhancing hospital performance through perioperative services. *Physician Executive*, *30*(6), 26–31. PMID:15597828

PwC Health Research Institute. (2012). The Future of the Academic Medical Center: Strategies to Avoid a Meltdown. Retrieved from http://www.pwc.com/us/en/health-industries/publications/the-future-of-academic-medical-centers.jhtml#

Raghupathi, W., & Tan, J. (2002). Strategic IT applications in healthcare. *Communications of the ACM*, *45*(2), 56–61. doi:10.1145/585597.585602 PMID:12238525

Ranjan, J. (2009). Data mining in pharma sector: Benefits. *International Journal of Health Care Quality Assurance*, *22*(1), 82–92. doi:10.1108/09526860910927970 PMID:19284173

Rockart, J. (1979). Chief executives define their own data needs. *Harvard Business Review*, *57*(2), 81–93. PMID:10297607

Ryan, J., Doster, B., Daily, S., & Heslin, M. (2008). Soft innovation as data-driven process improvement exploited via integrated hospital information systems. *Proceedings of the 41st Hawaii International Conference on System Sciences*, Waikoloa, HI, USA. 10.1109/HICSS.2008.405

Ryan, J., Doster, B., Daily, S., & Lewis, C. (2011a). Analyzing block scheduling heuristics for perioperative scheduling flexibility: A case study perspective. *Proceedings of the 44th Hawaii International Conference on System Sciences*, Kauai, HI, USA. 10.1109/HICSS.2011.64

Ryan, J., Doster, B., Daily, S., & Lewis, C. (2011b), Perioperative patient transparency and accountability via integrated hospital information systems. *Proceedings of the 17th Americas Conference on Information Systems*, Detroit, MI, USA. AISel.

Ryan, J., Doster, B., Daily, S., & Lewis, C. (2012), Evaluating and improving the perioperative process: Benchmarking and redesign of preoperative patient evaluations. *Proceedings of the 45th Hawaii International Conference on System Sciences*, Maui, HI, USA. Computer Society Press. 10.1109/HICSS.2012.250

Ryan, J., Doster, B., Daily, S., & Lewis, C. (2014a). A business process management approach to perioperative supplies/instrument inventory and workflow. *Proceedings of the 47th Hawaii International Conference on System Sciences*, Waikoloa, HI, USA. 10.1109/HICSS.2014.359

Ryan, J., Doster, B., Daily, S., & Lewis, C. (2014b). A balanced perspective to perioperative process management aligned to hospital strategy. *International Journal of Healthcare Information Systems and Informatics*, *9*(4), 1–19. doi:10.4018/ijhisi.2014100101

Ryan, J., Doster, B., Daily, S., Lewis, C., & Glass, R. (2013). A phased approach to implementing radio frequency identification technologies within the perioperative process. *Health Technology*, *3*(1), 73–84. doi:10.100712553-013-0054-7

Ryan, J., Doster, B., Daily, S., Ryan, R., & Lewis, C. (2015). Perioperative patient transparency and accountability via integrated hospital information systems. *Proceedings of the 21st Americas Conference on Information Systems*, Puerto Rico.

Schubnell, T., Meuer, L., & Bengtson, R. (2008). Improving surgical services performance through changing work culture. *AORN Journal, 87*(3), 575–583. doi:10.1016/j.aorn.2008.02.017 PMID:18328278

Silver, M., Markus, M., & Beath, C. (1995). The information technology interaction model: A foundation for the MBA core course. *Management Information Systems Quarterly, 19*(3), 361–391. doi:10.2307/249600

Silverman, D., & Rosenbaum, S. (2009). Integrated assessment and consultation for the preoperative patient. *The Medical Clinics of North America, 93*(5), 963–977. doi:10.1016/j.mcna.2009.05.010 PMID:19665614

Tarantino, D. (2003). Process redesign part 1: Process selection. *Physician Executive, 29*(6), 71–73. PMID:14686251

Tenner, A., & DeToro, I. (1997). *Process redesign: the implementation guide for managers.* Upper Saddle River, NJ: Prentice-Hall, Inc.

Tuomi, I. (2000). Data is more than knowledge: Implications of the reversed knowledge hierarchy for knowledge management and organizational memory. *Journal of Management Information Systems, 16*(3), 103–117. doi:10.1080/07421222.1999.11518258

Turban, E., Sharda, R., Aronson, J., & King, D. (2008). *Business Intelligence: A Managerial Approach.* Upper Saddle River, NJ: Prentice Hall.

Udell, J. (2014). Playing with data. *InfoWorld, 26*(41), 34.

Utzolino, S., Kaffarnik, M., Keck, T., Berlet, M., & Hopt, U. (2010). Unplanned discharges from a surgical intensive care unit: Readmissions and mortality. *Journal of Critical Care, 25*(1), 375–381. doi:10.1016/j.jcrc.2009.09.009 PMID:19914795

van Deursen, A. (1999). Software renovation. *ERCIM News, 36*(1), 13–14.

Walton, M. (1986). *The Deming Management Method.* New York: Dodd-Mead.

Wears, R. L., & Berg, M. (2005). Computer technology and clinical work: Still waiting for Godot. *Journal of the American Medical Association, 293*(10), 1261–1263. doi:10.1001/jama.293.10.1261 PMID:15755949

Weber, R. (2004). The rhetoric of positivism versus interpretivism. *Management Information Systems Quarterly, 28*(1), iii–xii.

Weissman, C., & Klein, N. (2008). The Importance of differentiating between elective and emergency postoperative critical care patients. *Journal of Critical Care, 23*(3), 308–316. doi:10.1016/j.jcrc.2007.10.039 PMID:18725034

Wickramasinghe, N., & Schaffer, J. (2006). Creating knowledge-driven healthcare processes with the intelligence continuum. *International Journal of Electronic Healthcare, 2*(2), 164–174. doi:10.1504/IJEH.2006.008830 PMID:18048242

Witten, I. H., & Frank, E. (2005). *Data Mining: Practical Machine Learning Tools and Techniques* (2nd ed.). San Francisco: Morgan Kaufmann Publishers.

Wright, J., Roche, A., & Khoury, A. (2010). Improving on-time surgical starts in an operating room. *Canadian Journal of Surgery*, *53*(3), 167–170. PMID:20507788

Yin, R. K. (2003). *Case study research: Design and methods* (3rd ed.). Thousand Oaks, California: Sage Publications.

Zani, W. M. (1970). Blueprint for MIS. *Harvard Business Review*, *48*(6), 85–90.

This research was previously published in the International Journal of Healthcare Information Systems and Informatics (IJHISI), 11(3); edited by Joseph Tan and Qiang (Shawn) Cheng; pages 19-41, copyright year 2016 by IGI Publishing (an imprint of IGI Global).

Chapter 4

A Soft Computing Approach for Data Routing in Hospital Area Networks (HAN)

Rakhee
Birla Institute of Technology and Science Pilani, India

M. B. Srinivas
Birla Institute of Technology and Science Pilani, India

ABSTRACT

This paper proposes an alternative model to deliver vital signs of patients in a hospital indoor environment where a large number of patients exist and the traffic generated rapidly changes over time using Body Area Network (BAN). The methodology for finding an optimal path includes a meta-heuristic that combines ANT Colony Optimization (ACO). The authors propose an ACO based framework for monitoring data originating from a BAN to improve network life, energy and load balancing of the overall network. Since the traffic generated by BANs on the network changes with time, finding a shortest path is important for Hospital Area Network. In this paper, the authors implemented an ACO based method and have carried out simulations using OMNeT++ to prove that the proposed method can find a better solution than conventional methods.

INTRODUCTION

Ant colony optimization (ACO) is a meta-heuristic search algorithm for problem solving that takes inspiration from the behavior of real ants. The basic idea of ACO lies on the fact that communication among individuals in ant colony happens based on the pheromone trails that are used for communication to other ants. It has been a combinatorial optimization problem by (Dorigo et al., 1996), for many applications. Many studies on ACO have been performed using traveling salesman problem and prove to be superior when compared with other meta-heuristic approaches.

DOI: 10.4018/978-1-7998-2451-0.ch004

Copyright © 2020, IGI Global. Copying or distributing in print or electronic forms without written permission of IGI Global is prohibited.

In this paper, the authors deal with Hospital Area Network where continuous data is being transferred from indoor hospital environment to the destination where a number of nodes exist in the network and the traffic on the network rapidly changes with time because of the critical nature of the data transfer. This scenario reflects where a particular instance typical traffic congestion happens during a network without affecting the network life time and energy consumption.

This paper deals with the finding shortest path without time delay and deliver the crucial data within time. Conventional problem solving methods are difficult because when the traffic changes rapidly, the information obtained from an old search may not be helpful because it carries a critical data of the patients. Hence, finding a shortest path solution helps in handling these issues.

In this paper, the researchers propose an evolution strategy method to solve the above issues using ACO. The proposed protocol makes an optimal use of the network energy and increases the network lifetime across the network.

RELATED WORK

Wireless Body Area Networks (WBAN) (Figure 1) together with HAN have created a high impact on the health care because of ageing population due to its sedentary lifestyle and poor diet resulting in an increase in number of people with chronic disease which requires continuous monitoring of the patient. Wireless sensor network technology offers a large scale and cost-effective solutions to this problem. It has become necessity for providing the quality health care timely by using Wireless Body Area Network technology. Authors in (ZK.et.al 2013), for an indoor hospital scenario, it uses centralized and distributed mode of communicating the BAN data packets which are sensitive and critical packets. Communication of the data packets plays a vital role in WBAN, since it consumes energy of the sensor node and that can be optimized by finding the best route to address all important issues concerned with latency, throughput.

Figure 1. General WBAN architecture

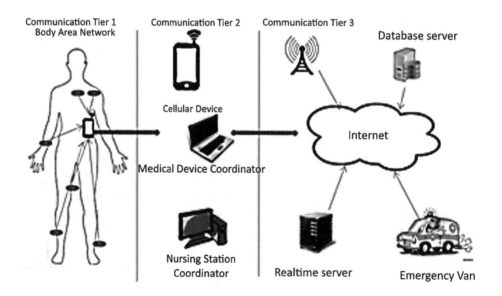

The challenges related to the management of patient's medical information and an intelligent continuous monitoring of BAN data in hospital environment is discussed (Chen et al. 2010). Many researchers (Wood et al., 2006, Chen et al., 2009; Huang and Fang, 2008; Liang et al., 2008; Razzaque et al., 2008, Curtis et al., 2008; Gao et al., 2007; Agarwal et al., 2010, ZKhan et al., 2013, Ugolotti et al., 2013; Amoretti et al., 2013) have proposed BAN network architecture by combining or splitting the BAN in inter-BAN communication but they failed to address the real time display of BAN data in indoor hospital environment using soft computing approach

PROPOSED ENERGY EFFICIENT OF WBAN USING ANT COLONY OPTIMIZATION TECHNIQUE

The proposed algorithm ANT based optimization is inspired by ant food foraging intelligence, where routing is done for exploration and updating of pheromones through locally and globally. When a source node wants to send data to the destination node i.e. NSC, it sends its ants like packets locally to find its new paths. During this process, they update their information in the pheromone and routing table regarding the most visited nodes and also the information regarding the pheromone and energy values of the visited nodes. This helps in laying down the communication links between adjacent nodes by making the paths stronger to send reliable data to the sink.

General Procedure

The general procedure of the proposed method is shown Algorithm 1. The shortest path from source to destination includes all the BANs and MDCs. When the ants move, the search is repeated.

Constructing a Tour by ACO

In the proposed method, the route of visiting BANs and MDCs is constructed and the paths between BANs are planned by ACO algorithm. Since ACO is superior to all other meta-heuristics algorithms, it is widely used as path constructing method.

Algorithm 1 shows the general procedure of ACO, where i is a current node of a path and Visited List (VL) is a set of visited nodes by the ants. Ants start from the current node location of the network and construct a route to the destination MDC or NSC. When the ant k is at the node j in constructing a route, next hop is selected based on the probabilities for all neighbor nodes which is calculated by using following formula:

$$P_{ij} = \frac{\left(\tau_{ij}\right)^a \left(\eta_{ij}\right)^\beta}{\sum_{l \in U} \left(\tau_{il}\right)^a \left(\eta_{il}\right)^\beta} \tag{1}$$

τ_{ij}: Pheromone trail of combination (i,j)

η_{ij}: Local heuristic of combination (i,j)

P_{ij}: Transition probability of combination (i,j)

α: Relative importance of pheromone trail

β: Relative importance of local heuristic

q_0: Determines the relative importance of exploitation versus exploration

ρ: Trail persistence

In conventional methods, paths connecting each pair of sensor nodes are calculated before the algorithm. In proposed method, we calculate the paths individually when they initiate for the first time. The ACO algorithm procedure helps in updating the candidate lists which includes the promising neighbors to participate, thus reducing the minimum number of nodes to participate, hence balancing the load among the nodes which helps in increasing the network lifetime of the network. This proposed ACO method is employed for BAN communication with MDC's in hospital environment. The main objective is to find a path between a BAN and an MDC taking into consideration the following two factors 1. minimal BAN energy consumption 2. Optimal path.

The procedure is shown in the algorithm 1, BAN network is initialized with a constant pheromone trail τ_{ij} on each connection between BAN's. MDC's are selected based on the probabilistic function based on their pheromone and energy values at each node. Whichever node has highest probabilistic value that node is chosen as next hop. Source BAN is designated as 's' and Destination MDC as 'd'. α, β are initialized with standard ACO values where the heuristic values are greater than 0. 'm' is the number of ants started at source BAN. Each ant from the current BAN 'i' hops to the next MDC 'j' according to the probability function given by equation 1. 'L' is a list carried by each ant which contains the BAN ID's of devices in the path traversed by it, keeping track of visited devices in list 'VL'. 'l' is the length of path.

When all ants have completed the tour, the optimal path is the best of all paths taken by all ants after a few iterations. The list 'SL' is initialized with shortest path found based on the minimum cost function from equation 2. Then the pheromone trials on the path are updated according to the procedures-*pheromoneLocalUpdate* and *pheromoneGlobalUpdate* which are discussed in following section. The outer loop controlled by NC is iterated until it reaches a user defined maximum number of cycle's parameter NCmax or all ants make the same tour which is called stagnation behavior. For every iteration, the shortest path is updated. Thus, the message from source BAN is communicated with MDC in optimal shortest path given by List 'SL'.

$$\text{Cost (i,j)} = \min \Sigma\{VL\} \tag{2}$$

ALGORITHM: *General Procedure of ACO in WBAN*

```
Procedure ACO(s, d, α, β, NCmax)
Initialization:
For every edge (i, j), τ_ij=c for trail intensity and Δτ_ij=0. // edges are ini-
tialized with some constant trial
Initialize each ants visited nodes list 'VL' with 1 for source BAN 's' and 0
for other nodes(BAN'S, MDC'S)
L={s}; // for each ant
SL={s};
NC=1, Slen=0,l=0;
while((NC <NCmax) || (stagnation not behavior observed))do
     for(k=1 to m) do    // m is number of ants started from source BAN 's'
          while((current node!='d') || (neighbor nodes of current node are 1
in list 'VL')
do
ant at current node 'i'(BAN or MDC) chooses next node 'j' (MDC) with probabil-
ity p^k_ij given in equation 1
          add node 'j' to a list 'L'
               Update the list VL
          end while
          if(current node ==d) then // required MDC or NSC is reached
               pheromoneLocalUpdate(k,L,l);
               updateShortestPath(SL,SLen,L,l);
          end if
     end for
     pheromoneGlobalUpdate();
     NC ←NC + 1;
     Nullify the updates of list 'L' of each ant;
     Nullify the updates of list 'VL' of each ant;
     For every edge (i,j) set Δτ_ij=0
end while
end procedure
```

Algorithm 1: General Procedure of ACO Using Probabilistic Function for WBAN

The following pheromoneLocalUpdate procedure updates the pheromone trials on the connections of devices given by the list 'L' for each ant. Pheromone trial is updated according to the algorithm 2. This operation makes the shortest path more probable for the next ant to choose. In the procedure pheromoneGlobalUpdate, the evaporation of pheromone trail along the connections in the network is imposed according to the algorithm 3, where ρ is the evaporation constant. In the procedure updateShortestPath, for every shortest path found, its length is compared with 'Slen,' the length of path formed by list 'SL' nodes, and 'SL' list is updated.

```
procedurepheromoneLocalUpdate(k,L,l)
initialization:
l← length of path formed by list 'L'
for ( every edge (i,j) of path ) do
```

$$\Delta \ddot{A}_{ij}^{*}$$

$$= \frac{1}{l} \left\{ \text{if} \left(i, j\right) \text{ is in the path described by list } 'L' \right\}$$

$$= 0 \text{ otherwise}$$

$$\Delta \ddot{A}_{ij} = \Delta \ddot{A}_{ij} + \Delta \ddot{A}_{ij}^{*}$$

```
end for
end procedure
```

Algorithm 2: *Pheromone Local Update*

```
procedureupdateShortestPath(SL,SLen,L,l)
if (SLen>l) then
        update list 'SL' as list 'L' of ant
        update Len to 'l'
end if
end procedure
```

```
procedurepheromoneGlobalUpdate()
for every edge (i,j) // in the network
τ_{ij} = ρ.τ_{ij} + Δτ_{ij}
end procedure.
```

Algorithm 3: Pheromone Global Update

The proposed algorithm helps in calculating the optimal path from routing table with lowest cost function. The neighbor selection is based on the probabilistic function. In this way load balancing is achieved by the intermediate nodes in the network. The effect of pheromone trail helps in finding the path proactive whenever traffic congestion occurs at NSC and also whenever position of the nodes keeps changing.

PERFORMANCE EVALUATION

The OMNeT++ based simulator is used to perform the experiments of ACO for WBAN for our proposed protocol (Table 1). We used two cases for our experiments. In scenario 1, authors deployed seven nodes with stationary BAN coordinators (BANCs) with fixed packets as shown in the below screen shots. The transmit power used in our experiments is -25dBm, -15dBm and -10dBm for all two cases. In Scenario 2, authors deployed 49 nodes in the network, as shown in the screen shots in Figures 2 through 5 below, in order to measure the following parameters. The successful transmission rate, overall energy consumption, traffic load, number of packets received, are measured for all the two scenarios.

Table 1. Simulation parameters information

Deployment	Area	10 m * 9 m
	Deployment type	Cases 1 : Fixed Packets Case 2 : Variable Packets
	Number of nodes	7 nodes (3 BANs, 3 MDCs, 1 NSC)
	Initial node energy	18720 J (2 AA batteries)
	Buffer size	32 packets
	Transmit power	-25dBm, -15dBm, -10dBm
Task	Application type	Event-driven
	Max. packet size	80K packets
	Traffic type	CBR (Constant Bit Rate)
MAC	IEEE 802.15.4	Default values
Simulation	Time	1000 seconds (average of 5 iterations)

Simulation Parameters Information

In both the scenarios, if the node B_2 sends a total of 10k artificial packets. The artificial packets return the tour and send real packets to the destination MDCs or NSC. On successful transmission of the packets at destination the end-to-end path reliability by using the probabilistic function of ACO it overcomes the issues related to redundant paths to ensure the requested reliability is met. The path selection of source depends upon the energy at each node at every interval of few seconds and pheromone deposit between to the nodes. Thus it ensures the link reliability between the nodes from source to destination.

The following Tables 2 and 3, gives the results made by proposed algorithm with and without ACO in terms of number of message count received at destination node i.e. NSC and network lifetime.

The following screen shots represent the test-bed set up for the BAN network for our proposed model. In our experiment, equal weight is given to the parameters α and β which represents the importance of pheromone delay and delay respectively.

The number of packets forwarded by the intermediate nodes BAN or MDC before reaching the destination in proposed method using ACO approach when the transmit power is -25dBm, -15 dBm and -10dBm. In comparison to the conventional methods, there are 2500, 2900 and 4,000 packets are forwarded by intermediate nodes for various transmit powers respectively. Due to the reduced number of broadcast packets and fewer packets by intermediate nodes i.e. BAN or MDCs, the results in reduced

Table 2. WBAN without ACO technique

No. of Nodes	Message Count	Network Lifetime(msec)
7	40	31.07
49	92	30.033

Table 3. WBAN with ACO technique

No. of Nodes	Message Count	Network Lifetime(msec units)
7	46	34
49	1193	35

Figure 2. Deployment of 7 nodes

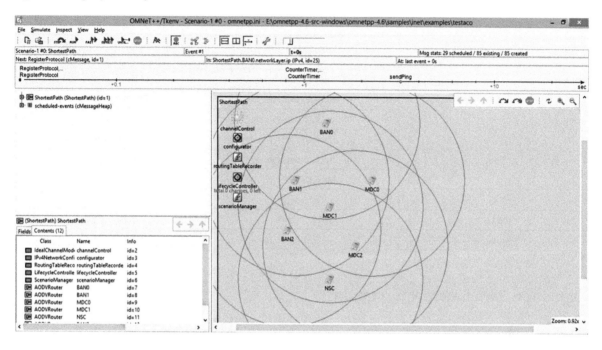

Figure 3. Broadcasting of Hello Packets within 7 nodes

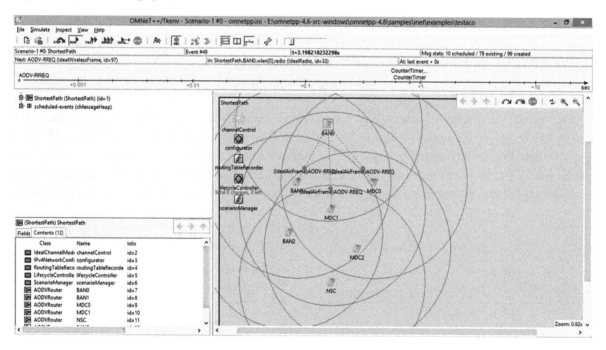

Figure 4. Deployment of 49 nodes

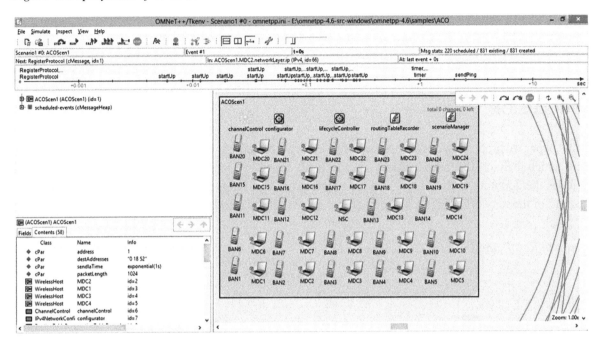

Figure 5. Broadcasting of hello packets from NSC

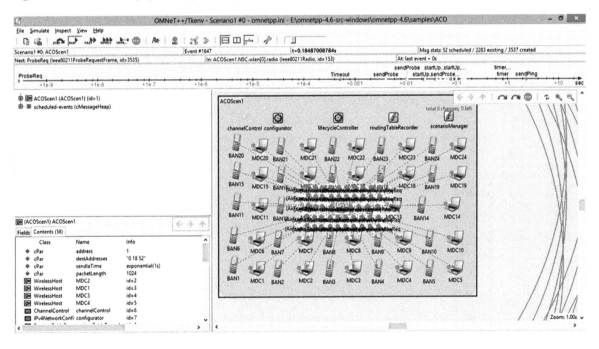

overall energy consumption and network traffic load as shown in Figures 6 through 8 respectively. The saved energy by all nodes in proposed method is better than the conventional methods. The amount of data packets received by the destination is shown in Figure 6 through 8. When compared to the conventional methods it is increased by 5, 10, 12% for various transmit powers respectively.

CONCLUSION

In this paper we proposed a novel approach of monitoring patient for the indoor hospital WBAN environment which includes the meta-heuristic approach ANT Colony Optimization technique. This technique includes the updating of local and global pheromones, which helps in finding the shortest path to route the data in the network. This technique helps in choosing the next hop based on the residual energy at

Figure 6. Result analysis of WBAN using ACO

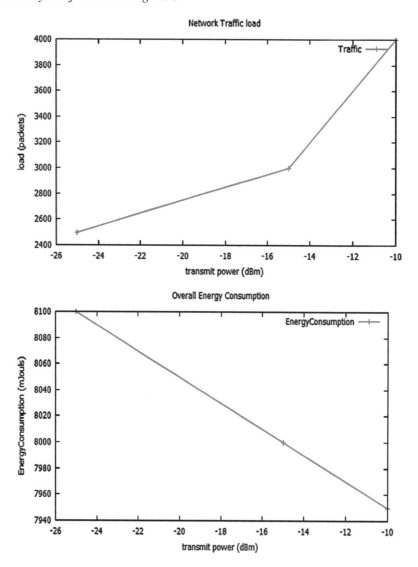

Figure 7. Result analysis of WBAN using ACO (continued)

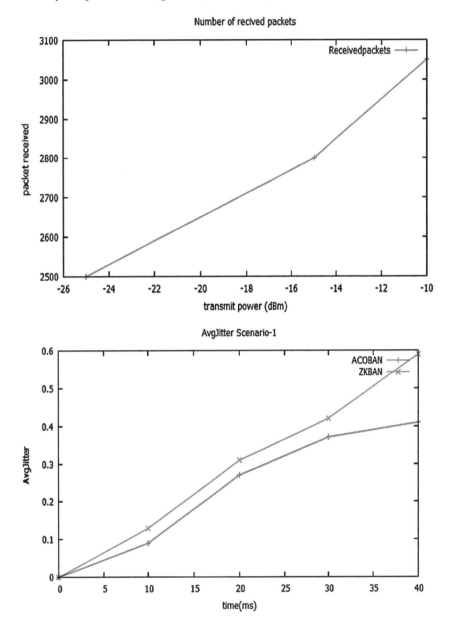

the node and the pheromone values deposited between the nodes, hence reducing the energy consumption by balancing the load on the network and reducing the traffic load. The routing is built based on the more energy at each node hence resulting in balancing the network and thereby increasing the network lifetime. We have performed extensive simulations using OMNeT++ simulator for these cases to test our proposed routing protocol. These results prove that our proposed routing protocol has better performance when compared to similar conventional protocols.

Figure 8. Result analysis of WBAN using ACO (continued)

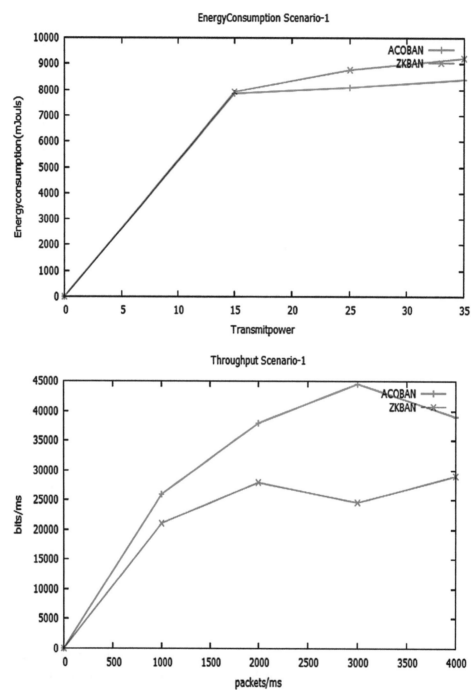

REFERENCES

Amoretti, M., Copelli, S., Wientapper, F., Furfari, F., Lenzi, S., & Chessa, S. (2013). Sensor data fusion for activity monitoring in the PERSONA ambient assisted living project. *J. Ambient Intell. Human Comput.*, *4*(1), 67–84.

Anton, P., Munoz, A., Mana, A., & Koshutanski, H. (2010). Security enhanced ambient assisted living supporting school activities during hospitalization. *J. Ambient Intell. Human Comput.*, *3*(3), 177–192.

Babu, B. R., Poojary, M., & Renuka, B. (2012). Application of hybrid ant colony optimization algorithm for solving capacitated vehicle routing problem. *International Journal of Computer Science and Information Technologies*, *3*(2).

Chen, M., Kwon, T., & Choi, Y. (2006, January). Energy-efficient differentiated directed diffusion (EDDD) in wireless sensor networks. *Computer Communications*, *29*(2), 231–245. doi:10.1016/j.comcom.2005.05.019

Chen, M., Kwon, T., Mao, S., Yuan, Y., & Leung, V. C. (2008). Reliable and energy-efficient routing protocol in dense wireless sensor networks. *Int. J. Sensor Networks*, *4*(1-2), 104–117.

Curtis, D., Shih, E., Waterman, J., Guttag, J., & Bailey, J., … Ohno-Machado, L. (2008). Physiological signal monitoring in the waiting areas of an emergency room. *Proceedings of ICST '08*.

Dorigo, M., Maniezzo, V., & Colorni, A. (1996). The Ant System: Optimization by a Colony of Cooperating Agents. *IEEE Transactions systems*, *26*(1), 29-41.

Jiang, S., Cao, Y., Iyengar, S., Kuryloski, P., Jafari, R., Xue, Y., ... Wicker, S. (2008, March). CareNet: an integrated wireless sensor networking environment for remote healthcare. *Proceedings of the ICST 3rd international conference on Body area networks*.

Khan, Z. A., Sivakumar, S., Phillips, W., Robertson, B., & Javaid, N. (2012). QPRD: QoS-aware Peering Routing Protocol for Delay Sensitive Data in hospital Body Area Network Communication. *Proceedings of IEEE BWCCA*, *12*, 178–185.

Ugolotti, R., Sassi, F., Mordonini, M., & Cagnoni, S. (2013). Multi-sensor system for detection and classification of human activities. *J. Ambient Intell. Human Comput.*, *49*(1), 27–41.

Wood, A., Virone, G., Doan, T., Cao, Q., Selavo, L., … Stankovic, J. (n. d.). ALARM-NET: Wireless sensor networks for assisted living and residential monitoring.

Xiangning, F., & Yulin, S. (2007, October). Improvement on LEACH protocol of Wireless Sensor Network. *Proceedings of the International Conference on Sensor Technologies and Applications* (pp. 260-264). IEEE.

This research was previously published in the International Journal of Business Data Communications and Networking (IJBDCN), 12(2); edited by Zoubir Mammeri; pages 16-27, copyright year 2016 by IGI Publishing (an imprint of IGI Global).

Chapter 5
Categorize Readmitted Patients in Intensive Medicine by Means of Clustering Data Mining

Rui Veloso
University of Minho, Portugal

José Machado
University of Minho, Portugal

Filipe Portela
University of Minho, Portugal

António da Silva Abelha
University of Minho, Portugal

Manuel Filipe Santos
University of Minho, Portugal

Fernando Rua
Centro Hospitalar do Porto, Portugal

Álvaro Silva
Centro Hospitalar do Porto, Portugal

ABSTRACT

With a constant increasing in the health expenses and the aggravation of the global economic situation, managing costs and resources in healthcare is nowadays an essential point in the management of hospitals. The goal of this work is to apply clustering techniques to data collected in real-time about readmitted patients in Intensive Care Units in order to know some possible features that affect readmissions in this area. By knowing the common characteristics of readmitted patients it will be possible helping to improve patient outcome, reduce costs and prevent future readmissions. In this study, it was followed the Stability and Workload Index for Transfer (SWIFT) combined with the results of clinical tests for substances like lactic acid, leucocytes, bilirubin, platelets and creatinine. Attributes like sex, age and identification if the patient came from the chirurgical block were also considered in the characterization of potential readmissions. In general, all the models presented very good results being the Davies-Bouldin index lower than 0.82, where the best index was 0.425.

DOI: 10.4018/978-1-7998-2451-0.ch005

Copyright © 2020, IGI Global. Copying or distributing in print or electronic forms without written permission of IGI Global is prohibited.

INTRODUCTION

This study was based on two previous studies in this thematic. One for predicting readmissions in Intensive Care Units (ICU) (Braga et al., 2014) and another about the use of clustering to understand the variables that can influence readmissions and non-readmission in ICU (Veloso et al., 2014). The attained results with the first study did not allow for an efficient patient's characterization. The second one using clustering proved that it was possible to characterize patients that are likely to be readmitted or non-readmitted. This third study arises as an improvement of the earlier studies, adopting new data and adding other variables that may contribute to the characterization of readmitted patients. The objective was to identify and declare features that influence and they are important to analyze at the moment of discharge in order to reduce the readmissions rate. In this study, it is used only readmitted patient data, being the main goal to classify readmitted patients and understand which group of variables / values can help to predict a further readmission. This study presented very interesting results being the best Davies-Bouldin index equal to 0.425, which means that it was possible to create a group of variables very well separated in the space. At the same time, it was possible to identify the variables platelets count, bilirubin and PaO2/FIO2 as the ones that mostly contribute to predict future readmissions.

This article is divided in five sections. The first one, Introduction, presents the basis for this work. The second one will define the problem and present the theory behind the work and his concepts. The third section describes the methods and tools used, business and data understanding, data preparation and evaluation. On the fourth section, Discussion, are presented some points of view on the results obtained with this study. In the last section are presented the achieved conclusions and launched the basis for further work.

BACKGROUND

Intensive Medicine

In the field of Medicine there is a particular area having as main goal to diagnose and treat patients with serious illnesses and restore them to their previous health condition (Silva et al., 2008), namely Intensive Medicine (IM). This type of patients is usually admitted to intensive care units (ICU). In ICU, the patients can maintain their physiological functions through various life-support devices. In these units, the patients are normally mechanical ventilated and the vital functions are continuously monitored as well as the status of each of the organic systems: neurological, respiratory, hepatic, hematological, cardiovascular and renal. In order to ensure the life and patient condition these functions can be supported through therapeutic plans, clinical procedures or by mechanical means until the patient has again its functions independently (Ramon et al., 2007). An interesting definition of intensive medicine can be: a multidisciplinary area that addresses specifically three moments, the prevention, diagnose and therapy of patients and physiopathology conditions potentially reversible that threaten or present the failure of one or more vital functions (Silva, 2007).

Clinical Analysis

Clinical Analysis consists in the use of data from laboratories. These data include results from blood and urine test analysis and microscopic studies like the analysis of tissues.

These analysis results are very important in the moment of diagnose and make a decision about treatments. Bilirubin is a fluid produced by the human liver. Tests to this substance are important to identify potential liver and gallbladder problems (Berk & Korenblat, 2011).

Another common analysis to perform in medicine is blood or urine test to obtain Creatinine values. This substance appears through the breakdown of creatine phosphate in the muscles. Testing this substance is important to assess kidney and muscle problems, problems during pregnancy and loss of blood fluids. Platelets are blood cells that prevent bleeding through the formation of blood clots. The test is useful to identify bleeding problems, bone marrow disease and excessive clotting or bleeding.

The Lactic Acid is a substance produced in the cells of the muscles and in red blood cells. The analysis of this substance is very important. Abnormal results indicate that the tissues are not receiving enough oxygen what may represent heart failure, liver and lung problems as also the presence of severe infections (Seifter, 2011). The white blood cells (leucocytes) are cells of the immune system being very important to the body protection. The count of leucocytes in blood is helpful to identify infectious and inflammatory processes, leukemia and lymphoma as also bone marrow disorders.

Readmissions

Readmissions theme is nowadays an important point of interest in healthcare area because of the costs associated to them. Readmissions work as a quality indicator of the healthcare service provided. The ageing of the world's population also contributes to the rise on readmission rates, being these readmissions directly related to bad application of therapies and lack of monitoring at home (Benbassat & Taragin, 2000)

In the ICU, bad decisions taken by the intensivist at the time of discharge are directly related to an unplanned readmission for the patient. Nowadays the ability of predicting a relapse in the patient after the discharge is limited (Gajic et al., 2008). It is considered a readmission when a patient is admitted to the same unit where he/she was earlier within thirty days after the discharge with the same diagnosis (ACSS, 2012). The number of readmitted patients in ICU is significant, having according to the literature review, in North America and Europe, an average rate around 7% (Rosenberg & Watts, 2000).

Analyzing the costs perspective, non-planned readmissions represent an issue because it represents a high cost to the hospital. The readmissions rate is high in many cases because the hospitals need to reduce the patient's length of stay to reduce the healthcare costs (Araújo & Pontes, 2002).

Clustering

Clustering is inserted in the group of Data Mining problems. Cluster analysis divides the dataset into groups that have sense, are helpful or the booth. The groups are the objective and the clusters should capture the natural structure of the data. Unlike other techniques, the classification criteria is not defined by the analyst but it is discovered along the process of clustering. The clusters are characterized by a great internal homogeneity and external heterogeneity (Tufféry, 2011).

The cluster analysis represent an important role in many areas like psychology and social sciences, biology, statistics, pattern recognition, information recovery, machine learning and data mining (Tan et al., 2005).

There are a large number of cluster algorithms and the choice of the methods to be adopted depends on the type of the data as well on the purpose and intended application. The majority of the clustering methods are included into five categories.

The Partition Methods build a set of partitions on the data, where each partition represents a cluster. The hierarchical methods execute a hierarchical decomposition of the data. These methods can be agglomerative or divisive. The agglomerative methods start with singular objects to form an isolated group. Then successively the groups or objects are merged until only one group left. Divisive methods behave the other way. The density-based methods are useful to filter outliers or to discover with arbitrary form. Grid-based methods restrict the space of objects to a finite number of cells that form a grid structure. The Model-based methods formulate a model hypothesis for each cluster and find the best fit of the data to the model (Han et al., 2006).

The evaluation of clustering results can be done laying on two factors: compactness and separability. The compactness is a property that expresses how much the cluster elements are close. Lesser the variance value greater will be the compactness of the cluster. The calculation of the intra cluster distance is very useful to assess this characteristic. The separability evaluates how diverse the clusters are. This can be assessed by the inter-cluster distance that will be the greater possible so the clusters are better (Cios, 2007). To this work the partition methods (k-means, k-medoids, x-means) were used.

INTCare

INTCare is a research project giving origin to an Intelligent Decision Support System (IDSS). This IDSS is deployed in the ICU of the CHP and it is in constant development and test.

INTCare is based on intelligent agents (Santos et al., 2011) and it aims to support the decision-making process by monitoring patient condition and predicting clinical events as is patient organ failure (cardiovascular, respiratory, renal, hepatic, neurological and hematologic), patient outcome (Portela et al., 2013a), readmissions, medical diseases, critical events, barotrauma among others. This work is framed in the goal of creating clusters of readmitted patients. Regarding to the predictions made, the system is able to suggest procedures, treatments and therapies.

This system is based in four autonomous subsystems (data acquisition, knowledge management, inference and interface) using intelligent agents to perform their actions in real-time (data processing, data transformation, data mining models induction and others) (Portela et al., 2013a; Portela et al., 2012).

SWIFT

With the goal of predicting readmission there are several models or mathematical techniques that can help the intensivists to predict the probability of a patient be readmitted in an ICU. In order to find the most viable and accurate model a study was conducted to develop and validate a numerical index called Stability and Workload Index for Transfer (SWIFT) [6].

Using SWIFT there are some variables that can be used to estimate the probability of unplanned ICU readmissions like the patient length of stay (LOS) in the ICU, measured in days, the source of patients admission, Glasgow Coma Scale (GCS), the ratio between partial pressure of oxygen in arterial blood (PaO2) and fraction of inspired oxygen (FIO2) and the evaluation of nursing care for respiratory problems (PCO2).

These variables are then scored taking into account the information available at hospital discharge time. Table 1 presents the SWIFT Variables and the scores to be assigned.

Table 1. SWIFT variables

Variables	Score
Original Source of ICU Admission	
Emergency Department	0
Transfer from a ward or outside hospital	8
Total ICU Length of Stay (in days)	
Lesser than 2	0
Between 2 and 10	1
Bigger than 10	14
Last measured PaO2/FIO2 ratio	
Bigger than 400	0
Lesser than 400 and bigger or equal to 150	5
Lesser than 150 and bigger or equal to 100	10
Lesser than 100	13
Glasgow Coma Scale at the time of ICU	
Greater than 14	0
Between 11-14	6
Between 8-10	14
Lesser then 8	24
Last arterial blood gas PaCO2	
Lesser than 45 mm Hg	0
Bigger than 45 mm Hg	5

Related Work

Included in the INTCare project, two studies have been made to understand the ICU readmission phenomena. The first one had as objective to study and define the variables that most influence the patient readmission and to develop Data Mining models to predict readmission. SWIFT method was used to create classification models to predict if a patient will be readmitted or not. The results were very satisfactory, obtaining 98.91% of accuracy. However, these results only have been possible due to the use of oversampling. More information about the study done and the results achieved using data mining models to predict patient's readmission in an ICU is available in the first work (Braga et al., 2014). In order to make a deeper data exploration and improve the previous results, a second study was developed (Veloso et al., 2014). This second study had as main goal to explore clusters in order to characterize possible readmitted patients and identify features that influence readmission and non-readmissions. That study revealed good results (Davies-Bouldin Index equal to 0,503) and two groups of variables were identified, so that at the time of discharge if the patient have variables that are framed with these two groups the patient is a potential case of readmission. In order to improve the characterization of the groups this new study has been conducted. This new study included new results from clinical analysis and new variables like the one that identifies if the patient came from the operating block when he needed from intensive healthcare. A new dataset and more recent data were also used.

STUDY DESCRIPTION

Methods and Tools

As data mining methodology, the Cross Industry Standard Process for Data Mining (CRISP-DM) was followed. Crisp-DM is divided in six phases: business understanding, data understanding, data preparation, modeling, evaluation, and deployment. The work presented follows the CRISP-DM phases. In terms of tools Oracle was used for data analysis, understanding and preparation and RapidMiner was used to build clustering scenarios. A benchmark analysis has been carried out comparing the following algorithms: k-means, k-means with kernels, k-means fast, k-medoids, x-means, expectation maximization clustering, top down clustering, DBSCAN, support vector clustering, random clustering and flatten clustering. From these techniques, the ones that suited better (in terms of statistical and domain criteria) were k-means, k-medoids and x-means, therefore considered in this work.

Business Understanding

This work presents as main goal the categorization (creation of clusters) of readmitted patients in an ICU. The idea is giving new knowledge to the intensivist by providing information about if a patient has clinical characteristics of readmitted patients, i.e., if he belongs or not to the clusters achieved in this work. The Data Mining goal encompasses a characterization of patient groups readmitted in ICU. Clinically, these models will support clinical decisions as well improve the quality of service and consequently it can contribute to decrease the number of readmissions.

Data Understanding and Data Preparation

This process is iterative and it was performed as many times as necessary to ensure the data quality. The data comes from three tables. The first one contains the data from the patient admission like age, sex, admission, and discharge date. The second table contains additional information about the patient like if he came from the emergency room or another ward of the hospital and if he was at the surgery block when there was the needed to transfer him to ICU. The third table contains analysis results from the patients. So, the following variables were considered in order to acquire the data necessary for the models:

- **Episode**: This variable identifies the clinical case of a patient;
- **Date of Birth**: This variable was later derived to originate the age variable that represents the age of the patient in years;
- **Date of Discharge and Date of Admission**: These variables were considered in order to derivate the length of stay of inpatient calculating the difference between the two dates;
- **Number of Process**: Using this variable and the date of discharge and admission it was possible to create a new attribute, called readmission indication if a patient corresponds to an unplanned readmission or not. All patients admitted before 30 days from the last discharge were considered readmission;
- **Emergency Room and Surgery**: These variables were pulled in order to know if a patient came from the emergency room or other ward and if the patient was on the surgery block when needed intensive cares;

- **Results, Exam and Validation Dates**: Were acquired the results and validation dates from the analysis relative to exams of Lactic Acid, Leucocytes, Bilirubin, Platelets and Creatinine.

Using PaO2 and FIO2 results it was possible to calculate the ratio PaO2/FIO2. Once this work is dealing with readmissions, it was considered the results of PaO2, FIO2, Leucocytes, Lactic Acid, Bilirubin, Creatinine and Platelets closest to the discharge date. The data to use on the models considers then 16 variables: age, sex, length of stay in the ICU (in days), emergency room (indicates if the patient came from the emergency room or if the patient was admitted from other hospital), PaO2/FIO2 (the ratio between the partial pressures of oxygen in blood and fraction of inspired oxygen), PaCO2 (partial pressures of carbon dioxide in blood), the scores relative to emergency room, length of stay, PaO2/FIO2 ratio, PaCO2 and the laboratory results of the quantity of lactic acid, leucocytes, bilirubin, platelets and creatinine. Table 2 presents some statistics for each dataset variable.

Notice that this study used real data acquired from the CHP databases. The data was collected from the patient clinical process and laboratory results. The data used is from April 23th, 2012 to December 10th, 2014 and corresponds to 1072 cases (patients). The number of readmission cases verified throughout this period is 45 (about 4.2% episodes). Being the base of this work use data provided by the readmitted patients, it was only used the data associated to the 45 readmission cases.

Table 2. Variables considered

Variable	Distinct Values	Average	Minimum Value	Maximum Value
Age	82	63.93	27.00	83.00
Sex	2 (1 or 2)	-	-	-
Length of Stay	38	6.60	1.00	43.00
Emergency Room	2 (0 or 1)	-	-	-
Surgery	2 (0 or 1)	-	-	-
PaO2/FIO2 Ratio	754	273.42	60.30	838.10
PaCO2	325	39.78	24.70	56.90
Bilirubin	687	2.22	0.20	20.67
Platelet	390	202.80	25.00	531.00
Creatinine	278	1.27	0.14	4.63
Lactic Acid	220	2.28	0.40	16.00
Leucocytes	766	11.68	0.92	43.42
PaO2/FIO2 Ratio Score	4 (0; 5; 10 or 13)	-	-	-
PaCO2 Score	2 (0 or 5)	-	-	-
Emergency Room Score	2 (0 or 8)	-	-	-
Length of Stay Score	3 (0; 1 or 14)	-	-	-
Readmission	2 (Yes or No)	-	-	-

MODELING

The modeling phase was focused on getting models to translate business goals through the application of clustering techniques. The modelling was done using Rapid Miner Studio 6.3. This tool is an integrated environment for data mining, machine learning, text mining, predictive and business analysis. It allows the development of many type of data mining works, being clusters one of them. In order to achieve the goals defined, several models using twelve scenarios and considering four main groups of variables were developed:

- Target Class = Readmission;
- Normal (N) = {emergencyroom, length_of_stay, PCO2, PaO2_FIO2_ratio, surgery};
- Scores (S) = {PCO2_Score, PaO2_FIO2_ratio_score, emergencyroom_score, length_of_stay_score};
- Case Mix (CM) = {sex, age};
- Lab Results (LR) = {lactic_acid, leucocytes, bilirubin, platelet, creatinine}.

The division of the variables on groups was made in order to conjugate different scenarios for the models.

Normal group is composed by the majority of the variables and it is formed by the values (in a continuous form) necessary for the SWIFT plus the indication if the patient was being submitted to a surgery in the moment that he needed an intensive care.

The Scores group contains the scores obtained by the application of the values defined by the SWIFT Table.

Case Mix is composed by non-clinical attributes associated to patients receiving healthcare on a unit or hospital.

Lab Results group contains the absolute result for the five clinical substances considered (lactic acid, leucocytes, bilirubin, platelets and creatinine).

The variable readmission was not considered in these groups because it was the target for the clustering models. So, with these groups 12 different scenarios (Table 3) were encoded.

These 12 scenarios originated 84 models:

$$M_n = \{S_i; TDM_y\}.$$

These models were obtained from the conjugation of the 12 scenarios (S_i) and 7 different clustering techniques (TDM_y) (the target is always the same), but from the 84 models only 36 models have been analyzed in this study – those representing points of interest from the clinical data results. Many of the 84 models induced presented interesting statistically results, however from the clinical domain and the defined objectives they are not useful.

To evaluate the models and to choose which models can be considered valid in the clinical domain it was need to make some meetings with the ICU medical staff. In these meetings, the models that had interest for them in a clinical point of view were selected. To each one of the models was associated a scenario, a target and a clustering technique. As above mentioned: k-means, k-medoids and x-means were the algorithms that demonstrated the best results.

Table 4 allows to see the settings defined for these three algorithms.

X-Means algorithm calculates an optimal number of clusters (k) for the running but k-Means and k-medoids did not calculate it. For those techniques, Davies-Bouldin Index was used to find the most

Table 3. Scenarios

Scenarios	Used Variables
S1	Normal
S2	Normal + Case Mix
S3	Normal + Case Mix + Scores
S4	Normal + Case Mix + Scores + Lab Results
S5	Scores
S6	Case Mix
S7	Lab Results
S8	Normal + Scores
S9	Normal + Lab Results
S10	Scores + Case Mix
S11	Scores + Lab Results
S12	Case Mix + Lab Results

correct number of clusters (the more lower the value is a better separation of the clusters and tightness inside clusters occur) and evaluated the Elbow method by observing the variations of the average within cluster distance (observe how the average within cluster distance varies from k to k and select the k where the natural progression of the measure dominates de structure). Table 5 demonstrates the optimal

Table 4. Algorithms settings

Algorithm	Setting	Value
k-means	K	2 to 8
	Max Runs	10
	Max Optimization Steps	100
	Measures Type	Numerical Measures
	Numerical Measure	Euclidean Distance
k-medoids	K	2 to 8
	Max Runs	10
	Max Optimization Steps	100
	Measure Types	Numerical Measures
	Numerical Measure	Euclidean Distance
x-means	K Min	2
	K Max	60
	Measure Types	Numerical Measures
	Numerical Measure	Euclidean Distance
	Clustering Algorithm	KMeans
	Max Runs	10
	Max Optimization Steps	100

Table 5. Optimum number of clusters for k-means and k-medoids

Model	Algorithm	Number of Clusters	Davies-Bouldin Index	Average within in cluster distance
M1	k-means	4	0.425	1745.845
	k-medoids	6	0.434	1217.740
M2	k-means	4	0.469	1945.538
	k-medoids	6	0.674	1837.016
M3	k-means	4	0.475	1980.688
	k-medoids	6	0.685	1890.749
M4	k-means	4	0.743	11514.016
	k-medoids	7	0.816	7351.339
M5	k-means	5	0.483	6.372
	k-medoids	5	0.557	12.267
M6	k-means	3	0.427	24.957
	k-medoids	5	0.588	19.956
M7	k-means	4	0.493	1201.265
	k-medoids	4	0.502	1376.468
M8	k-means	4	0.431	1780.995
	k-medoids	5	0.462	2409.784
M9	k-means	6	0.682	5818.096
	k-medoids	7	0.793	6937.805
M10	k-means	2	0.648	108.935
	k-medoids	3	0.686	186.311
M11	k-means	4	0.505	1233.572
	k-medoids	2	0.516	6243.052
M12	k-means	4	0.556	1400.639
	k-medoids	2	0.590	7563.608

number of clusters considered for each model taking into account the Davies-Bouldin Index and the Elbow Method (returning the average within cluster distance for the elbow).

Evaluation

This phase was focused first on the assessment of the results provided by the use of k-means, x-means and k-medoids and then the results were compared with the initial goals of the project. Analyzing the achieved results and considering the Davies-Bouldin index, it was evident that the technique that achieved the worst results was k-medoids. Although the difference between the results obtained with the use of k-means and x-means was not expressive, k-means got the best results. These results were expected since the x-means is based on k-means. Some models obtained interesting values for Davies-Bouldin index, unfortunately they do not achieve the lower limit imposed in this domain. Table 6 represents the cluster segmentation for the best models.

Analyzing in more detail the model 1 it is possible to observe that the majority of the readmission cases is distributed by C1, C2 and C3 with 18, 16 and 10 cases respectively. Exploring the results obtained in model 1 and observing Figure 1 it is possible to observe that the PaO2/FIO2 ratio is the feature that mostly influencing the clustering, where it is possible to observe three well-defined segment clusters

Table 6. Results for the best models

Model	Algorithm + Number of Clusters	Davies-Bouldin Index	Clusters	Number of Readmission Cases
M1 (N)	k-means with 4 clusters	0.425	C0	1
			C1	18
			C2	16
			C3	10
M2 (N+CM)	k-means with 4 clusters	0.469	C0	18
			C1	1
			C2	16
			C3	10
M3 (N+CM+S)	k-means with 4 clusters	0.475	C0	18
			C1	16
			C2	10
			C3	1
M4 (N+CM+S+LR)	k-means with 4 clusters	0.743	C0	1
			C1	13
			C2	16
			C3	15
M5 (S)	k-means with 5 clusters	0.483	C0	4
			C1	6
			C2	3
			C3	8
			C4	24
M6 (CM)	k-means with 3 clusters	0.427	C0	24
			C1	2
			C2	1
M7 (LR)	k-means with 4 clusters	0.493	C0	9
			C1	13
			C2	6
			C3	17
M8 (N+S)	k-means with 4 clusters	0.431	C0	1
			C1	16
			C2	18
			C3	10

continued on following page

Table 6. Continued

Model	Algorithm + Number of Clusters	Davies-Bouldin Index	Clusters	Number of Readmission Cases
M9 (N+LR)	k-means with 6 clusters	0.682	C0	1
			C1	4
			C2	9
			C3	7
			C4	9
			C5	15
M10 (S+CM)	k-means with 2 clusters	0.648	C0	29
			C1	16
M11 (S+LR)	k-means with 2 clusters	0.516	C0	28
			C1	17
M12 (CM+LR)	k-means with 2 clusters	0.613	C0	28
			C1	17

Figure 1. Distribution of readmission cases by clusters in PaO2/FIO2 Ratio, PaCO2 and Length of Stay for Model 1

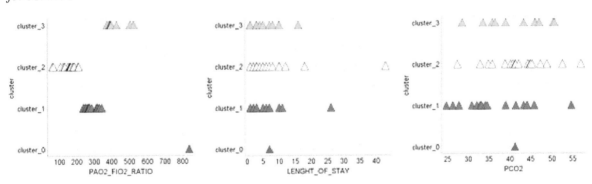

(total separation of the values). Cluster 1 with values between 238 and 344, cluster 2 between 66 and 210 and cluster 3 between 374 and 525.

In terms of the Lenght of Stay variable the readmission cases are equaly distributed by the clusters excluding cluster 0 that only have one case of readmission. On the feature PaCO2 it is possible to observe some distribution with cluster 1 obtaining the majority of the cases with PaCO2 values being below than 37 and cluster 2 having the bigger part of cases where PaCO2 value is above 39.

Surgery feature revealed some interesting results where the great part of readmissions was on the patients that came from operating block (cluster 2), being the patients that were not submitted to surgery presented on cluster 3. The feature Emergency Room did not demonstrate any relevant segmentation.

Observing the distribution of the features related with the laboratorial analysis by the clusters (model 7 and Figure 2) it is easily seen that the platelets, bilirrubin and lactic acida results are well segmented by the different clusters.

Figure 2. Distribution of readmission cases by clusters for Laboratorial Results

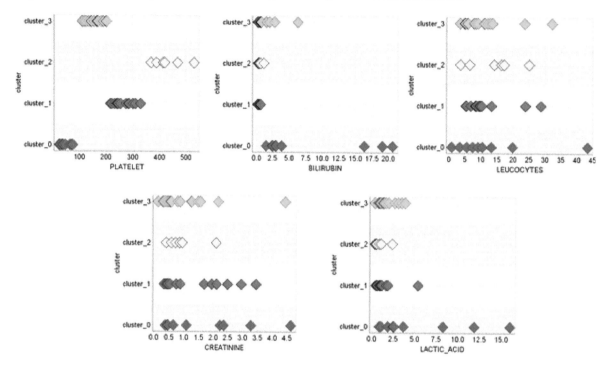

Analysing the results of the Case Mix group (model 6) it is possible to observe that the sex is not preponderant on the segmentation of readmission cases, however age contributes for the cluster separability.

For last, the scores (evidenced in model 5 results) did not revealed to be preponderant for the segmentation of the clusters, being the PaO2/FIO2 ratio the feature with most significance.

DISCUSSION

After making the evaluation and analysis of the models two global clusters were created to better represent the characteristics of future readmitted patients. Table 7 presents these groups and the correspondent attributes and values.

The Emergency Room, Creatinine, Leucocytes, Scores and Sex did not have much impact on the groups. The great majority of the patients came from wards outside the hospital so this feature is not much segmented. Creatinine and Leucocytes have the results very well distributed so the segmentation is low. The Scores are a direct characterization of the Normal group values using SWIFT so it was expected to not segment the readmissions in groups. Sex attribute also should not have been considered because the original dataset was well balanced between man and woman.

Table 7. Relevant information about groups of patient readmitted

Variable	Cluster 1	Cluster 2
PaO2/FIO2 Ratio	60 to 265	238 to 505
PaCO2	32 to 56	24 to 45
Length of Stay	2 to 20	1 to 10
Lactic Acid	0.8 to 3.9	0.4 to 1.9
Bilirubin	0.23 to 0.76	0.49 to 3.04
Platelets	112 to 254	243 to 531
Age	58 to 83	27 to 63

CONCLUSION

When compared this work with the related work presented in the section two, the main difference was in the dataset used, being in this case only considered data provided by readmitted patients. Consequently, all the analysis and achieved results are totally different in both levels: scientific and clinical.

In a unit of this type, the number of clinical variables for each patient is enormous so the set of possibilities is really big, however this work provided to be very useful helping to characterize readmitted patients. The clusters developed cannot ensure which patients will be readmitted but they give information about which type of patients the physicians should consider in terms of clinical situation before performing their discharge. With this work, new variables should be considered at the time of discharge to prevent a potential readmission. The platelets count and bilirubin value are variables that potentially influence the readmission of a patient. Once again it was confirmed the importance of variables like PaO2/FIO2 ratio, PaCO2, LOS, age and lactic acid have in identifying readmission patients.

The clusters created with these groups revealed to be an improvement to the ones developed in early works, since they consider the addition of new variables and the main criteria of evaluation for each cluster. Davies-Bouldin index was even better being lesser in the models created in this work, and the lesser the index is the better the cluster model is.

Councils with clinical experts and analysis of results obtained can be a good starting point. In the future, the information obtained with these models will be integrated in the decision support system at the time of discharge to start to help reducing the readmission rates. It is an interesting possibility to have some visual information on the patient's clinical data file that alerts for some values of features that are in the ranges presented by this study. So, that the intensivist can make a bigger post ICU accompaniment or schedule earlier visits from the patient to the hospital to monitor again some of the features.

ACKNOWLEDGMENT

This work has been supported by FCT – Fundação para a Ciência e Tecnologia in the scope of the project: UID/CEC/00319/2013. The authors would like to thank FCT for the financial support through the contract PTDC/EEI-SII/1302/2012 (INTCare II).

REFERENCES

ACSS. (2012). Administração Central do Sistema de Saúde, Circular Normativa n° 33/2012.

Araújo, D., & Pontes, M. (2002). *Comissões de Ética: das bases teóricas à atividade quotidiana. Em Doenças Crónicas*. Coimbra: Gráfica de Coimbra.

Benbassat, J., & Taragin, M. (2000). Hospital Readmissions as a Measure of Quality of Health Care: Advantages and Limitations. *Archives of Internal Medicine*, *160*(8), 1074–1081. doi:10.1001/archinte.160.8.1074 PMID:10789599

Berk, P. D., & Korenblat, K. M. (2011). Approach to the patient with jaundice or abnormal liver test results. In L. Goldman & D. Ausiello (Eds.), *Cecil Medicine* (24th ed.). Philadelphia, Pa: Saunders Elsevier.

Braga, P., Portela, F., Santos, M.F., Rua, F. (2014). Data Mining Models to Predict Patient's Readmission in Intensive Care Units. SCITEPRESS - Science and Technology Publications. doi:10.5220/0004907806040610

Chenhui, Z., Huilong, D., & Xudong, L. (2008). An Integration Approach of Healthcare Information System. *Proceedings of the 2008 International Conference on BioMedical Engineering and Informatics* (Vol. 1, pp. 606–609). IEEE. 10.1109/BMEI.2008.109

Cios, K., Swiniarski, R., Pedrycz, W., & Kurgan, L. (2007). Supervised Learning: Statistical Methods. In A Knowledge Discovery Approach (pp. 307–386). Springer US. doi:10.1007/978-0-387-36795-8_1

Gajic, O., Malinchoc, M., Comfere, T. B., Harris, M. R., Achouiti, A., Yilmaz, M., ... Farmer, J. C. (2008). The Stability and Workload Index for Transfer score predicts unplanned intensive care unit patient readmission: Initial development and validation. *Critical Care Medicine*, *36*(3), 676–682. doi:10.1097/CCM.0B013E318164E3B0 PMID:18431260

Han, J., & Kamber, M. (2000). *Data Mining: Concepts and Techniques*. San Francisco, CA, USA: Morgan Kaufmann Publishers Inc.

Israni, A. K., & Kasiske, B. L. (2011). Laboratory assessment of kidney disease: filtration rate, urinalysis, and proteinuria. In M. W. Taal, G. M. Chertow, P. A. Marsden, & ... (Eds.), *Brenner and Rector's The Kidney* (9th ed.). Philadelphia, Pa: Elsevier Saunders.Koh, H. C., & Tan, G. (2005). Data mining applications in healthcare. *Journal of Healthcare Information Management : JHIM*, *19*(2), 64–72. Retrieved from http://www.ncbi.nlm.nih.gov/pubmed/15869215 PMID:15869215

Portela, F., Pinto, F., & Santos, M. F. (2012). Data Mining Predictive Models For Pervasive Intelligent Decision Support In Intensive Care Medicine. *Proceedings of the International Conference on Knowledge Management and Information Sharing KMIS '12*.

Portela, F., Santos, M. F., Silva, Á., Machado, J., Abelha, A., & Rua, F. (2013a). Pervasive and Intelligent Decision Support in Critical Health Care Using Ensembles. *ITBAM*, *2013*, 1–16.

Portela, F., Santos, M. F., Silva, Á., Machado, J., Abelha, A., & Rua, F. (2013b). Data Mining for Real-Time Intelligent Decision Support System in Intensive Care Medicine. *Proceedings of the International Conference on Agents and Artificial Intelligence ICAART '13* (pp. 270–276).

Ramon, J., Fierens, D., Güiza, F., Meyfroidt, G., Blockeel, H., Bruynooghe, M., & Van Den Berghe, G. (2007). Mining data from intensive care patients. *Advanced Engineering Informatics, 21*(3), 243–256. doi:10.1016/j.aei.2006.12.002

Rosenberg, A. L., & Watts, C. (2000). Patients Readmitted to ICUs. *Chest, 118*(2), 492–502. doi:10.1378/chest.118.2.492 PMID:10936146

Santos, M. F., Portela, F., & Vilas-Boas, M. (2011). INTCARE -Multi-agent Approach for Real-time Intelligent Decision Support in Intensive Medicine. *Proceedings of the International Conference on Agents and Artificial Intelligence ICAART '11* (pp. 364–369).

Seifter, J. L. (2011). Acid-base disorders. In L. Goldman & A. I. Schafer (Eds.), *Cecil Medicine* (24th ed.). Philadelphia, Pa: Saunders Elsevier.

Silva, A. (2007). *Modelos de Inteligência Artificial na análise da monitorização de eventos clínicos adversos, Disfunção/Falência de órgãos e prognóstico do doente*. Universidade do Porto.

Silva, Á., Cortez, P., Santos, M. F., Gomes, L., & Neves, J. (2008). Rating organ failure via adverse events using data mining in the intensive care unit. *Artificial Intelligence in Medicine, 43*(3), 179–193. doi:10.1016/j.artmed.2008.03.010 PMID:18486459

Tan, P.-N., Steinbach, M., & Kumar, V. (2005). *Introduction to Data Mining* (1st ed.). Boston, MA, USA: Addison-Wesley Longman Publishing Co., Inc.

Tufféry, S. (2011). Cluster Analysis. In Data Mining and Statistics for Decision Making (pp. 235–286). John Wiley & Sons, Ltd. doi:10.1002/9780470979174.ch9

Veloso, R., Portela, F., Santos, M. F., Silva, Á., Rua, F., Abelha, A., & Machado, J. (2014). A Clustering Approach for Predicting Readmissions in Intensive Medicine. *Procedia Technology, 16*, 1307–1316. doi:10.1016/j.protcy.2014.10.147

This research was previously published in the International Journal of E-Health and Medical Communications (IJEHMC), 8(3); edited by Joel J.P.C. Rodrigues; pages 22-37, copyright year 2017 by IGI Publishing (an imprint of IGI Global).

Chapter 6
The Evolution of Comorbidities in Hospital Administrative Databases:
A 15-Year Analysis

Alberto Freitas

Faculty of Medicine of the University of Porto (FMUP), Portugal & Center for Health Technology and Services Research (CINTESIS), Portugal

Isabel Garcia Lema

Faculty of Medicine of the University of Porto (FMUP), Portugal & Center for Health Technology and Services Research (CINTESIS), Portugal

Altamiro Costa-Pereira

Faculty of Medicine of the University of Porto (FMUP), Portugal & Center for Health Technology and Services Research (CINTESIS), Portugal

ABSTRACT

The analysis of inpatient comorbidities is important for hospital management, epidemiological studies, and health services research and planning. This paper aims to study the evolution of coded comorbidities in a nationwide administrative database. Specifically, data from Portuguese hospitals over the period 2000-2014 was used. Secondary diagnoses, coded with ICD-9-CM, were used to identify comorbidities in 9,613,563 inpatient episodes, using both the Elixhauser and the Charslon/Deyo methods. A description of comorbidities evolution over years, including an analysis of the associated principal diagnosis, was carried out. Results clearly evidence a positive association between the number of secondary diagnoses and coded comorbidities. It can be argued that the increased number of comorbidities over time is mostly related to an increase in the quality of coded data, and not so much to an increase in the severity of treated patients. Data analysts, researchers and decision makers should be alert to possible data quality bias, such as completeness, when using administrative databases.

DOI: 10.4018/978-1-7998-2451-0.ch006

Copyright © 2020, IGI Global. Copying or distributing in print or electronic forms without written permission of IGI Global is prohibited.

INTRODUCTION

Comorbidity is a secondary diagnosis, i.e., a disease condition, other than the principal diagnosis, already present at the time patient is admitted. The presence of comorbidities may have consequences at various levels as, for instance, mortality, quality of life, utilization of health resources and treatment strategies.

Several studies showed that there is a relation between specific patient comorbidities and an increase (or decrease) in hospital costs, hospital mortality and length-of-stay (Deyo, Cherkin, & Ciol, 1992; Elixhauser, Steiner, Harris, & Coffey, 1998; Zhu & Hill, 2008). In fact, due to this association with health outcomes, the study, and assessment of comorbidities assumes particular importance for health services research, for epidemiological and clinical studies, and also for financing and health care planning.

Comorbidities are patient preexisting conditions that should be controlled when using administrative data (Deyo et al., 1992; Kuwabara et al., 2008). In administrative databases, comorbidities can be identified using ICD-9-CM (International Classification of Diseases, Ninth Revision, Clinical Modification) codes associated with secondary diagnoses (Southern, Quan, & Ghali, 2004).

In this context, the quality and the volume of the data coded can naturally have influence in the proportion of identified comorbidity conditions. That is especially important for the study of trends or any analysis over time. Comorbidities should also be used in risk-adjustment of health outcomes (e.g., mortality) to induce, for instance, a fairer comparison between health institutions.

The study of the number of coded secondary diagnoses is critical to understand the evolution in the proportion of identified comorbidities (Iezzoni et al., 1992). This number is increasing over years, and consequently, the number of identified comorbidities is also continuously increasing. This evolution is not necessarily related to an increase in the severity of patients treated.

This paper aims to study the evolution of comorbidities over time using administrative data, and was carried out under the CUTEheart project, Comparative use of technologies for coronary heart disease, an international partnership between the Harvard Medical School and the Faculties of Medicine from the Universities of Lisbon and Porto in Portugal. This paper extends authors' previous work (Freitas, Lema, & Costa-Pereira, 2016) with an update of the inclusion criteria and the inclusion of new analyses over a larger, updated, dataset.

Administrative Data

Administrative data (also known as billing or claims data) is routinely collected, commonly available, relatively inexpensive, and involves large amounts of data. Although with some data quality problems (Freitas et al., 2012; Peabody, Luck, Jain, Bertenthal, & Glassman, 2004), administrative data is a valuable source for measuring the quality of care. It has a standard format and can be used for many purposes, such as research or public reporting (Price, Estrada, & Thompson, 2003). This dataset typically contains demographic data (e.g., age, gender), "administrative data" (length of stay, type of admission, payer, discharge status, Diagnosis-Related Group – DRG) and ICD-9-CM codes for clinical data (diagnostics, procedures, external causes) (Iezzoni, 1997).

Comorbidity Classification Systems

Comorbidity scores are often used for epidemiological studies and health service research (de Groot, Beckerman, Lankhorst, & Bouter, 2003). These scores can be calculated using different data sources, such as ICD-9-CM data, as in the Elixhauser (1998) and Charlson indexes (Charlson, Pompei, Ales, & MacKenzie, 1987), and pharmacy claims, as in the RxRisk-V score (Fishman et al., 2003). These three examples are the most commonly used methods for measuring comorbidities. Next these methods are briefly described, with particular emphasis given to the two approaches that use administrative data (ICD-9-CM).

Charlson et al. (1987) defined a weighted index to classify comorbidity conditions associated with an increased risk of mortality. In the original definition, the index was calculated using 19 conditions with different assigned weights for each condition (1, 2, 3 or 6), considering the risk of death from each condition. For instance, 'congestive heart failure' had a weight of 1, 'leukemia' had a weight of 2, and 'AIDS' had a weight of 6. There are many variations of this index, including one of the most used, the Deyo et al. adaptation for use with ICD-9-CM administrative databases (Deyo et al., 1992).

The method proposed by Elixhauser et al. (1998) also used ICD-9-CM codes in the definition of a list of 30 comorbidity conditions. The performed study showed that the developed measures were associated with a remarkable increase in the length of stay, hospital charges, and hospital mortality. After that, several studies pointed out that Elixhauser method has better mortality prediction than the Charlson method (Dominick, Dudley, Coffman, & Bosworth, 2005; Southern et al., 2004).

The RxRisk-V is a comorbidity index based on computerized data from hospital pharmacies with good results in the prediction of total health costs (Sales et al., 2003).

Because different measures provide different identified comorbidities, and with various levels of agreement for common comorbidities, it is important to understand and use them appropriately in any epidemiological study and case-mix analysis (Inacio, Pratt, Roughead, & Graves, 2015).

METHODS

The analysis of this work was based on data from hospitalizations in acute care public hospitals, related to discharges between years 2000 and 2014. This dataset included inpatient episodes (outpatient episodes were excluded) in all Portuguese acute care hospitals, representing nearly 85% of all hospitalizations in Portugal. The access to the data was provided by the Ministry of Health's Central Authority for Health Services.

Similarly, to other comorbidity studies, for example in the study performed by Elixhauser et al. (1998), pediatric (age below 18 years) and obstetrical episodes (Major Diagnostic Category – MDC – 14, "Pregnancy, Childbirth, and the Puerperium" and MDC 15, "Newborns and Other Neonates with Conditions Originating in the Perinatal Period", considering All Patient Diagnosis Related Groups – AP-DRG 21 – grouper) were excluded. Patients discharged to another institution (discharge status "Discharged/ Transferred to a Short-term General Hospital for Inpatient Care") or transferred to other hospitals were also excluded. The initial dataset contained 22,167,646 (inpatient and outpatient) episodes and, after applying the exclusion criteria, 9,613,563 episodes remained for analysis.

Comorbidities were identified using the two most widely used comorbidity approaches, the Elixhauser (1998) and the Charslon/Deyo methods (Deyo et al., 1992). Specifically, the updated version (enhanced ICD-9-CM) proposed by Quan et al. was the used comorbidities definition (Quan et al., 2005). ICD-9-CM codes for the definition of these two methods can be seen in Appendix A. Secondary diagnoses (up to 19 available ICD-9-CM coded variables for each episode) were used to determine the absence or presence of each one of the comorbidities. The final score was the sum of existing comorbidities for the Elixhauser method and a weighted score for the Charlson/Deyo Comorbidity Index (Deyo et al., 1992).

Due to the extension of ICD-9-CM (over 14,000 diagnosis codes) the 2014 update of the Agency for Healthcare Research and Quality's Clinical Classifications Software (CCS) for ICD-9-CM was used to group principal diagnosis into a small number of clinically meaningful diagnosis groups. Then, changes between years 2000 and 2014 were calculated for the main diagnoses with higher volume.

Statistical analysis was performed using IBM SPSS Statistics for Windows, Version 24, Armonk, NY: IBM Corp.

RESULTS

Table 1 and 2 presents the proportion of identified comorbidities in inpatient episodes with discharges in years 2000, 2007 and 2014, the percentage of comorbidities increase between 2000 and 2014, and also the adjusted percentage considering the average number of secondary diagnoses, for both Elixhauser and Charlson/Deyo methods. As can be seen, the majority of comorbidities significantly increased throughout the study period, from the year 2000 to the year 2014. Some of them increased more than 100%, especially 'Hypothyroidism' with an increase of 702%, 'Depression' with 451%, 'Obesity' with 449%, and 'Hypertension, complicated' with 375%. The average comorbidity increase was 154% for the Elixhauser method and 96% for the Charslon/Deyo method. On the other hand, some comorbidities continuously decreased during this period of eleven years. For instance, 'Blood loss anemia' decreased 30% and 'AIDS/H1V' decreased 14%.

The average number of Elixhauser comorbidities continuously increased from 0.70 in 2000 to 1.79 in 2014 (154% more). For Charslon/Deyo the increase was 96%, from 0.66 in 2000 up to 1.30 in 2014. Figure 1 shows that this continuous increase is clearly associated with the increase in the number of secondary diagnoses. On average, in 2000, 1.71 secondary diagnoses were coded in each inpatient episode (in a maximum of 19, limited by the number of available variables) while, in 2014, this proportion was of 5.30 (209% more). In fact, in the year 2000, the percentage of episodes with at least one coded secondary diagnoses was 65% and, 15 years later, this proportion was 88%. If adjusted to the average number of secondary diagnoses, the majority of the comorbidities present a decrease in the studied period.

Table 3 presents the top 10 principal diagnoses (grouped by CCS) with a higher number of inpatient episodes and the evolution of the average number of secondary diagnoses and comorbidities scores. 'Non-hypertensive Congestive Heart Failure' is the principal diagnosis with the highest number of secondary diagnosis (mean of 9.0 in 2014), while 'Osteoarthritis' is on the opposite side with 2.9 in average. The principal diagnosis 'Pneumonia (except that caused by tuberculosis or sexually transmitted disease)' is the one with the smallest increase in the mean number of comorbidities, between 2000 and 2014, with 72%.

DISCUSSION

The results presented in this paper underline a continuous increase in the number of collected and coded secondary diagnoses in hospital administrative databases. This increase obviously leads to a general increase in the number of identified comorbidities, as seen for the two used comorbidities methods. In this context, any analysis or interpretation of administrative data, particularly when using data from secondary diagnoses or any other, not obligatory data (for instance, medical or surgical procedures), should always consider these possible limitations.

Table 1. Comparison of the proportion of identified Elixhauser comorbidities in episodes with discharges in 2000, 2007 and 2014

Elixhauser comorbidities	2000	2007	2014	2000-2014 Increase (%)	2000-2014 Adjusted Increase (%)*
Congestive heart failure	4.5	6.1	10.2	127.0	-27
Cardiac arrhythmias	6.0	9.2	15.2	154.6	-18
Valvular disease	1.5	2.2	4.1	179.1	-10
Pulmonary circulation disorders	0.7	0.9	1.5	128.5	-26
Peripheral vascular disorders	1.0	1.4	2.5	158.5	-16
Hypertension, uncomplicated	12.8	22.7	34.5	170.6	-13
Hypertension, complicated	1.5	2.9	7.3	375.2	54
Paralysis	0.7	0.8	2.3	216.3	2
Other neurological disorders	1.8	3.1	5.3	191.1	-6
Chronic pulmonary disease	4.0	5.5	9.0	125.0	-27
Diabetes, uncomplicated	6.2	10.9	16.3	160.1	-16
Diabetes, complicated	2.4	2.1	3.0	22.2	-60
Hypothyroidism	0.4	1.2	3.5	701.5	159
Renal failure	2.6	3.7	8.9	238.7	9
Liver disease	2.4	2.9	4.3	78.9	-42
Peptic ulcer disease excluding bleeding	0.4	0.4	0.4	-0.1	-68
AIDS/H1V	0.3	0.2	0.2	-13.5	-72
Lymphoma	0.4	0.5	0.7	67.6	-46
Metastatic cancer	3.2	3.7	4.8	51.7	-51
Solid tumor without metastasis	3.5	3.9	4.5	28.4	-59
Rheumatoid arthritis/collagen vascular diseases	0.6	0.8	1.3	124.1	-28
Coagulopathy	0.7	1.2	2.4	257.5	16
Obesity	1.5	3.6	8.4	449.1	77
Weight loss	0.8	0.9	1.6	92.1	-38
Fluid and electrolyte disorders	3.6	5.6	11.1	206.6	-1
Blood loss anemia	0.8	0.9	0.6	-30.0	-77
Deficiency anemia	1.1	1.3	2.3	105.8	-33
Alcohol abuse	2.8	3.3	5.0	75.5	-43
Drug abuse	0.7	0.6	0.9	28.4	-59
Psychoses	0.3	0.4	0.6	146.2	-20
Depression	1.1	2.5	6.2	451.4	78

* The proportion of increase is adjusted to the average number of secondary diagnoses coded (1.71 in 2000 and 5.30 in 2014)

The comorbidities are associated with greater use of hospital resources and, in 2014, 71% of analyzed episodes had at least one identified Elixhauser comorbidity, i.e., there is an important role of comorbidities in hospital admissions.

Table 2. Comparison of the proportion of identified Charlson/Deyo comorbidities in episodes with discharges in 2000, 2007 and 2014

Charlson/ Deyo comorbidities	2000	2007	2014	2000-2014 Increase (%)	2000-2014 Adjusted Increase (%)*
Myocardial infarction	1.0	1.6	3.2	211.2	1
Congestive heart failure	4.5	6.1	10.2	127.0	-27
Peripheral vascular disease	1.0	1.4	2.5	158.5	-16
Cerebrovascular disease	4.0	5.2	7.3	84.3	-40
Dementia	1.0	1.7	2.9	185.5	-8
Chronic pulmonary disease	4.0	5.5	9.0	125.0	-27
Rheumatic disease	0.4	0.6	1.1	191.8	-6
Peptic ulcer disease	0.7	0.6	0.6	-18.9	-74
Mild liver disease	1.8	2.4	3.8	114.8	-31
Diabetes without chronic complication	7.7	11.7	16.6	115.5	-30
Diabetes with chronic complication	1.0	1.4	2.7	171.7	-12
Hemiplegia or paraplegia	0.8	1.0	2.7	219.1	3
Renal disease	2.7	3.8	8.9	233.5	8
Any malignancy, including lymphoma and leukemia, except malignant neoplasm of skin	4.1	4.7	5.5	34.2	-57
Moderate or severe liver disease	0.9	1.0	1.2	30.0	-58
Metastatic solid tumor	3.2	3.7	4.8	51.7	-51
AIDS/HIV	0.3	0.2	0.2	-13.5	-72

* The proportion of increase is adjusted to the average number of secondary diagnoses coded (1.71 in 2000 and 5.30 in 2014)

Figure 1. Average number of secondary diagnoses and of comorbidity indexes (Elixhauser and Charslon/ Deyo), per hospital inpatient episode, per discharge year

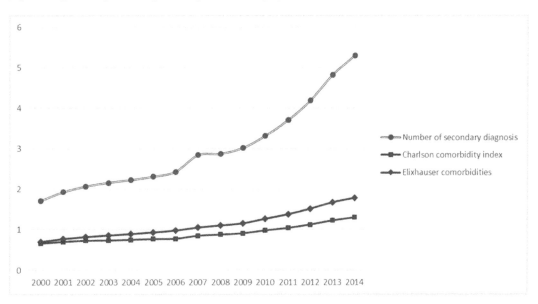

Table 3. Principal diagnosis in the period 2000-14, grouped by CCS (top 10)

Principal diagnosis grouped by CCS	Episodes 2000-14	Nbr secondary diagnoses			Charlson index			Elixhauser comorbidities		
		Mean, 2000	Mean, 2014	Increase (%)	Mean, 2000	Mean, 2014	Increase (%)	Mean, 2000	Mean, 2014	Increase (%)
Pneumonia (except that caused by tuberculosis or sexually transmitted disease)	480,167	3.00	7.87	162.8	1.14	1.95	71.8	1.42	2.83	99.7
Acute cerebrovascular disease	357,340	2.73	7.88	188.9	0.86	2.15	148.7	1.37	2.90	112.0
Biliary tract disease	340,666	1.12	3.70	229.2	0.23	0.66	183.6	0.44	1.30	193.8
Abdominal hernia	280,628	0.79	3.09	292.1	0.14	0.45	223.1	0.32	1.11	252.9
Coronary atherosclerosis and other heart disease	207,756	2.36	5.29	123.9	0.62	1.17	89.1	1.10	2.02	83.0
Congestive heart failure; nonhypertensive	207,013	3.11	9.00	189.7	0.87	2.00	131.1	1.48	3.62	144.9
Urinary tract infections	181,146	2.97	8.09	172.5	0.98	1.91	94.1	1.16	2.57	121.0
Osteoarthritis	169,020	0.79	2.89	264.3	0.12	0.31	170.6	0.32	1.18	272.3
Acute myocardial infarction	155,257	2.87	6.87	138.9	0.69	1.35	95.5	1.30	2.45	88.9
Fracture of neck of femur (hip)	149,860	1.23	3.70	201.8	0.33	0.71	115.8	0.53	1.42	169.6
…	…									
Total	9,613,563	1.71	5.30	209.4	0.66	1.30	95.9	0.70	1.79	154.1

The proportion of episodes with Elixhauser comorbidities increased from 42.3% to 71.0% in the period between 2000 and 2014. As stated, the number of coded secondary diagnoses is associated with this increase but this may not be the only factor responsible for this fact. A high variability in the proportion of comorbidities was found, the emphasis was given to difference evolutions in different comorbidities, and was also shown that, for some comorbidities, the proportion decreased over time.

The sub-analysis for the principal diagnoses with a higher volume of episodes, considering the average number of secondary diagnosis and average comorbidity scores, can also be necessary for specific diseases studies based on administrative data.

CONCLUSION

In this article, the evolution of comorbidities was examined using the most common, widely used, methods for administrative data. Results showed that the number of secondary diagnoses and, consequently, the number of identified comorbidities is continuously increasing. Authors argue that the amount of the increase of comorbidities be mostly related to more, and possibly better, coded data (secondary diagnoses coded with ICD-9-CM), and not necessarily due to a real increase in the number of comorbidities associated with hospital patients. That is, there is not necessarily such a high increase in the severity of treated patients.

Any statistical or epidemiological analysis over this data, specifically over secondary diagnoses, needs to consider both the evolution of the coding system and the daily coding practices. In fact, the increase in a specific comorbidity score, or of a particular comorbidity, is mostly associated with the increase in the number of coded secondary diagnoses. Also, one must bear in mind the possible changes over time in the scope of the collected data (for instance, the inclusion of ambulatory data in the administrative database), variations in the data collection/coding protocols, and the annual revision of ICD-9-CM codes with inclusion of new codes and possible exclusion of other codes.

Data analysts and decision makers should be aware of potential data quality problems, such as completeness and accuracy. Administrative data is a useful, cost-effective source of information, and is increasingly being used for several purposes, for instance, for performance evaluation, hospital financing, and to evaluate the impact of healthcare policies. However, much work is still needed to develop health information systems and increase the quality of this routinely collected data.

Expert domain knowledge about all the steps related to data collection, processing, and analysis must be considered when using and analyzing healthcare data. All the steps involved in the process of healthcare delivery should be adequately understood in order to analyze data and interpret results correctly.

ACKNOWLEDGMENT

This work was supported by FEDER through Programa Operacional Factores de Competitividade – COMPETE and by National Funds through FCT – Fundação para a Ciência e a Tecnologia within the research project "Comparative Use of Technologies for Coronary Heart Disease", reference HMSP-ICT/0013/2011. The authors also wish to thank the Portuguese Ministry of Health's Authority for Health Services (Administração Central do Sistema de Saúde I. P. – ACSS) for providing access to national hospitalizations data.

REFERENCES

Charlson, M. E., Pompei, P., Ales, K. L., & MacKenzie, C. R. (1987). A new method of classifying prognostic comorbidity in longitudinal studies: Development and validation. *Journal of Chronic Diseases*, *40*(5), 373–383. doi:10.1016/0021-9681(87)90171-8 PMID:3558716

de Groot, V., Beckerman, H., Lankhorst, G. J., & Bouter, L. M. (2003). How to measure comorbidity. a critical review of available methods. *Journal of Clinical Epidemiology*, *56*(3), 221–229. doi:10.1016/S0895-4356(02)00585-1 PMID:12725876

Deyo, R. A., Cherkin, D. C., & Ciol, M. A. (1992). Adapting a clinical comorbidity index for use with ICD-9-CM administrative databases. *Journal of Clinical Epidemiology*, *45*(6), 613–619. doi:10.1016/0895-4356(92)90133-8 PMID:1607900

Dominick, K. L., Dudley, T. K., Coffman, C. J., & Bosworth, H. B. (2005). Comparison of three comorbidity measures for predicting health service use in patients with osteoarthritis. *Arthritis and Rheumatism*, *53*(5), 666–672. doi:10.1002/art.21440 PMID:16208675

Elixhauser, A., Steiner, C., Harris, D. R., & Coffey, R. M. (1998). Comorbidity measures for use with administrative data. *Medical Care, 36*(1), 8–27. doi:10.1097/00005650-199801000-00004 PMID:9431328

Fishman, P. A., Goodman, M. J., Hornbrook, M. C., Meenan, R. T., Bachman, D. J., & OKeeffe Rosetti, M. C. (2003). Risk adjustment using automated ambulatory pharmacy data: The RxRisk model. *Medical Care, 41*(1), 84–99. doi:10.1097/00005650-200301000-00011 PMID:12544546

Freitas, A., Lema, I., & Costa-Pereira, A. (2016). Comorbidity Coding Trends in Hospital Administrative Databases. In Á. Rocha, A. M. Correia, H. Adeli, L. P. Reis, & M. M. Teixeira (Eds.), *New Advances in Information Systems and Technologies* (Vol. 445, pp. 609–617). doi:10.1007/978-3-319-31307-8_63

Freitas, A., Silva-Costa, T., Lopes, F., Garcia-Lema, I., Teixeira-Pinto, A., Brazdil, P., & Costa-Pereira, A. (2012). Factors influencing hospital high length of stay outliers. *BMC Health Services Research, 12*(1), 265. doi:10.1186/1472-6963-12-265 PMID:22906386

Iezzoni, L. I. (1997). Assessing quality using administrative data. *Annals of Internal Medicine, 127*(8 Pt 2), 666–674. doi:10.7326/0003-4819-127-8_Part_2-199710151-00048 PMID:9382378

Iezzoni, L. I., Foley, S. M., Daley, J., Hughes, J., Fisher, E. S., & Heeren, T. (1992). Comorbidities, complications, and coding bias. Does the number of diagnosis codes matter in predicting in-hospital mortality? *Journal of the American Medical Association, 267*(16), 2197–2203. doi:10.1001/jama.267.16.2197 PMID:1556797

Inacio, M. C., Pratt, N. L., Roughead, E. E., & Graves, S. E. (2015). Comparing co-morbidities in total joint arthroplasty patients using the RxRisk-V, Elixhauser, and Charlson Measures: A cross-sectional evaluation. *BMC Musculoskeletal Disorders, 16*(1), 385. doi:10.118612891-015-0835-4 PMID:26652166

Kuwabara, K., Imanaka, Y., Matsuda, S., Fushimi, K., Hashimoto, H., Ishikawa, K. B., ... Fujimori, K. (2008). The association of the number of comorbidities and complications with length of stay, hospital mortality and LOS high outlier, based on administrative data. *Environmental Health and Preventive Medicine, 13*(3), 130–137. doi:10.100712199-007-0022-9 PMID:19568897

Peabody, J. W., Luck, J., Jain, S., Bertenthal, D., & Glassman, P. (2004). Assessing the accuracy of administrative data in health information systems. *Medical Care, 42*(11), 1066–1072. doi:10.1097/00005650-200411000-00005 PMID:15586833

Price, J., Estrada, C. A., & Thompson, D. (2003). Administrative data versus corrected administrative data. *American Journal of Medical Quality, 18*(1), 38–45. doi:10.1177/106286060301800106 PMID:12583643

Quan, H., Sundararajan, V., Halfon, P., Fong, A., Burnand, B., Luthi, J. C., ... Ghali, W. A. (2005). Coding algorithms for defining comorbidities in ICD-9-CM and ICD-10 administrative data. *Medical Care, 43*(11), 1130–1139. doi:10.1097/01.mlr.0000182534.19832.83 PMID:16224307

Sales, A. E., Liu, C. F., Sloan, K. L., Malkin, J., Fishman, P. A., Rosen, A. K., ... Todd-Stenberg, J. (2003). Predicting costs of care using a pharmacy-based measure risk adjustment in a veteran population. *Medical Care*, *41*(6), 753–760. doi:10.1097/01.MLR.0000069502.75914.DD PMID:12773841

Southern, D. A., Quan, H., & Ghali, W. A. (2004). Comparison of the Elixhauser and Charlson/Deyo methods of comorbidity measurement in administrative data. *Medical Care*, *42*(4), 355–360. doi:10.1097/01.mlr.0000118861.56848.ee PMID:15076812

Zhu, H., & Hill, M. D. (2008). Stroke: The Elixhauser Index for comorbidity adjustment of in-hospital case fatality. *Neurology*, *71*(4), 283–287. doi:10.1212/01.wnl.0000318278.41347.94 PMID:18645167

This research was previously published in the International Journal of Reliable and Quality E-Healthcare (IJRQEH), 6(2); edited by Anastasius Moumtzoglou; pages 29-39, copyright year 2017 by IGI Publishing (an imprint of IGI Global).

APPENDIX

Table 4. ICD-9-CM codes for the identification of Elixhauser comorbidities

Elixhauser comorbidities	Enhanced ICD-9-CM codes
Congestive heart failure	398.91, 402.01, 402.11. 402.91, 404.01, 404.03, 404.11, 404.13, 404.91, 404.93, 425.4–425.9, 428.x
Cardiac arrhythmias	426.0, 426.13, 426.7, 426.9, 426.10, 426.12, 427.0–427.4, 427.6–427.9, 785.0, 996.01, 996.04, V45.0, V53.3
Valvular disease	093.2, 394.x–397.x, 424.x, 746.3–746.6, V42.2, V43.3
Pulmonary circulation disorders	415.0, 415.1, 416.x, 417.0, 417.8, 417.9
Peripheral vascular disorders	093.0, 437.3, 440.x, 441.x, 443.1–443.9, 447.1, 557.1, 557.9, V43.4
Hypertension, uncomplicated	401.x
Hypertension, complicated	402.x–405.x
Paralysis	334.1, 342.x, 343.x, 344.0, 344.6, 344.9
Other neurological disorders	331.9, 332.0, 332.1, 333.4, 333.5, 333.92, 334.x–335.x, 336.2, 340.x, 341.x, 345.x, 348.1, 348.3, 780.3, 784.3
Chronic pulmonary disease	416.8, 416.9, 490.x–505.x, 506.4, 508.1, 508.8
Diabetes, uncomplicated	250.0–250.3
Diabetes, complicated	250.4–250.9
Hypothyroidism	240.9, 243.x, 244.x, 246.1, 246.8
Renal failure	403.01, 403.11, 403.91, 404.02, 404.03, 404.12, 404.13, 404.92, 404.93, 585.x, 586.x, 588.0, V42.0, V45.1, V56.x
Liver disease	070.22, 070.23, 070.32, 070.33, 070.44, 070.54, 070.6, 070.9, 456.0–456.2, 570.x, 571.x, 572.2–572.8, 573.3, 573.4, 573.8, 573.9, V42.7
Peptic ulcer disease excluding bleeding	531.7, 531.9, 532.7, 532.9, 533.7, 533.9, 534.7, 534.9
AIDS/H1V	042.x–044.x
Lymphoma	200.x–202.x, 203.0, 238.6
Metastatic cancer	196.x–199.x
Solid tumor without metastasis	140.x–172.x, 174.x–195.x
Rheumatoid arthritis/collagen vascular diseases	446.x, 701.0, 710.0–710.4, 710.8, 710.9, 711.2, 714.x, 719.3, 720.x, 725.x, 728.5, 728.89, 729.30
Coagulopathy	286.x, 287.1, 287.3–287.5
Obesity	278.0
Weight loss	260.x–263.x, 783.2, 799.4
Fluid and electrolyte disorders	253.6, 276.x
Blood loss anemia	280.0
Deficiency anemia	280.1–280.9, 281.x
Alcohol abuse	265.2, 291.1–291.3, 291.5, 291.9, 303.0, 303.9, 305.0, 357.5, 425.5, 535.3, 571.0–571.3, 980.x, V11.3
Drug abuse	292.x, 304.x, 305.2–305.9. V65.42
Psychoses	293.8, 295.x, 296.04, 296.14, 296.44, 296.54, 297.x, 298.x
Depression	296.2, 296.3, 296.5, 300.4, 309.x, 311

Adapted from: Quan H, et al. Coding algorithms for defining Comorbidities in ICD-9-CM and ICD-10 administrative data. Med Care. 2005 Nov; 43(11):1130-9.

Table 5. ICD-9-CM codes for the identification of Charlson/Deyo comorbidities

Charlson/ Deyo comorbidities	Enhanced ICD-9-CM codes
Myocardial infarction	410.x, 412.x
Congestive heart failure	398.91, 402.01, 402.11, 402.91, 404.01, 404.03, 404.11, 404.13, 404.91, 404.93, 425.4–425.9, 428.x
Peripheral vascular disease	093.0, 437.3, 440.x, 441.x, 443.1–443.9, 47.1, 557.1, 557.9, V43.4
Cerebrovascular disease	362.34, 430.x–438.x
Dementia	290.x, 294.1, 331.2
Chronic pulmonary disease	416.8, 416.9, 490.x–505.x, 506.4, 508.1, 508.8
Rheumatic disease	446.5, 710.0–710.4, 714.0–714.2, 714.8, 725.x
Peptic ulcer disease	531.x–534.x
Mild liver disease	070.22, 070.23, 070.32, 070.33, 070.44, 070.54, 070.6, 070.9, 570.x, 571.x, 573.3, 573.4, 573.8, 573.9, V42.7
Diabetes without chronic complication	250.0–250.3, 250.8, 250.9
Diabetes with chronic complication	250.4–250.7
Hemiplegia or paraplegia	334.1, 342.x, 343.x, 344.0–344.6, 344.9
Renal disease	403.01, 403.11, 403.91, 404.02, 404.03, 404.12, 404.13, 404.92, 404.93, 582.x, 583.0–583.7, 585.x, 586.x, 588.0, V42.0, V45.1, V56.x
Any malignancy, including lymphoma and leukemia, except malignant neoplasm of skin	140.x–172.x, 174.x–195.8, 200.x–208.x, 238.6
Moderate or severe liver disease	456.0–456.2, 572.2–572.8
Metastatic solid tumor	196.x–199.x
AIDS/HIV	042.x–044.x

Adapted from: Quan H, et al. Coding algorithms for defining Comorbidities in ICD-9-CM and ICD-10 administrative data. Med Care. 2005 Nov; 43(11):1130-9.

Chapter 7
Data Quality and Critical Events in Ventilation:
An Intensive Care Study

Filipe Portela
Universidade do Minho, Portugal

Manuel Filipe Santos
Universidade do Minho, Portugal

António da Silva Abelha
Universidade do Minho, Portugal

José Machado
Universidade do Minho, Portugal

Fernando Rua
Centro Hospitalar do Porto, Portugal

ABSTRACT

The data quality assessment is a critical task in Intensive Care Units (ICUs). In the ICUs the patients are continuously monitored and the values are collected in real-time through data streaming processes. In the case of ventilation, the ventilator is monitoring the patient respiratory system and then a gateway receives the monitored values. This process can collect any values, noise values or values that can have clinical significance, for example, when a patient is having a critical event associated with the respiratory system. In this paper, the critical events concept was applied to the ventilation system, and a quality assessment of the collected data was performed when a new value arrived. Some interesting results were achieved: 56.59% of the events were critical, and 5% of the data collected were noise values. In this field, Average Ventilation Pressure and Peak flow are respectively the variables with the most influence.

DOI: 10.4018/978-1-7998-2451-0.ch007

Copyright © 2020, IGI Global. Copying or distributing in print or electronic forms without written permission of IGI Global is prohibited.

INTRODUCTION

Mechanical Ventilation is an artificial process of helping a patient to breathe. In an Intensive Care Unit (ICU), the patients are in a weak condition, and they need to be continuously monitored through bed-side monitors (vital signs and ventilation). The ventilators are an essential support for these patients as they suffer from organ failure. When the ventilator is connected to the hospital network, it is possible to obtain several patient results (e.g. Support Pressure, Compliance Dynamic (CDYN), Plateau Pressure, Positive End Expiratory Pressure (PEEP), Respiratory Rate and others). Transcription errors normally arise when the values are manually recorded. In the case of the values being automatically collected there is a set of problems that can be verified. The patient sensors can be wrongly placed and therefore being responsible for collecting noise values. To minimize this problem, a trigger was designed. This trigger assesses all the received values according to the values and rules defined by the ICU. The critical events rules are defined using the collected values. With this new concept, it is possible to know the value / variable significance. In this work, an analysis was made to attest the data quality and observe the number of Critical Events (CE). This study was part of the INTCare project, and it was conducted in the ICU of Centro Hospitalar do Porto, Hospital Santo António. For this work, a huge volume of data provided by the ventilator was analysed. All the information was collected from the ICU in real-time. In this study, it was possible to observe that 2% of the values collected were noise values and 50% represented a Critical Event. This study is a sequel of a study previously conducted where the Critical Events concept was applied to mechanically ventilated patients (Portela et al., 2016).

Finally, the paper is divided into six sections. After the introduction, the main concepts associated with this work are presented. Section 3 presents the data acquisition and data quality process and their architecture. Section 4 presents the data quality analysis and Section 5 the critical events analysis, and some conclusions are drawn.

BACKGROUND

Mechanical Ventilation

A patient needs to be connected to a ventilator when he cannot breathe. In this work, the mechanical ventilation (artificial) is used. Mechanical ventilation in Intensive Care Units is considered an essential, life-saving therapy for patients with critical illness and respiratory failures (Prevention, 2015). According to Evans (Evans et al., 2005), the ventilators were also developed to generate alarms when a patient becomes disconnected, or the ventilation values are critical. Despite these innovations, the ventilator is not capable of determining if a value is valid or not, i.e., if the patient presents a normal value or a noise value or how critical is the collected value. A valid analysis requires some human observations. However, the humans can only see the collected values, and it is tough to analyse several values in a few minutes. To minimize this problem a set of intelligent procedures, able to detect the data quality, can be defined. These procedures are usually based on the use of intelligent agents (Cardoso et al., 2014). In this field, a set of experiments was made to define and detect critical events in the respiratory system (Portela, Gago, Santos, Silva, & Rua, 2012; Portela, Gago, et al., 2013; Portela et al., 2016).

Intensive Medicine and Intensive Care Units

Intensive Medicine is a field of medicine where patients with critical illness and organ failure are treated. This area of medicine is applied in Intensive Care Units (ICUs). The ICUs has as main goal the treatment of a patient to recover him/her to the previous condition (Silva, Cortez, Santos, Gomes, & Neves, 2008). This type of patient needs continuing medical attention to avoid organ failure.

The respiratory diseases are one of the most common causes of ICU admission (Hoo, 2009). In the ICU, 75% of the patients need mechanical ventilation (Hoo, 2009). However, despite their benefits, these procedures might have some serious drawbacks, like contributing to the lung's injury.

Mechanical ventilation can have adverse effects, and its mortality rate ranges from 41% to 65% (Fauci, 2008). The number of reintubations varies from 2% to 25% (Tehrani, 2008). An automatic control of the mechanical ventilation can significantly improve the patient care in the ICUs, reduce the mortality and morbidity rates associated with the provision of inappropriate ventilator treatments and reduce healthcare costs.

Critical Events in Ventilation

In a previous work, the Critical Event concept (Portela, Gago, et al., 2012; Silva et al., 2008) was applied to mechanical ventilation patients (Portela et al., 2016). The critical event ranges were defined by analysing the literature and the use of expert knowledge provided by the intensivists (Intensive Medicine professionals). The critical event is defined when a value is out of the normal range for a pre-defined period of a specific variable. Table 1 presents a set of variables, and the values used to define critical events. The Min Normal and Max Normal column represents the normal values (range) possible in the ICU. The columns Min and Max value are used to validate the values, i.e., it is the minimum and maximum value that a ventilator can monitor. After a single value is considered as critical or not, the gateway will use the quality agent to, at the same time, assess if the value is valid or not. After the value is considered valid, the CE calculation process starts. The time (in minutes) is used to define an event as critical. The pre-processing agent is responsible for calculating the CE time. This agent will use the

Table 1. Ventilation critical events definition

Variable	ID	Units	Min Normal	Max Normal	Min Value	Max Value	Time (minutes)
Average Ventilation Pressure (AVP)	039	cmH2O	6	25	0	40	10
Compliance Dynamic (CDYN)	065	mL/ cmH2O	21	43	0	250	30
Flow	012	litters per minute	20	80	20	250	10
Peak Pressure	038	cmH2O	8	50	0	100	10
PEEP	015	cmH2O	5	15	0	20	10
Plateau Pressure	040	cmH2O	8	30	0	100	10
Respiratory Rate	010	breaths per minute	8	25	1	200	10
Support Pressure	026	cmH2O	6	26	1	100	10

range table (Table 1) to perform its tasks and decide if a set of values can represent or not a critical event. For example, in the case of Compliance Dynamic (CDYN an event is considered critical when a patient has a valid CDYN value (higher than 0 and lower than 250), and lower than 21 or upper than 43 for a period more than 30 minutes.

INTCare System

The INTCare system was designed to work in critical health units as the ICU. This system is a result of a research project with the same name. This system is composed of two platforms: monitoring and decision support (Portela, Santos, et al., 2014). The architecture is based on intelligent agents (Santos et al., 2011) which perform the main tasks automatically and in real-time. The INTCare system provides new insights during the decision process. It uses artificial intelligence techniques like Data Mining to predict clinical events. To achieve good results, it is essential to have quality datasets. It is also crucial to ensure the data quality in order to define procedures and design solutions which can monitor the data quality during the acquisition process. One of the cases is the respiratory system, where the data provided by the ventilator can have wrong values. In this field, INTCare can predict a plateau pressure value, barotrauma (Oliveira et al., 2015; Oliveira et al., 2015a, 2015b) and help the physicians to decide the best extubate time. This study contributes to understanding how many values are noise and what set of values can be considered a critical event (Portela, Gago, et al., 2012; Portela, Gago, et al., 2013). The use of critical incidents, based on data, improves the sensitivity of the data mining models (Portela, Pinto, & Santos, 2012; Portela, Oliveira, Santos, Abelha, Machado, Silva & Rua, 2014; Braga, Portela, & Santos, 2014; Portela, Santos, Machado, Abelha, & Silva, 2013) while the system provides a continuous assessment process (Aguiar et al., 2013; Portela, Aguiar, Santos, Silva, & Rua, 2013; Portela, Aguiar, et al., 2014; Portela, Santos, Silva, et al., 2013).

DATA ACQUISITION AND DATA QUALITY PROCESS

Data Acquisition Process

The acquisition process uses data streaming to collect the data from the ventilator. An architecture based on intelligent agents (Figure 1) was developed to support the acquisition process. The use of intelligent agents allows automatizing the tasks (Cardoso et al., 2014; Marins et al., 2014). In this architecture, the gateway receives the entire patient data (ventilation) monitored in real-time (a continuous process started by the ventilator). Then the gateway creates an HL7 message (Hooda, Dogdu, & Sunderraman, 2004) and sends it to the Ventilation Acquisition Agent (VAA). The VAA is responsible for analysing the message and store the message in the database. During the process, the patient identification (PID) is validated by the agent. This task ensures a correct patient identification, i.e., the values received are from the patient bed. After the data (HL7_DATA) are stored, a pre-processing agent is activated. This agent assesses all the values received to guarantee the data quality.

Figure 1. Data acquisition architecture

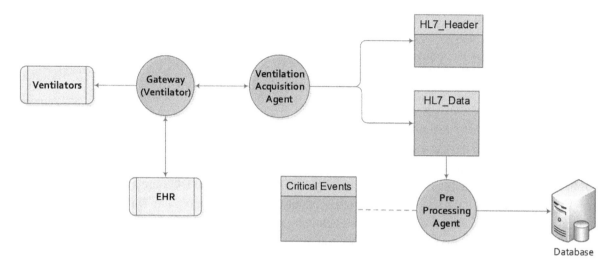

Data Quality Process

After the data collection, a data quality analysis was made. The first analysis had in consideration all the collected values. The second analysis considered only the critical values. In both analyses, it is important to note that, in the case of the time variable, some of the values were not considered. That happened when a patient was discharged and during this process, the ventilator was not disconnected. This process sends the wrong result about the event time because the gateway continued to receive values even if a patient had not been admitted. The process started when a new value arrived. For each value, the pre-processing agent will execute quality tasks with the goal to assess the results. The agent will consult the range values for each variable (Table 1), and it will fill two columns. The first column presents valid (1) or not (0) values; the second column presents critical (1) or not (0) values. It is also possible to know the number of data correctly collected and which values represent critical events using these two columns,

The analysis made in this study had in consideration the data collected from January 1 to June 30, 2015. These data come from 67 ventilated patients.

DATA QUALITY ANALYSIS

In the analysis process, two more variables were considered in addition to the critical events variables. Tidal volume setting in liters (011) and Exhaled tidal volume in liters (035) were the new variables considered.

Table 2 presents the number of values collected (total) and how many values are normal (i.e., values that did not require patient observation, out of range (out) and critical (Max and Min). In this table, it is also possible to observe the total number of occurrences by each variable and their percentage. In the Case of CDYN, 146580 records were collected. From this dataset, all the values were considered normal (they can be collected). However, 47621 of the values present a higher value and 22603 a lower value.

Table 2. Data quality analysis

Variables	ID	Total	Normal	Out	Max	Min
Dynamic compliance (CDYN) in mL/cmH2O*	065	146589	76365	0	47621	22603
End inspiratory pressure in cmH2O	040	150522	139585	1041	8218	1678
Exhaled tidal volume in litters	035	150565	0	17	0	150548
Maximum circuit pressure in cmH2O	038	150508	146158	119	3964	267
Mean airway pressure in cmH2O	039	150540	149273	47	56	1164
O2% setting	013	150764	150764	0		0
Peak flow setting in litters per minute	012	150781	114474	35456	851	0
PEEP or PEEP Low (in BILEVEL) setting in cmH2O	015	150733	125339	0	1	25393
Pressure support setting in cmH2O	026	150679	43925	106136	567	51
Respiratory rate setting in breaths per minute	010	150820	109392	39077	2333	18
Tidal volume setting in litters	011	150805				150805
Total		1653306	1055275	181893	63611	352527
% of Total		100%	64%	11%	4%	21%

In both cases, they represent critical events. For example, in the case of O2% all the values are normal. The ratios of values are presented in Figure 2.

Figure 2 presents the maximum and minimum value collected for each variable and the percentage of cases for each value type (normal, out of range minimum and out of range maximum). The chart presented in Figure 2 uses the values of the columns Min Value and Max Value defined in Table 1. For example, in the case of PEEP (015) the values collected range from 0 and 20. In this case, all the values belong to the normal range.

Figure 2. Data analysis distribution

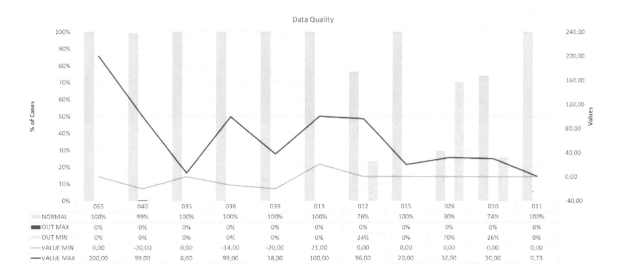

After thE analysis, the values' duration and if the critical values can represent a critical event were studied. In the critical events column, there is the number of events categorized as 1 (critical).

CRITICAL EVENTS ANALYSIS

In Figure 3, it is possible to observe the events distribution: Normal (0), Critical (1) or severe (2). A critical event arises when a patient has an abnormal value that can be considered critical. It is important to note that the regular events (values between the normal ranges) are identified as Ev_Type – 0.

For example, analysing variable 026 – support pressure, it is possible to observe that 53.06% of the events are normal, 17.35% of the events are critical, and the remaining (16.67%) are severe. For this variable, it is also possible to see the average time of each event by the patient. In the case of the normal events, the average duration is 73864 seconds. A critical event normally has a length of 71018.76 seconds and a severe value in average has duration of 107595 seconds. These values mean that, in average, when a patient starts an event, independent of their type, he/she will be in the same incident for an extended period. The variable which presents more common events is Tidal volume. On the opposite side, it is the Average Ventilation Pressure (AVP). Regarding the critical events, the most important variable is PEEP. Patients showed the worst values in the AVP variable. This type of analysis can be done for each one of the eleven variables presented in this study.

Figure 3. Critical Events analysis distribution

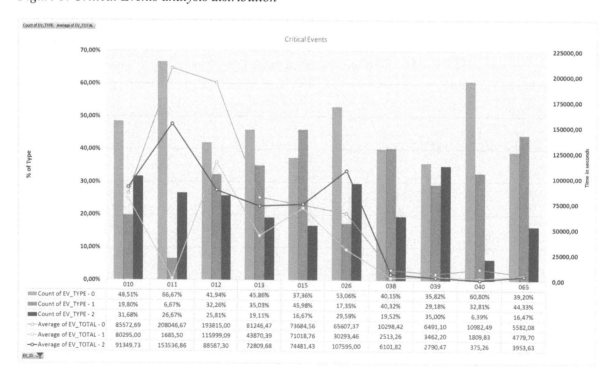

	010	011	012	013	015	026	038	039	040	065
Count of EV_TYPE - 0	48,51%	66,67%	41,94%	45,86%	37,36%	53,06%	40,15%	35,82%	60,80%	39,20%
Count of EV_TYPE - 1	19,80%	6,67%	32,26%	35,03%	45,98%	17,35%	40,32%	29,18%	32,81%	44,33%
Count of EV_TYPE - 2	31,68%	26,67%	25,81%	19,11%	16,67%	29,59%	19,52%	35,00%	6,39%	16,47%
Average of EV_TOTAL - 0	85572,69	208046,67	193815,00	81246,47	73684,56	65607,37	10298,42	6491,10	10982,49	5582,08
Average of EV_TOTAL - 1	80295,00	1685,50	115999,09	43870,39	71018,76	30293,46	2513,26	3462,20	1809,83	4779,70
Average of EV_TOTAL - 2	91349,73	153536,86	88587,30	72809,68	74481,43	107595,00	6101,82	2790,47	375,26	3953,63

CONCLUSION

The work was based on a data analysis study. In this study, a set of values collected from the ventilation system of an Intensive Care Unit was analysed. The Critical Event concept was adopted to understand the significance of the values better. This study only represents one of the analyses.

The work helps the intensivists to look at certain variables in a different way. The values which presented most values out of the normal range or variables where there is the probability of a patient to have a critical event should be closely monitored. At the same time, the analysis can help the research team to improve their work. This type of analysis also can be done by using, for example, the results collected from the patient tracking system (Oliveira, Portela, Santos, Abelha & Machado, 2015).

After the data analysis, this work can provide the community an overview of ICU reality. The variables most propitious to collecting noise values and the variables which can represent critical events can be identified. As a result, the intensivist can look at this work as an advisor, and they should take into account the identified variables. Finally, this work does not exclude any clinical analysis; it only provides new information to help the patient monitoring and decision process.

ACKNOWLEDGMENT

This work has been supported by FCT - Fundação para a Ciência e Tecnologia within the Project Scope UID/CEC/00319/2013. The authors would like to thank FCT (Foundation for Science and Technology, Portugal) for the financial support through the contract PTDC/EEI-SII/1302/2012 (INTCare II).

REFERENCES

Aguiar, J., Portela, F., Santos, M. F., Machado, J., Abelha, A., Silva, A., & ... . (2013). Pervasive Information Systems to Intensive Care Medicine Technology Acceptance Model. *Proceedings of the 15th International Conference on Enterprise Information Systems* (Vol 1, pp. 177-184).

Braga, P. Portela, F., & Santos, M. F. (2014). Data Mining Models to Predict Patient's Readmission in Intensive Care Units. *Paper presented at the ICAART - International Conference on Agents and Artificial Intelligence*, Angers, France.

Cardoso, L., Marins, F., Portela, F., Santos, M., Abelha, A., & Machado, J. (2014). The Next Generation of Interoperability Agents in Healthcare. *International Journal of Environmental Research and Public Health*, *11*(5), 5349–5371. doi:10.3390/ijerph110505349 PMID:24840351

CDC. (2015). *Ventilator-Associated Event (VAE)*. Retrieved from http://www.cdc.gov/nhsn/PDFs/vae/Draft-Ventilator-Associate-Event-Protocol_v6.pdf

Evans, R. S., Johnson, K. V., Flint, V. B., Kinder, T., Lyon, C. R., Hawley, W. L., ... Thomsen, G. E. (2005). Enhanced notification of critical ventilator events. *Journal of the American Medical Informatics Association*, *12*(6), 589–595. doi:10.1197/jamia.M1863 PMID:16049226

Fauci, A. S. (2008). Harrison's Principles of Internal Medicine. Silverchair Science: Minion.

Hoo, G. W. S. (2009). *Barotrauma and Mechanical Ventilation* (p. 24). Medscape.

Hooda, J. S., Dogdu, E., & Sunderraman, R. (2004). Health Level-7 compliant clinical patient records system.

Marins, F., Cardoso, L., Portela, F., Santos, M. F., Abelha, A., & Machado, J. (2014). Improving High Availability and Reliability of Health Interoperability Systems. In *New Perspectives in Information Systems and Technologies* (Vol. 2, pp. 207–216). Springer. doi:10.1007/978-3-319-05948-8_20

Oliveira, S., Portela, F., Santos, M. F., Machado, J., Abelha, A., Silva, Á., & ... . (2015). Predicting Plateau Pressure in Intensive Medicine for Ventilated Patients. In *New Contributions in Information Systems and Technologies* (pp. 179–188). Springer. doi:10.1007/978-3-319-16528-8_17

Portela, F., Pinto, F., & Santos, M.F. (2012). Data mining predictive models for pervasive intelligent decision support in intensive care medicine. *Proceedings of the international Conference on Knowledge Management and Information Sharing KMIS*, Barcelona.

Portela, F., Aguiar, J., Santos, M. F., Abelha, A., Machado, J., Silva, Á., & Rua, F. (2014). Assessment of Technology Acceptance in Intensive Care Units. *International Journal of Systems and Service-Oriented Engineering*, *4*(3), 26–45. doi:10.4018/ijssoe.2014070102

Portela, F., Aguiar, J., Santos, M. F., Silva, Á., & Rua, F. (2013). Pervasive Intelligent Decision Support System - Technology Acceptance in Intensive Care Units. In Advances in Intelligent Systems and Computing. Springer.

Portela, F., Gago, P., Santos, M. F., Machado, J., Abelha, A., Silva, Á., et al. (2013). Pervasive real-time intelligent system for tracking critical events in intensive care patients.

Portela, F., Gago, P., Santos, M. F., & Silva, Á., & Rua, F. (2012). Intelligent and Real Time Data Acquisition and Evaluation to Determine Critical Events in Intensive Medicine. *Paper presented at the International Conference on Health and Social Care Information Systems and Technologies HCist'12*, Portugal. 10.1016/j.protcy.2012.09.079

Portela, F., Santos, M. F., Machado, J., Abelha, A., & Silva, Á. (2013). Pervasive and Intelligent Decision Support in Critical Health Care Using Ensembles. In *Information Technology in Bio-and Medical Informatics* (pp. 1–16). Berlin Heidelberg: Springer . doi:10.1007/978-3-642-40093-3_1

Portela, F., Santos, M. F., Machado, J., Abelha, A., Silva, Á., & Rua, F. (2014). Pervasive and intelligent decision support in Intensive Medicine–the complete picture. In *Information Technology in Bio-and Medical Informatics* (pp. 87–102). Springer. doi:10.1007/978-3-319-10265-8_9

Portela, F., Santos, M. F., Machado, J., Abelha, A., Silva, Á., & Rua, F. (2016). Critical Events in Mechanically Ventilated Patients. In *New Advances in Information Systems and Technologies* (pp. 589–598). Springer International Publishing. doi:10.1007/978-3-319-31307-8_61

Portela, F., Santos, M. F., Silva, Á., Rua, F., Abelha, A., & Machado, J. (2013). Adoption of Pervasive Intelligent Information Systems in Intensive Medicine. *Procedia Technology*, *9*, 1022–1032. doi:10.1016/j.protcy.2013.12.114

Portela, F., Oliveira, S., Santos, M., Machado, J., & Abelha, A. (2015). A Real-Time Intelligent System for tracking patient condition. In Ambient Intelligence for Health, LNCS (Vol. 9456).

Portela, F., Veloso, R., Santos, M. F., Machado, J. M., Abelha, A., Silva, Á., ... & Oliveira, S. M. C. (2014). Predict hourly patient discharge probability in Intensive Care Units using Data Mining. *ScienceAsia Journal.*

Santos, M. F., Portela, F., Vilas-Boas, M., Machado, J., Abelha, A., & Neves, J. (2011). INTCARE - Multi-agent approach for real-time Intelligent Decision Support in Intensive Medicine. *Paper presented at the 3rd International Conference on Agents and Artificial Intelligence (ICAART)*, Rome, Italy.

Sérgio Oliveira, F. P. Manuel Filipe Santos, José Machado, António Abelha, Álvaro Silva and Fernando Rua. (2015a). Characterizing Barotrauma Patients in ICU - Clustering Data Mining using ventilator variables.

Sérgio Oliveira, F. P. Manuel Filipe Santos, José Machado, António Abelha, Álvaro Silva and Fernando Rua. (2015b). Intelligent Decision Support to predict patient Barotrauma risk in Intensive Care Units. In Procedia Technology Healthy and Secure People HCIST 2015. Elsevier.

Silva, Á., Cortez, P., Santos, M. F., Gomes, L., & Neves, J. (2008). Rating organ failure via adverse events using data mining in the intensive care unit. *Artificial Intelligence in Medicine, 43*(3), 179–193. doi:10.1016/j.artmed.2008.03.010 PMID:18486459

Tehrani, F. T. (2008). Automatic control of mechanical ventilation. Part 2: The existing techniques and future trends. *Journal of Clinical Monitoring and Computing, 22*(6), 417–424. doi:10.100710877-008-9151-y PMID:19020981

This research was previously published in the International Journal of Reliable and Quality E-Healthcare (IJRQEH), 6(2); edited by Anastasius Moumtzoglou; pages 40-48, copyright year 2017 by IGI Publishing (an imprint of IGI Global).

Chapter 8

An Online Neonatal Intensive-Care Unit Monitoring System for Hospitals in Nigeria

Peter Adebayo Idowu
Obafemi Awolowo University, Nigeria

Franklin Oladiipo Asahiah
Obafemi Awolowo University, Nigeria

Jeremiah Ademola Balogun
Obafemi Awolowo University, Nigeria

Olayinka Olufunmilayo Olusanya
Tai Solarin University of Education, Nigeria

ABSTRACT

This paper presents an online monitoring system for the storage and retrieval of physiological data from neonates admitted into the Neonatal intensive care units (NICU) of Obafemi Awolowo University Teaching Hospital, Ile-Ife, Nigeria. In order to develop this system, the requirements of the proposed system were identified and analyzed as system and user requirements independently and the requirements were designed using the Unified Modeling Language (UML) tools. The system was implemented using Web 2.0 technologies such as, the hypertext markup language (HTML), the cascading styling sheets (CSS), PHP and MySQL. With the system, storage and retrieval of information by the nurses and any authorized users will be easy.

INTRODUCTION

A neonatal intensive care unit (NICU), also known as an intensive care nursery (ICN), is an intensive care unit specializing in the care of ill or premature newborn infants. The first newborn intensive care unit located in the United States was designed by Louis Gluck in October 1960 at Yale–New Haven Hospital

DOI: 10.4018/978-1-7998-2451-0.ch008

Copyright © 2020, IGI Global. Copying or distributing in print or electronic forms without written permission of IGI Global is prohibited.

in New Haven, Connecticut (Gluck, 1985). A NICU is typically directed by one or more neonatologists and staffed by nurses, nurse practitioners, pharmacists, physician assistants, resident physicians, respiratory therapists, and dietitians (Whittfield et al., 2004). Many other ancillary disciplines and specialists are available at larger units. The term neonatal comes from neo, new, and natal, pertaining to birth or origin (Harper, 2010). Neonatal nurse practitioners are advanced practice nurses that care for premature babies and sick newborns in intensive care units, emergency rooms, delivery rooms and special clinics. Prematurity is a risk factor that follows early labour, a planned caesarean section or pre-eclampsia—a condition in pregnancy regarding high blood pressure.

Continuous health monitoring for neonates provides crucial parameters such as cessation of breathing, heart rhythm disturbances and drop in blood oxygen saturation etc. More than 50% premature infants show deficits in their further developments such as developmental delay, speech and language delay, behavioral, attention and learning problems. Medical conditions including chronic lung disease, apnea and bradycardia, transient thyroid dysfunction, jaundice and nutritional deficiencies are potential contributing factors (Perlman, 2001; Perlman, 2003).

Newborn babies who need intensive medical attention are often admitted into the NICU. The NICU combines advanced technology and trained healthcare professionals to provide specialized care for the tiniest patients. NICUs may also have intermediate or continuing care areas for babies who are not as sick, but do need specialized nursing care. About 10% of all newborn babies require care in a NICU. Vital parameters of clinical relevance for neonatal monitoring include body temperature, electrocardiogram (ECG), respiration, and blood oxygen saturation (Polin and Fox, 1992). Body temperature is monitored with adhesive thermistors; ECG and respiration are obtained by adhesive skin electrodes. The oxygen saturation of the blood is monitored by a pulse oximeter with the sensor applied on the foot or palm of the neonate.

Continuous health monitoring is crucial for the survival of the ill and fragile infants admitted at NICUs through the collection and identification of vital signs information. The process of monitoring and collecting information from the medical sensors attached to infants placed at NICUs by nurses at times may prove very challenging with additional problems associated with keeping constant and up-to-date information of the state of infants monitored at any time from remote locations by doctors.

There is presently no system available to make information monitored by nurses during regular wards rounds at NICU stored and accessible by other medical practitioner assigned to the NICU at any time ad from any remote location using the Internet. There is the need for the development of a web-based monitoring system capable of storing and making infants vital signs recorded at the NICU available to other medical staffs as and when due. This paper presents a web-based monitoring system for the storage and retrieval of vital signs information captured from neonates admitted into the NICU and made available to other authorized medical personnel.

Related Work

A number of published works exists which are focused on the development of monitoring systems for neonatal monitoring systems alongside other health-related monitoring systems. Following are a number of related works considered in the review of literature.

Joshi et al. (2013), developed a wireless monitoring embedded system for neonatal monitoring system for NICU. This system provided that same environment as that of the baby's mother does. The system deploys a set of suitable sensors for the system development. The analogue signals from the sensors are processed using a peripheral interface controller (PIC) microcontroller and further transmitted towards the receiving end with the help of Global system for mobile communications (GSM) using application terminal (AT) commands.

Suresh et al. (2014), developed a neonatal monitoring system using a combination of hardware components for measuring and monitoring various vital signs on neonates attended to in NICUs. The prototype system developed could monitor various vital signs such as: electrocardiogram (ECG), blood oxygen saturation, body temperature etc. using various sensors and hardware devices connected to various parts of the baby. The system made use of three (3) electrodes placed on the baby's chest to monitor the baby's ECG and the respiratory monitoring. The challenges encountered with this system is with the sensors placed on the baby's body which cause the baby further discomfort and lack of sleep hindering the baby's development.

Zhuhia et al. (2015), focused on the development and fusion of wearable sensing technologies, wireless communication techniques and a low energy-consumption microprocessor with high performance data processing algorithms. As a clinical tool applied in the constant monitoring of physiological parameters of infants, wearable sensor systems for infants are able to transmit the information obtained inside an infant's body to clinicians or parents. Future work is aimed at performing extensive and complex analysis of the variables monitored using the wearable devices.

METHODS

In order to develop the neonatal monitoring system, the system development life cycle of software development approach was applied to the development of the proposed information system for monitoring the vital signs of neonates. Figure 1 shows the conceptual diagram of the process used in this study for the development of the monitoring system and shows the different stages of the methodology process.

The development of the neonatal monitoring system began with the identification of the problem associated with the existing system following which the review of related works was performed in order to identify the body of knowledge surrounding the development of monitoring system for the vital signs of neonates at the ICUs. Following this process, the user requirements of the proposed system was evaluated using structured interview and observation methods to gather necessary information from staffs of the hospital (OAUTHC) while the system requirements were also identified based on the security requirements and structure of the hospital's organization.

The design process of the system was achieved using the object-oriented analysis and design methodology thus, use-case was used to design the user requirements while the system requirements design were defined using the class and sequence diagrams. The data model of the database was also achieved using the object-oriented design which was used to define the structure of the database using the contextual, conceptual and logical views of the data model.

Web 2.0 technologies, namely: hypertext markup language (HTML), PHP and cascading styling sheets (CSS) were used to implement the web layout of the information system of the proposed monitoring system while the structured query language (SQL) was used to implement the data model design proposed for the system. Finally, the implemented system was tested for functionality and user-friendliness by the proposed users of the system.

Figure 1. Conceptual diagram of development process of monitoring system

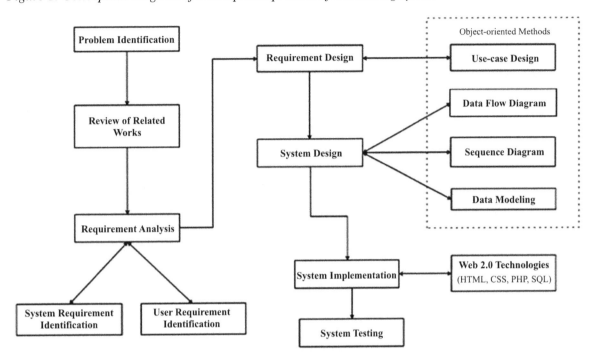

Problem Identification

This study is focused at the development of an information system for monitoring the vital signs of neonates that are put in the ICU of OAUTHC, Ile-Ife. The existing system uses a paper-based system for recording and storing the readings of vital signs of neonates using the machines attached to them whenever they are placed in the ICU for monitoring.

New-born babies who need intensive medical attention are often admitted into the NICU of the Obafemi Awolowo University Teaching Hospital (OAUTHC), Ile-Ife, Nigeria located in south-western Nigeria. Most of these babies are premature (born before 37 weeks of pregnancy), have low birth-weight (less than 2.5kg) or have a medical condition that requires special care also, twins/triplets and other multiples are often admitted as they tend to be born earlier and smaller than single babies alongside babies with certain medical conditions such as heart problems, infections or birth defects. Vitals signs monitored in babies include their respiration rate, heart rate, oxygen saturation levels, baby's skin and bones, body heat etc.

Most of the times these babies are monitored using special types of machines connected to them while they are placed in their respective beds using sensors connected to special parts of their body where the necessary information is required. The challenge has been able to consistently monitor the baby's vital sign in real time and from remote locations. Also, historical records of the vital signs of the babies are very difficult to track unless such files are collected from the shelves and the process of extracting such information is usually a tedious and hectic activity. Also, another challenge is for nurses to consistently monitor the vital signs of babies remotely even when they have to attend to an emergency especially if the sensors attached to the babies are turned off or are not attached to the baby properly or whenever the vital sign monitored shows unpleasant readings.

The proposed system is expected to solve the problem of real-time monitoring of the vital signs of the babies from remote locations especially by doctors who are not in the confines of the hospitals but need to know the state of babies located in the NICU. For this reason, a web-based information system was proposed which could be used by nurses and doctors alike to monitor the vital signs read from babies using sensors which can also be accessed by registered nurses and doctors alike remotely via access to the Internet.

The summary of the limitations of the existing system are as follows:

- Difficulty accessing neonatal vital signs from remote access by doctors
- Difficulty tracking neonatal vital signs by nurses
- Difficulty in storage and retrieval of neonatal vital signs by nurses and doctors
- Difficulty identifying and allocating space to newly admitted neonates by nurses

After the identification of these limitations facing the existing systems, the following paragraphs focus on the requirements of the proposed neonatal monitoring system for the intensive care unit (ICU).

Requirement Analysis of Neonatal Monitoring System

In software engineering, requirement analysis encompasses those tasks that go into determining the needs or conditions to meet for a new or altered product or project, taking into account of the possibly conflicting requirements of the various stakeholders, analyzing, documenting, validating and managing software requirements. It was very critical to the success or failure of the proposed system. It composed of three (3) important aspects, namely:

- Eliciting requirements – via business process documentation or in the case of this study with the use of interview
- Analyzing requirements – resolving any apparent conflicts
- Recording requirements – achieved using use-case diagrams as in this study

Non-Functional Requirements of Neonatal Monitoring System

In systems engineering and requirements engineering, a non-functional requirement is a requirement that specifies criteria that can be used to judge the operation of a system, rather than specific behaviors. They are contrasted with functional requirements that define specific behavior or functions. The plan for implementing functional requirements is detailed in the system design. Broadly, functional requirements define what a system is supposed to do and non-functional requirements define how a system is supposed to be. For the purpose of the development of the development of the neonatal monitoring system, the non-functional requirements are as follow:

- The system shall be able to recognize all required data that are needed in the management of the neonatal monitoring system required for performing the necessary activities by each respective users of the system
- The system shall be able to recognize all personal information with respect to each individual's part played in the system alongside the respective activities/process to be performed with such data

- The system shall provide a timely response to any request by users
- The system shall be able to restrict unauthorized access to personal information with the use of usernames and passwords for authorized users
- The system shall make information requested by users available as when due
- The system shall be able to provide security protection to passwords so as to protect users' access in the case of database intrusion attacks using encryption methods

Following the identification of the non-functional requirements of the proposed system, the next paragraph is focused at looking into the functional requirements of the system.

Functional Requirements of Neonatal Monitoring System

In Software engineering and systems engineering, a functional requirement defines a function of a system or its component. A function is described as a set of inputs, the behavior, and outputs. Functional requirements may be calculations, technical details, data manipulation and processing and other specific functionality that define what a system is supposed to accomplish. Following are the functional requirements of the system:

- The system must allow new users (doctors and nurses) to be created by the system administrator;
- The system must require new users to log into the system before being able to perform any necessary activities needed to be performed
- The system must allow nurses to create profiles for newly admitted neonates
- The system must allow information about vital signs of each neonates stored by nurses to be stored and accessible to doctors and nurses alike
- The system must allow doctors or nurses alike to query the system for the vital signs' information of neonates stored in the system

Part of the functional requirements to be understood are the behavioural and structural requirements of the system which were analyzed and designed using the use-case, data flow and sequence diagrams.

User Requirement Analysis of Neonatal Monitoring System

The user requirements define the basic actors (user objects) of the proposed monitoring system alongside their respective functions. It also defines the interaction that exists among the system users and their respective functions. Following is a list of the actors alongside their specific functions after which use case scenarios and use case diagrams were used to model the requirement's design process.

A. System Administrator

The system administrator is the super-user of the proposed system; the administrator is responsible for creating the profiles of any authorized user of the system (doctors/nurses). The system administrator provides default username and passwords to respective health officer, namely: hospital administrative officer, nurse and doctors;

B. Nurses

The nurses use the username and passwords provided to them by the administrator to register their personal information into the system, namely: first name, last name, address and gender following which the system generates an identification number after confirming details. The nurses are responsible for registering the newly admitted neonates and also updating the neonates' vital signs as the nurses perform their ward-rounds in the neonates' ICU. The neonate's information provided at the point of registration include: names (in full), registration number, blood group, gender, age, packed cell volume (PCV), temperature, respiration rate, heart rate and random blood sugar.

C. Doctors

The doctors also use the username and passwords provided to them by the administrator to register their personal information into the system, namely: first name, last name, address and gender following which the system generates an identification number after confirming details. The doctors can only search for a neonate and view the vital signs for the interested neonates. There are two (2) criteria proposed for retrieving neonates, namely: by name and by registration number – which follows the format NEO/ "year of entry"/number.

System Design of Neonatal Monitoring System

Following the full investigation of the problem with the existing system there is a need for a solution proposed to the problems identified in line with the functional and non-functional requirements of the proposed monitoring system. The design of the proposed system emphasizes a conceptual solution that fulfills the specified requirements, rather than its implementation which will follow afterwards. It is also the process of separating data descriptions from procedures and thus models them separately.

The purpose of the method of object-oriented (OO) design was to define the classes (alongside their relationships) which were needed for meeting the specified requirements contained in the systems requirements specification mentioned earlier. The Unified Modeling Language (UML) is, at its most fundamental, an information systems modeling language. The most common use of UML is in the analysis and design of software solutions/applications; in short, it is the collection of conceptual tools with which the design of a system is done. The major goals of using the UML include the following:

- Identifying key usage scenarios for the system (from the perspective of different users)
- Describing the interactions between users and system in the execution of usage scenarios
- Assigning responsibilities for the outcomes to the most appropriate objects in the system

Use Case Modeling of Neonatal Monitoring System's Requirements

Use-Case diagrams are a requirements discovery technique first introduced in the Objectory method. In its simplest form, a use-case identifies the actors (users) involved in an interaction and the names and the types of the interactions involved. These use case scenarios were used to present the system requirements of the proposed neonatal monitoring system with the use-case diagrams giving a graphical representation of those requirements. Using the scenarios afforded the opportunity to obtain the realistic description of the flow of information and processes of the system giving an explicit description of the actions of each user.

For the purpose of this study, the use-case was used to model the user requirements of three (3) actors – administrator, doctor and the nurse alongside their basic functions and how they interact with each other. The use-case model uses a *"stick-man"* to represent an actor, *"arrows"* to represent inheritance among actors, *"ovals"* to define use-cases (actions) and the *"edges"* between ovals to represent relationships.

Table 1. Data Insertion Use Case Scenario Table

Use Case Name	Data Insertion
Description	Scenario to illustrate the data insertion requirements of the neonatal monitoring system
Actors	Administrator, Doctor and Nurse
Scenarios	1. Administrator creates username and password for new users – doctors and nurses 2. Doctors/Nurses alike must update the personal profile information following login using the username and passwords provided by administrator 3. Nurses register new neonates by providing personal information and vital sign information 4. Nurses update the vital signs' information of neonates following regular word-rounds

Figure 2. Use case for data insertion requirements

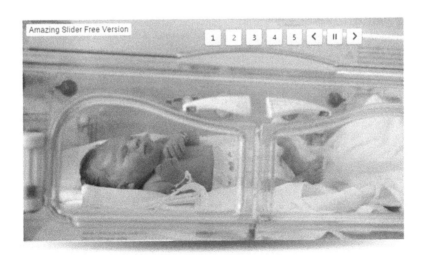

Table 1 shows a representation of the data insertion use-case scenario describing the user requirements for each user of the neonatal monitoring system's data insertion (Figure 2). In the data insertion table, the following are permitted:

- Administrators can create usernames and passwords for authorized intending users of the proposed system
- Primary users (the doctors and nurses) can update their personal profiles by providing personal information
- Nurses can register a neonate
- Nurses can also update the vital signs' information for a specified neonate

Table 2 shows a representation of the data query use-case scenario describing the requirements for each user of the proposed system (Figure 3). In the data query table, the following are permitted:

- Doctors can query the vital signs' information of any neonate by name; and
- Doctors can query the vital signs' information of any neonate by hospital number.

Table 2. Data Query Use Case Scenario Table

Use Case Name	Data Query
Description	Scenario to illustrate the data query requirements of the neonatal monitoring system
Actors	Doctor and Nurse
Scenarios	1. System checks for user identification provided by administrator for login details: • If user is valid then system displays menu for actions to be performed; else • If user is invalid then the system rejects the user's access. 2. Doctor/Nurse can retrieve neonate by using the name or the hospital number 3. Doctor/Nurse can view the vital signs' information of interested neonates.

Figure 3. Use case for data query requirements

DEVELOPMENT OF A NEONATAL MONITORING SYSTEM FOR INTENSIVE CARE UNIT (ICU)

PATIENT REGISTRATION DETAILS
First Name
Last Name
Home Adddress
SELECT GENDER ▾
Age In Weeks
telephone number
Registration Number

REGISTER

OR REGISTER NEW USER

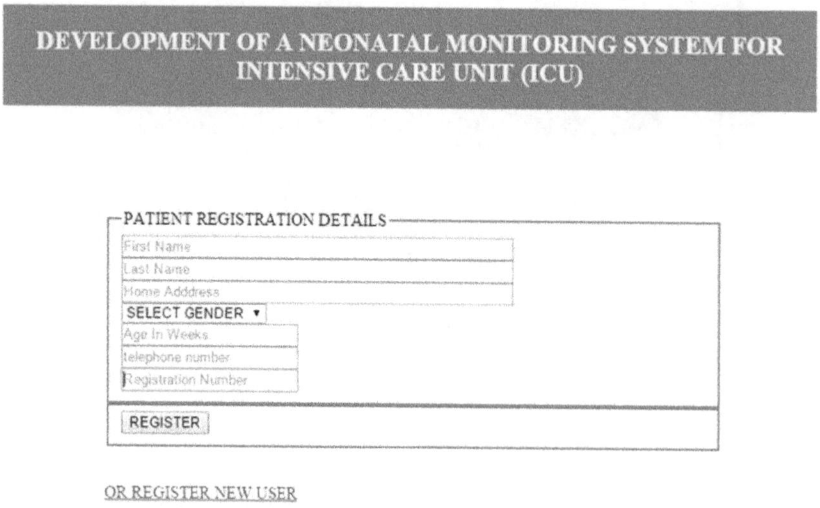

Data Flow Diagram (DFD) of Neonatal Monitoring System

Data flow diagram (DFD) is a graphical representation of the flow of data through an information system like the proposed system in this study with the aim of modeling its process aspects. It is a way of giving a description of the structural requirements of the system. This is a preliminary step to create an overview of the system by showing the kind of information that will be input to and output from the system, where the data will come from and go to, and to where the data will be stored. A DFD can't give information about the timing of process or information about whether processes will operate in sequence or in parallel. They are generally used as technical descriptors for the following reasons:

- DFDs are easier to understand by technical and non-technical audiences;
- DFDs can provide a high-level system overview, complete with boundaries and connections to other systems; and
- DFDs can provide a detailed representation of system components.

Figure 4 shows a description of the flow of data within the proposed system which starts form the creation of usernames and passwords for the primary user by the administrator following which, the primary users can then update their personal information using the username and passwords provided. The nurses can also register new neonates and also update the database after regular ward rounds at the intensive care unit (ICU) with information about the vital signs of neonates recorded. The doctors/nurses can search for neonates in order to view the vital signs' information of neonates as required.

Figure 4. Data flow diagram of neonatal monitoring system

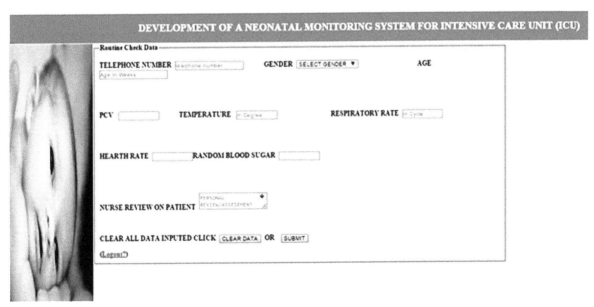

Sequence Diagram of Neonatal Monitoring System

Sequence diagram was used in this study to represent the interaction between objects and how they operate with one another and in what order. It can also be referred to as a construct of a Message Sequence Chart. A sequence diagram shows object interactions arranged in time sequence. It depicts the objects and classes involved in the scenario and the sequence of messages exchanged between the objects needed to carry out the functionality of the scenario. Sequence diagrams are typically associated with use case realizations in the Logical View of the system under development. Sequence diagrams are sometimes called event diagrams or event scenarios.

Figure 5 shows the sequence diagram that describes the sequence of actions that are required for the process of registering a newly admitted neonatal into the intensive care unit by nurse following the process of querying the database for the vital signs' information of an existing neonate. The sequence diagrams shows the user (nurse) logging into the system using the username and password provided by the administrator at the point of pre-registration after which the user can then access his/her user profile screen. From the user's profile, the user can then register a newly admitted neonate by providing the personal information of the neonate which includes the name of the neonate, the registration number of the neonate, the sex of the neonate, the blood group of the neonate followed by the age of the neonate.

Figure 5. Sequence diagram of neonatal monitoring system

DEVELOPMENT OF A NEONATAL MONITORING SYSTEM FOR INTENSIVE CARE UNIT (ICU)

Patient with Low PCV

Patient with High or Low Temperature

Patient with High or Low Respiratory Rate

Patient with High or Low Hearth Rate

Patient with High or Low Random Blood Sugar

Search Category: [Select category ▼]

Criteria to search: [criteria to search]

[submit]

Search Using Hospital Number [E.g. NEO/2016/Hospitan N]

[submit]

(Logout?)

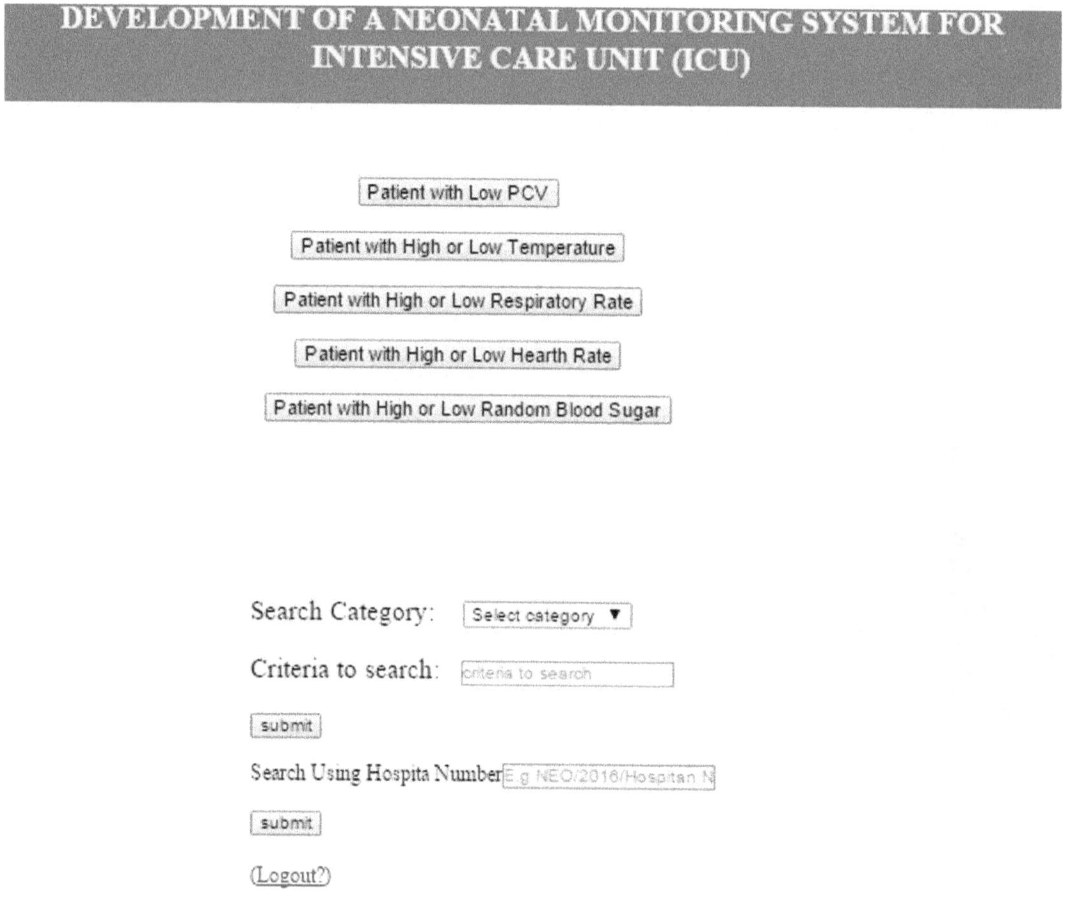

Following this, the vital signs' information at the first ward round visit is provided which consists of the packed cell volume (PCV), temperature, respiration rate, heart rate and random blood sugar. Information regarding any neonate stored in the database could be retrieved using the hospital number or name of the neonate in order to monitor the values of the vital signs stored by the monitoring system.

Data Modeling of Neonatal Monitoring System's Database

Data modeling is an important aspect of database design. It is not only the first step in database design; it is also used for many other purposes. This ranges from high level conceptual data models to physical data models. It allows the database designers to be able to visualize how each data item is related and how the designers will be able to represent, visualize and present data. It is the analysis of data objects that are used to identify the relationships within data objects. The process of a data model is an attempt to capture the essence of things both concretely and abstractedly in the problem domain.

In literature, there are three stages involved in developing a data model. These stages include: The conceptual data model, the logical data model and the physical data model stages. But this study included a fourth stage in its model development; the purpose was to have a more reliable, flexible, complete, usable and efficient data model for any system (Idowu and Adagunodo, 2010); which is called the contextual data model. The physical data model on the other hand, is the implementation of the data model as the database of the neonatal monitoring system.

The first stage of the development of the data model is to design the contextual data model which is needed to clearly state the users and organization's requirements. The subject area in this case, which is known as a package or the core component of a data model, is a way of grouping related classes into

Figure 6. Contextual data model of neonatal monitoring system

DEVELOPMENT OF A NEONATAL MONITORING SYSTEM FOR INTENSIVE CARE UNIT (ICU)

Telephone	PCV	Nurse Review	Firstname	Address
0803884	44	the patient is doing very fine	segun	villa
0147	56	lekan file	okmola	ohrm
0147	54	very good patient	okmola	ohrm
0147	54	very good patient	okmola	ohrm
	0			
	0			

(Go Back)
(Logout)

DEVELOPMENT OF A NEONATAL MONITORING SYSTEM FOR INTENSIVE CARE UNIT (ICU)

Telephone	TEMPERATURE	Nurse Review	Firstname	Address
0803884	453	the patient is doing very fine	segun	villa
0147	66	lekan file	okmola	ohrm
08055	40	jerry will soon be discharged	Bologun	moveta
0147	56	very awesome patient	okmola	ohrm
0147	11	very good patient	okmola	ohrm
0147	11	very good patient	okmola	ohrm

(Go Back)

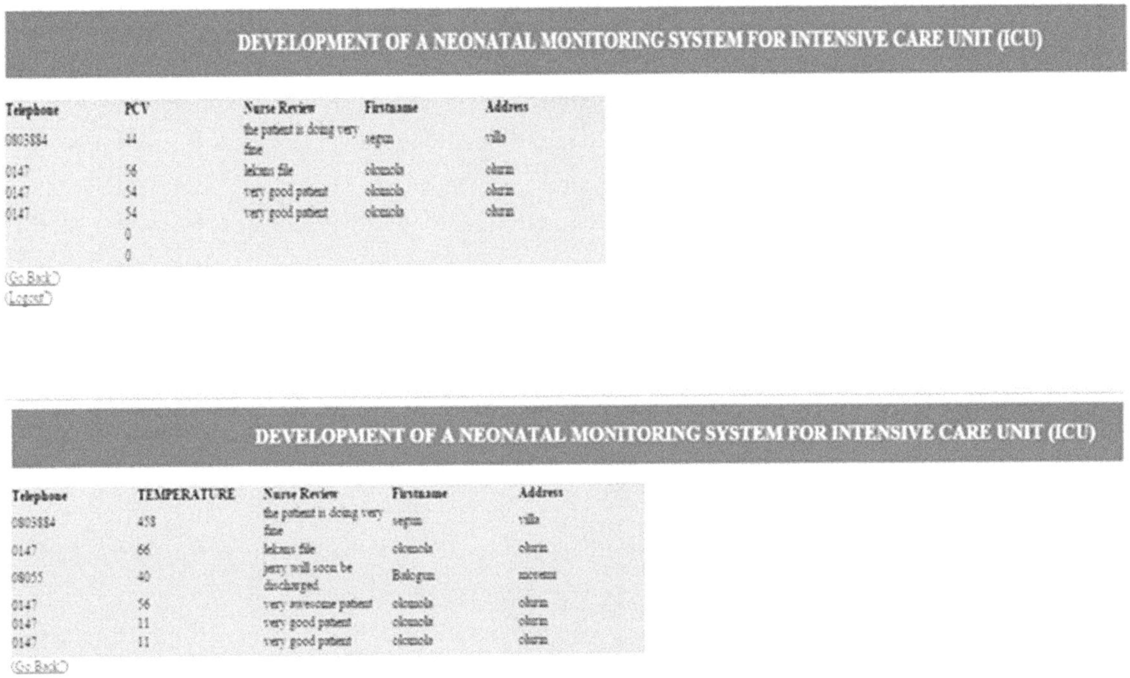

higher level of the units within the data model (Idowu and Adagunodo, 2010). As a result of this, three groups of entities were defined – Activities, Location and Parties. The activity component covers the different activities that can be performed in the system by users; these activities were classified into two groups: user information activities which include registering a user, updating a user profile the other, neonatal information activities which includes registering a newly admitted neonate, updating the information of an existing neonate and searching for the information of a neonate.

The party component includes information regarding the user entities identified in the system, which includes: the neonate, doctor and nurses – these information can be classified into the user component and patient component. The location component contains information regarding the position/location of objects within the system. Two components were identified for the location, namely: the electronic which can include e-mail addresses and phone numbers while the other called the physical can contain information like the address of an entity or the postal address of an entity (Figure 6).

The conceptual data model is the second stage in the data modeling development process. During the course of the development of the data model, a relationship association was used to depict the relationship between two entities, which are associated with each other. The relationship association in the developed data model was also used to show the type of relationship that exists between the super type class and sub-type class. Relationships were featured with the use of cardinality such as one to one $(1 – 1)$, many to one $(* - 1)$, many to many $(* - *)$ and one to many $(1 - *)$. The relationships in the

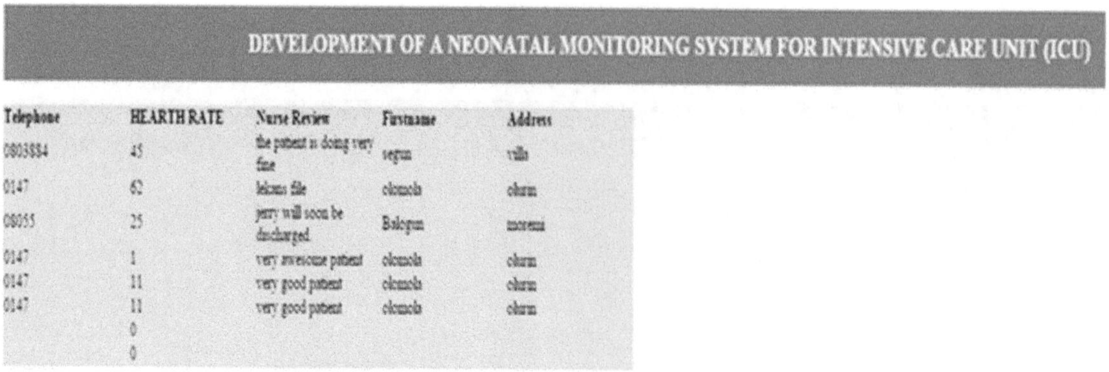

Figure 7. Conceptual data model of neonatal monitoring system

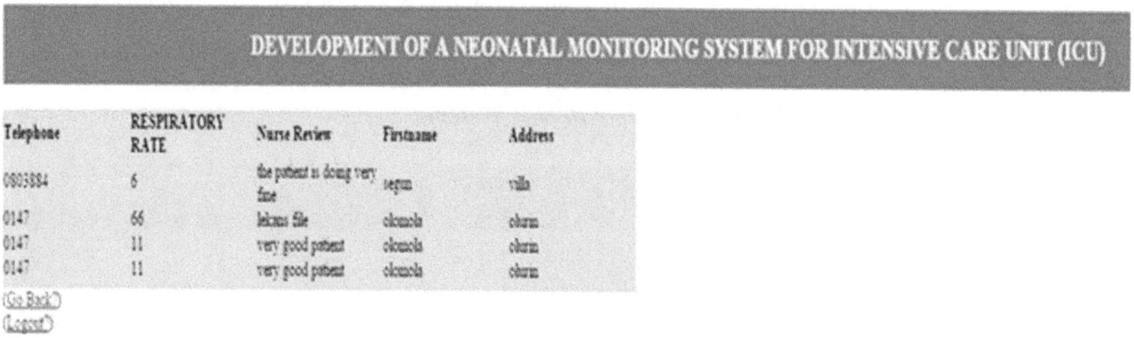

models are represented with classes which have a relationship with the three subject areas namely: party relationship, activity relationship and location relationship.

The party relationships are those relationships that exist between two or more parties in the activity relationship. One example is the relationship that exists between a nurse and a neonate been registered into the system or the relationship that exist between a doctor and a search for a neonate information stored on the system in order to retrieve the vital signs' information of the neonate in the ICU. A location relationship provides information about the relationship that exists between locations in the health; for example, the relationship between the locations where a doctor can be reached. An activity relationship is the relationship between a patient and his/her neonatal vital signs' information stored or that which exists between a doctor/nurses and their personal information. Figure 7 shows a description of the conceptual data model for the relationship that exists in the data model for the neonatal monitoring system.

Neonatal Monitoring System Architecture

Following the design of the system's requirements – the system architecture of the proposed monitoring system was proposed in order to describe how the different components of the system are interconnected for both users and communication components. In this study, the multi-tier architecture (also called the n-tier architecture) was proposed, it is also called a client-server architecture in which the presentation, application processing and data management functions are physically separated. It provides a model by which developers can create flexible and reusable applications; thus, it is easy to modify or add specific layers instead of re-working the entire application. The components of the 3-tier architecture proposed in this study consist of the presentation layer, a domain logic tier (business logic) and the data storage layer.

In the 3-tier architecture proposed in this study for the development of the neonatal monitoring system, the user interface for each system user (presentation layer), functional process logic layer (business logic) of the behaviour and process involved in neonatal monitoring alongside the computer data storage and data access layers were managed as independent modules/platforms. This has an advantage of allowing room for upgrades or replacements when necessary in response to changes in requirements and/or technology. Figure 8 shows a description of the 3-tier architecture of the neonatal monitoring system proposed for the system's architecture for the neonatal monitoring system in this study.

The presentation layer which is the top-most level of the application, displays information related to services as browsing merchandise, registration pages and information access and updates pages. It communicates directly with the tiers using the browser/client tier and all other tiers in the network. In short, this layer allows the system uses to access the system's functionality via a web-page on an operating

Figure 8. Neonatal monitoring system architecture

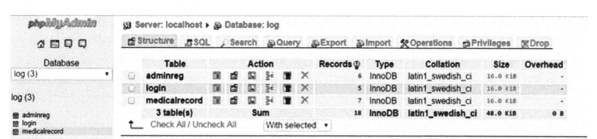

systems graphical user interface (GUI). The application layer is pulled from the presentation layer and it controls the functionality of the neonatal monitoring system by performing all the necessary functionalities required. The data tier includes the data persistent mechanisms (database servers, file shares etc.) and the data access layer that encapsulates the mechanisms and exposes the data. This layer provides an application programming interface (API) to the application tier that exposes methods of managing the stored data without exposing or creating dependencies on the data storage mechanisms. Avoiding these dependencies on the storage mechanisms allows for updates or changes without the application tiers' clients being affected by or even aware of the changes taking place.

RESULTS

Results of Prototype Implementation

As discussed earlier, the system implementation was performed using standard Web 2.0 technologies, namely: HTML, CSS, PHP and SQL for the front-end (client side) and back-end (server side) components of the neonatal monitoring system. As discussed in the system architecture earlier, the presentation tier component of the system was presented using graphical user interfaces (GUI) which were implemented as a collection of web-pages.

The web application was implemented as a set of web-pages each representing different aspects of the neonatal monitoring system's business logic layer. The primary page of the system implementation was the home page which was defined as the index of the web application – the first page that is viewed by all users accessing the system. Following is a presentation of the result of the implementation of the interfaces used to present the presentation layer of the neonatal monitoring system.

Results of the Allocation of Username and Password

Figure 9 shows the page where the administrator creates username and passwords to potential users of the neonatal monitoring system. The username is stated alongside the password which is written twice so as to confirm that the password presented by the user is consistent. Furthermore, the administrator selects the description of the user be it a nurse or a doctor. The figure shows the registration of a doctor with the name Olumuyiwa as a user of the neonatal monitoring system.

Result of the Login Page for Users of the System

Figure 10 shows the homepage of the neonatal monitoring system which is provided for the administrator, doctor and the nurses who intend to perform any data retrieval and insertion on the neonatal monitoring system. The page uses a lock screen that needs to authenticate the user that have privilege to data retrieval or data insertion based on the users access level during the point of registration provided by the system administrator. Each user accesses the system using the username and password provided to them by the system administrator at the point of their registration into the neonatal monitoring system.

Figure 9. Interface for user authentication

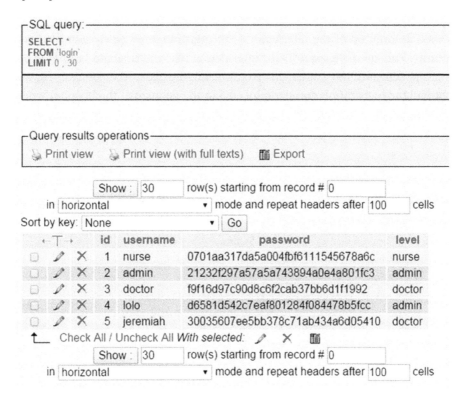

Figure 10. Login page for users of the system

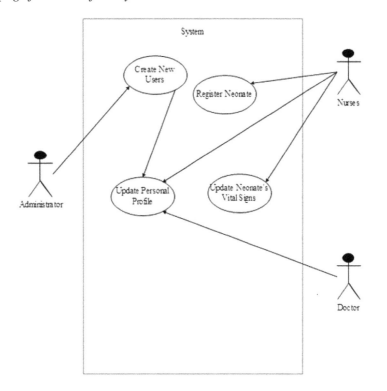

Result of the Registration Page of Newly Registered Neonates

Figure 11 shows a description of the interface for the registration of newly admitted neonate into the intensive care units. The interface requests for information like, the first and last name of neonates, the home address of the neonates, the gender (male or female), the age of the neonates (in weeks), parent's contact number and the registration number allocated to the neonate at the hospital where the neonate is registered. Following the completion of the information provided in this interface, the nurse can then submit the information so that such information can be stored in the database of the neonatal monitoring system.

Figure 11. Registration page of newly registered neonates by nurses

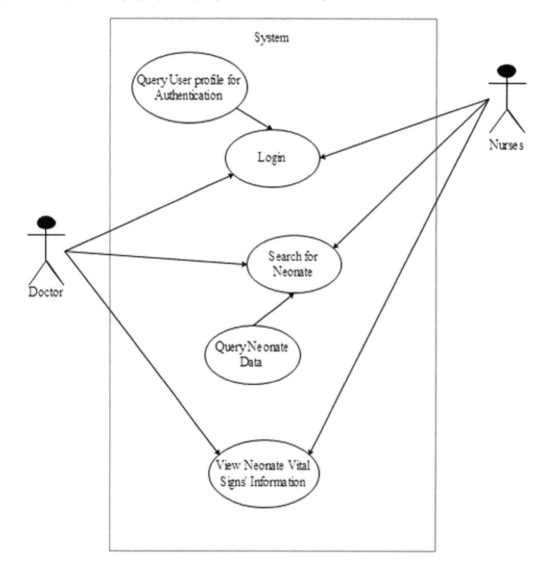

Figure 12. Insertion of neonates' vital signs' information by nurses

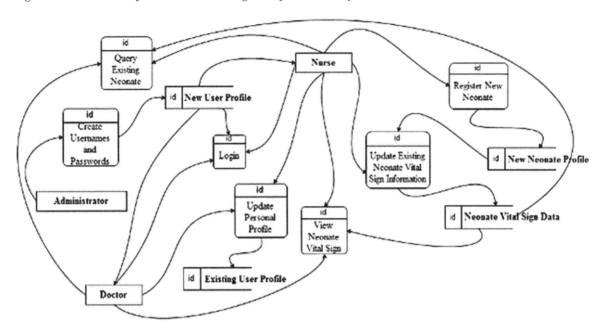

Result of the Insertion of Neonates' Vital Signs' Information By Nurses

Figure 12 shows a description of the interface for the data insertion module of the neonates' vital signs' information following the ward rounds conducted by the nurse on duty. Following the nurses' registration into the neonatal monitoring system, the interface shown in Figure 12 is displayed. The nurse is expected to provide the registration number of the neonates in question followed by information about the vital signs recorded during the regular ward rounds conducted by the nurse. The information inserted by the nurse includes: the neonates' random blood sugar, the packed cell volume (PCV), the heart rate, the temperature, respiratory rate alongside the nurses' review of the patient in question based on the observation made during the regular ward rounds conducted. If the information provided is not satisfactory, then the information can be removed else the information is submitted and loaded into the system's database.

Results of the Data Retrieval Module for Monitoring Neonates

Figure 13 shows a description of the data retrieval module through which the doctors can be able to monitor the vital signs information of the neonates stored in the system's database. Through this interface, the doctors can be able to view the information regarding neonates either as a group or as an individual. If the search is made as group then the doctors can easily decide to select any of the icons identifying the specific vital sign to be monitored – these icons can be seen on the top-centre of Figure 13. The doctor can also decide to retrieve the neonates' vital signs' information specifically suing the name of the neonate or the hospital number of the neonate using the search located on the bottom-centre of the interface.

If the doctor decides to view the neonates' information as a group using the top-centre icons on Figure 13 then he will be displayed the interfaces in Figures 14 and 15. Figure 14 shows the group results of the neonates who have high and low PCV (top in Figure 14) and high and low temperatures (bottom

Figure 13. Data retrieval module for monitoring neonates

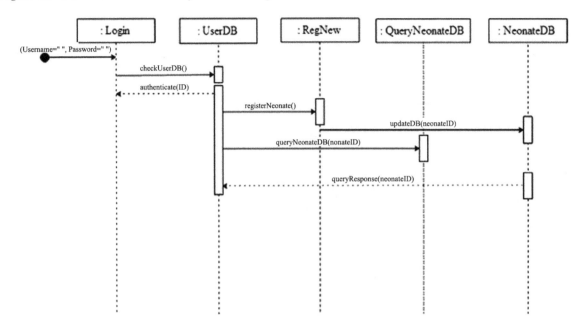

Figure 14. Results of data retrieval for neonates' PCV (above) and temperature (below)

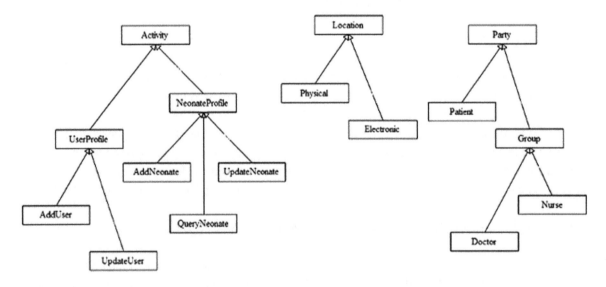

in Figure 14) while Figure 15 show the group of neonates who have high and low respiratory rate (top in Figure 15) and high and low heart rates (bottom in Figure 15). The information in the figures shows the registration number of the neonates followed by the value of the vital sign, their full names, address and the nurses' comments during the regular ward rounds conducted in the intensive care unit (ICU).

Figure 15. Results of data retrieval for neonates' respiratory rate (above) and heart rate (below)

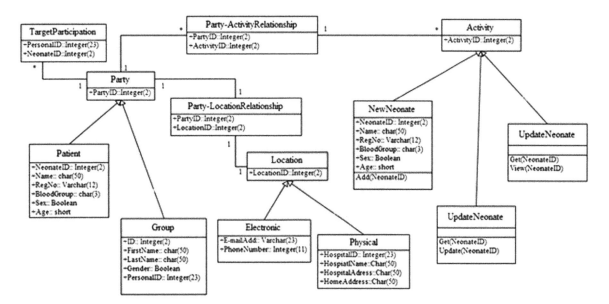

Results of the Implementation of the Physical Data Model of the Neonatal Monitor System

The neonatal monitoring system's database was implemented using the structured query language (SQL). The system's database was titled log with three (3) tables defined, namely: login, adminreg and the medical record. The login table stores information regarding the username and passwords of new users registered into the system by the administrator subject to the point of completing their personal profile, as discussed earlier to be used by each user to log into the system from the homepage. The adminreg table stores information regarding the personal profile of each registered user of the system, such details which include: their first and last names, job description (doctor or nurses), e-mail address, contact number, address and registration number. The medical record table stores information regarding the neonates' vital sign information collected and stored by the nurses during their regular ward rounds. This information is used to display the result of the search for the vital sign information of the neonates in question either as an individual or as a group (see Figure 16).

In the case of the login table, the information stored regarding the passwords were encrypted using encryption algorithm in order to provide additional security mechanisms to the personal information of the users and the neonates stored in the database from illegal access by hackers. Thus, whenever the administrator creates the username and passwords which are assigned to each user at the point of registration then the password is encrypted immediately it is stored into the database table that stores the login information for each user. Figure 17 shows the table login within which the password values for each user is replaced with the encryption results.

Figure 16. Neonatal monitoring system's database showing tables

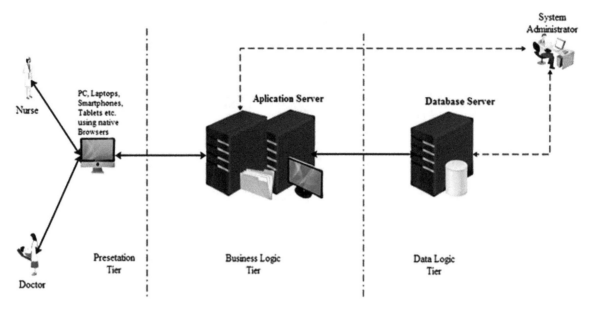

Figure 17. Table login showing the encryption results of user's passwords

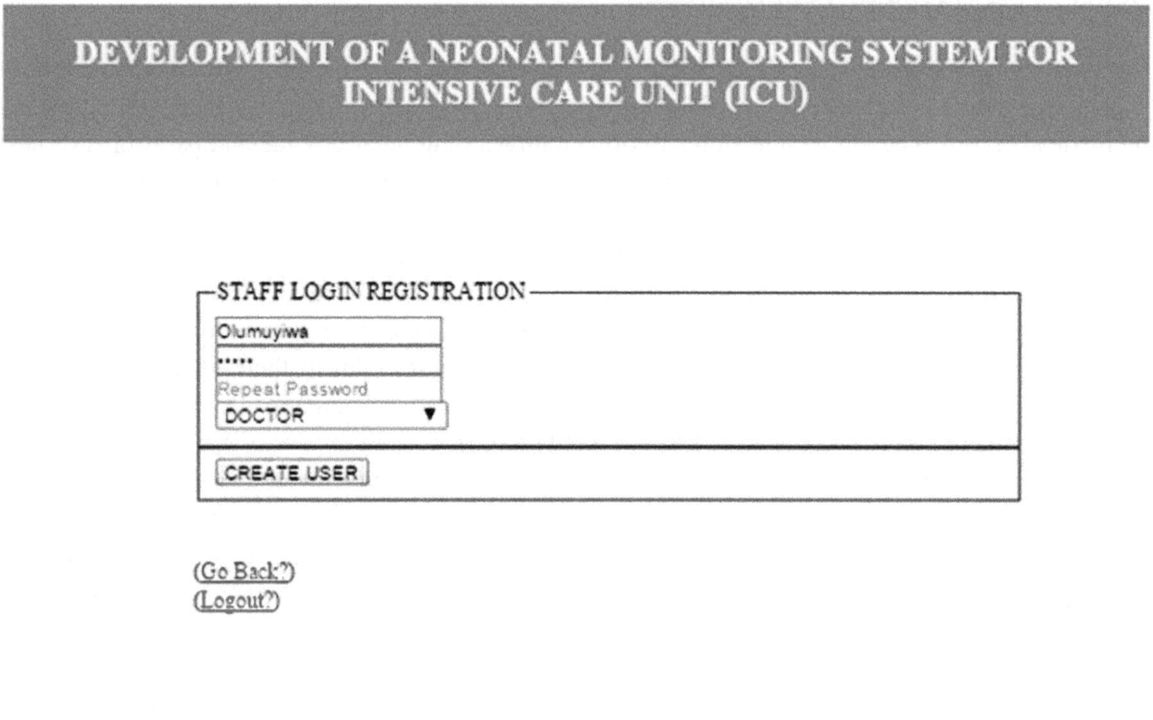

DEVELOPMENT OF A NEONATAL MONITORING SYSTEM FOR INTENSIVE CARE UNIT (ICU)

STAFF LOGIN REGISTRATION

Olumuyiwa

•••••

Repeat Password

DOCTOR ▼

CREATE USER

(Go Back?)
(Logout?)

DISCUSSIONS

The results of the implementation of the neonatal monitoring system proposed for neonates that are admitted into the intensive care units (ICU) of Obafemi Awolowo University teaching Hospital Complex (OAUTHC), Ile-Ife has been presented. The system architecture presented showed that the proposed system will support the access of system's resource by any intended user from any remote location as long as the user has access to internet connection provided by a service provider. The results also showed that the proposed system has the capacity to perform effectively and efficiently for the storage and retrieval of neonates vital signs' information due to the separation of concern taking place within the system using the three-tier architecture proposed in this study. Although, the results of this study was limited to deploying the system on a localhost, it is believed that the framework will be able to sustain increasing number of users and concurrent accessibility which is a functionality common with hospital management where multiple users may intend to access similar information at the same time.

The results of the implementation of the neonatal monitoring system using the Web 2.0 technologies show also how portable and scalable today's web technologies are at the implementation of web-based application required for the real-time analysis of information provided and accessed from remote location irrespective of location and device limiting barriers. The system's user interface was implemented using simple design patterns with illustrations reflecting the neonatal concern using graphical pictures of healthy babies alongside babies placed in intensive care units.

CONCLUSION

The developed neonatal monitoring system can be used by workers in the neonatal intensive care unit (NICU) tasked with the responsibility of monitoring and taking care of babies admitted into the NICU of OAUTHC. The system developed was able to perform the requirements proposed by the users of the system – the nurses and the doctors. The system was able to store and retrieve information provided by the nurses during data entry and such information was made accessible to authorized users as and when due. The system was also able to protect the vital login information provided by the administrator to each user using encryption algorithms for the safety of information and for ensuring the confidentiality of private information stored on the system.

REFERENCES

Gluck, L. (1985). *Conceptualization and initiation of a neonatal intensive care nursery in 1960. Neonatal intensive care: a history of excellence*. National Institute of Health.

Harper, D. (2010). *Neonatal*. Online Etymology Dictionary.

Idowu, P. A., & Adagunodo, E. R. (2010): A Spatial Conceptual Public Health Data Model for Nigeria. In *Proceedings of the 5th International Conference on Application if Information and Communications Technology for Training, Research and Administration (AICTTRA)* (pp. 11-23).

Joshi, N. S., Kamar, R. K., & Galkwad, P. K. (2013). Development of Wireless Monitoring System for Neonatal Intensive Care Unit. *International Journal of Advanced Computer Research, 3*(11), 2277–7970.

Perlman, J. M. (2001). Neurobehavioral deficits in premature graduates of intensive care -Potential medical and environmental risks factors. *Pediatrics, 108*(6), 1339–1348. doi:10.1542/peds.108.6.1339 PMID:11731657

Perlman, J. M. (2003). The genesis of cognitive and behavioural deficits in premature graduates of intensive care. *Minerva Pediatrica, 55*, 89–101. PMID:12754453

Polin, R. A., & Fox, W. W. (1992). *Sensors in neonatal monitoring: Current practice and future trends. Technology and Health Care, Fetal and Neonatal Physiology*. W.B. Saunders Company.

Suresh, L., Anju, L., Rama, M., Tanveer, A., & Jyothi, B. (2014). Neonatal Monitoring System. *Int. Journal of Engineering Research and Applications, 4*(7), 12–16.

Whitfield, J. M., Peters, B. A., & Shoemaker, C. (2004). Conference summary: a celebration of a century of neonatal care. Proceedings of Baylor University Medical Center, 17(3), 255–258. PMID 16200108.

Zhihua, Z., Tao, L., Guangyi, L., Tong, L., & Yoshio, I. (2015). Wearable sensor systems for infants. *Sensors (Basel, Switzerland), 15*(2), 3721–3749. doi:10.3390150203721 PMID:25664432

This research was previously published in the International Journal of Biomedical and Clinical Engineering (IJBCE), 6(1); edited by Natarajan Sriraam; pages 1-22, copyright year 2017 by IGI Publishing (an imprint of IGI Global).

Section 2
Information Systems

Chapter 9
Effect of Information Service Competence and Contextual Factors on the Effectiveness of Strategic Information Systems Planning in Hospitals

Shin-Yuan Hung
National Chung Cheng University, Taiwan

David C. Yen
SUNY at Oneonta, USA

Wei-Min Huang
National Chung Cheng University, Taiwan

She-I Chang
National Chung Cheng University, Taiwan

Chien-Cheng Lu
National Chung Cheng University, Taiwan

ABSTRACT

Many hospitals in Taiwan have started to encounter new and fierce competition as a result of the enactment of the National Health Insurance Policy in 1995. Hospitals should strive to use information technology (IT) strategically to improve their competitive advantage and meet the dynamic challenges in this competitive environment. This study adopts the Technology-Organization-Environment framework to understand the effects of contextual factors (e.g., environmental uncertainty and information intensity) and information service competence on the effectiveness of strategic information systems planning (SISP) to improve hospital management efficiency. A field survey was conducted using questionnaires distributed to accredited hospitals that serve patients from different regions/districts and with academic teaching qualifications/capabilities. These hospitals represent approximately a quarter of all hospitals in Taiwan. The findings show that the environmental unpredictability and business competence of IS executives are negatively related to the two SISP constructs: IT participation in the hospital planning and alignment of the IT plan with the comprehensive hospital plan. In addition, the findings demonstrate

DOI: 10.4018/978-1-7998-2451-0.ch009

Copyright © 2020, IGI Global. Copying or distributing in print or electronic forms without written permission of IGI Global is prohibited.

that information intensity has a significantly positive relation to both aforementioned SISP constructs. Finally, both constructs justify the significant positive correlations with the use of IT in increasing competitive advantages and improving the satisfaction of customers and end users. This research intends to guide the healthcare industry in raising competitive advantages to improve the operational efficiency of hospital management in today's highly digitalized environment.

1. INTRODUCTION

Information technology (IT) and increasing Internet usage has made the exchange and sharing of information and knowledge more convenient and timely. Moreover, the advent of the knowledge-based economy has made knowledge rather than traditional production elements the most important resource for businesses (Drucker, 1993). American firms allocate approximately 50 percent of their capital investment to IT (Morris et al., 2002) because IT serves as a key tool in acquiring, disseminating, and utilizing knowledge in such a competitive environment. Information systems (IS) planning must be incorporated into the strategic planning function of the businesses and implemented in the entire organization to realize its business objectives and improve competitive advantages through IT. For this reason, strategic IS planning (SISP) is important at the information management level in various industries.

The healthcare industry needs to apply SISP because healthcare organizations have faced a continuous challenge to reduce overhead costs while maintaining quality care amidst increasing demand for data exchange, information sharing, and better quality reporting. Technologies advance every day; thus, the IT adopted in hospitals has either reached the end of its useful life or is a candidate for contract renewal (Hitachi Consulting, 2001). Moreover, the medical treatment and healthcare policy of a government plays a decisive role in influencing the business operation of the medical sector. For example, US healthcare providers were required to use electronic health records and follow strict data coding standards, which forced them to increase their IT budgets (Terry, 2012). According to Anderson (2005), the UK spent more money on health IT than any other country in Europe, with approximately €2.4 billion out of €8 billion in total in the EU. In addition, the global healthcare budget system in Taiwan places some restrictions on the annual growth of medical expenses, creating more uncertainties and thus establishing a highly competitive environment for the capital-, labor-, and knowledge-intensive medical industry. Thus, hospitals must spend additional time and extra effort to properly utilize the available resources, actively minimize growing expenditure, and aggressively improve performance. From this perspective, many studies have shown that introducing IT can help reduce operating costs, improve performance, and facilitate the differentiation of products and services toward a strengthened competitive advantage (Neo, 1988; Clemons, 1991; Clemons and Row, 1991; Silva and Hirschheim, 2007; Zubovic et al., 2014).

Furthermore, the level of information service in an enterprise hierarchy is an important indicator of IT application utilization. A higher level in the organizational hierarchy for the IT function/department within a hospital can certainly increase the recognized importance of information service level and, hence, make its strategic role more critical. As such, information service competence is a key factor in terms of the strategic role of IS in the healthcare industry and has an immediate influence on the success or failure of strategic objectives using IT. Premkumar and King (1994) and Vitale, Ives and Beath (1986) suggested that organizational performance can be improved if fitness can be kept within the operating strategy, environment, and IS, in accordance with the concept of Technology-Organization-Environment framework. In addition, environmental uncertainty and information intensity are two external factors that affect the role of IT in improving the competitive advantages of enterprises (Johnston and Carrico, 1988; Wilkin1 and Cerpa 2012). Kearns and Lederer (2004) also found that companies with higher information intensity pay closer attention to IT applications in environments with greater uncertainty. Consequently, senior management tends to implement SISP formally in these environments (Chen et al., 2010).

Previous studies have seldom focused on the influence of information service competence on SISP and its actual performance in a manner unique to the healthcare industry (Clemons, 1991; Clemons and Row, 1991; Kearns and Lederer, 2004; Chi et al., 2005; Chen et al., 2010). None of these aforementioned studies have shown that investment in task-critical systems can improve the performance of an organization under the conditions of environmental uncertainty and information intensity. Large amounts of labor, time, and capital are required for SISP; as such, competitive opportunities may be completely lost in the event of any failure, and these can also lead to a waste of resources and investments (Raghunathan and King, 1988). However, previous studies on SISP have mainly focused on exploratory analyses on common enterprises or governmental bodies rather than on the capital-, labor-, and knowledge-intensive medical industry (Kearns and Lederer, 2004; Chi et al., 2005; Ravishankar et al., 2011; Hovelja et al., 2013). As a result, one of the major contributions of this paper is to bridge the gap in this subject field to perform a study in the medical industry.

SISP has been used widely in many enterprises and governmental institutions to oversee daily business operations and carry out the defined organizational plans and objectives (Lee and Pai, 2003). SISP is also indispensable for the healthcare industry because recent technological changes in medicine have been a major cause of rising healthcare expenditures in many countries. Since the enactment of the National Health Insurance Policy in 1995, the medical industry in Taiwan has been experiencing increasing technological changes in the areas of physician services, hospital care, and prescription drugs (Hsieh and Sloan, 2008). Local hospitals must strive to maintain the balance between their healthcare budget and the quality of their services (Hsieh and Sloan, 2008; Lin and Chang, 2010) because the healthcare budget exponentially increases annually to provide and maintain better medical services for the public. Therefore, hospitals in Taiwan must adopt SISP to manage the required information service competence internally in an organization and the changing environmental factors existed externally in a more effective and systematic way. Well-organized SISP management can enhance efficiency and competitiveness to help domestic hospitals survive under the increasingly competitive healthcare industry in Taiwan (Lin and Chang, 2010).

Based on the above discussion, this paper aims to guide hospitals in Taiwan as they strive to establish a more efficient organizational management via SISP. To this end, hospitals can increase their relative competitive advantages under the rapidly changing environment. In other words, by analyzing the influences of environmental factors and information service competence to improve related performance and competitive advantages associated with SISP, the healthcare industry can align its objectives with the implementation of IT. Moreover, in addition to benefiting the hospitals in Taiwan, all healthcare industries worldwide can gain additional insights that produce better management as a result of analyzing the following issues:

- Influence of environmental uncertainty and information intensity on the IT dependency of hospitals;
- Influence of information service competence on the IT dependency of hospitals;
- Influence of environmental uncertainty and information intensity on hospital SISP;
- Influence of information service competence on hospital SISP; and

- Influence of SISP on the performance of hospitals under various environmental factors and internal variables.

This paper is organized as follows: Section 2 discusses related literature. Section 3 presents the research method. Section 4 provides the data analysis and results. Section 5 concludes this paper and provides suggestions.

2. LITERATURE REVIEW

2.1. Environmental Uncertainty and Information Intensity

Among the external factors, environmental uncertainty and information intensity are the most important and influential factors that affect the creation of competitive advantages through IT utilization (Johnston and Carrico, 1988; Hovelja et al., 2013), system planning, and IT investment capability (Kearns and Lederer, 2004). Moreover, these factors are significantly correlated with the success of strategic IT investment (Reich and Benbasat, 1990). Environmental uncertainty includes attributes such as dynamism, heterogeneity, and hostility (Teo and King, 1997). Dynamism is the speed and unpredictability of external environment transformation, and heterogeneity is the complexity caused by diversified products and market orientations (Miller and Friesen, 1983; Hovelja et al., 2013). Hostility is the availability of resources and competition.

Environmental uncertainty may play an important role in terms of strategy management and organizational performance (Miller et al., 1991; Mohdzain and Ward, 2007).When evaluating the fitness from a matching perspective, Miller et al. (1991) uncovered that the fitness of environment and strategy positively correlates with organizational performance. However, when evaluating fitness from the perspective of profile deviation, Venkatraman and Prescott (1990) argue that fitness may have a positive effect on performance. Furthermore, uncertainty expands the role of SISP and thus increases the requirement associated with organizational structure and integration (Khandwalla, 1973). To this end, IS may be greatly affected by environmental uncertainty in an unsettled company environment (Lederer and Mendelow, 1990). Thus, assuming that hospitals, which have been increasingly dependent on IT, may have a strong necessity to improve their performance and management to increase their competitive advantages is reasonable.

Although environmental uncertainty has become one of the important variables of IT and organizational structure fitness, relevant research findings still vary in this subject field. For instance, Teo and King (1997) state that environmental uncertainty has an insignificant effect on the combination of enterprise planning and SISP. In addition, the influence of environmental uncertainty on enhancing competitive advantage through IT may not differ from that of SISP (Karagozoglu, 1993). However, Choe et al., (1997) argue that external factors such as environmental variability and competitive hostility make becoming involved with the enterprise strategy planning (Bergeron et al., 2001) difficult for the initiators of strategic IS, such as chief information officers (CIOs). As a result, proper assessment of environmental uncertainty is helpful in realizing the objectives of SISP (Chi et al., 2005).

Information intensity is defined as the dependency of companies' products, services, and business operations on information collection and processing, which are part of value chain exchange activity (Porter, 1985; Porter and Millar, 1985; Glazer, 1991). Industries in a dynamic business environment with higher information intensity focus on IT investments to improve their respective competitive advantages. Companies in information-intensive environments attempt to provide quick feedback (Cusmano and Selby, 1997) due to the decreasing life cycle of products. In such cases, the business process should be kept flexible so that it can be adjusted to meet changes in customer requirements for products and services. For this reason, companies often resort to concurrent engineering, iterative enhancement, and modular design to enhance their competitive edge (Boehm, 1988).

Due to the variability and chaos in information-intensive environments, enterprises require more IT applications to guarantee a quick response and to coordinate different tasks (Glazer, 1991), which leads to demanding information processing requirements and increased IT dependence. The industry's information intensity probably affects the implementation of SISP (Earl, 1993). For example, compared with the service in manufacturing industries, service companies are inclined to invest more in SISP in the hopes of improving their service planning capacity (Lederer and Salmela, 1996).Similarly, hospitals, which provide medical service that seems to be quite different from industries that manufacture products or offer general service, may still face some dynamic challenges while using SISP in response to fierce and increasing medical competition and growing public awareness of and demand for higher medical quality.

2.2. Information Service Competence

IT application and information service competence critically influence the improvement of the competitive advantages of modern enterprises (Neo, 1988). Information service competence refers to information service-related expertise and the knowledge capability of enterprises, including systems planning capability and SISP proficiency measured using the cognition capacity of insiders, and the relative capability of the system compared with peers and competitors. Therefore, indexes of IS capability include common knowledge in the industries, extensive application of computer systems in an organization, service reliability and efficiency of an IS, the IT manager's familiarity with the business process, and the IT manager's competence in prior planning and identifying challenges (Teo and King, 1997). Teo and King (1997) further divide IS competence into expertise and knowledge ability of enterprises, which suggests that a positive correlation exists between information managers' knowledge ability and IT planning together with the consistency of business planning.

System planning capability refers to system fostering, control, and innovation. Nolan (1979) suggests that IS should be planned more flexibly such that the IS process can properly respond to new opportunities, thereby resulting in fostered and balanced innovative capability through a proper control system. Raghunathan and Raghunathan (1991) investigated how five key dimensions, namely, planning systems capability, link to organizational concerns, internal consideration, organization's environmental considerations, and general environmental considerations, affect IS planning. Moreover, the key variable of system planning capability was found to be significantly correlated with planning efficiency. Therefore, this paper will examine the information service competence of Taiwan hospitals, which have relied heavily on IT and experienced IT changes, according to Hsieh and Sloan (2008).

2.3. Strategic Information System Planning

SISP is defined in the literature as the computer-aided process that assists organizations in implementing plans and realizing objectives (Lederer and Sethi, 1988). Specifically, it is defined as the process of deciding or choosing the correct portfolio of IS and the objectives for organizational computing as well as identifying potential computer applications that the organization should implement (Doherty et al., 1999; Doherty and Fulford, 2006; Abdisalam et al., 2011; Wilkin1 and Cerpa 2012). Organizations can prioritize the IS they are using and proceed with planning (Doherty et al., 1999) using SISP. Given that it starts by identifying organizational strategic information needs (Abdisalam et al., 2011), SISP is regarded as a tool to help change the development orientation of core organizational activities. Doing so enables executives to reconsider the amendment of their enterprises' strategy and redefine their enterprises' framework. Consequently, business managers and CIOs consider improving SISP a crucial element of their management system (Niederman et al., 1991).

Lederer and Sethi (1996) point out that the functions of SISP include such items as matching business requirements with IT, obtaining competitive advantages with IT, providing latest and real-time application as well as strategic application systems, increasing the support of executives for IS, improving the communication between users and information, and predicting the resource requirements to develop the IS. The contributions of SISP to the business operation include developing valuable IS with SISP, assisting enterprises in implementing business strategies, realizing business objectives via the IS, and assisting enterprises in updating applicable strategies and IT policies for consistency.

In the study of Raghunathan et al. (1991), the key dimensions of SISP and strategy planning include organizing systems capability and considering environmental factors toward the efficiency of SISP. The dependency of enterprises on IT in terms of core activities, the involvement of IT in business planning, and the alignment of IT with business planning (Kearns and Lederer, 2004)clearly demonstrate the relationship between an organization and IT applications. To this end, IT must be efficiently used to support company objectives and contribute to building the consensus between IS and enterprise strategy (Lederer and Mendelow, 1989). As an important strategic resource, IT is one of the major tools in modifying priority levels in IT planning (Lederer and Mendelow, 1990). In the process of conducting remote business planning, CIOs should evaluate SISP in detail (Chi et al., 2005; Mohdzain and Ward, 2007) and improve the innovation and flexibility of planning in response to the uncertainty and complexity of the external environment.

Although past studies have measured SISP performance using quantifiable indexes, such as return on investment, pre-tax income, sales increase, profitability, and price–earnings ratio, few positive conclusions have been reached due to the large number of influential factors (Kearns and Lederer, 2004; Tallon and Pinsonneault, 2011). Byrd, Lewis, and Bryan (2006) point out the possibility of utilizing increased operating performance when IS strategy is implemented according to enterprise strategy. With higher target consistency, the performance of IT investment is improved, which demonstrates that IS contributes more to improving organizational performance (Bechor et al., 2010; Johnson and Lederer, 2010; Velcu, 2010; Teo and King, 1996). However, the influences of IS competence on the efficiency of SISP are not yet validated (Hung et al., 2001). For this reason, this paper also covers information service competence and the factors that influence the efficiency of SISP in the context of Taiwan hospitals.

3. RESEARCH MODEL, HYPOTHESES AND METHOD

3.1. Definition and Measurement of Research Variables

This research model includes eight dimensions: (1) environmental uncertainty, which represents external environmental factors; (2) IS competence; (3) information intensity representing internal environmental factors; (4) IT dependency of hospitals; (5) involvement of IT in the strategy planning of hospitals; (6) alignment of IT planning with hospital planning that represents the process of SISP; (7) efficiency of SISP involved in improving competitive advantage; and (8) satisfaction with the use of IT (the items and scales are referenced and provided in Table 6 of the Appendix):

1. **Environmental Uncertainty:** Environmental uncertainty includes dynamism, heterogeneity, and hostility (Miller and Friesen, 1983; Sabherwal and King, 1992; Teo and King, 1997). This paper constructs the items and associated scales of environmental uncertainty from these three aforementioned studies based on the scale developed by Teo and King (1997);

2. **Information Intensity:** Information intensity refers to the dependency of a company's products, services, and business operations on information collection and processing, which comprise part of the value chain activity (Porter and Miller, 1985; Glazer, 1991). Information intensity can be measured by the availability of information, frequency of information updating, accuracy of information, and dependency of business operation on information. In this study, the items and scales of information intensity are adopted based on the scale of Kearns and Lederer (2004);

3. **Information Service Competence:** Information service competence is defined as IT expertise and knowledge capability in relation to information service. In this paper, information service competence is measured comparatively through recognized competence and scale proposed by Teo and King (1997);

4. **IT Dependency of Hospitals:** Higher IT dependency represents the core activity of an organization accomplished with the help of the relevant IS. In this paper, the items and scales of IT dependency of hospitals are based on the scale developed by Kearns and Lederer (2004);

5. **Involvement of CIOs in Hospitals' Strategy Planning:** This refers to the process and level of CIO's involvement in strategy planning with the aim to provide relevant opinions and realize the operating objectives of strategies (Kearns and Lederer, 2004). According to Kearns and Lederer (2004), the involvement of IT managers in strategy planning is categorized as formal and informal. The items and scales for the involvement of CIOs in hospital planning were developed subsequently;

6. **Alignment of SISP with Hospital Planning:** This refers to the level and results of the alignment of the IS strategy with the overall business strategy (Baets, 1992; Henderson and Venkatraman, 1993). This study proposes new items and scales based on those developed by Kearns and Lederer (2004);

7. **Improving the Competitive Advantages of Hospitals by IT:** IT is considered a powerful tool for improving competitive advantage (Parsons, 1983; Porter and Millar, 1985; Bakos et al., 1986; Clemons, 1986; Neo, 1988; Clemons, 1991; Clemons and Row, 1991). Through the application of IT, obtaining financial benefits as well as reducing production cost and product differentiation while assisting enterprises in improving the resulting performance and efficiency is possible (Kearns and Lederer, 2004). In this study, the items and scales are adopted based on the scale developed by Kearns and Lederer (2004);

8. **Satisfaction:** Satisfaction refers to the degree of satisfaction of the interested parties. Customer satisfaction can be improved by combining enterprise planning and SISP (Teo and King, 1994). In this study, the items and scales are based on the study by Premkumar and King (1994) and developed by Teo and King (1999).

3.2. Research Model

The purpose of this study is to understand how environmental uncertainty, information service competence and information intensity can be applied to improve the management efficiency in hospitals through SISP. In addition, it also aims at studying the correlation of these aforementioned factors associated with SISP and their influences to improve the efficiency of SISP. Based on Technology-Organization-Environment framework, the process by which a firm implements various technological innovations may be influenced by such attributes as the technological context, the organizational context, and the environmental context (Tornatzky and Fleisher, 1990; Kuana and Chau, 2001; Baker, 2011).

After comprehensively analyzing the relevant SISP literature and taking industry characteristics of hospitals into consideration, this paper adopted the Technology-Organization-Environment framework and selected those three important variables to develop the research model (Chen et al., 2010; Hovelja et al., 2013; Silva and Hirschheim, 2007; Wilkin and Cerpa, 2012). In the hospital context, environmental uncertainty was selected as the influencing factor in the environment dimension. Further, information intensity was selected as the critical one in the organization dimension while information service competence was selected as the important one in the technology dimension. In addition, IT dependency of hospitals, involvement of CIOs in hospitals' strategy planning and the alignment of SISP with hospital planning were selected as the influencing factors in the strategy dimension. Finally, improving the competitive advantages of hospitals by IT and satisfaction attributes were selected as the dependent variables in the performance dimension. As per earlier discussion, the proposed research model is thus presented in Figure 1.

3.3. Research Hypotheses

An IS executive must take internal and external environmental factors into account simultaneously to plan SIS in the hospitals efficiently. In the past decades, environmental uncertainty and information

Figure 1. Research model

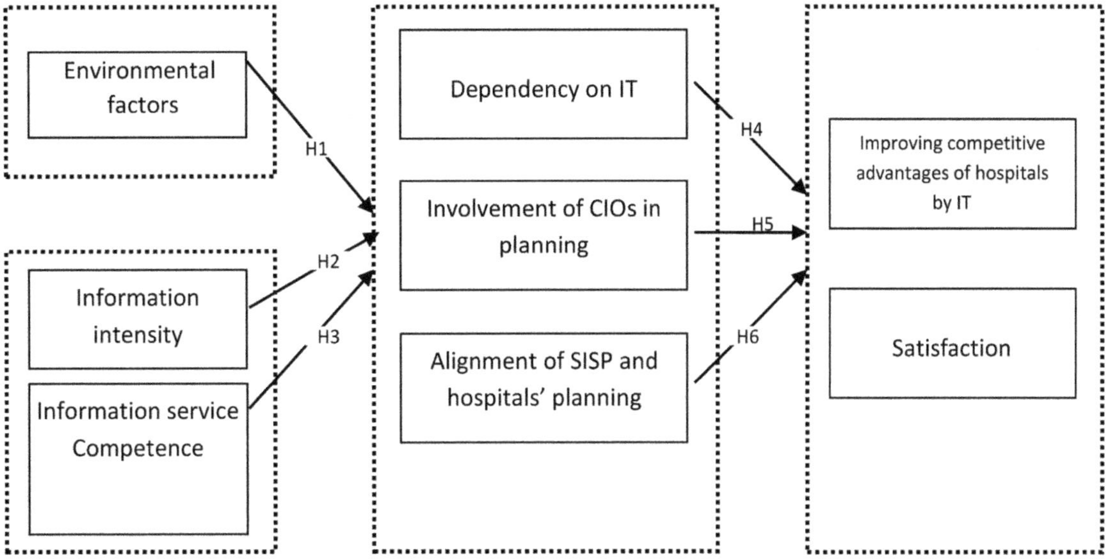

intensity have been identified as two critical contextual factors that affect IT in improving the competitive advantage of enterprises (Johnston and Carrico, 1988; Kearns and Lederer, 2004; Chen et al., 2010; Hovelja et al., 2013). Moreover, information service competence is deemed an important factor when planning SIS (Teo and King, 1997). To plan the SIS of hospital efficiently, IT managers should have the required expertise and knowledge of hospital to support the relevant activities and goals of the hospital at every level. Thus, the proposed hypotheses are provided as follows (the relational diagram is provided in Table 1):

H1: Environmental uncertainty has a significantly positive influence on the SISP of hospitals.
H2: Information intensity has a significantly positive influence on the SISP of hospitals.
H3: Information service competence has a significantly positive influence on the SISP of hospitals.

Moreover, due to the diverse nature of environmental uncertainty, hospitals require a more sophisticated information system to reduce its uncertainties and maintain its competitive advantage (Teo and King, 1997; Silva and Hirschheim, 2007; Wilkin and Cerpa, 2012). To this end, hospitals depend increasingly on IT to respond to these uncertainties. However, planning a SIS for a hospital is a complex job because it strengthens the request for the involvement of IT managers. As noted, IT managers play a key role in planning SIS and integrating SIS and business planning (Kearns and Lederer, 2004; Teo and King, 1999; Wilkin and Cerpa, 2012). To meet this end and ensure that IT resources are allocated adequately to support the core activities of hospitals, the SISP must be kept in line with the business strategy of the hospital to sustain its competitive advantage. Hence, this study proposed the following hypotheses:

H1a: Environmental uncertainty has a significantly positive influence on the IT dependency of hospitals.
H1b: Environmental uncertainty has a significantly positive influence on the involvement of CIOs in hospital planning.
H1c: Environmental uncertainty has a significantly positive influence on the alignment of SISP with hospital planning.

Enterprises with higher information intensity may support the related core activities and take advantage of the strategic opportunities provided by IT (Bergeron et al., 1991). Higher information intensity means an increasingly important role for rendering an information service (Porter and Millar, 1985). Hospitals are filled with various high information-intensity services and activities every day. To respond to the various challenges encountered in this information-intensity environment, a hospital actually depends more on IT applications (Glazer, 1991). To this end, CIOs should be more involved with the planning of hospital SIS, meeting with other managers, and providing expertise for developing future planning. In addition, due to the complex nature of high information-intensity services and activities associated with the hospital, IT strategies should be aligned with the business strategies in particular to keep its competitive advantages (Kearns and Lederer, 2004; Chen et al., 2010; Wilkin and Cerpa, 2012). Hence, this paper proposes the requirements for the alignment of information planning with business planning. The proposed hypotheses are provided as follows:

H2a: Information intensity has a significantly positive influence on the IT dependency of hospitals.
H2b: Information intensity has a significantly positive influence on the involvement of CIOs in hospital planning.

H2c: Information intensity has a significantly positive influence on the alignment of SISP with hospital planning.

When a company has a stronger information service, it is more likely to improve its competitive advantage through the employment of IT applications (Neo, 1988). Information service competence is a crucial element to the users and senior management in preparing strategic IS as well as in ensuring the necessary communication and coordination (Teo and King, 1997). Information service competence in a hospital may include not only software and hardware technologies but also factors such as the IT manager's familiarity with hospital processes, knowledge of medical industry, and expertise in planning SIS of the hospital. CIO should provide his/her knowledge and expertise to integrate SISP with the hospital business planning (Chen et al., 2010; Hovelja et al., 2013; Leidner et al., 2010). Doing so ensures that information service competence may improve the competitive position of a hospital over other competitors. Thus, the proposed hypotheses are provided as follows:

H3a: Information service competence has a significantly positive influence on the IT dependency of hospitals.

H3b: Information service competence has a significantly positive influence on the involvement of CIOs in hospital planning.

H3c: Information service competence has a significantly positive influence on the alignment of SISP with hospital planning.

Hospitals depend more heavily on IT with the increasing complexity of handling the associated activities and services in hospitals (Gordon et al., 1998). Hospitals search for various IT innovations to differentiate its services, establish entry barriers in the medical market, and create switching costs (Porter, 1985). IT has become a competitive weapon for hospitals to create and sustain its competitive advantage (Kim and Michelman, 1990; Leidner et al., 2010). To sustain their competitive advantage, hospitals must keep track of the performance of IT investments. To this end, two important indicators can be used to evaluate the performance of IT investments: user satisfaction and customer satisfaction (or patient satisfaction). User satisfaction implies the success or effectiveness of using information systems (Baroudi and Orlikowski, 1988; Chen et al., 2010; Wilkin and Cerpa, 2012). Customer satisfaction reflects the level to which patients are satisfied with the medical services of the hospital. Greater customer satisfaction may lead to returning customers, which results in more profit. Therefore, hospitals depend more on IT to provide better services which, in turn, improve the satisfaction of users and customers. Thus, the following hypotheses are proposed:

H4: Hospital IT dependency has a significantly positive influence on SISP efficiency.

H4a: Hospital IT dependency has a significantly positive influence on improving competitive advantage.

H4b: Hospital IT dependency has a significantly positive influence on satisfaction.

Information sharing and operational performance can be improved if the CIO becomes more involved with enterprise planning (Premkumar and King, 1994). Hospital CIOs provide technical suggestions as well as a vision of how to use IT to improve hospital performance (Kearns and Lederer, 2004). Increased participation of the CIO in the business planning of a hospital corresponds to increased information sharing (Kearns and Lederer, 2004), enhanced mutual understanding between CIO and CEO, more alignment of

SISP with the hospital business planning, better quality of care for patients, and better services for users (Leidner et al., 2010; Zubovic and Khan, 2014). Therefore, this study proposes the following hypotheses:

H5: The involvement of CIOs in the strategy planning of the hospital has a significantly positive influence on the efficiency of SISP.

H5a: The involvement of CIOs in the strategy planning of the hospital has a significantly positive influence on improving competitive advantage.

H5b: The involvement of CIOs in the strategy planning of the hospital has a significantly positive influence on satisfaction.

The objectives of the enterprises can be realized through the alignment of SISP with enterprise planning (Lederer and Mendelow, 1989; Chen et al., 2010; Hovelja et al., 2013; Silva and Hirschheim, 2007; Wilkin and Cerpa, 2012). Hospitals can benefit from IT investment only under the alignment of SISP with business planning (Kearns and Sabherwal, 2006/2007). The alignment of SISP with hospital planning may assure the support of IT, lead to the same strategic direction, and increase the competitive advantage of a hospital. Consequently, IT can be used to provide better services for users and customers. Thus, the following hypotheses are proposed:

H6: The alignment of SISP with hospital planning has a significantly positive influence on the efficiency of SISP.

H6a: The alignment of SISP with hospital planning has a significantly positive influence on improving competitive advantage.

H6b: The alignment of SISP with hospital planning has a significantly positive influence on satisfaction.

Table 1. Proposed hypotheses and their relationships

	Mediating Variables			Dependent Variable	
	IT Dependency of Hospitals	Involvement CIO in SP	Alignment	Improving Advantages	Satisfaction
Independent Variables					
Environmental uncertainty	H1a (+)	H1b (+)	H1c (+)		
Information intensity	H2a (+)	H2b (+)	H2c (+)		
Information service competence	H3a (+)	H3b (+)	H3c (+)		
Mediating Variables					
IT dependency of hospitals				H4a (+)	H4b (+)
Involvement CIO in SP				H5a (+)	H5b (+)
Alignment				H6a (+)	H6b (+)

3.4. Questionnaire Design and Distribution

The structured questionnaire was designed based on a five-point Likert's scale that includes the following items: (1) "Strongly disagree," (2) "Disagree," (3) "Fair," (4) "Agree," and (5) "Strongly agree." The measures of good reliability and validity used in previous studies were translated. Furthermore, to improve the reliability and validity of the questionnaire, a panel of seven CIOs, executives, and information management experts from various medical centers were invited to conduct a pre-test. The questionnaire was reviewed and amended based on the extensive reviews and feedback. Furthermore, the personnel information of reputable hospitals was verified/checked, and the questionnaire was further tested to verify the alignment of content difficulty with the items in the dimensions. In addition, a pilot test with 20 practitioners with related working experience and expertise was conducted to ensure the practicability and reliability of the questionnaire. Analysis of the responses of 20 random respondents revealed limited problems with the survey design, and proper actions were taken. Finally, the questionnaire samples were mailed to the CIOs of the hospitals that serve patients at the regional or higher levels, as approved and published by the Health Department. The questionnaires were collected after two weeks.

4. DATA ANALYSIS AND RESULTS

The questionnaire samples were sent to the CIOs or executives of the hospitals at the regional or higher levels. Out of 125 hospitals listed by the Taiwan Joint Commission on Hospital Accreditation, 19 were

Table 2. Profile of the respondents

Item	Count	Percentage	Cumulative Percentage
Title			
CIO	76	75.2%	75.2%
Manager of management center	4	4.0%	79.2%
Others	20	19.8%	99.0%
Unknown	1	1.0%	100.0%
Educational degree			
Junior college	53	52.5%	52.5%
Master	43	42.6%	95.0%
Doctor	3	3.0%	98.0%
Unknown	2	2.0%	100.0%
Track record in medical industry			
Below three years	8	7.9%	7.9%
4–6 years	14	13.9%	21.8%
7–12 years	33	32.7%	54.5%
13–20 years	30	29.7%	84.2%
21 years above	12	11.9%	96.0%
Unknown	4	4.0%	100.0%

medical centers, 66 were regional hospitals, and 40 were local hospitals. A total of 101 valid samples were returned, including 18 from medical centers, 53 from regional hospitals, and 30 from local hospitals. Data were justified as homogeneous because these were collected from medical centers, regional hospitals, and local hospitals. A follow-up procedure was used to fix/remedy incomplete data and missing data issues to complete the survey process.

Table 2 shows the basic data distribution of the respondents. Most respondents showed familiarity with the medical and IT industries in terms of the educational degree and track record of CIOs.

4.1. Reliability and Validity Analysis

In terms of construct validity, principal component analysis was conducted to extract factors with an eigenvalue of>1 to represent all observation variables by minimum factors (Hair et al., 2006). The factors were analyzed, and the results are listed in Table 3. Good construct validity can be derived from the results of factor analysis. The items of environmental dynamism can be further divided into variability (items 1–2) and unpredictability (items 3–4), which are consistent with the research findings of Teo and King (1997).Meanwhile, the items of IS competence comprise technical capacity (items 1–4) and medical knowledge ability of CIOs (items 5–6). Subsequent statistical analysis and hypotheses validation were conducted by taking these four factors as independent variables of the proposed research framework.

Reliability analysis aims to evaluate the reliability of the entire scale. In this paper, Cronbach's α was used to measure the reliability of the questionnaire as an index of the internal consistency of measurement items. The values of the Cronbach's α of heterogeneity and IT capability were 0.608 and 0.604, respectively. Those of other dimensions fell within the range of 0.7–0.909. These findings show that the research questionnaire has good reliability and consistency (Hair et al., 2006)). In addition to the aforementioned manipulative control, proper analytical control, such as information auditing using additional interviews, was used in this study.

Table 3. Factor analysis results

Dimension	Item	Factor Loading	Eigenvalue	Cumulative Explained Variance %
Hostility	Q1_9	0.843	3.322	25.06
	Q1_8	0.840		
	Q1_11	0.741		
	Q1_10	0.700		
	Q1_12	0.691		
Heterogeneity	Q1_6	0.777	2.081	39.92
	Q1_7	0.701		
	Q1_5	0.684		
Unpredictability (dynamism)	Q1_4	0.898	1.443	54.35
	Q1_3	0.832		
Variability (dynamism)	Q1_2	0.864	1.343	68.25
	Q1_1	0.824		

continued on following page

Table 3. Continued

Dimension	Item	Factor Loading	Eigenvalue	Cumulative Explained Variance %
IT capability (IS competence)	Q3_3	0.689	3.523	22.16
	Q3_2	0.678		
	Q3_1	0.651		
	Q3_4	0.512		
Information intensity	Q2_4	0.816	1.704	42.94
	Q2_1	0.751		
	Q2_2	0.613		
	Q2_3	0.400		
Medical knowledge ability (IS competence)	Q3_5	0.880	1.026	62.53
	Q3_6	0.854		
Alignment of SISP with hospitals' planning	Q6_3	0.851	7.742	17.28
	Q6_2	0.812		
	Q6_1	0.811		
	Q6_5	0.782		
	Q6_4	0.738		
Involvement of CIO in hospitals' strategy planning	Q5_3	0.843	2.445	33.47
	Q5_1	0.814		
	Q5_4	0.788		
	Q5_5	0.787		
	Q5_2	0.708		
Improving hospitals' competitive advantage by IT	Q7_4	0.826	2.128	48.49
	Q7_3	0.786		
	Q7_2	0.762		
	Q7_5	0.742		
	Q7_1	0.577		
IT dependency of hospitals	Q4_1	0.796	1.697	60.07
	Q4_4	0.778		
	Q4_2	0.686		
	Q4_5	0.606		
	Q4_3	0.513		
Satisfaction	Q8_1	0.815	1.253	69.38
	Q8_2	0.802		

4.2. Hypotheses Testing

Structural equation modeling (SEM) is generally used to validate the interdependency of two or more groups of variables as well as to discuss the causal relationship model among the variables (Hair et al., 2006). Consequently, SEM is used in this study to learn the causal relationship among variables and verify the research hypotheses presented earlier.

Following the analytical method proposed by Anderson and Gerbing (1988), this study calculated the composite scores as well as the goodness-of-fit (GOF) of SEM by using AMOS 5.0 package software. Table 4 shows the results of the model GOF as recommended by Hair et al. (2006). The results that comply with the criterion demonstrate the satisfactory GOF of this research model. The analytical results of the structural model are provided in Figure 2, and the explanatory power (R^2) of each dependent variable is provided in Table 5.

Table 4. Results of the goodness-of-fit of the model

Fit Index	Recommended Criteria	Results in this Study
χ^2 /d.f.	<3.00	1.41
GFI	>0.90	0.96
CFI	>0.90	0.97
RMSEA	<0.08	0.06
RMR	<0.05	0.02

Figure 2. Structural equation modeling (including path coefficient)

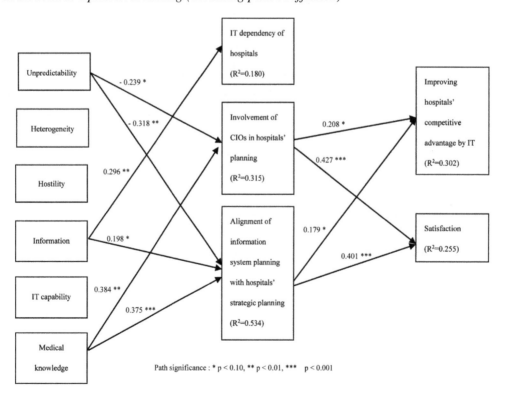

Table 5. Dependent variables and their corresponding explanatory power (R2)

Dependent Variable	Explanatory Power (R^2)
IT dependency of hospitals	0.180
Involvement of CIOs in hospital planning	0.315
Alignment of SISP with hospital planning	0.534
Improving the competitive advantages of hospitals by IT	0.302
Satisfaction	0.255

According to the path analysis results of SEM (Figure 2), environmental uncertainty converged into environmental variability and environmental unpredictability. Moreover, IS competence converged into IT capability and medical knowledge ability. In this study, the increased factors were incorporated to validate the relationship with the dependent variables.

4.3. Results and Discussion

The test results of the research hypothesis are presented below.

4.3.1. H-1: Environmental Uncertainty has a Significantly Positive Influence on the SISP of Hospitals

Among the 12 hypotheses on environmental uncertainty, the analytical results of only two hypotheses are significant, which indicates that their validity is as follows: Path 1: unpredictability →involvement of CIOs in hospital planning, path coefficient = -0.239, p = 0.009; and Path 2: unpredictability →alignment of SISP with hospital planning, path coefficient = -0.318, p<0.001, thus reaching a significant level.

In other words, this paper studies the influences of environmental uncertainty on the SISP of hospitals by dividing environmental uncertainty into four variables (i.e., variability, unpredictability, heterogeneity, and hostility). The finding shows that IT has greater importance if the senior management of hospitals perceives decreased unpredictability in the business environment. Lower environmental unpredictability denotes a higher degree of CIO involvement in hospital planning and alignment of SISP with the hospital planning. This result is consistent with the findings of Sabherwal and King (1992), which also indicates that IT is still considered a supportive tool in dealing with the medical service process. At the same time, some relevant measures, such as the involvement of CIOs in hospital planning and the alignment of SISP with hospital planning, are considered part of business tasks and objectives. In practice, environmental uncertainty may result from the policy making decisions of the various national health departments and other healthcare bureaus.

4.3.2. H-2: Information Intensity has a Significantly Positive Influence on the SISP of Hospitals

Among these three hypotheses on information intensity, the analytical results of the two hypotheses are significant, which indicates that their validity is as follows. Path 1: information intensity →IT dependency of hospitals, path coefficient = 0.296, p = 0.006; and Path 2: information intensity →alignment of SISP with hospital planning, path coefficient = 0.198, p = 0.014, thus reaching a significant level.

This finding shows that higher information intensity in the value chain activity of hospitals indicates a higher IT dependency. At the same time, the alignment of SISP with hospital planning is higher because IT also demonstrates higher importance. Therefore, this paper concludes that hospitals intend to conduct SISP aligned with the hospital planning by relying on IT employment, which is consistent with the proposition by Kearns and Lederer (2004). Aligning SISP with the hospital planning is possible, but only if the information is extensively used in medical services with a higher accuracy and timeliness.

4.3.3. H-3: Information Service Competence has a Significantly Positive Influence on the SISP of Hospitals

Among these six hypotheses of information service competence, the analytical results of only two hypotheses are significant, which indicates that their validity is as follows. Path 1: medical knowledge ability →involvement of CIO in hospital planning, path coefficient = 0.384, p<0.001; and Path 2: medical knowledge ability →alignment of SISP with hospital planning, path coefficient = 0.375, p<0.001, thus reaching a significant level.

This fact indicates that although CIOs have abundant medical expertise, the senior managers would likely provide them with more opportunities to participate in the strategy planning and assist in realizing higher alignment of SISP with hospital planning. In addition, the test result on the hypotheses related to IT capacity is insignificant, which shows the importance of the medical expertise of CIOs, which is consistent with the results found by Teo and King (1997). However, the empirical results of IT capability have not been supported, which indicates that IT may have gradually widespread applications available in hospitals. Consequently, IS department/function may have more opportunities to communicate with an increasing number of other operational units inside and with users outside the hospital. Sufficient medical knowledge can foster better communication and facilitate smooth operations in such cases. Senior managers should understand the value of the strategies employed by CIOs, which will offer more opportunities for any further involvement in the areas of business planning and information planning.

4.3.4. H-4: The IT Dependency of Hospitals has a Significantly Positive Influence on the SISP of Hospitals

These two hypotheses specific to the IT dependency of hospitals had p values of 0.726 and 0.776, respectively, which are not significant. Thus, H-4$_a$ and H-4$_b$ are rejected.

4.3.5. H-5: The Involvement of CIOs in Hospital Strategy Planning has a Significantly Positive Influence on the SISP of Hospitals

These two hypotheses specific to the involvement of CIOs in hospital planning are significant (p<0.10), which indicates that their validity is as follows: Path 1: involvement of CIO in hospital planning →improving the competitive advantages of hospitals by IT, path coefficient = 0.208, p = 0.022; and Path 2: involvement of CIOs in hospital planning →satisfaction, path coefficient = 0.179, p = 0.055.

This result indicates that the increased involvement of CIOs in hospital strategy planning results in easier access to the business strategy and objectives of hospitals. Moreover, the senior management has more opportunities to improve the competitive advantages of hospitals using IT. Given the higher level of involvement of CIOs in hospital strategy planning, IT can now improve the competitive advantage of the hospital and the satisfaction of customers and users, which is consistent with the findings of Kearns and Lederer (2004). CIOs can greatly contribute to organizational performance through proper IT investment by enhancing the relevant medical knowledge with a deeper understanding of strategy and process (Armstrong and Sambamurthy, 1999). Hence, senior managers and hospital CIOs should complement each other through formal and informal contacts and/or maintain close interactions to positively enhance competitive advantages and increase the satisfaction of users and customers.

4.3.6. H-6: The Alignment of SISP with Hospital Planning has a Significantly Positive Influence on the SISP of Hospitals

These two hypotheses specific to the alignment of SISP with hospital planning are extremely significant. Thus, the validity of these two hypotheses is as follows: Path 1: alignment of SISP with hospital planning →improving the competitive advantages of hospitals through IT, path coefficient = 0.427, p<0.001; and Path 2: alignment of SISP with hospital planning →satisfaction, path coefficient = 0.401, p<0.001.

The higher alignment of SISP with hospital planning indicates a higher possibility of reflecting the missions and objectives of business planning and providing additional insights into the competitive pressure of the external environment. The alignment of SISP with the hospitals' strategy planning has a significantly positive influence on improving the competitive advantages of hospitals through IT, which is consistent with the findings of Kearns and Lederer (2004). Furthermore, IT applications can be used to increase differential services and enhance the service capacity for customers and users, thereby improving the competitive advantage of hospitals and their capability to draw higher levels of user satisfaction. Improving the competitive advantage of hospitals is an important objective of IT application development. Enhancing customer satisfaction is one of the critical objectives of improving the efficiency of business operations. The higher alignment of SISP with overall planning of hospitals indicates that the senior managers can better understand the implications of using IT applications and, hence, promote better collaboration of IT planning and adoption with the support from CIOs.

5. CONCLUSION AND SUGGESTIONS

Nowadays, healthcare industries worldwide are changing their management practice due to the diverse nature and various perspectives of related problems. Since the implementation of the National Health Insurance Policy in 1995, hospitals in Taiwan have had to determine how to reduce medical expenses and in the meantime raise the quality of service to meet the demands of all citizens with the onset of information challenges. Furthermore, given that Medicare is granted only to certain groups of people, many Americans continue to view it as a universal national health insurance program (Fischer, 2006). The US has the most technologically intensive medical practice (Chernichovsky and Leibowitz, 2010). Thus, it is expected to receive great benefits from SISP in the early stage of healthcare reform since its implementation in March 2010. In the case of Taiwan, with government and public support, the results of this paper shows that factors such as environmental uncertainty, information intensity, information service competence, involvement of CIOs, and the alignment of SISP with hospital planning all have a significantly positive influence on the implementation of SISP in hospitals. Hospitals worldwide can work more efficiently with the implementation of SISP because it can assist organizations in terms of constructing plans as well as determining and identifying objectives.

According to the concept of external validity by Tsang and Williams (2012), this study gathered data from healthcare industry in Taiwan, which, per force, limits the generality of the results. SISP aims at developing a top-priority and sustainable IS. Thus, researchers should make the long-term assessments, develop the comparisons at different times, and then determine if the influence of environmental factors on SISP varies in different time periods and locations in the future. Researchers may also need to investigate the managers of other industries, such as finance, to obtain different insights and thus strengthen the reliability of the results. The National Health Insurance policy was enacted in Taiwan in March 1995, and the revamped payment system had a decisive effect onto the business management strategy of hospitals. It also became a factor that causes the environmental uncertainty. This change has led to variations in healthcare payment systems, regulations, and requirements with different mediums and various claim processes. These results have created several complex effects on the healthcare insurance cards and the electronic medical record implementation of IT applications. The results of this study indicate that, in the case of lower environmental unpredictability, senior management considers the use of IT applications to benefit their SISP as more important.

This study guides further discussion and research in this academic field because the influence of information service competence on SISP and how it can benefit the healthcare industry were seldom addressed in past research. The results of this study also indicate a possible avenue by which SISP can be employed to improve management efficiency in the healthcare industry. Prior to preparing/drafting important health policies, starting a complete communication with all relevant stakeholders is essential. Policies must only be fully implemented after a consensus is reached. Doing so reduces the possibility of unpredictability, thereby creating a favorable situation in improving the competitive advantages of hospitals. Moreover, the implementation of global budget systems and the gradual increase of information budgets can raise significant concerns to the senior management level with regard to the effectiveness of information investment, which can offset accompanying costs. The involvement of CIOs in hospital planning and the alignment of SISP with the overall planning also help improve competitive advantage and the satisfaction of medical customers and users. To this end, senior management should strongly support and provide further insights in to the employment of IT applications while assisting CIOs in strengthening their medical knowledge for overall development. Furthermore, SISP should align with hospital planning to improve competitive advantage and enhance the satisfaction of customers and users, provided that CIOs have a strong medical knowledge and are actively involved with overall planning. Consequently, CIOs should not pay attention only to enhancing their IT capability, but also to enriching their medical knowledge so they can make better contributions to their respective hospitals.

REFERENCES

Abdisalam, I. S., Sharif, L., & Ahmed, M. (2011). Strategic Information Systems Planning as the Centre of Information Systems Strategies. *International Journal of Research and Reviews in Computer Science*, 2(1), 156–162.

Anderson, J. C., & Gerbing, D. W. (1988). Structural equation modeling in practice: A review and recommended two-step approach. *Psychological Bulletin, 103*(3), 411–423. doi:10.1037/0033-2909.103.3.411

Anderson, R. (2006). *Healthcare IT in Europe and North America.* National Audit Office.

Armstrong, C. P., & Sambamurthy, V. (1999). Information technology assimilation in firms: The influence of senior leadership and IT infrastructures. *Information Systems Research, 10*(4), 304–327. doi:10.1287/isre.10.4.304

Baets, W. (1992). Aligning information systems with business strategy. *The Journal of Strategic Information Systems, 1*(4), 205–213. doi:10.1016/0963-8687(92)90036-V

Baker, J. (2011). The Technology–Organization–Environment Framework. *Series of Integrated Series in Information Systems* (Vol. 28, pp. 231-245).

Bakos, J. Y., & Brynjolfsson, E. (1993). Information technology, incentives, and the optimal number of suppliers. *Journal of Management Information Systems, 10*(2), 37–53. doi:10.1080/07421222.1993.11517999

Bechor, T., Neumann, S., Zviran, M., & Glezer, C. (2010). A contingency model for estimating success of strategic information systems planning. *Information & Management, 47*(1), 17–29. doi:10.1016/j.im.2009.09.004

Bergeron, F., Buteau, C., & Raymond, L. (1991). Identification of strategic information systems opportunities: Applying and comparing two methodologies. *Management Information Systems Quarterly, 15*(1), 89–104. doi:10.2307/249439

Bergeron, F., Raymond, L., & Rivard, S. (2001). Fit in strategic information technology management research: An empirical comparison of perspectives. *Omega, 29*(2), 125–142. doi:10.1016/S0305-0483(00)00034-7

Boehm, B. W. (1988). A spiral model of software development and enhancement. *IEEE Computer, 5*, 61-72.

Byrd, T. A., Lewis, B. R., & Bryan, R. W. (2006). The leveraging influence of strategic alignment on IT investment: An empirical examination. *Information & Management, 43*(3), 308–321. doi:10.1016/j.im.2005.07.002

Case Study: Steven Hospital. (2001Hitachi Consulting. Strategic Information Systems Planning.

Chen, D. Q., Mocker, M., Preston, D. S., & Teubner, A. (2010). Information Systems Strategy: Reconceptualization, Measurement, and Implications. *Management Information Systems Quarterly, 34*(2), 233–259.

Chernichovsky, D., & Leibowitz, A. A. (2010). Integrating Public Health and Personal Care in a Reformed US Health Care System. *American Journal of Public Health, 2*(100), 205–211. doi:10.2105/AJPH.2008.156588 PMID:20019310

Chi, L., Jones, K. G., Lederer, A. L., Li, P., Newkirk, H. E., & Sethi, V. (2005). Environmental assessment in strategic information systems planning. *International Journal of Information Management, 25*(3), 253–269. doi:10.1016/j.ijinfomgt.2004.12.004

Choe, J.-M., Lee, Y.-H., & Park, K.-C. (1997). The relationship between the influence factors and the strategic applications of information systems. *European Journal of Information Systems, 7*(2), 137–149. doi:10.1057/palgrave.ejis.3000297

Clemons, E. K. (1986). Information systems for sustainable competitive advantage. *Information & Management, 11*(3), 131–136. doi:10.1016/0378-7206(86)90010-8

Clemons, E. K. (1991). Competition and strategic value of information technology. *Journal of Management Information Systems, 7*(2), 5–8. doi:10.1080/07421222.1990.11517886

Clemons, E. K., & Row, M. C. (1991). Sustaining IT advantage: The role of structural differences. *Management Information Systems Quarterly, 15*(3), 275–294. doi:10.2307/249639

Cusmano, M. A., & Selby, R. W. (1997). How Microsoft builds software. *Communications of the ACM, 40*(6), 53–61. doi:10.1145/255656.255698

Doherty, N.F., Marples, C.G., & Suhaimi, A. (1999). The relative success of alternative approaches to strategic information systems planning: an empirical analysis. *Strategic Information Systems, 8*, pp. 263-283.

Drucker, P. E. (1993). *Post-Capitalist Society*. New York: Harper Business Press.

Earl, M. J. (1993). Experiences in strategic information systems planning. *Management Information Systems Quarterly, 17*(1), 1–24. doi:10.2307/249507

Fischer, J. E. (2006). Surgical practice and medicine in the USA. *The Surgeon, 4*(1), 267–271. doi:10.1016/S1479-666X(06)80003-X PMID:17009545

Glazer, R. (1991). Marketing in an information-intensive environment: Strategic implications of knowledge as an asset. *Journal of Marketing, 55*(4), 1–19. doi:10.2307/1251953

Hair, J. F., Black, W. C., Babin, B. J., Anderson, R. E., & Tatham, R. L. (2006). *Multivariate Data Analysis* (6th ed.). New Jersey: Prentice Hall.

Henderson, J. C., & Venkatraman, N. (1993). Strategic alignment: Leveraging information technology for transforming organizations. *IBM Systems Journal, 32*(1), 4–16. doi:10.1147j.382.0472

Hovelja, T., Vasilecas, O., & Rupnik, R. (2013). A model of influences of environmental stakeholders on strategic information systems planning success in an enterprise. *Technological and Economic Development of Economy, 19*(3), 465–488. doi:10.3846/20294913.2013.818591

Hsieh, C. R., & Sloan, F. A. (2008). Adoption of Pharmaceutical Innovation and the Growth of Drug Expenditure in Taiwan: Is It Cost Effective? *Value in Health, 11*(2), 334–344. doi:10.1111/j.1524-4733.2007.00235.x PMID:18380646

Johnson, A. M., & Lederer, A. L. (2010). CEO/CIO mutual understanding, strategic alignment, and the contribution of IS to the organization. *Information & Management, 47*(3), 138–149. doi:10.1016/j.im.2010.01.002

Johnston, R. H., & Carrico, S. R. (1988). Developing capabilities to use information strategically. *Management Information Systems Quarterly, 12*(1), 37–48. doi:10.2307/248801

Karagozoglu, N. (1993). Environmental uncertainty, strategic planning, and technological competitive advantage. *Technovation, 13*(6), 335–347. doi:10.1016/0166-4972(93)90075-7

Kearns, G. S., & Lederer, A. L. (2004). The impact of industry contextual factors on IT focus and the use of IT for competitive advantage. *Information & Management, 41*(7), 899–919. doi:10.1016/j.im.2003.08.018

Khandwalla, P. N. (1973). Effect of competition on the structure of top management control. *Academy of Management Journal, 16*(2), 285–310. doi:10.2307/255329

Kuana, K. K. Y., & Chau, P. Y. K. (2001). A perception-based model for EDI adoption in small businesses using a technology–organization–environment framework. *Information & Management, 38*(8), 507–521. doi:10.1016/S0378-7206(01)00073-8

Lederer, A. L., & Mendelow, A. L. (1989). Coordination of information systems plans with business plans. *Journal of Management Information Systems, 6*(2), 5–19. doi:10.1080/07421222.1989.11517854

Lederer, A. L., & Mendelow, A. L. (1990). The impact of the environment on the management of information systems. *Information Systems Research, 1*(2), 205–222. doi:10.1287/isre.1.2.205

Lederer, A. L., & Salmela, H. (1996). Toward a theory of strategic information systems planning. *The Journal of Strategic Information Systems, 5*(5), 237–253. doi:10.1016/S0963-8687(96)80005-9

Lederer, A. L., & Sethi, V. (1988). The implementation of strategic information systems planning methodologies. *Management Information Systems Quarterly, 12*(3), 444–461. doi:10.2307/249212

Lederer, A. L., & Sethi, V. (1996). Key prescriptions for strategic information systems planning. *Journal of Management Information Systems, 1*(13), 35–62. doi:10.1080/07421222.1996.11518111

Lee, G. G., & Pai, J. C. (2003). Effects of organizational context and inter-group behavior on the success of strategic information systems planning: An empirical study. *Behaviour & Information Technology, 4*(22), 263–280. doi:10.1080/0144929031000136548

Lin, C. T., & Chang, H. F. (2010). Performance Evaluation for Medical Industry in Taiwan: Applying Grey Situation Decision Making. *Journal of Grey System, 3*, 219–226.

Miller, C. C., Glick, W. H., Wang, Y. D., & Huber, G. P. (1991). Understanding technology-structure relationships: Theory development and meta-analytic theory testing. *Academy of Management Journal, 34*(2), 370–399. doi:10.2307/256447

Miller, D., & Friesen, P. H. (1983). Strategy-making and environment: The third link. *Strategic Management Journal, 4*(4), 221–235. doi:10.1002mj.4250040304

Mohdzain, M. B., & Ward, J. M. (2007). A study of subsidiaries' views of information systems strategic planning in multinational organisations. *The Journal of Strategic Information Systems, 16*(4), 324–352. doi:10.1016/j.jsis.2007.02.003

Morris, S. A., Clark, J., Holmes, J., Clark, C., & Gambill, S. (2002). IT investment planning: The best hospitals. *Journal of Healthcare Information Management, 16*(2), 62–65. PMID:11941924

Neo, B. S. (1988). Factors facilitating the use of information technology for competitive advantage: An exploratory study. *Information & Management, 15*(4), 191–201. doi:10.1016/0378-7206(88)90045-6

Newkirk, H. E., Lederer, A. L., & Johnson, A. E. (2008). Rapid business and IT change: Drivers for strategic information systems planning. *European Journal of Information Systems, 17*(3), 198–218. doi:10.1057/ejis.2008.16

Niederman, F., Brancheau, J. C., & Wetherbe, J. C. (1991). Information systems management issues for the 1990s. *Management Information Systems Quarterly, 16*(4), 474–500.

Nolan, R. L. (1979). Managing the crisis in data processing. *Harvard Business Review, 57*(2), 115–126.

Parsons, G. L. (1983). Information technology: A new competitive weapon. *Sloan Management Review, 25*(1), 3–14.

Porter, M. (1985). Technology and competitive advantage. *The Journal of Business Strategy, 5*(6), 60–78. doi:10.1108/eb039075

Porter, M., & Miller, V. E. (1985). How information gives you competitive advantage. *Harvard Business Review, 63*(4), 149–160.

Prela, C. M., Baumgardner, G. A., Reiber, G. E., McFarland, L. V., Maynard, C., Anderson, N., & Maciejewski, M. (2009). Challenges in Merging Medicaid and Medicare Databases to Obtain Healthcare Costs for Dual-Eligible Beneficiaries. *PharmacoEconomics, 27*(2), 167–177. doi:10.2165/00019053-200927020-00007 PMID:19254049

Premkumar, G., & King, W. R. (1994). Organizational characteristics and information systems planning: An empirical study. *Information Systems Research, 5*(2), 75–109. doi:10.1287/isre.5.2.75

Preston, D. S., & Karahanna, E. (2009). Antecedents of IS Strategic Alignment: Analogical Network. *Information Systems Research, 20*(2), 159–179. doi:10.1287/isre.1070.0159

Raghunathan, B., & Raghunathan, T. S. (1991). Information Systems Planning and Effectiveness: An Empirical Analysis. *Omega, 19*(*2/3*), 125–135. doi:10.1016/0305-0483(91)90022-L

Raghunathan, T. S., & King, W. R. (1988). The impact of information systems planning on the organization. *Omega, 16*(2), 85–93. doi:10.1016/0305-0483(88)90039-4

Ravishankar, M. N., Pan, S. L., & Leidner, D. E. (2011). Examining the Strategic Alignment and Implementation Success of a KMS: A Subculture-Based Multilevel Analysis. *Information Systems Research, 22*(1), 39–59. doi:10.1287/isre.1080.0214

Reich, B. H., & Benbasat, I. (1990). An empirical investigation of factors influencing the success of customer-oriented strategic systems. *Information Systems Research, 1*(3), 325–347. doi:10.1287/isre.1.3.325

Sabherwal, R. (1989). *Strategic Utilization of Information Resources: A Contingency Approach* [Ph. D. Dissertation]. University of Pittsburgh.

Sabherwal, R., & King, W. R. (1992). Decision Processes for Developing Strategic Applications of Information Systems: A Contingency Approach. *Decision Sciences, 23*(4), 917–943. doi:10.1111/j.1540-5915.1992.tb00426.x

Silva, L., & Hirschheim, R. (2007). Fighting against windmills: Strategic information systems and organizational deep structures. *Management Information Systems Quarterly*, *31*(2), 327–354.

Tallon, P., & Pinsonneault, A. (2011). Competing Perspective on the Link between Strategic Information Technology Alignment and Organizational Agility: Insights from a Mediation Model. *Management Information Systems Quarterly*, *35*(2), 463–486.

Teo, T. S. H., & King, W. R. (1996). Assessing the impact of integrating business planning and IS planning. *Information & Management*, *30*(6), 309–321. doi:10.1016/S0378-7206(96)01076-2

Teo, T. S. H., & King, W. R. (1997). Integration between business planning and information systems planning: An evolutionary-contingency perspective. *Journal of Management Information Systems*, *14*(1), 185–214. doi:10.1080/07421222.1997.11518158

Teo, T. S. H., & King, W. R. (1999). An empirical study of the impacts of integrating business planning and information systems planning. *European Journal of Information Systems*, *8*(8), 200–210. doi:10.1057/palgrave.ejis.3000334

Terry, K. (2012, November 15). EHR adoption: U.S. remains the slow poke. *Information Week*. Retrieved from http://www.informationweek.com/healthcare/electronic-medical-records

Tornatzky, L. G., & Fleischer, M. (1990). *The Processes of Technological Innovation*. Lexington, Massachusetts: Lexington Books.

Tsang, E. W., & Williams, J. N. (2012). Generalization and induction: Misconceptions, clarifications, and a classification of induction. *Management Information Systems Quarterly*, *36*(3), 729–748.

Velcu, O. (2010). Strategic alignment of ERP implementation stages: An empirical investigation. *Information & Management*, *47*(3), 158–166. doi:10.1016/j.im.2010.01.005

Venkatraman, N., & Prescott, J. E. (1990). Environment-strategy coalignment: An empirical test of its performance implications. *Strategic Management Journal*, *11*(11), 1–23. doi:10.1002mj.4250110102

Vitale, M. R., Ives, B., & Beath, C. M. (1986). Linking information technology and corporate strategy: an organizational view. *Proceedings of the 7th International Conference on Information Systems*, San Diego (pp. 265-276).

Wilkin, C.L., & Cerpa, N. (2012). Strategic Information Systems Planning: An Empirical Evaluation of Its Dimensions. *Journal of Technology Management & Innovation*, 7(2), 52-62.

Zubovic, A., Pita, Z., & Khan, S. (2014, June 24-28). A Framework for Investigating the Impact of Information Systems Capability on Strategic Information Systems Planning Outcomes. *Proceedings of Pacific Asia Conference on Information Systems 2014*, Chengdu, China.

This research was previously published in the Journal of Global Information Management (JGIM), 24(1); edited by Zuopeng (Justin) Zhang; pages 14-36, copyright year 2016 by IGI Publishing (an imprint of IGI Global).

APPENDIX

Table 6. Sources of items and scale of variables

Research Variable	Source of Scale	Item
Environmental Uncertainty		
Dynamism	Teo and King (1997)	1. Your medical service mode is outdated or phased out very quickly. 2. Your hospital's know-how is quickly applied to medical services. 3. Your senior management can predict the future orientation of the competitors. 4. Your senior management can predict the changing requirements on medical services.
Heterogeneity	Teo and King (1997)	1. There is a big difference in hospitalization habits for patients. 2. There is a big difference in the nature of competition between your hospital and other competitors. 3. There is a big difference in the medical services offered by your hospital.
Hostility	Teo and King (1997)	1. Insufficient staff will pose a threat to the normal operation and survival of your organization. 2. Insufficient material supply will pose a threat to the normal operation and survival of your organization. 3. Serious price-cutting competition will pose a threat to the normal operation and survival of your organization. 4. Strict medical services' quality competition will pose a threat to the normal operation and survival of your organization. 5. Strict medical services' differentiation competition will pose a threat to the normal operation and survival of your organization.
Information Intensity		
Value chain specific information intensity	Kearns and Lederer (2004)	1. Information is widely applied to your medical services. 2. Information for the medical services is frequently updated. 3. Information for the medical services is extremely accurate. 4. Different information must be used often during the medical services.
Information Service Competence		
Information service competence	Teo and King (1997)	1. Your hospital fully ignores the know-how associated with the information system. 2. Your hospital is equipped with a number of computer equipment. 3. Your hospital boasts of leading information system technology in the medical care sector. 4. The services delivered by your information system are often unreliable. 5. Your CIO has abundant medical knowledge. 6. Your CIO can identify future business challenges and plans.
IT Dependency of Hospitals		
IT dependency of hospitals	Kearns and Lederer (2004)	1. Any shutdown of the existing information system will lead to serious consequences. 2. Any program mistake of the existing information system will seriously affect the patients' satisfaction. 3. Temporary manual operation is not feasible in case of malfunction of the computer specific to the existing information system. 4. The routine operation of your hospital depends greatly on the existing information system. 5. The existing information system has many indispensable online, real-time transaction, or batch processing functions.
Involvement of CIO in Hospital Planning		
Involvement of CIO in planning	Kearns and Lederer (2004)	1. Your CIO can attend the business planning meeting regularly. 2. Your CIO contributed to the drafting of the hospital's business objectives. 3. Your CIO regularly keeps informal contact and liaises with the executives of your hospital. 4. Your CIO can easily call the director of your hospital. 5. Your CIO regularly keeps in contact and liaises with the director of your hospital.

continued on following page

Table 6. Continued

Research Variable	Source of Scale	Item
Alignment of SISP with Hospitals' Planning		
Alignment of SISP with hospital planning	Kearns and Lederer (2004)	1. Your SISP can reflect the mission of your business planning. 2. Your SISP can reflect the objective of your business planning. 3. Your SISP can support your business strategy. 4. Your SISP can help identify the competitive pressure of external environment. 5. Your SISP can reflect the restrictions of resources in the planning.
Improving Competitive Advantage by IT		
Improving competitive advantage by IT	Kearns and Lederer (2004)	1. Your hospital can apply IT to create competitive advantages by reducing cost or increasing service differentiation in terms of core medical services, major customer groups, and suppliers. 2. Your hospital can apply IT to establish electronic links with the suppliers and customers in terms of core medical services, major customer groups, and suppliers. 3. Your hospital can apply IT to add barriers in market access against the competitors in terms of core medical services, major customer groups, and suppliers. 4. Your hospital can apply IT to make the patients alter their decisions and transfer to your hospital in terms of core medical services, major customer groups, and suppliers. 5. Your hospital can apply IT to strengthen the unique service capability in terms of core medical services, major customer groups, and suppliers.
Satisfaction		
User satisfaction	Premkum-ar and King (1994)	1. How can your information system contribute to user satisfaction?
Customer satisfaction	Teo and King (1999)	1. How can your information system contribute to customer satisfaction?

Chapter 10
Lessons Learned from the Implementation of an Emergency Department Information System

Paraskevas Vezyridis
University of Nottingham, UK

Stephen Timmons
University of Nottingham, UK

Heather Wharrad
University of Nottingham, UK

ABSTRACT

Clinical information systems are increasingly used in emergency departments across the English National Health Service. The implementation outcome is unpredictable and success is not guaranteed. This study identifies facilitating social and technical factors for implementing an Emergency Department Information System. This is a qualitative study, using interviews with 28 emergency department clinicians, administrators and managers. Project management documents, user guides, design blueprints and internal reports were also analysed. Lessons learned include the importance of acquiring an established, customised and user-friendly system, attracting funding, establishing communication channels between stakeholders, developing detailed implementation plans and tailored training programmes, investing in peer-support, and analysing the workflow impact of the system. Socio-technical factors, both in and out of the hospital, influenced the success of the implementation. By being systematic in addressing these socio-technical factors certain implementation barriers can be overcome.

DOI: 10.4018/978-1-7998-2451-0.ch010

Copyright © 2020, IGI Global. Copying or distributing in print or electronic forms without written permission of IGI Global is prohibited.

INTRODUCTION

Emergency departments (EDs) require sophisticated information technology (IT) for managing their complex operations. Despite a rather low adoption rate (Landman, Bernstein, Hsiao, & Desai, 2010), introducing such clinical information systems can assist EDs in the provision of quality care (Aronsky, Jones, Lanaghan, & Slovis, 2008). EDs are thus well equipped to improve their efficiency (Baumlin & Richardson, 2006) through more accurate forecasting of demand and better resource allocation (Stuart, 2004). This is particularly true as patient volume, crowding and acuity continue to rise (Shapiro et al., 2010), whilst the number of inpatient beds decreases (Baumlin et al., 2010).

However, the outcome of the implementation of a clinical information system in practice is often unpredictable and success is not always guaranteed. Even in cases where failure in the process of deploying a system is attributed to specific technical inconsistencies or deficiencies, there are always issues and parameters outside the sphere of influence of IT staff that need to be considered; issues that are rooted in the organisation or in the surrounding social environment in which the system is designed to operate (Berg, 1998). There is also the issue of time. Hillestad et al. (2005) assert, for example, that for a system to prove its efficiency a widespread adoption is required. Only after a certain period of time, process changes, and resource reduction will the potential cost effectiveness or quality improvements become clear. Thus, it is necessary to consider both technology and the organisation as concepts that intertwine with one another to produce something new. Despite technology's capacity to act as an agent for change, organisational change is often a prerequisite for the deployment of new technologies (Grimson & Grimson, 2002). This is because it is the established organisational norms and values that provide the context of this interaction and, often, determine the outcome of the implementation (Berg, 2001).

In this chapter, the authors attempt to contribute to an increasing body of knowledge around the lessons that can be learned from these types of programmes. They studied an Emergency Department Information System (EDIS) for patient registration and tracking in an ED of a large University NHS hospital in England: the first clinical information system that was successfully implemented under the National Programme for Information Technology (NPfIT). They have previously identified clinical users' initial reactions and interacting concerns with EDIS (Vezyridis, Timmons, & Wharrad, 2012). Here, by adopting a qualitative approach, based on interviews and document analysis, the study evolved around the identification and analysis of the *wider* social, technical, economic and policy factors, conditions and processes that have impacted upon its initial diffusion. The particular research questions were:

- Why was this particular system selected for deployment? Was the selection of this system internal or external to the organisation process?
- How was this project initiated and how did this implementation proceed?
- What are the practical lessons that can be learned from this implementation?

BACKGROUND

Emergency Department Information Systems

First pioneered in Australia in 1994 (New South Wales Department of Health [NSW DH], 1998), Emergency Department Information Systems can provide EDs with computing capabilities for electronic *registration* and *triage*, real-time patient flow and care *tracking*, *charting* (time-stamped patient care documentation and continuity, remuneration, benchmarking and critical pathways), *referencing* (information about medications, interactions, diagnoses, treatments and best practices), *prescribing, order entry* and finally *discharging* (clinical and non-clinical information for discharge, follow-up instructions and recommendations) (DeWoody & Loadman, 1999; Righini, 2002; Rowe et al., 2006; Shapiro et al., 2010). A fully functional EDIS may also provide access to past medical history, follow-up notes and electronic imaging, transmission of prescriptions to pharmacies and decision support (Landman et al., 2010). Therefore, it can be used as an effective set of tools for managing workload, forecasting demand and allocating resources (Stuart, 2004); improving all aspects of care, from throughput and turnaround times (Weiner, Baumlin, & Shapiro, 2007) to satisfaction for patients and staff alike (Wiler et al., 2010).

In the US, the implementation and use of EDIS is thought to improve workflows with quick (3-6 months) return on investment (ROI) (Rogoski, 2002), particularly for cost savings (coding, dictation, transcription, paper use, medication errors) and revenue captures (charges, reimbursement, increased patient visits) (Fisher & Tibbs, 2003; Anderson, 2005). Other cost, time, performance and satisfaction benefits claimed (due to automation) include (Neal, 2003; Fisher & Tibbs, 2003; Garvie, 2004; Anderson, 2005; Bouchard, 2005; Berghoef, 2006):

- Elimination of illegible prescriptions, lost patient records, duplications and *bottlenecks*.
- Improved clinical documentation for patient registration and tracking.
- Increased time for direct patient care.
- Increased clinical accountability and improved evaluation of clinical performance.
- Improved patient data protection.
- Reduced average length of stay for patients and, increased patient satisfaction and staff morale.

Challenges and Barriers of EDIS Implementation

However, although these systems claim to reduce expenditures, by replacing the costly paper record with technology, few cost-benefit analyses are available in the market for purchasers to make evidence-based decisions (Milbank Memorial Fund, 2000). Their methods and outcome measures, and also the accuracy and completeness of the information they collect (Coonan, 2004), are often questionable (Wiler et al., 2010). Numerous studies have highlighted reasons why these and other clinical information systems, despite their supposed potential, have not been widely accepted or fully integrated into health systems around the world.

For example, there can be certain features of the system or certain characteristics of the hospital that may have a negative impact on the implementation, such as multiple departments within the hospital with different cultures and work practices, adequacy of communication between vendors and hospital managers, the financial circumstances of the hospital, performance ratings, existing information technology infrastructure and timetables for replacement of existing systems (Hendy, Reeves, Fulop, Hutchings, & Masseria, 2005). There are also issues of high cost, a lack of mature products, the complexity of the clinical setting, users' computer competence and data input that challenge their deployment (Burton, Anderson, & Kues, 2004; Hier, Rothschild, Lemaistre, & Keeler, 2005). Other studies have found perceived implementation costs for training, change management, loss of revenue, operational control, disruption to practice, negative impact on clinician-patient relationship and work pressure as substantial barriers to the computerisation of clinical tasks (for more see Johnston, Leung, Wong, Ho, & Fielding,

2002). Importantly, clinicians' data privacy concerns around security breaches and tampering of patients' records are thought to negatively impact adoption (Yoon, Chang, Kang, Bae, & Park, 2012; Inokuchi et al., 2014). Since most of these systems have been developed for the Anglophone healthcare IT market, the system's language has also been identified as a significant barrier (Inokuchi et al., 2013).

Especially in the user context, factors include age, gender and personality characteristics, specialty and experience, expectations and interests, computer literacy, emotions and attitudes towards health informatics and, commitment of clinical leadership (Young, 1984; Anderson, Jay, Schweer, & Anderson, 1986; Cork, Detner, & Friedman, 1998; O'Connell, Cho, Shah, Brown, & Shiffman, 2004). A lack of clarity amongst the users about the advantages of such systems has also been identified (Sujansky, 1998). These user aspects have been identified in several theories, such as the technology acceptance model (TAM), the unified theory of acceptance and use of technology (UTAUT), the innovation diffusion theory (IDT), the theory of planned behaviour (TPB) and the theory of reasoned action (TRA). However, as Najaftorkaman, Ghapanchi, Talaei-Khoei, & Ray (2014) note in their systematic literature review these theories, while they identify most of the *individual*, *psychological* and *behavioural* factors in healthcare IT adoption, they tend to ignore other, sometimes equally important, *financial* (start-up and on-going costs, ROI), *legal* (security, privacy, liability, policies and standards), *environmental* (job security, vendor efforts, prior experience), *organisational* (age, size and type of practice, experience, ownership, workflows) and *technical* (system customisability, reliability and usability) factors.

Other experts such as Eason (2005) assert that clinical information systems will be abandoned if a user-centred, local design approach is not rolled out. He goes on to suggest that only by understanding local ambitions, studying sociotechnical design, establishing local planning teams and constantly reviewing systems' implications and users' experiences can the system be saved from failure. The selection of an appropriate system relies heavily upon issues of intuitiveness, user-friendliness and comprehensiveness, in order to persuade users to input the data (Rogoski, 2002) as well as on the system's ability to be integrated to existing IT infrastructures (Neal, 2003). The majority of successful stories of implementing an EDIS refer to the need of establishing a strategic interdisciplinary committee, consisting of nurses, physicians, clerical staff, information technologists, finance officers and departmental administrators, for selecting the system and leading the change management (Bouchard, 2005; Anderson, 2005; Taylor, 2006; Berghoef, 2006; Wickramasinghe, Tumu, Bali, & Tatnall, 2007). From there, the transition to computing usually begins by marketing the system internally and preparing for big learning curves. This is achieved by a *phased implementation* (Wickramasinghe, et al. 2007), where modules and core components are gradually installed and integrated to the main system, providing staff with time to get accustomed to new workflows and developing competent *super users* for training, demonstrating and assisting the other users around the system (Garvie, 2004; Taylor, 2006).

METHODS

Case Study Profile

The study was conducted in the ED of a large university NHS hospital in England. It serves a local population of 650,000 and treats approximately 400 attendees per day (60% discharged, 25% admitted and 15% referred as outpatients). With around 14-18 nurses, 6-7 doctors and 6 emergency department assistants (EDAs), all of various grades and experience, on duty at any given time and across its six sections (Areas 1, 2 & 3, paediatric, X-ray and Emergency Nurse Practitioners' offices), it is now one of the busiest in the UK.

The EDIS studied was implemented in October 2004 through a *phased implementation* (Wickramasinghe et al., 2007) and under the Projects in Controlled Environments (PRINCE2) integrated project management framework (Office of Government Commerce [OGG], 2012). Previously, patient registration was completed by clerical staff at the reception desk using the hospital's main Patient Administration System (PAS), while nurses and physicians were using a single, three-page, paper form to record and store observations, investigations, clinical notes and drug prescriptions. Now, after (the electronic) registration at the reception desk by EDAs, clinicians can use EDIS to enter triage details, observations, clinical notes, consultations, prescribed medicines and investigations, view alerts and track patients around the ED. This *first phase* of the implementation also involved the interfacing to the trolley wait system and to PAS as well as the rollout of the module for the production of General Practitioners (GPs) letters. For accessing EDIS, there are password-protected desktop terminals in each staff station, the reception desk, the Sisters' office and the doctors' writing room, while 13 wall-mounted workstations were installed inside the cubicles. The system's hardware requirements were scoped at 100-150 concurrent users.

Data Collection

Data were collected through semi-structured interviews (approximately 4.5 years after implementation), while potential participants were recruited via purposive, snowball sampling. The only selection criterion was that participants had started working in the ED for at least a year before the implementation of EDIS. Each interview was 30 minutes long on average (15 hours in total) and all but two of them were digitally audio-recorded. Participants were asked to recall and describe their experience with EDIS implementation. Written materials about the implementation were also examined, including; project management documents (implementation planning study, project initiation, site specific tasks, project review), user guides, reference manuals, business cases, paper forms, contingency plans, minutes, policy documents, and financial reports. In this way, views and assumptions from people closer to the implementation and from the organisational viewpoint were collected, while the project management documents contributed to an understanding of the organisational and professional context of the implementation process.

Data Analysis

These documents and the interview transcripts were then organised and analysed with the use of Computer Assisted Qualitative Data Analysis Software (QSR NVivo 8). Through a thematic analysis (Dixon-Woods, Agarwal, Jones, Young, & Sutton, 2005), prominent, recurrent and inclusive thematic categories were identified. Then, these thematic headings and coding categories were cross-referenced for relevance, consistency and relationships. Careful consideration was given so as not to exclude activities, processes or accounts that offer limited explanatory value, however semi-statistical constructions like *most of the users* were used as to highlight stronger and prevalent themes.

The study was approved by the local Research Ethics Committee. Participants were given an information sheet and individual written consent was obtained. Data were stored securely, and all findings reported anonymously.

FINDINGS

Participants

Twenty-eight participants (23 female and 5 male), mainly ED clinicians, were interviewed for this study: 1 system administrator, 1 change manager, 2 EDAs, 1 operational services coordinator, 4 ENPs, 4 charge nurses (NICs), 15 nurses of various grades and experience.

Lesson 1: Timing

This study highlights the importance of choosing the right moment when implementing EDIS. By this, we mean building and maintaining a positive momentum by converging the interests and commitment of relevant stakeholders (ED, ICT teams and vendor).

This includes being alert for IT procurement funding and waiting until the system of choice is available. Here, the hospital's clinical, operational and strategic management had been investigating systems for 4 years and had identified this EDIS as their system of choice. However, cost was prohibiting its acquisition. With the advent of the NPfIT, the ED was finally able to acquire the system free of charge and with adequate technical and legal support under the Local Service Providers (LSP) scheme (Brennan, 2005). Yet, contracts with the LSP were still under central negotiation and the rollout was not planned until the next year (2005). To overcome this obstacle, the hospital's Director of ICT had the NPfIT and the LSP to agree to a tactical early adoption of the system. Sometimes, however, this momentum can be strengthened further by new requirements imposed on the ED from outside the hospital. In this particular case, there were several additional requirements that acted as an impetus for this implementation, since:

- From January 2005, it had to formally report to the DH on waiting times and achieve the 4hr wait target (DH, 2004).
- At the same time, investigations, consultations, special treatments, diagnostics and admissions had to be accurately recorded for correct payments, under the Payments by Results (PbR) financial scheme.
- From 2005, the Commissioning Data Set (CDS) was being mandated.
- Each December-March, it always faces *winter pressures*.
- At the end of 2004, the vendor's time slot to fully concentrate on this implementation was expiring and no onsite support would have been available afterwards.

In addition, following specific recommendations by NHS Estates (2003; 2004), a major refurbishment of the ED had been completed one year before implementation. The department now featured 9 resuscitation bays, compared to the previous 4, and 26 adult treatment cubicles for minor and major illnesses/injuries, compared to the previous 12.

The department layout changed radically...it's compartmentalised so without EDIS I don't think the new actual department layout and accommodation would have been as practical and as useful as it is now.

Therefore, as the working environmental, clinical, service and informational needs of the department changed drastically, the use of a clinical information system became a necessity. In fact, a key factor in the acceptability of EDIS was that it challenged the efficacy of existing, hand-written, systems for time-sensitive information management. For example, the traditional whiteboard and the paper records have limited calculative and sharing capabilities, making it difficult to handle patient tracking with pen and paper or magnetic strips in an ED which had recently doubled its capacity to treat patients.

We'd always been keen to have a new system for the new department because we knew by expanding it physically it was going to become more difficult to manage it practically...we needed a new way of managing the information that we had about patients with all the targets that have come in since...

I suspect that if we had to go back to the whiteboard and relying on a nurse's memory as to where a patient was at any given time, I think we would soon start to see a lot more four hour breaches...actually being able to track times of patients to see how we are doing and where the weak points are, that's a big advantage.

By securing additional funding for hardware upgrades to support the new software, and by making this project a high priority for the hospital, in March 2004 a tight (6-month) timescale for the implementation of EDIS was set.

Lesson 2: Project Management

The EDIS was, at the time, quite popular within the NHS, with several hospitals having implemented it already[1]. This was important, as it had already been modified, to a certain extent, to NHS practice. Therefore, the hospital project team had the opportunity to visit other sites and learn from their experience. It also meant that the hospital did not have to spend additional resources on in-house development of EDIS.

However, the hospital did not have a desired plan of action for this implementation. The Implementation Planning Study (IPS), devised by the vendor in collaboration with the hospital's project team, provided this detailed plan of how the implementation should be organised, what each member of the team had to do and what tasks and actions had to be carried out. In particular, it defined objectives, scopes and benefits, personnel and resources, hardware and software requirements, training, delineation of roles and responsibilities as well as risks and contingencies. It was, therefore, well received by the hospital implementation team.

... the idea of an implementation planning study was absolutely spot on, it was brilliant, it's the sort of thing that I wish we adopted more in that for three days we lived and breathed how we were going to do EDIS.

From there, four implementation teams, each with a project manager, were established. One team from the vendor and one from the hospital were responsible for the implementation until the go-live date, with the other two (again, one from the vendor and one from the hospital) assuming their responsibilities after that day. The vendor and ED project managers were responsible for developing the project management documents so that a plan was agreed and followed by both teams. The ED project manager was responsible for measuring whether the project was managed successfully and that an acceptable product was delivered.

While the whole of implementation on the *shop floor* was organised by the project managers and the above two teams, a hospital project board dealt with the overall management of the project at a higher level. This board had the overall responsibility, accountability and authority to provide direction and management for the success of the project. It consisted of a *Senior User* (an ED Consultant), the *Senior Supplier* (the hospital's Director of ICT) and a *Project Sponsor* (Executive member of the hospital). This structure, by taking advantage of the rapid deployment of EDIS, was found to be beneficial in the development of direct communication channels and, therefore, of a better working relationship with the vendor.

Importantly, *Clinical Leads* had a fundamental role in the implementation of EDIS and in change management. The authors have previously reported that clinical users' initial reactions to EDIS implementation evolved around issues of technology integration and transition to paperless practices, computer-based information provision as well as issues of computer literacy and system availability (Vezyridis et al., 2012). The Clinical Leads, as experienced clinicians, constituted the link between the shop floor, the vendor of the system and the project board, representing users' views during project team meetings, communicating to the users the organisational and technical processes to be followed, while actively advocating and promoting the system's benefits among their more apprehensive colleagues. They were also involved in user training and support. Lastly, they provided the vendor with detailed departmental workflows so as to analyse the system's organisational impact and make it compatible with the department's work practices.

One of the key things that I did was almost like a patient process looking at where each of the patients would go through, which gave the software team an understanding of how our Department worked... Once the software had been installed ..we were then involved in setting up all the various EDIS pages and settings and entering various diagnostic codes and things like that, in conjunction with the ICT teams as well..

However, the more configurations the systems had to undergo the more likely it was for the project to hit difficulties with severe deployment delays. A balance had to be reached. In the end, it was decided that the two subsequent phases, with more advanced and site-specific modifications, (e.g. interfaces to other hospital main systems and departments) could be completed later (under a maintenance and support services agreement) as the users and the department acquired greater working knowledge of the system. The first crucial phase concentrated on EDIS basic capabilities for patient registration and tracking, and tracking of tariff-based investigations, such as configuring modules (clinical workflow, task management, clinical documentation, orders, prescribing, alerts, allergies), interfacing to PAS and the trolley wait system, producing GP letters, web linking to Pathology and Radiology and, regional and site-specific code setting (diagnosis, minimum data set). Despite this, EDIS was unable to meet the hospital's reporting requirements and the department had to make its own arrangements for ad hoc reporting via a third party application.

Lesson 3: Training

Particularly in big departments, training all potential users is not an easy task. In this ED, approximately 275 members of staff, with a further 100 non-ED staff, were identified for training. After the vendor's recommendations, a *Train the Trainer* methodology was adopted. The vendor trained 8 core trainers who then trained 30 *super users*. Training sessions and documentation were organised by the vendor who also assisted in the delivery of training by the core trainers to the front users. Three two-hour training slots for each clinician-user were arranged 3-4 months before the go-live day, in a dedicated (close to the ED) computer room with around 15 workstations in place. Users were also encouraged to spend any available time playing with the system at their own pace.

The training programme included development of both basic Microsoft Windows and EDIS functionality skills. This was important as users were expected to navigate themselves between the various computer screens with two new devices (keyboard and a mouse) so as to locate, from an array, several *text boxes*, to *move* patients on the *map* area of the system, to *save* the cubicles for a patient that had gone for an x-ray or electronically discharge a particular patient and to *save* data input once they completed typing. At the same time, this increased attention to the development of keyboard and navigation skills was adding to the users' fear of mishandling the system and making mistakes that could not be rectified later on, affecting the quality of the information electronic patient records hold. In fact, one thing that users immediately realised, to their great disappointment, was that what gets *saved* it stays for good. While on paper they could write something down and later rub it or cross it out, in EDIS nothing could be deleted or even spell-checked. Therefore, all data entry and reporting had to be completed accurately, affecting speed of use.

In the end, the tight timescale for the implementation and the lack of adequate funding to buy out work time resulted in only a handful of super users being trained and ready for the go live day. Also, while pocket-sized user guides and manuals were developed to guide users through the system, their uptake was limited as their linear structure and technical language were abhorred by most clinicians without previous exposure to computer use.

Lesson 4: Support

During the crucial first weeks after go-live, support involved overstaffing the ED and placing computer competent clinical users, hospital IT staff and the clinical leads within the department to help those less competent. Initially they focused on the reception desk to support clerical staff in registering new patients via EDIS. *Handhold* sessions were also in place particularly for the clinical areas and for certain periods, talking staff though the use of the system.

Just being there really, I spent a lot of hours that week we went live here in the department, about 80, 85 hours actually physically present in the department, hand holding, showing them how to do things, making sure things were running smoothly.

Importantly, users who managed to grasp the system quickly were sharing information and knowledge with their colleagues about filling in text boxes, navigating through screens and menus, moving patients through the system, 'saving' clinical notes and rectifying data entry mistakes (Vezyridis et al., 2012). This additional support was very helpful particularly during those difficult hours when the department was experiencing immense pressures while opportunities to bleep the IT Helpdesk or the software trainers were not available (out-of-hours).

Lots of people were finding little ways around things, by working it out on the computer and then telling you, you know, I've found this, this is how you do it and you make it quicker. So you know, as we found little things we all just told each other.

… so you did have support if you were unsure about something and people were quite patient, you know, with people that are a bit stupid!

Implementation teams should also consider the issue of seniority and how it correlates with age and computer competence. This is important because these users not only had to familiarise themselves with a new, technologically mediated practice, but were also expected to provide technical support to other, junior members of staff. As professional seniority may be related to a bigger EDIS learning curve, this new role may not be embraced as expected, as the system disturbs their relationships with junior staff and displaces them from the centre of clinical network within the ED:

You've perhaps got a charge nurse or a sister…very experienced…can lead the whole department and has been the nurse in charge for years… and then suddenly they are put in EDIS and they were put way out of their comfort zones and people were looking to them to help them and they were frightened of it…

The role of the *system administrator* was also developed for departmental autonomy regarding training of new users, basic support, maintenance, user account management and reporting. From there, the system administrator (an EDA) could also liaise further with the hospital ICT team and the vendor for issues such as downtime resolution, scheduled upgrading and software modification.

Lastly, while wall-mounted EDIS terminals were also installed inside the cubicles for users to directly input clinical notes during patient assessment, these were not widely used. For most of the times, clinicians expressed their preference for paper note-taking at the bedside, particularly those who were feeling embarrassed by their lack of computing typing skills and speed. Also, there were times when these terminals were obstructed by medical equipment. Other reasons for not using these terminals included their fixed position on the wall which was not always ergonomically convenient for users of different heights, occasions when clinicians had to turn their back to a patient who seemed to be agitated or when it was preferable to keep certain information more confidential (e.g. domestic violence, mental health issues) and not having patients looking over their shoulders as they typed in their notes. This, however, resulted in congestion at the main staff desk as clinicians were trying to find an available desktop to work on.

DISCUSSION

The implementation of EDIS was completed successfully within a tight, but realistic, timescale. The 4hr wait time target acted as an impetus for several changes to take place. Before the system was introduced, the built environment and the reconfiguration of patient flows were drastically reconfigured, challenging traditional information management artefacts (dry-erase whiteboard, paper records), but causing overcrowding around computer terminals by clinicians waiting to get access to them for data input. A multidisciplinary hospital project team of enthusiastic and motivated members attracted adequate funding and, with the vendor's help, set out a detailed plan of action to carry out the implementation, including working out EDIS's impact on current workflows. Early adoption allowed for some customisation of the system to meet local requirements. Despite the preparation of a good number of super users and user manuals, adoption by users was facilitated by an inspiring and consistent clinical leadership as well as by intensive peer support post go-live. A summary of key recommendations for implementing EDIS follows:

Healthcare Organisation

- Ensure an active project board
- Accurately identify all stakeholders and involved personnel (ICT, ED, vendor), and assign specific roles
- Assemble two project teams, one from the hospital and one from the vendor
- Assemble an experienced and mixed hospital project team (clinical and ICT)
- Perform work and information flows analyses to determine organisational impact and resolve issues
- Train project teams on hospital's procurement procedures
- Develop and practice downtime contingency plans before going live
- Develop adequate interfaces with any legacy hospital systems (e.g. trolley wait, PAS)
- Perform extended testing/piloting (including usability testing) for user acceptance
- Attract additional financial resources for supportive software and hardware (e.g. printers and printing material, spare equipment for breakdowns)
- Expect delays in cabling the ED, ordering workstations and printers, development of local specifics and interfaces
- Maintain open communication channels between ED and hospital ICT
- Continuously monitor and evaluate data quality (from day one)

System Vendor

- Experienced in ED implementations in the context of NHS
- Provides an Implementation Planning Study
- Agree on regular ED visits, meetings and (de)briefings with hospital project team for onsite feedback and progress
- Agree on specific communication channels between project teams
- Provides advice and support on hardware acquisition (e.g. servers, cabling, terminals, network) and training programme
- Clarify level of involvement and relationships between vendor, LSP and hospital
- Clarify framework and level of technical support
- Open and flexible to customise EDIS and develop interfaces to existing systems according to requirements
- Clarify timescale for full concentration on implementation
- Clarify framework and level of support after go-live, particularly on working hours

User Training

- Clarify training requirements with vendor and tailor programme to audience
- Work on getting majority of staff trained and buy-out ED staff time
- Locate a computer room, with demo software installed on terminals, close to (or within) the ED
- Widely advertise training sessions across staff and provide flexible training hours
- Develop repeated short sessions for each user rather than few long ones
- Follow a *Train the Trainer* approach within the ED for autonomy
- Identify computer proficient core trainers
- Assign core training in software and in hardware use to EDIS vendor
- Balance Microsoft Windows and mouse skills set across user base
- Include training on workarounds and shortcuts (with caution)
- Invest in super-user training
- Be prepared to extend training as technical delays unfold

User Support

- Identify experienced and enthusiastic Clinical Leads and provide them with time and resources to be present in the ED, but be prepared for their burn out
- Prepare hospital ICT team to step in when vendor becomes slow to respond
- Rely more on face-to-face (e.g. meetings) and less on read communication
- Engage middle management and staff
- Make provisions for on call and out-of-hours ICT helpdesk
- Invest in *handholding* and peer support for longer than expected
- Raise awareness across the whole hospital of what is happening in the ED and why
- Identify decision makers and problem solvers and place them on the *shop floor*
- Identify skilled super-users and arrange a good number of them in each shift, but expect their limited, incremental contribution during first weeks after go-live
- Develop user guides to fit staff's pockets, but expect an incremental reliance on them
- Expect reduced departmental performance during the first weeks after going live

Some of these results have also been found by other researchers who examined barriers to successful IT implementations in similar settings (see Khalifa, 2013). For example, Avgar, Litwin, & Pronovost, (2012) believe an organisation is more likely to adopt health IT if the specific solution serves its strategic (performance) objectives and reinforces its organisational practices, the department has the operational capacity to innovate and the frontline staff has the necessary set of skills and involvement in the implementation process. Handel, Wears, Nathanson, & Pines, (2011), in their consensus paper, identified the analysis of "patient flow and integration into clinical work" (p. e47) and usability testing as crucial steps to determine the impact of the system on the delivery of care and to increase system's user-friendliness. Clayton et al. (2005) suggest that extended testing/piloting can determine user acceptance and number of concurrent users the system can sustain, while Ash, Stavri, Dykstra, & Fournier, (2003b) add high-level integration with legacy systems for speed and continuity of care. For all this, Dinh and Chu (2006), and Inokuchi et al., (2014) emphasise the importance of adequate funding, not only for software and hardware but also for on-going maintenance. It is also important to set realistic timescales (Handel & Hackman, 2010) to avoid disappointment and loss of enthusiasm by people on the *shop floor*.

In any case, contracting a suitable vendor, specialised in EDIS development and with a system open to modifications, is essential to a successful outcome. Da've (2004) considers an experienced, resourceful and financially healthy vendor to be better in guiding the implementation with minimum delays, adequate communication and support in the long run (Inokuchi et al., 2014). Also, the American College of Emergency Physicians [ACEP] (2009) seems to be more favourable of vendors knowledgeable of the ED clinical reality as they are more likely to have a system that meets the specific ED requirements. The vendor's role in EDIS implementation may extend further into the training of users and ACEP notes that this important and often neglected process has financial implications that should be equally addressed. They also suggest identifying competent core trainers for delivering repeated, short and flexible training sessions (ACEP 2009), while Clayton et al. (2005) emphasise the buy-out of as much staff time as possible to encourage participation.

For wider support, Ash et al. (2003a; 2003b) emphasise the importance of identifying active multidisciplinary project teams (clinicians, technologists and leaders) and, generally, having *special people* in all levels of leadership and support (administrative, clinical and technological). Handel and Hackman (2010) highlighted the need for recruiting experienced and enthusiastic Clinical Leads, characterised, as Ash et al. (2003b) have found, by advanced social (positive, persistent, influential and understanding) skills. In fact, a systematic review by Ingebrigtsen et al. (2014) found that skilled and experienced, with IT project management, clinical leaders are more visionary and motivated to commit long-term to successful organisational and clinical outcomes from the implementation. Serving as liaisons between clinical, technical and hospital staff, these champions can "ensure safe and efficient EDIS operations" (Farley et al., 2013, p. 403).

During go-live, Ash et al. (2003a) suggest an extensive period of *handholding* and peer support on the *shop floor* for several weeks when reduced performance is expected (Meadors, Benda, Hettinger, & Ratwani, 2014; Handel & Hackman, 2010), while Fenton, Giannangelo, & Stanfill, (2006) suggest providing users with on call and out-of-hours ICT helpdesk access. Since unscheduled system downtimes (network infrastructure and servers failures, power outages) (Hoot, Wright, & Aronsky, 2003) is the harsh reality in a computerised practice, Handel and Hackman (2010) note that contingency plans need to be developed and practiced well in advance. Lastly, we too, in accordance with Svenson, Pollack, Fallat, & Drapeau, (2003) and Gordon, Flottemesch, & Asplin, (2008), emphasise continuous monitoring and validation of EDIS data from day one for avoiding misclassifications (e.g. discharge, admission) or incorrect timestamps of ED events. Without adequate training and supervision, the department might end up having its staff misinterpreting these reporting terms, which could result in the production of inaccurate information for process evaluation and performance improvement (Avgar et al., 2012).

Study Limitations

As the study was limited to a single clinical setting, implementing one commercial system, generalisations should be made with caution. Other EDs may benefit from alternative approaches due to differences in size, resources, procurement and contractual arrangements, workflows, infrastructure, built environment, leadership, staffing levels and workload. In addition, the sample, although small, was of the appropriate size for the nature of the topic, objectives, design, quality of data and, importantly, ED-specific conditions (high levels of workload and staff turnover) which made difficult the recruitment of participants who met selection criteria. While poor recall of prior experiences in participants is always an issue in individual interviews, we were able to collect more crystallised accounts about the implementation processes that have persisted over time. We also complemented these qualitative findings with information from several project documents. Lastly, although this study examined an implementation that occurred 8 years ago, its findings are still relevant today. While adoption rates of fully functional EDIS remain low (Landman et al., 2010), the market is steadily growing. Particularly in England, more hospitals acquire Emergency Department Information Systems than ever before (e.g. Mid Staffordshire, Blackpool, Morecambe Bay) as the NPfIT (now under the responsibility of the Health and Social Care Information Centre) is far from complete.

FUTURE RESEARCH DIRECTIONS

The literature on case studies from EDs that have implemented EDIS is very limited, as any lessons learned usually stay with the respective organisation. Given the facts that this EDIS was one of the first to go live under the NPfIT and NHS hospitals today still have to use the same project management framework (PRINCE2), the findings of this study are particularly illuminating. The authors hope that through this paper, they promote inter-organisational knowledge sharing. However, more similar studies are required to conduct cross-case comparisons (Sheikh et al., 2011) so as to facilitate the safe adoption of best practices. These can be enriched by observations during implementation to explicate the subtle details and fine nuances of the complex interactions not included in interviews and written materials. Lastly, they, too, suggest that a more sociotechnical approach to the examination of processes, concerning both the people and the technologies involved (Greenhalgh et al., 2010), will better incorporate the local circumstances of individual settings into project management planning.

CONCLUSION

The authors have presented some valuable lessons from one implementation of EDIS at a large university hospital that other EDs might find useful when deploying similar systems. EDIS is a technology that can improve documentation, clinical flows and, consequently, patient care. However, it takes time and effort before such systems can find their place in the ED. While performance indicators might create the necessary impetus, these kinds of projects are complex in nature and should not be treated as straightforward deployments. From the design and installation of the system to user training and support, relationships between staff and with the vendor, careful planning and motivated stakeholder involvement are required for a successful outcome.

REFERENCES

American College of Emergency Physicians. (2009). *EDIS: primer for emergency physicians, nurses, and IT professionals*. Irving, TX: ACEP SEMI.

Anderson, J. G., Jay, S. J., Schweer, H. M., & Anderson, M. M. (1986). Why doctors don't use computers: Some empirical findings. *Journal of the Royal Society of Medicine*, 79, 142–144. PMID:3701749

Anderson, P. (2005). Building on Success. *Health Management Technology*, 26(5), 32–34. PMID:15932071

Aronsky, D., Jones, I., Lanaghan, K., & Slovis, C. M. (2008). Supporting Patient Care in the Emergency Department with a Computerized Whiteboard System. *Journal of the American Medical Informatics Association*, 15(2), 184–194. doi:10.1197/jamia.M2489 PMID:18096913

Ash, J. S., Fournier, L., Stavri, P. Z., & Dykstra, R. (2003a). Principles for a Successful Computerized Physician Order Entry Implementation. In *AMIA Symposium Proceedings*. Washington, DC: American Medical Informatics Association.

Ash, J. S., Stavri, P. Z., Dykstra, R., & Fournier, L. (2003b). Implementing computerized physician order entry: The importance of special people. *International Journal of Medical Informatics*, 69(2-3), 235–250. doi:10.1016/S1386-5056(02)00107-7 PMID:12810127

Avgar, A. C., Litwin, A. S., & Pronovost, P. J. (2012). Drivers and barriers in health IT adoption: A proposed framework. *Applied Clinical Informatics*, 3(4), 488–500. doi:10.4338/ACI-2012-07-R-0029 PMID:23646093

Baumlin, K. M., & Richardson, L. D. (2006). Emergency Department Information System (EDIS) Success: EDIS Implementation Improves Documentation and Increases Charges and Revenue. *Academic Emergency Medicine, 13*(5Supplement 1), s61. doi:10.1197/j.aem.2006.03.138

Baumlin, K. M., Shapiro, J. S., Weiner, C. Gottlieb, B., Chawla, N., & Richardson, L. D. (2010). Clinical Information System and Process Redesign Improves Emergency Department Efficiency. *Joint Commission Journal on Quality and Patient Safety, 36*, 179-1AP.

Berg, M. (1998). Medical work and the computer-based patient record: A sociological perspective. *Methods of Information in Medicine, 37*, 294–301. PMID:9787631

Berg, M. (2001). Implementing information systems in health care organizations: Myths and challenges. *International Journal of Medical Informatics, 64*(2-3), 143–156. doi:10.1016/S1386-5056(01)00200-3 PMID:11734382

Berghoef, H. (2006). (Good) growing pains. Michigan ED automates patient tracking, nurse documentation and charge capture to maintain excellent customer service, increase efficiencies and boost revenue. *Health Management Technology, 27*(3), 30–35. PMID:16594517

Bouchard, M. (2005). What works. ED on Track With IT. *Health Management Technology, 26*(8), 28–31. PMID:16156525

Brennan, S. (2005). *The NHS IT project: the biggest computer programme in the world ever!* Abingdon: Radcliffe.

Burton, L. C., Anderson, G. F., & Kues, I. W. (2004). Using electronic health records to help coordinate care. *The Milbank Quarterly, 82*(3), 457–481. doi:10.1111/j.0887-378X.2004.00318.x PMID:15330973

Clayton, P. D., Narus, S. P., Bowes, W. A., III, Madsen, T. S., Wilcox, A. B., & Orsmond, G., ...Leckman, L. (2005). Physician use of electronic medical records: Issues and successes with direct data entry and physician productivity. In *AMIA Annual Symposium Proceedings*. Washington, DC: American Medical Informatics Association.

Coonan, K. M. (2004). Medical informatics standards applicable to emergency department information systems: Making sense of the jumble. *Academic Emergency Medicine, 11*(11), 1198–1205. doi:10.1111/j.1553-2712.2004.tb00705.x PMID:15528585

Cork, R. D., Detner, W. M., & Friedman, C. P. (1998). Academic physicians' use of, knowledge about, and attitudes toward computers: Measurement study and validation. *Journal of the American Medical Informatics Association, 5*, 164–176. doi:10.1136/jamia.1998.0050164 PMID:9524349

Da've, D. (2004). Benefits and barriers to EMR implementation. *Caring, 23*(11), 50–51. PMID:15633313

Department of Health. (2004). *Improving Emergency Care in England, Report by the Comptroller and Auditor General (HC 1075 Session 2003–2004)*. London: National Audit Office.

DeWoody, S., & Loadman, G. P. (1999). Implementing an Emergency Department Information System – How Complicated Can We Make This? *Journal of Healthcare Information Management, 13*(3), 19–30. PMID:10787597

Dinh, M., & Chu, M. (2006). Evolution of health information management and information technology in emergency medicine. *Emergency Medicine Australasia, 18*(3), 289–294. doi:10.1111/j.1742-6723.2006.00855.x PMID:16712540

Dixon-Woods, M., Agarwal, S., Jones, D., Young, B., & Sutton, A. (2005). Synthesising qualitative and quantitative evidence: A review of possible methods. *Journal of Health Services Research & Policy, 10*(1), 45–53B. doi:10.1258/1355819052801804 PMID:15667704

Eason, K. (2005). Exploiting the potential of the NPfIT: A local design approach. *British Journal of Healthcare Computing & Information Management, 22*, 14–15.

Estates, N. H. S. (2003). *The impact of the built environment on care within A&E departments: Key findings and recommendations*. London: The Stationery Office.

Estates, N. H. S. (2004). *A&E design evaluation. Evaluation of two proposed accident and emergency departments: Brent Emergency Care and Diagnostic centre at Central Middlesex Hospital, and an Exemplar Plan*. London: The Stationery Office.

Farley, H. L., Baumlin, K. M., Hamedani, A. G., Cheung, D. S., Edwards, M. R., Fuller, D. C., ... Pines, J. M. (2013). Quality and safety implications of emergency department information systems. *Annals of Emergency Medicine, 62*(4), 399–407. doi:10.1016/j.annemergmed.2013.05.019 PMID:23796627

Fenton, S. H., Giannangelo, K., & Stanfill, M. (2006). Essential people skills for EHR implementation success. *Journal of American Health Information Management Association, 77*, 60A–60D. PMID:16805302

Fisher, W., & Tibbs, E. W. (2003). What works. Three phases of EDIS. Installation of a comprehensive emergency department information system enables a Virginia IDN to revitalize its ED services. *Health Management Technology, 24*, 36–40. PMID:12647615

Garvie, D. (2004). Strategic Planning Supports ED Automation. *Health Management Technology, 25*(11), 34–36. PMID:15551708

Gordon, B. D., Flottemesch, T. J., & Asplin, B. R. (2008). Accuracy of staff-initiated emergency department tracking system timestamps in identifying actual event times. *Annals of Emergency Medicine, 52*(5), 504–511. doi:10.1016/j.annemergmed.2007.11.036 PMID:18313799

Greenhalgh, T., Stramer, K., Bratan, T., Byrne, E., Russell, J., & Potts, H. W. (2010). Adoption and non-adoption of a shared electronic summary record in England: A mixed-method case study. *BMJ (Clinical Research Ed.), 340*(jun16 4), c3111. doi:10.1136/bmj.c3111 PMID:20554687

Grimson, J., & Grimson, W. (2002). Health care in the information society: Evolution or revolution? *International Journal of Medical Informatics, 66*(1-3), 25–29. doi:10.1016/S1386-5056(02)00032-1 PMID:12453554

Handel, D. A., & Hackman, J. L. (2010). Implementing electronic health records in the emergency department. *The Journal of Emergency Medicine, 38*(2), 257–263. doi:10.1016/j.jemermed.2008.01.020 PMID:18790591

Handel, D. A., Wears, R. L., Nathanson, L. A., & Pines, J. M. (2011). Using information technology to improve the quality and safety of emergency care. *Academic Emergency Medicine, 18*(6), e45–e51. doi:10.1111/j.1553-2712.2011.01070.x PMID:21676049

Hendy, J., Reeves, B. C., Fulop, N., Hutchings, A., & Masseria, C. (2005). Challenges to implementing the national programme for information technology (NPfIT): A qualitative study. *BMJ (Clinical Research Ed.), 331*(7512), 331–336. doi:10.1136/bmj.331.7512.331 PMID:16081447

Hier, D. B., Rothschild, A., Lemaistre, A., & Keeler, J. (2005). Differing faculty and housestaff acceptance of an electronic health record. *International Journal of Medical Informatics, 74*(7-8), 657–662. doi:10.1016/j.ijmedinf.2005.03.006 PMID:16043088

Hillestad, R., Bigelow, J., Bower, A., Girosi, F., Meili, R., Scoville, R., & Taylor, R. (2005). Can Electronic Medical Record Systems Transform Health Care? Potential Health Benefits, Savings, And Costs. *Health Affairs, 24*(5), 1103–1117. doi:10.1377/hlthaff.24.5.1103 PMID:16162551

Hoot, N., Wright, J. C., & Aronsky, D. (2003). Factors contributing to computer system downtime in the emergency department. In *AMIA Annual Symposium Proceedings*. Washington, DC: American Medical Informatics Association.

Ingebrigtsen, T., Georgiou, A., Clay-Williams, R., Magrabi, F., Hordern, A., Prgomet, M., ... Braithwaite, J. (2014). The impact of clinical leadership on health information technology adoption: Systematic review. *International Journal of Medical Informatics, 83*(6), 393–405. doi:10.1016/j.ijmedinf.2014.02.005 PMID:24656180

Inokuchi, R., Sato, H., Nakajima, S., Shinohara, K., Nakamura, K., Gunshin, M., ... Yahagi, N. (2013). Development of information systems and clinical decision support systems for emergency departments: A long road ahead for Japan. *Emergency Medicine Journal, 30*(11), 914–917. doi:10.1136/emermed-2012-201869 PMID:23302505

Inokuchi, R., Sato, H., Nakamura, K., Aoki, Y., Shinohara, K., Gunshin, M., ... Nakajima, S. (2014). Motivations and barriers to implementing electronic health records and ED information systems in Japan. *The American Journal of Emergency Medicine, 32*(7), 725–730. doi:10.1016/j.ajem.2014.03.035 PMID:24792932

Johnston, J. M., Leung, G. M., Wong, J. F., Ho, L. M., & Fielding, R. (2002). Physicians' attitudes towards the computerization of clinical practice in Hong Kong: A population study. *International Journal of Medical Informatics, 65*(1), 41–49. doi:10.1016/S1386-5056(02)00005-9 PMID:11904247

Khalifa, M. (2013). Barriers to health information systems and electronic medical records implementation. A field study of Saudi Arabian hospitals. *Procedia Computer Science, 21*, 335–342. doi:10.1016/j.procs.2013.09.044

Landman, A. B., Bernstein, S. L., Hsiao, A. L., & Desai, R. A. (2010). Emergency Department Information System Adoption in the United States. *Academic Emergency Medicine, 17*(5), 536–544. doi:10.1111/j.1553-2712.2010.00722.x PMID:20536810

Meadors, M., Benda, N., Hettinger, A. Z., & Ratwani, R. M. (2014). Going Live Implementing an Electronic Health Record System in the Emergency Department. *Proceedings of the International Symposium of Human Factors and Ergonomics in Healthcare, 3*, 44-49. 10.1177/2327857914031006

Milbank Memorial Fund. (2000). *Better Information, Better Outcomes?: The Use of Health Technology Assessment and Clinical Effectiveness Data in Health Care Purchasing Decisions in the United Kingdom and the United States*. New York: Milbank Memorial Fund.

Najaftorkaman, M., Ghapanchi, A. H., Talaei-Khoei, A., & Ray, P. (2014). A taxonomy of antecedents to user adoption of health information systems: A synthesis of thirty years of research. *Journal of the Association for Information Science and Technology, 66*(3), 576–598. doi:10.1002/asi.23181

Neal, K. (2003). ROI in the ED. *Health Management Technology*, (November): 2003. PMID:14608714

NSW Department of Health. (1998). *Emergency Department Information System: Information Management and Technology Audit*. Sydney: NSW Department of Health.

O'Connell, R. T., Cho, C., Shah, N., Brown, K., & Shiffman, R. N. (2004). Take Note(s): Differential EHR Satisfaction with Two Implementations under One Roof. *Journal of the American Medical Informatics Association, 11*(1), 43–49. doi:10.1197/jamia.M1409 PMID:14527978

Office of Government Commerce. (2012). *PRINCE2*. Retrieved from http://www.prince-officialsite.com

Righini, N. (2002). *Information Systems in the Emergency Departments. HM 816: Healthcare Information System*. Boston University School of Management.

Rogoski, R. R. (2002). IT in the ED. The nature of emergency department medicine means specific and comprehensive IT needs for clinicians. *Health Management Technology, 23*, 14–16. PMID:11842574

Rowe, B. H., Bond, K., Ospina, M. B., Blitz, S., Schull, M., Sinclair, D., & Bullard, M. (2006). Data collection on patients in emergency departments in Canada. *Canadian Journal of Emergency Medicine, 8*, 417–424. PMID:17209491

Shapiro, J. S., Baumlin, K. M., Chawla, N., Genes, N., Godbold, J., Ye, F., & Richardson, L. D. (2010). Emergency Department Information System Implementation and Process Redesign Result in Rapid and Sustained Financial Enhancement at a Large Academic Center. *Academic Emergency Medicine, 17*(5), 527–535. doi:10.1111/j.1553-2712.2010.00720.x PMID:20536809

Sheikh, A., Cornford, T., Barber, N., Avery, A., Takian, A., Lichtner, V., ... Cresswell, K. (2011). Implementation and adoption of nationwide electronic health records in secondary care in England: Final qualitative results from prospective national evaluation in 'early adopter' hospitals. *BMJ (Clinical Research Ed.), 343*(1), d6054. doi:10.1136/bmj.d6054 PMID:22006942

Stuart, P. (2004). A casemix model for estimating the impact of hospital access block on the emergency department. *Emergency Medicine Australasia, 16*(3), 201–207. doi:10.1111/j.1742-6723.2004.00587.x PMID:15228462

Sujansky, W. V. (1998). The benefits and challenges of an electronic medical record: Much more than a "word-processed" patient chart. *The Western Journal of Medicine, 169*, 176–183. PMID:9771161

Svenson, J. E., Pollack, S. H., Fallat, M. E., & Drapeau, J. L. (2003). Limitations of electronic databases: A caution. *The Journal of the Kentucky State Medical Association*, *101*, 109–112. PMID:12674902

Taylor, C. (2006). The Waiting Room Is Closed. *Health Management Technology*, *27*(4), 24–28. PMID:16629252

Vezyridis, P., Timmons, S., & Wharrad, H. J. (2012). Implementation of an Emergency Department Information System: A Qualitative Study of Nurses' Attitudes and Experience. *Computers, Informatics, Nursing*, *30*, 540–546. PMID:23079482

Weiner, C., Baumlin, K. M., & Shapiro, J. S. (2007). Process redesign and emergency department information system implementation improve efficiency. *Academic Emergency Medicine*, *14*(5 Supplement 1), s72. doi:10.1197/j.aem.2007.03.901

Wickramasinghe, N., Tumu, S., Bali, R. K., & Tatnall, A. (2007). Using Actor Network Theory (ANT) as an analytic tool in order to effect superior PACS implementation. *International Journal of Networking and Virtual Organisations*, *4*(3), 257–279. doi:10.1504/IJNVO.2007.015164

Wiler, J. L., Gentle, C., Halfpenny, J. M., Heins, A., Mehrotra, A., Mikhail, M. G., & Fite, D. (2010). Optimizing Emergency Department Front-End Operations. *Annals of Emergency Medicine*, *55*(2), 142–160. doi:10.1016/j.annemergmed.2009.05.021 PMID:19556030

Yoon, D., Chang, B.-C., Kang, S. W., Bae, H., & Park, R. W. (2012). Adoption of electronic health records in Korean tertiary teaching and general hospitals. *International Journal of Medical Informatics*, *81*(3), 196–203. doi:10.1016/j.ijmedinf.2011.12.002 PMID:22206619

Young, D. W. (1984). What makes doctors use computers?: Discussion paper. *Journal of the Royal Society of Medicine*, *77*, 663–667. PMID:6481741

KEY TERMS AND DEFINITIONS

4hr Wait Target: From January 2005, the English Department of Health required 98% (now 95%) of patients to be treated, admitted or discharged in four hours from the time they enter the emergency department.

Commissioning Data Sets (CDS): A basic structure for accurate data collection and analysis of clinical activity, demand forecasting and commissioning on an on-going basis (e.g. discharges, elective and emergency daily admissions, demand profiles, causes of breaches, length of stay).

Early Adoption: This strategy of IT procurement, where a system is deployed at an early stage, while it exposes an organisation to many problems and risks, it can also attract additional resources, secure more time for testing and deployment, and increase an organisation's input in the shaping of the final system to meet particular requirements. It can also foster greater enthusiasm and commitment to the success of the project.

Local Service Provider: An industry partner responsible for delivering the English NPfIT to healthcare organisations across a geographical cluster under the guidance of the NHS IT Director and a ministerial team.

National Programme for Information Technology (NPfIT): Established in 2002 in England, as one of the largest healthcare IT projects in the world, this programme aspired a common national approach in the deployment of electronic patient records, electronic prescribing, broadband networking, electronic booking for appointments, Picture Archiving and Communications Systems (PACS), GP payments and a central email and directory service across the NHS.

PRINCE (PRojects IN Controlled Environments): A de facto, flexible, standard used by governments and the private sector to establish a common language between customers, users and suppliers by addressing planning, delegation, monitoring and control of the six variables involved in any project: costs, timescales, quality, scope, risk and benefits.

Payments by Results: A public policy instrument used in the English NHS to decentralise rewards and payments in an attempt to instil concepts of self-management and accountability in hospitals. It associates carefully recorded and measured clinical activity with payments based on specific investigation and treatment coding lists.

Shop Floor: The clinical workplace where all patient assessment, treatment and management takes place.

Super Users: Enthusiastic with information systems and computer competent senior clinical staff responsible for basic troubleshooting advice and support to front users, particularly for out-of-hours. After advance training in all aspects of the system, they also act as trainers for new personnel on an on-going basis.

Winter Pressures: During winter, the cold weather and influenza as well as healthcare system's inefficiencies drive up demand for hospital admissions and trolley wait space on emergency departments, due to an increase of mortality and morbidity in the elder, very young and chronically ill population.

ENDNOTE

[1]   The Australian-based vendor of the system had a successful record of implementations in more than 145 emergency departments in Australia, Canada and the UK, making it one of the leading actors in this market.

This research was previously published in Maximizing Healthcare Delivery and Management through Technology Integration edited by Arthur Tatnall and Tiko Iyamu; pages 237-256, copyright year 2016 by Medical Information Science Reference (an imprint of IGI Global).

Chapter 11
A Simulation Knowledge Extraction–Based Decision Support System for the Healthcare Emergency Department

Manel Saad Saoud
University of Bordj Bou Arreridj, Algeria

Abdelhak Boubetra
University of Bordj Bou Arreridj, Algeria

Safa Attia
University of Bordj Bou Arreridj, Algeria

ABSTRACT

Nowadays, healthcare systems services have become a serious concern for many countries across the world. Due to its complexity and Variability the Emergency Department (ED) is considered the most critical unit of the hospital and the healthcare systems in general. Increasing the patient satisfaction, reducing as much as possible the patient's waiting time and the patient's length of stay, and optimizing the resources utilization are the overriding preoccupation for any ED manager. To support the performance enhancement in the ED, simulation studies have profusely been involved. In this paper the authors describe a decision support system based on the combination of a simulation and a temporal knowledge extraction model for the operation improvement of the emergency department in the public hospital Lakhdar Bouzidi in Bordj Bou Arreridj (Algeria). Their methodology points out how agent-based modeling simulation can benefit from data mining analysis methods to provide a powerful decision support system that can help managers to improve the functioning of the ED.

DOI: 10.4018/978-1-7998-2451-0.ch011

Copyright © 2020, IGI Global. Copying or distributing in print or electronic forms without written permission of IGI Global is prohibited.

1. INTRODUCTION

Healthcare system is a sensitive and critical sector that has become a serious concern for most governments across the world. Accordingly, many researchers have become increasingly interested in modeling and improving the efficiency of such complex and dynamic systems. The efficiency of the healthcare systems has often been measured and related to the effectiveness of hospitals and their departments, more particularly the Emergency Department (ED), due to its complexity and variability compared to other hospital departments. Crowdedness, high demand (patient flow) for services, long waiting time and limited healthcare resources (doctors, nurses, equipment, space…) are the key problems that the emergency department managers must cope with. Furthermore, the emergency staff is required to adapt to those conditions and to provide a quick and appropriate care for all patients.

In order to improve the performance of the emergency department by reducing patients' waiting time, decreasing the patients' length of stay, optimizing the resources utilization, and increasing patients throughput (number of patient served), ED managers ought to have a good patient flow management and to find the optimal ED staff configurations. However, the unplanned and unpredictable nature of patients' arrival hinders the managers to achieve this task. Hence, developing decision support systems using computer simulation methods can be the best solution to anticipate and help ED managers choosing the adequate and efficient decision strategies and policies.

In recent years, simulation has profusely been used to model healthcare systems since it allows researchers to understand them better and analyze efficiently their functioning. Different simulation techniques have been presented in order to provide powerful systems that can help the managers to enhance the quality of services in the ED. A large portion of these studies have focused on the discrete event simulation (Evans, Gor, & Unger, 1996; Duguay & Chetouane, 2007; Konrad, et al., 2013) or the agent based modeling simulation (Cabrera, Taboada, Iglesias, Epelde, & Luque, 2012; Cabrera, Taboada, Iglesias, Epelde, & Luque, 2011; Jones & Evans, 2008).

Adopting simulation approaches facilitates the examination of different ''what-if'' scenarios and the evaluation of possible policies and changes in the system without making costly decisions and uncertain changes in the real one. Agent-based modeling is one of the most powerful simulation techniques that helps researchers to analyze a complex system such as the emergency department due to its ability to model systems close to the reality, to represent heterogeneous individuals and their interactions, to observe their behaviors and to understand their interrelations. In this paper, in addition to the choice of the multi-agent-based simulation model (programmable modeling environment Netlogo (Wilensky, 1999)), we used two data mining techniques (Pujari, 2001; Fayyad, Piatetsky-Shapiro, & Smyth, 1996; Hegland, 2001; Han, Kamber, & Pei, 2011) called respectively "preprocessing methods" and "linear regression", to design a decision support system for the improving operation of the emergency department in the public hospital Lakhdar Bouzidi in Bordj Bou Arreridj (Algeria) and help the ED managers to enhance the quality of care provided. The first technique was used to process the simulation inputs and the second one to investigate the relationship between the patients' arrival time and the acuity levels. Due to these latter techniques, we could find the optimal staff configurations and the simulation results showed that the average waiting time, the average length of stay and doctors' utilization have been consequently, improved considerably.

The remainder of this paper is organized as follows; Section two focus on the simulation within the healthcare. Section three describes how the emergency department is functioning. In Section four, the phases of design and development of the proposed simulation model using data mining techniques are displayed. The proposed system verification and validation is presented in the fifth section, while the model results and discussion are given in section six. Finally, the paper is closed with the conclusion and prospects.

2. BACKGROUND

Many simulation studies have been touched on the different ways to enhance the quality of care in the emergency department. The authors in (Evans, Gor, & Unger, 1996) proposed a simulation model using Arena software package, the model developed investigated various schedules for nurses, doctors and ED technicians in order to reduce the average patient time in the system. A discrete event simulation study of an emergency department was described in (Duguay & Chetouane, 2007). To reduce waiting times, the methodology was based on considering physicians, nurses, and examination rooms as control variables and modeling and simulation were performed using Arena software. In (Konrad, et al., 2013) a discrete event simulation model was built to support process improvement in ED. The authors presented a split-flow process and evaluated the impact of different splitting patient flow configuration through the simulation on the patient length-of-stay and patient congestion in the ED. In order to help emergency department heads in setting up management guidelines to improve the operation of EDs a decision support system (DSS) for healthcare EDs using an agent-based modeling simulation was presented (Cabrera, Taboada, Iglesias, Epelde, & Luque, 2012; Cabrera, Taboada, Iglesias, Epelde, & Luque, 2011). To find out the optimal ED staff configuration the authors used Exhaustive Search (ES) optimization. The study presented in (Jones & Evans, 2008) developed an agent-based simulation tool using NetLogo software to evaluate the impact of various physician staffing configurations on patient waiting times in the ED. In (Connelly & Bair, 2004) the authors developed and operated a new platform for computer simulation of ED activity named Emergency Department SIMulation (EDSIM). The EDSIM model was then used to compare the fast-track triage approach with an alternative acuity ratio triage (ART) approach.

The paper presented in (Rossetti, Trzcinski, & Syverud, 1999) discussed the use of computer simulation to test and analyze the impacts of alternative ED attending physician staffing schedules on patient throughput and resource utilization. The model also used to identify process inefficiencies and to evaluate the effects of staffing, layout, resource and patient flow changes on system performance. The authors in (Hoot, et al., 2008) focused on the forecast of emergency department crowding using discrete event simulation. The ForecastED simulation model was developed and validated to predict near-future ED operational measures. A case study of a discrete event simulation model of an Accident and Emergency Unit at a hospital in the UK. A novel approach to modeling the arrival pattern of patients was utilized which represented the random and deterministic nature of the arrivals. The simulation case study was performed using the MedModel simulation package (Meng & Spedding, 2008). The authors in (Laskowski, McLeod, Friesen, Podaima, & Alfa, 2009) applied both agent-based models (ABM) and queuing model (QM) techniques to investigate patient access and patient flow through emergency departments. The models were developed independently the ABM approach was applied to investigate scenarios for resource optimization within the operations of an ED (for example, staffing scenarios). The QM approach facilitates quantitative analysis of operational parameters in EDs (for example, wait times). A simulation model of the Emergency Department of Special Health Care at the Central Hospital of Jyväskylä, Finland has been developed in (Ruohonen, Neittaanmaki, & Teittinen, 2006) using the simulation package MedModel. A new operational method called the triage team method was presented.

The authors demonstrated the effects of this method on the effectiveness of the ED more precisely on the patient waiting times and patient throughput time.

A decision support tool for the operation of ED unit at a governmental hospital in Kuwait was presented (Ahmed & Alkhamis, 2009). The methodology combined simulation with optimization to identify the optimal staffing configuration and to evaluate the impact of various staffing on ED service efficiency, patient throughput and waiting time. An interactive simulation-based decision support framework for healthcare process improvement was presented in (Abo-Hamad & Arisha, 2013). The framework integrated balanced scorecard (BSC) as a performance management tool to support continuous and sustainable improvement by using strategic-linked performance measures and actions. The authors presented a simulation model for the operation in ED at Cooper Health Systems (Samaha, Armel, & Starks, 2003). This methodology helped to avoid costs and allowed Cooper Health System to focus on making only the changes that would provide the needed benefit reducing the length of stay within the Emergency Department. In (Komashie & Mousavi, 2005) the paper discussed the application of discrete event simulation for the operation of an emergency department. The model was developed as a tool for helping ED managers to understand the behavior of the system concerning hidden causes of excessive waiting times. A simulation-based decision support system (DSS) to prevent and predict strain situations in an ED was developed in (Kadri, Chaabane, & Tahon, 2014). A discrete-event simulation model was constructed to visualize the strain situations, examine the relationship between the strain situations and propose corrective actions. To reduce the average waiting time of the patient in the ED, improve the nurses' utilization, and increase the number of served patients a simulation study and Data Envelopment Analysis (DEA) were applied (Al-Refaie, Fouad, Li, & Shurrab, 2014).

In (Kuo, Rado, Lupia, Leung, & Graham, 2015)the paper presented a case study that used simulation to analyze patient flows in a hospital emergency department in Hong Kong. To obtain a good estimation of input parameters of the simulation model, the authors proposed a simulation–optimization approach (integrating simulation with meta-heuristics). The paper presented in (Masmoudi, Leclaire, Cheutet, & Casalino, 2014) described the modeling and simulation of the patient's stay process at the ED. The authors also presented a method of modeling doctors' availability in the emergency department taking into account their number and availability in trauma and medicine areas. In (Lim, Worster, Goeree, & Tarride, 2013) the authors presented an alternative approach where physicians and their delegates in the ED are modeled as a hierarchy of heterogeneous interacting pseudo-agents in a discrete event simulation (DES) and to compare it with the traditional approach ignoring such interactions.

Knowledge based systems and decision support systems have been widely adopted in many scientific areas, more especially in healthcare systems. A knowledge based system for the clinical information management system is presented in (Kalogeropoulos, Carson, & Collinson, 2003). In (Bose, 2003) a knowledge management-enabled health care management system is introduced. The research provided in one hand, a decision support infrastructure for clinical and administrative decision-making. In the other hand, it helped integrate clinical, administrative, and financial processes in health care through a common technical architecture. A fuzzy cognitive map medical decision support system for the hospital admission procedure of elderly patients is presented in (Georgopoulos & Stylios, 2013). A simulation based decision support model is used in (Oh, et al., 2016) in order to improve emergency department throughput.

Data mining techniques has exceedingly used in healthcare systems. Authors in (Yeh, Wu, & Tsao, 2011) presented a decision support system that combines temporal abstraction with data mining techniques to predict hospitalization of hemodialysis patients. A model that simplifies massive data of unknown characteristics in the triage database at a Taiwanese regional hospital using the cluster analysis and the rough set theory is built in (Lin, Wu, Zheng, & Chen, 2011). To analyze the forecasting model of patients' demand in the Emergency department (Yang, Lin, Chen, & Shi, 2009) data mining, classification and a decision tree were adopted. (Isken & Rajagopalan, 2002) demonstrated the application of K-means cluster analysis of data mining techniques to support the development of computer simulation models. In (Lin, et al., 2010) A model based on the application of the cluster analysis and the decision tree analysis on the abnormal diagnoses in an emergency department of a Taiwan Medical Center is built.

3. SYSTEM DESCRIPTION

The public hospital Lakhdar Bouzidi in Bordj Bou Arreridj (Algeria) has become a destination for many patients and injured, in view of the large demographic growth and the important strategic location of the state of Bordj Bou Arreridj, where it is considered as a connecting link between the east, west and south of Algeria.

Lakhdar Bouzidi emergency department is open 24 hours a day, seven days a week and receive an average of 470 patients daily with a variable inter-arrival time and various patients' condition and illness acuity.

3.1. Physical Layout

The ED is composed of; 4 waiting zones (consultation rooms' waiting area, laboratory's waiting area, X-ray's waiting area, and nursing room's waiting area), 3 consultation rooms (considered as the first contact between the doctor (physician) and the patient. It used to treat the patients arriving from the consultation rooms' waiting area), a laboratory(used just for medical analysis of patients arriving in ED), X-ray(ED X-ray room used just for ED patients), nursing room (used for injections, Cleansing and suturing of wounds, and bandages), observation unit (equipped and devoted to patients whose need a treatment and monitoring, The observation unit is composed of 3 rooms each room contains 4 equipped beds), a resuscitation room (used to treat the seriously and critically ill patients), and administration zone to register admitted patients to the hospital.

3.2. ED Staff and Shifts

To cover the high demand for services over the whole day and provide 24hours care for all patients arriving in the ED, different shifts are employed. Basically, there are three shifts distributed over the day; the morning shift (from 8.00 to 14.00), the evening shift (from 14.00 to 20.00), and the night shift (from 20.00 to 8.00).

Every shift is composed of:

- Three physicians distributed between the consultation rooms, the observation unit, and the resuscitation room (if the patient condition needs a specialist opinion an expert physician is requested).
- Six nurses distributed between the observation unit and the nursing room.
- Two technicians distributed between the X-ray and the laboratory (for the morning and the evening shifts four technicians employed).

Generally, after midnight the patient flow is decreased, hence, the night shift team is divided into 3 teams composed of ;1 physician and 3 nurses (if the patient flow is increased or an exceptional event happens, like the occurrence of an accident … etc. the full night shift team is requested).

3.3. Patient Flow

Patients arrive in ED either as walk-in patients or by ambulance. The critical patients arriving by ambulance or even by their personal vehicles are directly rushed to the resuscitation room to be treated immediately. Otherwise, the patients wait for the availability of a consultation room to be examined. The first arrived patient is often the first seen by the doctor, exceptionally, the patient who arrived by ambulance get carried directly into the consultation room to be promptly seen. After the consultation, the doctor assesses the acuity of patient's illness and decides to discharge him or the need for further tests such as the lab tests or X-ray. The patient needed additional tests was sent to the X-ray waiting room or the laboratory waiting room, after getting his tests the patient re-wait for a doctor consultation. After the physician evaluation of the patient's tests, the patient needed further treatment is sent to the observation unit (equipped unit) to provide him continued monitoring, diagnostic evaluation (request the opinion of an expert physician), and/or treatment prior to leaving the emergency department or be admitted to the hospital. The patient flow is illustrated in (Figure 1).

4. SIMULATION MODEL DESIGN AND DEVELOPMENT

4.1. Data Collection

To better understand the functioning of the emergency department, a previewing of the work process and a comprehensive study have been carried out. Unfortunately, the information system of Lakhdar Bouzidi emergency department is not yet computerized, which made the gathering data a very difficult task because we had to collect the data manually. All data necessary for building our model was collected, such as the number of patients arrived in ED, patient arrival rates, current schedules of doctors, nurses and technicians, the duration of each treatment …etc. A large portion of our data was derived from the patient consultation registry, patient observation registry, and the admission registry. The rest of data was obtained through the direct observation of the system, the interviews and the discussion with the medical and paramedical staff. The data collected and the information given by the hospital staff showed that 5% of patients arriving in ED, are the critical emergency cases with a high acuity level, 15% are the medium acuity level patients, and 80% are the non-urgent patients. Where 25% of patients are discharged after the initial consultation, the other 75% require additional tests (lab tests, x-ray, or a nursing care) only 40% of them are treated and monitored in the observation unit. Our dataset covers the information of patients who were present in Lakhdar Bouzidi emergency department during the period of January 1, 2013 to December 31, 2013. The patient information includes the personal information (name, sex, age, address), arriving time, leaving time, length of stay, waiting time, and acuity level.

Figure 1. Patient flow process

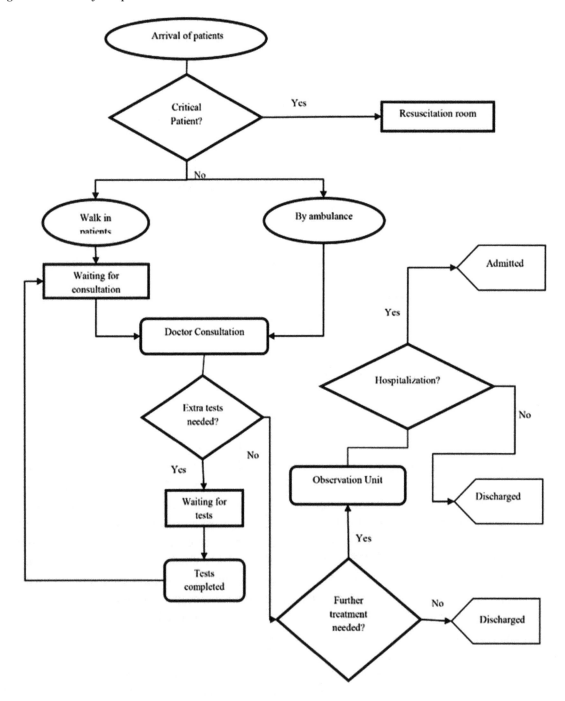

4.2. Data Preparation and Analysis

Due to the high demand for services and pressures within the ED, patient registries are often a lack of accuracy and coherence. Therefore, prior to using any of this data as un input of our simulation study, data mining techniques are required to extract the reliable data sets of that raw data as shown in (Figure

Figure 2. Data preparation and analysis process

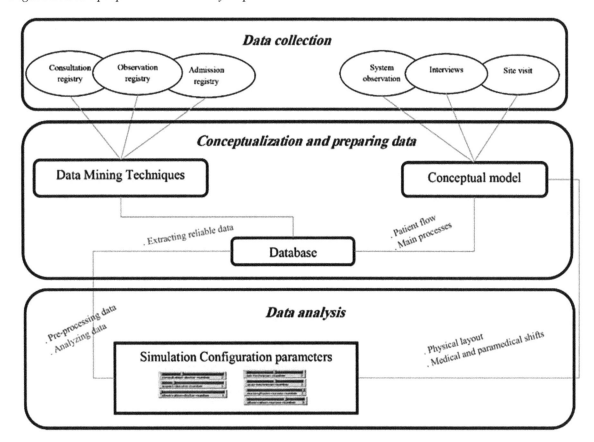

2). Afterward, the patient flow and the main processes are integrated into our database as well as the patients' data extracted from patients' registries to be preprocessed using the data preprocessing steps of the knowledge discovery process.

In order to get the best configuration parameters of our simulation and to develop a robust model, with a high level of details and similar to the real system, a thorough analysis of the preprocessed data is needed to discover valuable and useful patterns.

4.3. Simulation Model Development

A simulation model similar to the real system is built, with all the details including the physical layout, the patient flow, the treatment processes, the ED resources (doctors, nurses, technicians, beds...etc.), and the medical /paramedical shifts.

The model was implemented using the multi-agent programmable modeling environment Netlogo, a well-suited platform for modeling and developing complex systems composed of hundreds or thousands of agents all operating and acting in parallel and independently. Thus, it can be possible to explore the connection between the micro-level behavior of individuals and the macro-level patterns that emerge from their interaction.

Figure 3. System overview

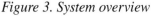

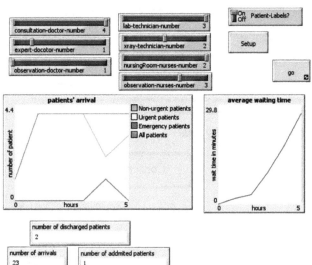

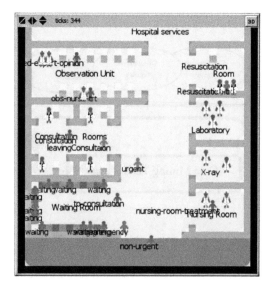

Our model includes the five primary areas of the ED as shown in (Figure 3); the waiting area, consultation /diagnostic area, observation and monitoring area, the resuscitation room and the further tests area, which includes the laboratory, the X-ray room and the nursing room. To model a dynamic environment such as the ED with full human interactions, two kinds of agents are implemented:

- Cognitive agents with the ability of thinking and reasoning to represent patients, doctors, nurses and technicians.
- Reactive agents to represent waiting chairs and beds where their state change (available/occupied).

Based on the interviews with the ED medical and paramedical staff, a site visit and a close system observation, a detail conceptual model is built, where the different actions and the behavior changes of agents are modeled using the state machines. Various types of doctors are implemented in our simulation:

- The consultation doctor installed initially in the consultation room receives patients who need diagnostic and assessment. The consultation doctor can leave his office to the resuscitation room if a critical patient is rushed there and no other doctor is monitoring him (Figure 4).
- The observation doctor installed initially in the observation unit monitors and treats serious patients assessed by the consultation physician. If the patient's state needs a specialized opinion, the observation doctor requests an expert doctor who decides whether an outpatient treatment or the patient's hospitalization (Figure 5).

Depending on the patient's state and symptoms, three patient acuity levels are presented in our simulation. Patients are classified in low-acuity (non-urgent patients), medium-acuity (urgent patients) and high-acuity (emergency and critical patients) (Figure 6).

Non-urgent patients arriving in the ED, may have to wait in one or more queues for medical services, as consultation doctor assessment, lab tests, nursing treatment, X-ray, or even to have a treatment in the

Figure 4. Consultation doctor state machine

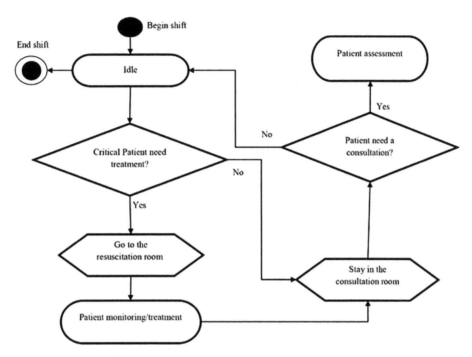

Figure 5. Observation doctor state machine

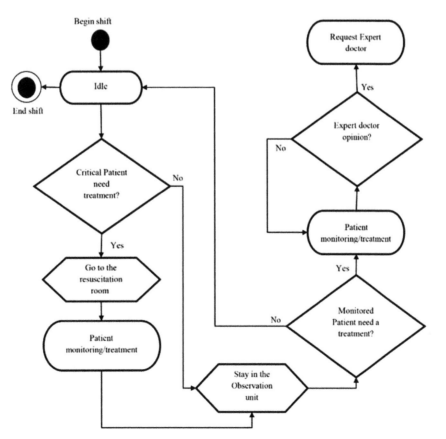

Figure 6. Patient acuity levels

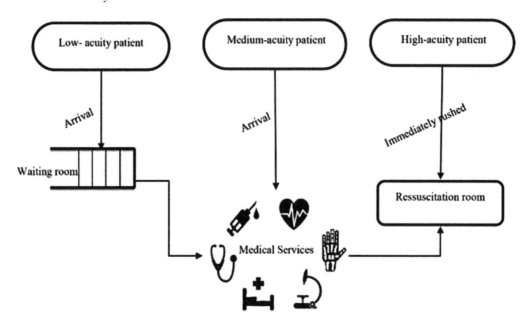

observation unit. To ensure the operation of the waiting lines as it is in the reality, a queueing system based on the queuing method FIFO is implemented and integrated with our simulator. The first non-urgent patient arrived is typically the first seen and diagnosed by the consultation doctor, exceptionally, the urgent patients who arrived by ambulance or by their means get carried directly into the consultation room to be promptly seen. The high-acuity patients are immediately rushed to the resuscitation room to be treated and monitored by the observation doctor or the consultation physician.

5. VERIFICATION AND VALIDATION

To ensure the model credibility and increase the accuracy of the simulation results, the verification, and the validation were carried out throughout all the conceptualization and the development phases of the ED, simulation model. Following the recommendation of Sargent (Sargent, 2005), after each development phase, the model was verified and reviewed with the involvement of the emergency department staff to ascertain that it behaves as intended and implements the assumptions correctly. To achieve that, the model's operational behavior has been displayed graphically using the animation and tracking the changes of the different parts and activities of system, as well as the movement of the patients and the medical and paramedical staff and their interactions. Various techniques have been applied to validate the results of our simulation model: face validity, historical data validation and model comparison. Face validity is carried out by the interviewing of the doctors and the nurses who have been heavily participated in all the progress steps of the project in order to validate and determine whether the model behaves like the real system or not. The second approach that was followed is historical data validation where our database has been divided into two parts, the first one is used to build the model and the rest of data is used to test objectively and validate the model performance by comparing it with the input data used to initialize and start the simulation process. Comparing the output of the simulation model with the real system output is a crucial point to prove the validity of the model. Under an identical configuration parameter of the actual system, the simulation has been executed many times where each execution represents 24 hours of activity. Three key performance indicators have been used to measure the performance of the system: number of patients arriving in the ED, the average Length of Stay (LOS) of discharged and admitted patients and the average waiting time(AWT). Simulated results are compared with the observed data and presented in (Figure 7), (Figure 8), and (Figure 9).

Figure 7. Average Length of Stay simulation results validation

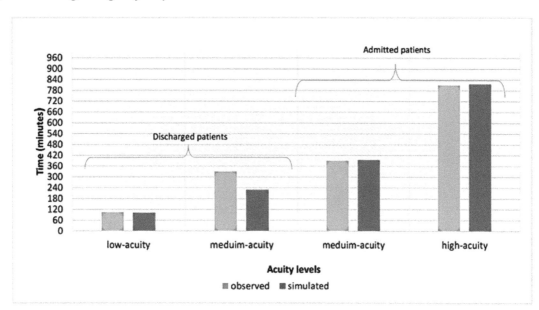

Figure 8. Average waiting time simulation results validation

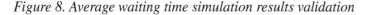

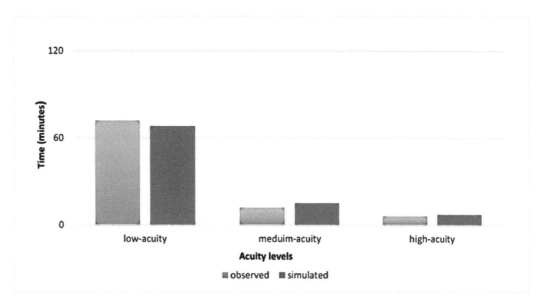

Figure 9. Validation of the patient arrival rate

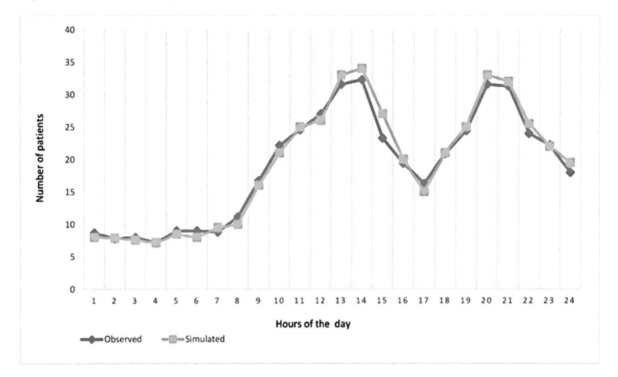

6. SIMULATION RESULTS AND DISCUSSION

6.1. Scenarios Design

To measure the performance of our ED model and evaluate the different changes in it, a series of simulation executions under different scenarios have been done. As inputs of the base scenario, we used identical configuration parameters of the real system as the staff schedule and patients' arrival distribution. Also, with the aim to reduce the average waiting time and the average Length of Stay, two other scenarios are tested. The first scenario we aim to confirm that adding one more doctor per shift in the consultation zone can help to reduce the patients' waiting time, especially for the low-acuity patients. In the second scenario, an extra doctor per shift was installed in the observation unit to decrease the Length of Stay of the medium-acuity and the high-acuity patients. The scenarios tested gave us acceptable results regarding the length of stay and the waiting time (Table 1) whereas, we faced another challenge that is considered one of the key performance indicators of the ED that is the medical resources utilization. Due to the unstable and changeable arrival rate of patients during the day, employing the same medical staff configuration in all the shifts and adding one more doctor to each shift, caused a decrease in the resources utilization especially the medical staff utilization. To deal with this problematic, a temporal knowledge extraction model used the concepts of data mining techniques and regression analysis is adopted.

Table 1. Simulation results of scenarios 1, and 2

	Base Scenario			Scenario 1: An additional doctor in the consultation room			Scenario 2: An additional doctor in the observation unit		
	Low-Acuity	Medium-Acuity	High-Acuity	Low-Acuity	Medium-Acuity	High-Acuity	Low-Acuity	Medium-Acuity	High-Acuity
Average length of stay (min	102	228	394	98	227	300	101	220	385
Average waiting time (min)	68	15	07	60	13	6	67	14	5

6.2. Temporal Knowledge Extraction Model

In order to increase the medical staff utilization and to get the optimal configurations to reduce the length of stay and the waiting time of patients, a reconfiguration of the ED shifts depending on the hourly patient flow and the acuity levels is carried out. Data mining regression analysis is performed on the patients' arrival pattern dataset derived from the patients' database where each pattern represents the patients' arrival time and his acuity level. Once we obtained the dataset prepared, the linear regression (linear correlation) algorithm was applied using TANAGRA software, to investigate the relationship among the patients' arrival time and the acuity levels. The different steps of the temporal knowledge extraction model are illustrated in (Figure 10).

Figure 10. Temporal knowledge extraction model steps

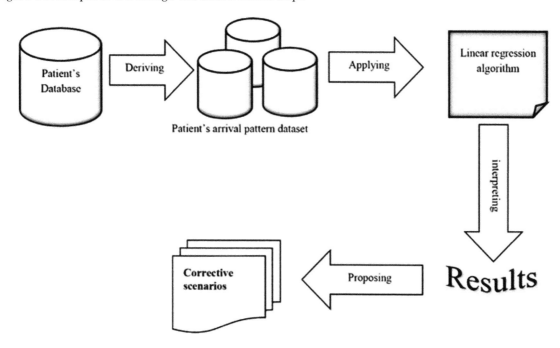

In order to analyze and to assess the correlation between patients' arrival and the acuity levels and to measure its strength and significance, a correlation coefficient ranges between -1 and +1 is estimated. The most significant coefficients that approximate to +1 (which means a strong positive correlation between the arrival time and the acuity level) will be the only accepted.

The analysis results showed that, there is a strong relationship among the patient's arrival rate from 11 am to 3 pm and the low acuity level, which indicates that the large number of patients arrive in the ED between 11 am and 3 pm are the non-urgent patients with a low acuity level. In the other hand, medium acuity and high acuity level are powerfully correlated with the patient's arrival rate from 6 pm and 11 pm. Thus, almost all the patients arrive in the ED between 6 pm and 11 pm are the urgent patients with a medium acuity level and the emergency patients with a high acuity level.

Results analysis of our temporal knowledge extraction model represent a crucial decision point that can help the ED managers of Lakhdar Bouzidi hospital to propose new staff configurations and then assessing their efficiency and their impact on the quality of care provided using the simulation model proposed.

6.3. Corrective Scenarios

Based on the analysis results of the temporal knowledge extraction model three scenarios are proposed:

Scenario A1: To avoid the overcrowding and the long waiting time before the doctor consultation, caused by the remarkable arrival of low-acuity patients between 11 am and 3 pm, we suggested to add a doctor in the consultation zone in that period.

Scenario A2: Adding a doctor in the observation unit to decrease the increased length of stay due to the augmented patients' arrival rate between 6pm and 11pm, especially for the medium and high acuity patients, who often need a continued monitoring in the observation unit.

Scenario A3: Is combined between the two scenarios aforementioned, where between 11 am and 3 pm a doctor is added in the consultation zone, and between 6 pm and 11 pm a doctor is added in the observation unit.

Table 2. Simulation results of scenarios A1, A2, and A3

	Scenario A1: An additional doctor in the consultation zone between 11am and 3pm			Scenario A2: An additional doctor in the observation unit between 6pm and 11pm			Scenario A3: Scenario A1 + Scemarop A2		
	Low-Acuity	Medium-Acuity	High-Acuity	Low-Acuity	Medium-Acuity	High-Acuity	Low-Acuity	Medium-Acuity	High-Acuity
Average length of stay (min)	96	220	370	80	200	290	70	180	270
Average waiting time (min)	52	09	03	57	11	05	48	07	03

Figure 11. Doctors utilization results of the scenarios proposed

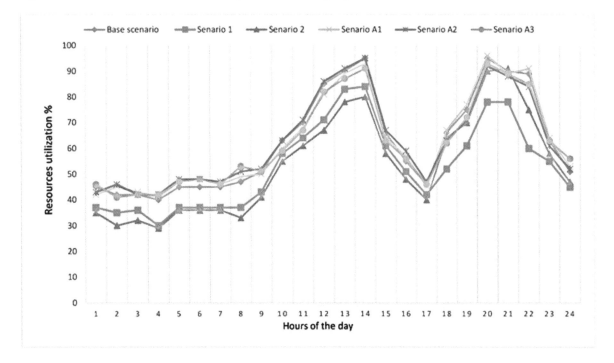

Table 2 summarizes the results of the average length of stay and the average waiting time of scenario A1, scenario A2, and scenario A3. It can be noted that scenario A1 contributed significantly to decreasing the average waiting time before the doctor consultation, mainly, for the low acuity patients. Where, the scenario A2 gave us better results, concerning the reducing of the average length of stay of the medium-acuity and high-acuity patients. It is clearly observed that the combination of the two scenarios in the scenario A3 provided the best results regarding the average length of stay and even the average waiting time.

6.4. A Comparative Study

A comparative study is carried out in order to test the performance of the scenarios proposed. Simulation results' comparisons of the medical resources utilization, the average length of stay, and the average waiting time are shown in (Figure 11), (Figure 12), and (Figure 13) respectively.

(Figure 11) illustrates the resources utilization results of the six scenarios proposed, more precisely the doctors' utilization results over the 24 hours of the day. It can be easily noted that, the scenario 1 and scenario 2 provided us the worst results, especially when the patient flow is decreased. Where the results of the other scenarios were close to each other.

(Figure 12) summarizes the results of the average length of stay of the low-acuity, medium-acuity, and high-acuity patient for each scenario. The length of stay of the low-acuity patients is decreased from 102 min of the base scenario to 98 min, 101 min, 96 min, 80 min, and 70 min for scenarios 1, 2, A1, A2, and A3 respectively. While the results of the medium-acuity patients were as follows; 228 min for the base scenario, 227 min, 220 min, 220 min, and 180 min for scenarios 1, 2, A1, A2, and A3 respectively.

Figure 12. Average length of stay results of the scenarios proposed

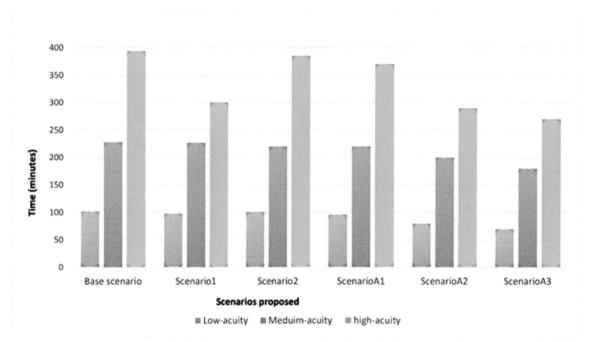

Figure 13. Average waiting time results of the scenarios proposed

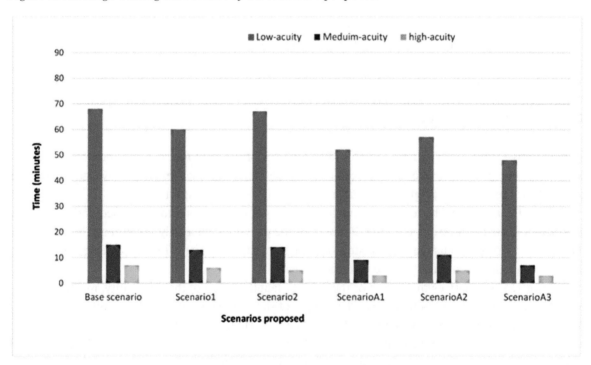

In comparison with the base scenario, high-acuity patients' sojourn in the ED is reduced by 94 min, 09 min, 24 min, 104 min, and 124 min for scenarios 1, 2, A1, A2, and A3 respectively.

According to (Figure 13), the results of the average waiting time of high-acuity patients is ranged between 07 min and 03 min. After applying, the scenarios suggested the average waiting time of the medium-acuity patients is reduced from 15 min of the base scenario to 13 min, 14 min, 9 min, 11 min, and 7 min for scenarios 1, 2, A1, A2, and A3 respectively. In comparison with the base scenario, the waiting time of the low-acuity patients is decreased by 8 min, one min, 16 min, 11 min, and 20 min for scenarios 1, 2, A1, A2, and A3 respectively.

To summarize, the implementation of the alternative corrective scenarios (A1, A2, A3) based on the results analysis of the proposed knowledge extraction model compared to scenarios (1, 2) without the contribution of data mining, presented many improvement including the average waiting time, the average length of stay, and doctors' utilization.

7. CONCLUSION

A decision support system for the operation of the emergency department in the public hospital Lakhdar Bouzidi in Bordj Bou Arreridj (Algeria) has been presented. The proposed framework integrates the agent-based modeling simulation with the data mining techniques to provide a powerful tool that can help managers to improve the functioning of the ED.

We developed an agent-based simulation model using the multi-agent programmable modeling environment Netlogo, to cope with the dynamic nature of the ED by creating a virtual system close to the reality, on one hand, and to test the different strategies and scenarios on the other hand. Prior to performing the simulation model, data mining preprocessing methods were applied on the collected dataset in order to get a reliable simulation inputs.

Besides, in order to improve the quality of care in the ED and to help the ED managers adopting the optimal staff configuration regarding the patient flow and patients' acuity levels, a temporal knowledge extraction model is implemented. The adopted model investigates the relationship between the patients' arrival time and the acuity levels, by applying the linear regression algorithm on the patients' arrival pattern dataset. Based on the analysis results of the proposed knowledge extraction model, various alternative corrective configurations of the ED medical staff depending on the diversified patient flow and acuity levels are tested. A comparative study between the results of the different scenarios proposed in our study has been carried out.

The simulation results showed that adopting the configurations of the ED medical staff based on the results analysis of the proposed knowledge extraction model outperformed on the classical configurations implemented without the contribution of data mining. Consequently, the average waiting time, the average length of stay, and doctors' utilization have been considerably improved.

While there is a clear benefit to integrating the agent-based modeling simulation and the data mining techniques, we plan to support our simulation model by integrating a patients' flow forecasting model. We will predict the hourly patients' arrival patterns using the artificial neural networks, in order to improve the quality of the simulation inputs. Similarly, reconfiguration the nurses' and technicians' schedules base on the analysis model proposed in this paper should be a focus of future work.

REFERENCES

Abo-Hamad, W., & Arisha, A. (2013). Simulation-based framework to improve patient experience in an emergency department. *European Journal of Operational Research, 224*(1), 154–166. doi:10.1016/j.ejor.2012.07.028

Ahmed, M. A., & Alkhamis, T. M. (2009). Simulation optimization for an emergency department healthcare unit in Kuwait. *European Journal of Operational Research, 198*(3), 936–942. doi:10.1016/j.ejor.2008.10.025

Al-Refaie, A., Fouad, R. H., Li, M.-H., & Shurrab, M. (2014). Applying simulation and DEA to improve performance of emergency department in a Jordanian hospital. *Simulation Modelling Practice and Theory, 41*, 59–72. doi:10.1016/j.simpat.2013.11.010

Bose, R. (2003). Knowledge management-enabled health care management systems: Capabilities, infrastructure, and decision-support. *Expert Systems with Applications, 24*(1), 59–71. doi:10.1016/S0957-4174(02)00083-0

Cabrera, E., Taboada, M., Iglesias, M. L., Epelde, F., & Luque, E. (2011). Optimization of healthcare emergency departments by agent-based simulation. *Procedia computer science, 4*, 1880-1889.

Cabrera, E., Taboada, M., Iglesias, M. L., Epelde, F., & Luque, E. (2012). Simulation optimization for healthcare emergency departments. *Procedia Computer Science, 9*, 1464–1473. doi:10.1016/j.procs.2012.04.161

Connelly, L. G., & Bair, A. E. (2004). Discrete event simulation of emergency department activity: A platform for system-level operations research. *Academic Emergency Medicine, 11*(11), 1177–1185. doi:10.1111/j.1553-2712.2004.tb00702.x PMID:15528582

Duguay, C., & Chetouane, F. (2007). Modeling and improving emergency department systems using discrete event simulation. *Simulation, 83*(4), 311–320. doi:10.1177/0037549707083111

Evans, G. W., Gor, T. B., & Unger, E. (1996). A simulation model for evaluating personnel schedules in a hospital emergency department. *Proceedings of the 28th conference on Winter simulation* (pp. 1205-1209). IEEE Computer Society. 10.1145/256562.256933

Fayyad, U., Piatetsky-Shapiro, G., & Smyth, P. (1996). From data mining to knowledge discovery in databases. *AI Magazine*, 37.

Georgopoulos, V., & Stylios, C. (2013). Fuzzy cognitive map decision support system for successful triage to reduce unnecessary emergency room admissions for the elderly. In Fuzziness and Medicine: Philosophical Reflections and Application Systems in Health Care (pp. 415-436). Springer Berlin Heidelberg. doi:10.1007/978-3-642-36527-0_27

Han, J., Kamber, M., & Pei, J. (2011). *Data mining: concepts and techniques*. Elsevier.

Hegland, M. (2001). Data mining techniques. *Acta Numerica, 2001*, 313–355.

Hoot, N. R., LeBlanc, L. J., Jones, I., Levin, S. R., Zhou, C., Gadd, C. S., & Aronsky, D. (2008). Forecasting emergency department crowding: A discrete event simulation. *Annals of Emergency Medicine*, *52*(2), 116–125. doi:10.1016/j.annemergmed.2007.12.011 PMID:18387699

Jones, S. S., & Evans, R. S. (2008). An agent based simulation tool for scheduling emergency department physicians. *AMIA ... Annual Symposium Proceedings / AMIA Symposium. AMIA Symposium*, *2008*, 338. PMID:18998871

Kadri, F., Chaabane, S., & Tahon, C. (2014). A simulation-based decision support system to prevent and predict strain situations in emergency department systems. *Simulation Modelling Practice and Theory*, *42*, 32–52. doi:10.1016/j.simpat.2013.12.004

Kalogeropoulos, D. A., Carson, E. R., & Collinson, P. O. (2003). Towards knowledge-based systems in clinical practice: Development of an integrated clinical information and knowledge management support system. *Computer Methods and Programs in Biomedicine*, *72*(1), 65–80. doi:10.1016/S0169-2607(02)00118-9 PMID:12850298

Komashie, A., & Mousavi, A. (2005). Modeling emergency departments using discrete event simulation techniques. *Proceedings of the 37th conference on Winter simulation* (pp. 2681-2685). 10.1109/WSC.2005.1574570

Konrad, R., DeSotto, K., Grocela, A., McAuley, P., Wang, J., Lyons, J., & Bruin, M. (2013). Modeling the impact of changing patient flow processes in an emergency department: Insights from a computer simulation study. *Operations Research for Health Care*, *2*(4), 66–74. doi:10.1016/j.orhc.2013.04.001

Kuo, Y.-H., Rado, O., Lupia, B., Leung, J. M., & Graham, C. A. (2015). Improving the efficiency of a hospital emergency department: a simulation study with indirectly imputed service-time distributions. *Flexible Services and Manufacturing Journal*.

Laskowski, M., McLeod, R. D., Friesen, M. R., Podaima, B. W., & Alfa, A. S. (2009). Models of emergency departments for reducing patient waiting times. *PLoS ONE*, *4*(7), e6127. doi:10.1371/journal.pone.0006127 PMID:19572015

Lim, M. E., Worster, A., Goeree, R., & Tarride, J.-É. (2013). Simulating an emergency department: The importance of modeling the interactions between physicians and delegates in a discrete event simulation. *BMC Medical Informatics and Decision Making*, *13*(1), 1. doi:10.1186/1472-6947-13-59 PMID:23692710

Masmoudi, M., Leclaire, P., Cheutet, V., & Casalino, E. (2014). Modelling and Simulation of the Doctors' Availability in Emergency Department with SIMIO Software. Case of Study: Bichat-Claude Bernard Hospital. In *Mechatronic Systems: Theory and Applications* (pp. 119–129). Springer International Publishing.

Meng, L. Y., & Spedding, T. (2008). Modelling patient arrivals when simulating an accident and emergency unit. *Proceedings of the Simulation Conference WSC '08* (pp. 1509-1515). IEEE. 10.1109/WSC.2008.4736231

Oh, C., Novotny, A., Carter, P., Ready, R., Campbell, D., & Leckie, M. (2016). *Use of a simulation-based decision support tool to improve emergency department throughput*. Operations Research for Health Care.

Pujari, A. K. (2001). *Data mining techniques.*

Rossetti, M. D., Trzcinski, G. F., & Syverud, S. A. (1999). Emergency department simulation and determination of optimal attending physician staffing schedules. *Proceedings of the Simulation Conference* (Vol. 2, pp. 1532-1540). IEEE. 10.1145/324898.325315

Ruohonen, T., Neittaanmaki, P., & Teittinen, J. (2006). Simulation model for improving the operation of the emergency department of special health care. *Proceedings of the Simulation Conference, 2006. WSC 06. Proceedings of the Winter* (pp. 453-458). IEEE. 10.1109/WSC.2006.323115

Samaha, S., Armel, W. S., & Starks, D. W. (2003). Emergency departments I: the use of simulation to reduce the length of stay in an emergency department. *Proceedings of the 35th conference on Winter simulation: driving innovation* (pp. 1907-1911).

Sargent, R. G. (2005). Verification and validation of simulation models. *Proceedings of the 37th conference on Winter simulation* (pp. 130-143).

Wilensky, U. (1999). *NetLogo.* Center for Connected Learning and Computer Based Modeling, Northwestern University. Retrieved from http://ccl.northwestern.edu/netlogo/

This research was previously published in the International Journal of Healthcare Information Systems and Informatics (IJHISI), 11(2); edited by Joseph Tan and Qiang (Shawn) Cheng; pages 19-37, copyright year 2016 by IGI Publishing (an imprint of IGI Global).

Chapter 12
Step Towards Pervasive Technology Assessment in Intensive Medicine

Filipe Portela
Universidade do Minho, Portugal

Manuel Filipe Santos
Universidade do Minho, Portugal

José Machado
Universidade do Minho, Portugal

António da Silva Abelha
Universidade do Minho, Portugal

Fernando Rua
Centro Hospitalar do Porto, Portugal

ABSTRACT

This paper presents the evaluation of a Pervasive Intelligent Decision Support System in Intensive Medicine making use of Technology Acceptance Model 3 (TAM3). Two rounds of questionnaires were distributed and compared. The work is based on a discursive evaluation of a method employed to assess a new and innovative technology (INTCare) using the four constructs of TAM3 and statistical metrics. The paper crosses the TAM3 constructs with INTCare features to produce a questionnaire to provide a better comprehension of the users' intentions. The final results are essential to validate the system and understand the user sensitivity. The paper validates a method to access technologies in critical environments and shows an example of how a questionnaire can be developed based on TAM3. It also proves the viability of using this method and advises that two rounds of questionnaires should be performed if we want to have better evidence on user satisfaction.

DOI: 10.4018/978-1-7998-2451-0.ch012

Copyright © 2020, IGI Global. Copying or distributing in print or electronic forms without written permission of IGI Global is prohibited.

INTRODUCTION

The process of implementing Information Systems needs to be carefully designed and well done. The success of implementation depends primarily on the type of the system, the characteristics of the environment, the users and their willingness to change. This process should be properly evaluated before the final implementation as it is fundamental in critical areas as is Intensive Care Units (ICU). ICUs are categorized as hospital units where the patients are in a serious condition which requires continuous treatments. In this type of environments, the arrival of a new technology can be incorrectly interpreted as compromising ICU tasks. In these cases and according to the ICU professionals there is a set of barriers to overcome: as the system cannot fail, it should require a low number of human tasks. Moreover, it cannot interfere with the normal activity of the service, and it should contribute to the patient's best care.

Pervasive Intelligent Decision Support Systems (PIDSS) in ICUs are crucial to support the decision-making process. ICUs are recognized to be critical environments where the patients are in weak conditions, usually with organ dysfunction and in a life-risk situation (Silva, Cortez, Santos, Gomes, & Neves, 2008). The adoption of PIDSS is a valuable asset for the users who want to improve their decisions (Lyerla, LeRouge, Cooke, Turpin, & Wilson, 2010; Varshney, 2009). Nowadays, this type of systems requires an environment change and an information system architecture redesign. After the system deployment, the use of a methodology to understand the usability of the PIDSS (intention and behaviour) by the ICU professionals (users) is fundamental. Evaluating the technology during the test phase becomes essential as this environment is complex. In the literature, there are many methodologies to assess technologies. In this case, the Technology Acceptance Model (TAM) 3 was chosen. TAM3 (Chooprayoon & Fung, 2010) was developed to evaluate the Perceived Ease of USE (PEOU), Perceived Usefulness (PU), Behaviour Intention (BI) and Use Behaviour (UB). This approach was applied to a real system called INTCare which was implemented in the ICU of Centro Hospitalar do Porto (CHP) – Hospital Santo António. To support the evaluation phase, a questionnaire covering all the system features and TAM constructs was introduced. This questionnaire was sent to the INTCare users in two separate phases. The first round was essential to understand the system's viability and user opinions. The second round was performed after resolving the issues reported in the first round. Its main goal was the final evaluation of the system.

This paper presents the study conducted, its conditions and the main result achieved in each round. The results allow understanding the degree of satisfaction denoted by the users and which features need to be improved. Beyond this introductory section, the paper contains seven sections. The second section presents the related concepts. The third section presents the TAM3 constructs, the questionnaire and their relation to system features. Section four presents the modifications done in the system after the first questionnaires. Section five and six present and discuss the attained results. Finally, some final conclusions are made, and the future work is described.

BACKGROUND

Intensive Care Units

Intensive Care Units (ICU) are a specialized hospital unit where intensive medicine treatments are applied. Intensive Medicine is concerned with the treatment of patients with complex problems. ICU is reserved to a patient in critical conditions with the failure of one or more organ systems according to Sequential Organ Failure Assessment (SOFA): cardiovascular, neurologic, hepatic, renal, respiratory and coagulation. The ICU professionals (nurses and physicians) work under constant pressure because they deal with human lives in critical condition.

The intensivists attest that the Decision Making Process (DMP) in this ICU is a vital process because it can save human lives. A wrong decision can result in a non-return situation to the patient. The decision needs to be made quickly and with a high level of accuracy. Currently, the decisions are based on the human knowledge due to the low number of existing decision support systems in the ICUs. INTCare brings a new technology able to support the DMP in real-time.

INTCare

INTCare is a Pervasive Intelligent Decision Support System (PIDSS) developed for Intensive Medicine. That is an innovative system which is not comparable with the similar solutions found in the literature review. INTCare is divided into two subsystems: monitoring and decision support. The monitoring subsystem is ensured by the Electronic Nursing Record (ENR), and it is interoperable with all hospital system (Electronic Health Record, Drugs System, Laboratory system, etc.). ENR can monitor in real-time: vital signs, therapeutic plan, fluid balance, scores and other clinical records. The decision subsystem can create, automatically and in real-time, relevant knowledge to support the decision makers anywhere and anytime. This subsystem includes Data Mining models (Dietterich, 2000) for predicting clinical events. The system is also able to send clinical alerts to the intensivists. Overall, INTCare system provides:

- Patient Clinical data (Vital Signs, Fluid Balance, Patient Scales Laboratory Results);
- Critical Events tracking (SPO2, Hear Rate, Blood Pressure, Urine Output and Temperature) (Portela, Gago, Santos, Silva, & Rua, 2012);
- ICU Medical Scores (SAPSII, SAPSIII, Glasgow SOFA, MEWS, and TISS) (Portela, Santos, Machado, et al., 2012);
- The probability an organ dysfunction occurring (Cardiovascular, Coagulation, Respiratory, Hepatic, and Renal) and the likelihood of a patient's death (Portela, Pinto, & Santos, 2012).

The results associated with the decision-making process were already evaluated in other study / work (Portela, Aguiar, Santos, Silva, & Rua, 2013). All the results obtain by INTCare system are included in a pervasive system (web platform), and the information / knowledge achieved is presented in the form of dashboards. These dashboards are divided into two modules, and they can be configured to present data from three points of view patient (individual), all patients and service.

TECHNOLOGY ACCEPTANCE MODEL 3

The success of the technology deployment stage can be directly associated with the way of how the new technology is evaluated. This process can be assessed by different forms or methodologies. The evaluation of a technology application is crucial to comprehend its suitability in a specific environment, and it also is fundamental to measure the satisfaction level of its users. One of the most commons approaches is the Technology Acceptance Model (TAM). "TAM is adapted from the Theory of Reasoned Action (TRA) model which describes human behaviours in a given situation" (Fishbein & Ajzen, 1975).

TAM presents, as its main goal, essentially the ease of use and usefulness of technology through the evaluation of external variables towards people's internal beliefs, attitudes, and intentions (Chooprayoon & Fung, 2010). In the current case, this model allows having an understanding of the acceptance of the PIDSS by the ICU professionals and how it can be useful in the course of their daily work. More recently Venkatesh & Bala (2008) set a model of perceived ease of use determinants (Venkatesh & Davis, 2000) and developed an integrated model of technology acceptance – TAM3. TAM3 is composed by four constructs: Perceived Ease of USE (PEOU), Perceived Usefulness (PU), Behaviour Intention (BI) and Use Behaviour (UB). This model was derived from another type of analysis as can be seen in figure 1 (Venkatesh & Bala, 2008). TAM 3 adds a few variables as influencing the perceived ease of use:

Figure 1. TAM 3 Model retrieved from (Venkatesh & Bala, 2008)

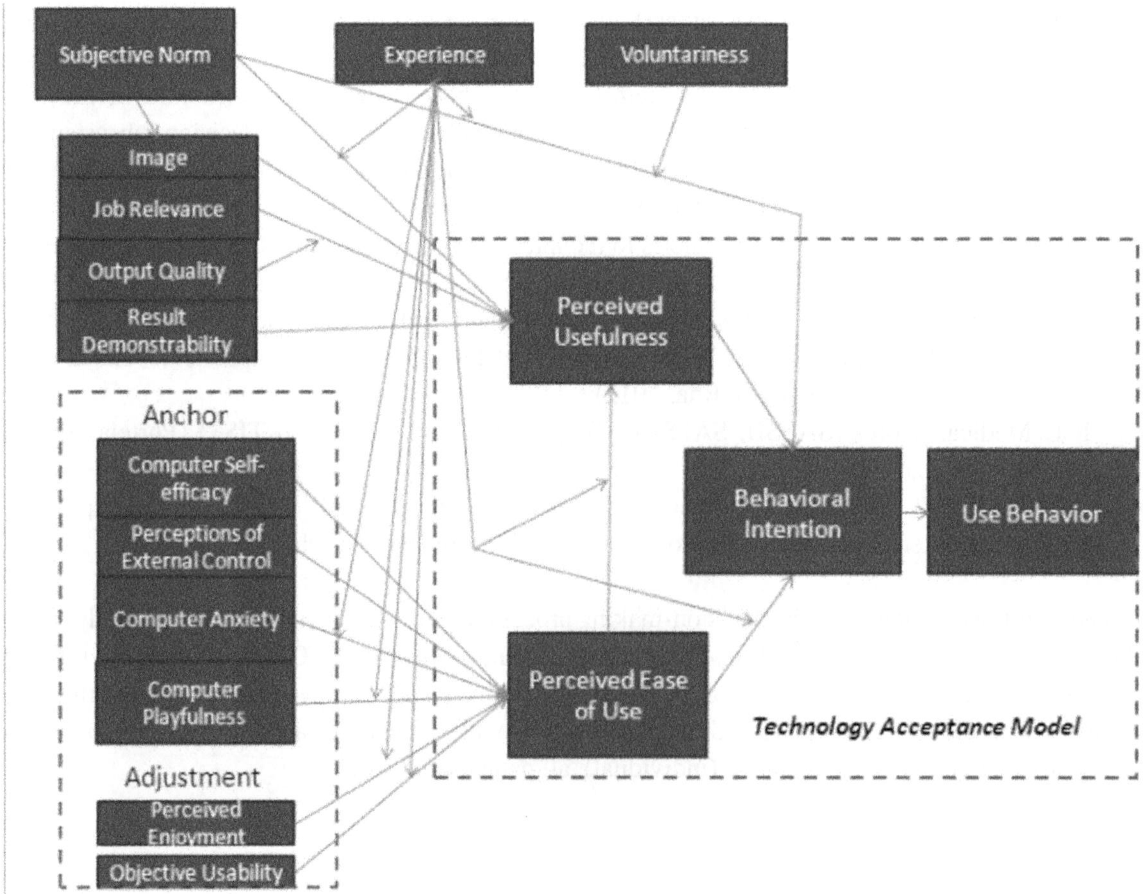

1. In ground or basis (self-efficacy in technological environment, perceptions of external control, computer anxiety, and enjoyment in technological environment);
2. In systematization (perceived enjoyment and actual usability).

This model was chosen because, scientifically, it is considered as one of the complete models to evaluate how a person can influence an information system; assess how he is affected by the system and evaluate its intention in using the system. At the same time, distinct technologies can be applied in different situations and under various controls.

METHODS

The use of questionnaires is fundamental to achieve the TAM3 goals. The four constructs of TAM3 (PEOU, PU, BI, UB) should be the questionnaire base. To have a better comprehension of the technology and user acceptance, the same questionnaire should be used in two rounds. The second questionnaire can have more questions than the first due to modifications we did after receiving the first questionnaire feedback. With the use of two rounds of questions, it is possible to have a better comprehension about the user opinion and their acceptance regarding the new technology developed. At the same time, the system can be improved between the two rounds. In this case study, the time gap between the two rounds was six months. In both cases, the questionnaires were distributed after deploying INTCare in the ICU (i.e. after the system fulfilled all the requirements, defined in each phase). The assessment process was performed during the testing phase. The questionnaires were disseminated electronically (online answering) after a brief discussion with the users. In most cases, the questionnaires were answered during working breaks. The respondents' group was chosen by the ICU director. During this process, 20 questionnaires were distributed to the nurses selected by the ICU director.

In this paper, only the answers provided by the nursing staff were considered. The questionnaires were distributed to the nurses because they are the main users of the system. They are responsible for validating and storing the results that will be used by the physicians in the decision process. All the questionnaires were delivered in the user's native language.

Constructs

The use of the TAM3 involves a set of tasks to understand the constructs and the user attitudes - individual's positive or negative feeling about performing a targeted behaviour (e.g., using a system). TAM3 is divided into four types of attitudes / constructs (Venkatesh & Bala, 2008):

- **Behavioural Intention (BI):** The degree in which a person has formulated conscious plans to perform or not perform some specified future behaviour;
- **Perceived Ease of Use (PEOU):** The level of ease associated with the utilization of the system;
- **Perceived Usefulness (PU):** The degree in which an individual believes that using the system will help him or her to attain gains in job performance;
- **Use Behaviour (UB):** The degree in which a person has formulated conscious plans to use the technology.

Questionnaire

The main goal of the questionnaire was to assess the adoption of a PIDSS in terms of its intrinsic features (Portela, Pinto, et al., 2012; Portela, Santos, et al., 2013; Portela, Gago, et al., 2012; Portela et al., 2011; Portela, Santos, Machado, et al., 2012; Portela, Santos, & Vilas-Boas, 2012; Santos et al., 2011) and the users' acceptance. A questionnaire was designed crossing TAM3 constructs with the features of the system in the study (INTCare). The questionnaire is presented in Supplementary Table 1 (Appendix). The first questionnaire was introduced to have the first perception of the user's acceptance and behaviour. The second questionnaire was essential to understand the real intention of the user and validate the solution, taking into account the feedback received in the first round.

To accomplish this task, the first questionnaire was composed of a total of 96 questions. The second questionnaires had the same 96 questions and five more questions (related to the introduction / removal of new contents). Both the questionnaires have been defined taking essentially into account the scientific literature related to similar technology; the environment particularities; PIDSS features and clinical knowledge.

To evaluate the results, the Likert Scale (Johns, 2010) concept was considered. This scale was chosen based on two principles:

1. The use of short scales can constrain results into closed type of answers such as a simple yes or no
2. Applying higher scales could lead to a dispersion of results and consequently into inaccurate results

The chosen scale followed a range from one to five, because it allowed having two points for each side and at the same time to find a neutral point (Johns, 2010). The considered levels were the following:

3. Not satisfied/in complete disagreement
4. Satisfied a bit/in some degree of disagreement
5. Satisfied/under some level of agreement
6. Satisfied a lot/strongly agreement
7. Satisfied completely/full agreement

To have better success in the questionnaires, it is imperative to appraise the conscious level of the respondents. To avoid this problem, some screening questions were added with the goal to understand the degree of the user's consciousness (Ex: two + two).

Analysis of the Answers

To obtain results of using TAM3, i.e., in the analysis of the questionnaires, a program called statistical data analysis by PAleontological STatistics (PAST) (Hammer, Harper, & Ryan, 2001) was used. To understand the correlation between the answers and respondents Kendall's tau technique (i.e. for each question it was evaluated if the replies given by the users are similar or disperse, trying to find convergence and divergence points in user opinions) was used. This technique uses a non-parametric correlation coefficient that can be used to assess and test correlations between non-intervals scaled ordinal variables. Kendall's tau (τ) (Bolboaca & Jantschi, 2006) is often used as a statistical test to determine if two variables can be considered as statistically dependent. In other words, the correlation coefficient should deliver a range of [-1, 1]. If the agreement between the two evaluations is perfect, the coefficient has a value (1). If the divergence between the two evaluations is perfect (inverse), the coefficient has a value (-1), but if the two evaluations are independent, the coefficient is zero (Bolboaca & Jantschi, 2006).

Modifications Made in the PIDSS between the Two Rounds

Between the two rounds of questionnaires, some improvements were made in the PIDSS taking into account the answers given by the users in the Questions 2.14 and 2.15:

2.14 - The users made some suggestions for mitigating the less positive aspects previously evaluated.
2.15 - The user presented some suggestions regarding the use of the system.

Some significant modifications were made with the objective to:

A. Improve the speed of the scheme – optimize the database and application process, source-code reducing
B. Implement a timer controller – used to understand if the application is being used or not to control the interface refreshing
C. Ensure that all data are stored – automatically save after recording a value
D. Improve the record and acquisition system
E. Modify the user interface aspect
F. Include some features required by the nurses (e.g. more charts, introduction of new variables and others)
G. Change aspects related to medication

RESULTS

The results presented in this work are related to the answers obtained from the questions contained in both questionnaires. Using this process, it was possible to make a comparison between each round of questionnaires and to understand the main differences related to technological features and user acceptance. The final goal of this task was to "attest" the platform's viability, i.e. if the users are familiar with the system and if it can be helpful in performing their jobs and if at the same time improves patients' condition. In the first round, 13 valid questionnaires were obtained and in the second round, ten questionnaires were validated. All the questions should be answered by the users for the questionnaire to be valid. At the same time, the user must answer all the screening questions.

Supplementary Table 2 (Appendix) presents the level of experience regarding information technology demonstrated by the respondents. Specifically, 40% of the second questionnaire respondents also participated in the first round of questions. The respondent's characteristics / typology are similar in the two rounds.

The following two tables (1 and 2 present statistical results (global and construct analyses) and the coefficient of correlation (Kendall) of the questionnaire. For example, the correlation level presented in

Table 1. TAM Results (Kendall)

Construct	Questionnaire I			Questionnaire II		
	Average	Min	Max	Average	Min	Max
Global	0.15	-0.33	0.93	0.17	-0.24	0.97
PU	0.19	-0.48	1.00	0.19	-0.23	1.00
PEOU	0.19	-0.48	1.00	0.18	-0.27	0.99
BI	0.18	-0.52	0.98	0.21	-0.22	0.95
UB	0.17	-0.51	0.99	0.18	-0.24	0.97

Table 2. TAM Results (Statistics)

Construct	Number Questions	Questionnaire I					Questionnaire II				
		Average	Standard Deviation	Median	25 percentile	75 percentile	Average	Standard Deviation	Median	25 percentile	75 percentile
Global	92	3.39	0.79	4.00	2.92	3.92	3.21	0.93	3.00	3.00	4.00
PU	49	3.35	0.78	3.00	2.88	3.92	3.12	0.91	3.00	3.00	4.00
PEOU	74	3.35	0.81	3.00	2.92	3.92	3.25	0.94	3.00	3.00	4.00
BI	42	3.48	0.74	4.00	3.08	4.10	3.09	0.93	3.00	3.00	4.00
UB	48	3.43	0.79	4.00	2.87	44.00	3.06	0.91	3.00	3.00	4.00

the second round was better, having an increase of 2% (from 0.1478 to 0.1674). This situation is essentially due to the rise verified by the answers given in the BI construct. In the other constructs, Kendall values are similar presenting variations around one point.

Analysing Table 2, it is possible to verify that the results of the second round are slightly worse. However, still being higher 3 points. The construct which presented the best results in the second round was Perceived Ease of Use (PEOU), with an average of 3.254. On the opposite side, it was Use Behaviour (UB), with a mean of 3.058.

DISCUSSION

The obtained results showed that the respondents agreed with most of the questions. Kendall was greater than 0 for all the constructs in the two rounds. That means, in general, the users approved the system's characteristics (i.e. the answers are more convergent than divergent). Overall, the majority of the questions were evaluated with three or more points, presenting an average more than 3 points. Questionnaires addressed all the features of the system, and the results were studied by answers' frequency and were organized in the relevant constructs. The charts of Figure 2 present the average (line) and mode (points) results for each of the questions. In Figure 2, it is possible to observe the answers by a question and questionnaire (Q1 and Q2).

Figure 2. General – Answers frequency in the two questionnaires

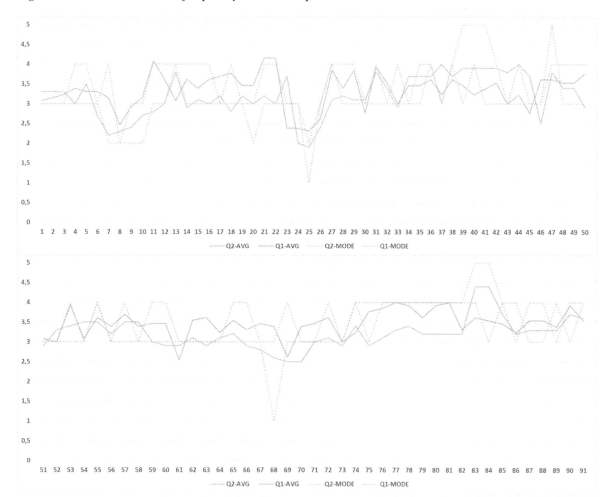

The questions which presented the highest differences between the two questionnaires were

23 - Did you receive any superior directive?
45- Metabolic Control?
84 - Utility of consulting information (hourly, daily, continuous)?
11 - Potentiates an improvement delivery of patient's health care?
22 - It allows an efficient use based on the available technical support?
46 - Others?

The average differences between Q2 and Q1 are significant for these questions, being respectively 1.32, 0.93, 0.86 and -1.28, -1.15, -1.12. Mode values for Q2 are between the minimum (1) and maximum (5), a fact not verified in Q1. These values indicate that users know which the best and worst system's features, and they have a firm opinion about that.

Table 3. Top 3 questions (highest and lowest evaluation)

Questionnaire I							
Construct	Global Mode	Highest Evaluation			Lowest Evaluation		
		Question	Mode	Average	Question	Mode	Average
PU	3	83	4	4.15	8	3	2.38
		84	4	4.15	18	2	2.46
		90	4	3.92	50	3	2.54
PEOU	4	31	4	4.08	8	3	2.38
		83	4	4.15	50	3	2.54
		84	4	4.15	51	4	2.61
BI	3	83	4	4.15	8	3	2.38
		84	4	4.15	24	2	2.31
		90	4	3.92	25	3	2.38
UB	3	76	4	3.77	8	3	2.38
		79	4	3.69	18	2	2.46
		90	4	3.92	24	2	2.31
Questionnaire II							
Construct	Global Mode	Highest Evaluation			Lowest Evaluation		
		Question	Mode	Average	Question	Mode	Average
PU	3	83	5	4.40	7	2	2.20
		84	5	4.40	8	2	2.30
		13	4	3.80	9	2	2.40
PEOU	3	84	5	4.40	7	2	2.20
		83	5	4.40	8	2	2.30
		44	3	4.40	9	2	2.40
BI	3	84	5	4.40	25	1	1.90
		23	3	3.70	24	3	2.00
		85	4	3.70	8	2	2.30
UB	3	83	5	4.40	25	1	1.90
		13	4	3.80	24	3	2.00
		90	3	3.70	8	2	2.30

Analysing Figure 2 and Table 3, we understand which features present better and worst results in the two questionnaires. The implemented modifications of the system resolved the reported problems because the worst results are different in the second questionnaire.

Some of the best results are related to the features of the two panels: vital signs and diary. The worst results are associated with functional characteristics and INTCare system relevance from the user's perspective. The users consider the system very useful (question 91 has an average of 3.6%). However, a problem remains: most of the nurses do not have time to operate the system because the patient requires their attention. Nevertheless, the system presents many benefits as can be verified by the answers given.

CONCLUSION AND FUTURE WORK

In this study, TAM3 was used to assess technology in a critical area (where, usually, the user is busy, with a multitude of tasks except information recording). In ICUs, the nurses have, as the main concern, the patient, and their main goal is to contribute to its recuperation. In this context, the use of four constructs allows having a real idea of the user perception of the deployed system.

The use of questionnaires to evaluate the four constructs turned out to be a good option because that way we assessed the quality of the system (the degree to which an individual believes that the system performs his or her job tasks appropriately) and to have a perception of the job relevance (individual's perception regarding the degree to which the targeted system is relevant for his or her job) (Venkatesh & Bala, 2008).

TAM3 advises that when the users are presented with new technology, some factors can influence their decision about how and when they will use it, particularly at the level of the four constructs. In this study, TAM3 was used to evaluate INTCare perception/adoption by ICU professionals and the users gave the system an average of 4 points to factors associated with patient monitoring (vital signs and some diary records). At the opposite direction (average less than 2.5) were the factors indirectly related to IN-TCare, i.e., factors associated with third-party systems and the data sources not controlled by INTCare.

Both questionnaires indicate that the user is sensitive to the system's features and its importance for the ICU. They consider INTCare, as a new system overriding prior systems. The results of the questions from Behaviour Intention showed that the high workload does not allow the use of multiple systems. The usefulness and importance of INTCare were verified by analysing the results associated with the constructs: Perceived Ease of USE and Perceived Usefulness. These questions showed that the system is a very useful tool for monitoring vital signs and for recording values that were previously recorded on paper.

The good results of Kendall (correlation level exceeding 0) allow concluding that this approach is likely to be used in ICUs since the degree of agreement among users for some answers is quite high. The increase of t, in the second round, demonstrates a better agreement, due to a better comprehension of the system. At the level of TAM, it was possible to observe that the user had a real perception of its behaviour and the system usability when the answers were distributed by user / group and construct.

After this study and according to the replies received in each questionnaire, it is possible to conclude that the system is very useful, and most of the problems previously identified were fixed. Further work includes the implementation of the information provided by the users. Combining TAM3, Kendall and two rounds of questionnaires to assess a technology represents a logical step to evaluate pervasive technologies in critical environments as is ICU. Finally, we proved that the use of an assessment mode can benefit ICU users and how TAM3 can be applied in this specific area of medicine.

ACKNOWLEDGMENT

This work has been supported by FCT - Fundação para a Ciência e Tecnologia within the Project Scope UID/CEC/00319/2013. The authors would like to thank FCT (Foundation for Science and Technology, Portugal) for the financial support through the contract PTDC/EEI-SII/1302/2012 (INTCare II).

REFERENCES

Bolboaca, S. D., & Jantschi, L. (2006). Pearson versus Spearman, Kendall's tau correlation analysis on structure-activity relationships of biologic active compounds. *Leonardo Journal of Sciences*, 5(9), 179–200.

Chooprayoon, V., & Fung, C.C. (2010). TECTAM: An Approach to Study Technology Acceptance Model (TAM) in Gaining Knowledge on the Adoption and Use of E-Commerce/E-Business Technology among Small and Medium Enterprises in Thailand.

Dietterich, T. (2000). Ensemble methods in machine learning. In *Multiple classifier systems*.

Fishbein, M., & Ajzen, I. (1975). *Belief, attitude, intention and behaviour: An introduction to theory and research*. Addison-Wesley.

Hammer, Ø., Harper, D.A.T., & Ryan, P.D. (2001). PAST-Palaeontological statistics. www.uv.es/~pardomv/pe/2001_1/past/pastprog/past.pdf

Johns, R. (2010). Likert Items and Scales. Survey Question Bank: Methods Fact Sheet.

Lyerla, F., LeRouge, C., Cooke, D. A., Turpin, D., & Wilson, L. (2010). A Nursing Clinical Decision Support System and potential predictors of Head-of-Bed position for patients receiving Mechanical Ventilation. *American Journal of Critical Care, 19*(1), 39–47. doi:10.4037/ajcc2010836 PMID:20045847

Portela, F. Filipe Pinto, & Santos, M. F. (2012). Data mining predictive models for pervasive intelligent decision support in intensive care medicine. *Proceedings of the international Conference on Knowledge Management and Information Sharing KMIS '12*.

Portela, F., Aguiar, J., Santos, M. F., Silva, Á., & Rua, F. (2013). Pervasive Intelligent Decision Support System - Technology Acceptance in Intensive Care Units. In Advances in Intelligent Systems and Computing. Springer.

Portela, F., Gago, P., Santos, M. F., & Silva, Á., & Rua, F. (2012). Intelligent and Real Time Data Acquisition and Evaluation to Determine Critical Events in Intensive Medicine. *Paper presented at the International Conference on Health and Social Care Information Systems and Technologies HCist'12*, Portugal. 10.1016/j.protcy.2012.09.079

Portela, F., Gago, P., Santos, M. F., Silva, A., Rua, F., Machado, J., ... (2011). Knowledge Discovery for Pervasive and Real-Time Intelligent Decision Support in Intensive Care Medicine. *Proceedings of International Conference on Knowledge Management and Information Sharing KMIS '11*, Paris, France (p. 12). Springer.

Portela, F., Santos, M. F., Machado, J., Silva, Á., Rua, F., & Abelha, A. (2012). Intelligent Data Acquisition and Scoring System for Intensive Medicine. In Information Technology in Bio- and Medical Informatics, LNCS (Vol. 7451). Springer. doi:10.1007/978-3-642-32395-9_1

Portela, F., Santos, M. F., & Vilas-Boas, M. (2012). A Pervasive Approach to a Real-Time Intelligent Decision Support System in Intensive Medicine. In Knowledge Discovery, Knowledge Engineering and Knowledge Management, CCIS (Vol. 272).

Portela, F., Santos, M. F., Machado, J. M., Abelha, A., Silva, Á., & Rua, F. (2013). Real-Time Decision Support in Intensive Medicine - An intelligent approach for monitoring Data Quality. *International Journal of Medical and Bioengineering*.

Santos, M. F., Portela, F., Vilas-Boas, M., Machado, J., Abelha, A., & Neves, J. (2011). INTCARE - Multi-agent approach for real-time Intelligent Decision Support in Intensive Medicine. *Paper presented at the 3rd International Conference on Agents and Artificial Intelligence (ICAART)*, Rome, Italy.

Silva, Á., Cortez, P., Santos, M. F., Gomes, L., & Neves, J. (2008). Rating organ failure via adverse events using data mining in the intensive care unit. *Artificial Intelligence in Medicine*, *43*(3), 179–193. doi:10.1016/j.artmed.2008.03.010 PMID:18486459

Varshney, U. (2009). *Pervasive Healthcare Computing: EMR/EHR, Wireless and Health Monitoring*. New York: Springer-Verlag. doi:10.1007/978-1-4419-0215-3

Venkatesh, V., & Bala, H. (2008). Technology acceptance model 3 and a research agenda on interventions. *Decision Sciences*, *39*(2), 273–315. doi:10.1111/j.1540-5915.2008.00192.x

Venkatesh, V., & Davis, F. D. (2000). A theoretical extension of the technology acceptance model: Four longitudinal field studies. *Management Science*, *46*(2), 186–204. doi:10.1287/mnsc.46.2.186.11926

This research was previously published in the International Journal of Reliable and Quality E-Healthcare (IJRQEH), 6(2); edited by Anastasius Moumtzoglou; pages 1-16, copyright year 2017 by IGI Publishing (an imprint of IGI Global).

APPENDIX

Table 4. Questionnaire

		Question	PU	PEOU	BI	UB
-	1.	**Level of experience in technology**				
-	1.1.	What is your experience in technology?				
-	1.1.1.	How much time you spend on the computer?	X	X		X
-	1.1.1.1.	Less than 2 hours/day	X	X		X
-	1.1.1.2.	Between 2 to 4 hours/day	X	X		X
-	1.1.1.3.	More 4 hours/day	X	X		X
-	1.2.	Type of User?				
-	1.2.1.	Full autonomy	X			X
-	1.2.2.	Rarely need technical support (less than 3 times/month)	X			X
-	1.2.3.	Need regular technical support	X			X
-	1.3.	Use computer preferably for?				
-	1.3.1.	Application of production stuff (email, word processing, spread sheet)	X	X	X	X
-	1.3.2.	Handling/Consulting administrative information	X	X	X	X
-	1.3.3.	Handling/Consulting clinical information	X	X	X	X
-	1.3.4.	Handling/Consult management information	X	X	X	X
-	2.	**System INTCare**				
-	2.1.	Functional Characteristics				
1	2.1.1.	It allows the efficient registration of the information?		X		X
2	2.1.2.	It allows obtaining efficient information for decision support?		X		X
3	2.1.3.	It is easy to operate?		X		X
4	2.1.4.	It shows the prevision of Adverse Effects in an efficacy way?		X	X	
5	2.1.5.	It shows usefulness when predicts the Scores?		X	X	
6	2.1.6.	It improves the proactive performance of the professionals?	X	X	X	X
7	2.1.7.	It allows tasks to be performed with greater precision?	X	X		
-	2.1.8.	Three + Two?				
8	2.1.9.	Can help to mitigate situations of an excessive workload?	X	X	X	X
9	2.1.10.	Can allow a major control of several tasks?	X	X		X
10	2.1.11.	Can help to have a better decision making based in best evidences?	X	X	X	X
11	2.1.12.	Potentiates an improvement delivery of patient's health care?	X	X		X
12	2.1.13.	It allows inquire and modify records from the previous day?	X	X		X
13	2.1.14.	It allows monitoring the patient's condition?	X	X		X
14	2.1.15.	It promotes automating tasks?	X	X		X
15	2.1.16.	It allows inquire the therapeutic plan for the next day?	X	X		X
16	2.1.17.	It allows answering with the appropriate information to perform the task?	X	X	X	X
-	2.2.	Technical Characteristics:				

Table 4. Continued

		Question	PU	PEOU	BI	UB
17	2.2.1.	Can promote quality of the information?	X		X	X
18	2.2.2.	Can access to information quickly?	X			X
19	2.2.3.	It allows access to information in a secure way (e.g. EHR)?	X	X		X
20	2.2.4.	Can operate simultaneously with other hospital systems?	X	X	X	X
21	2.2.5.	Can facilitate an operation by having a tactile interface beside to patient's beds?	X	X	X	X
22	2.2.6.	It allows an efficient use based on the available technical support?	X	X	X	X
-	2.3.	Relevance of the INTCare system from the user's perspective:				
23	2.3.1.	Did you receive any superior directive?			X	X
24	2.3.2.	Do you think that other nurses should use the system as well?			X	X
25	2.3.3.	Other professional colleagues think that you should use the system?			X	X
26	2.3.4.	The person who assesses your performance does think that you should use the system?			X	X
27	2.3.5.	The ICU chief board has been useful to implement the system?			X	X
28	2.3.6.	The CHP supports the utilization of the system?			X	X
29	2.3.7.	Do you believe the system influences your professional performance?			X	X
30	2.3.8.	It brings direct or indirect benefits to the patients?	X		X	X
-	2.4.	Individually evaluate the registration of each parameter presented on the Diary Panel				
31	2.4.1.	Monitoring of the patient?		X		
32	2.4.2.	Transfusions of the patient?		X		
33	2.4.3.	Medication of the patient?		X		
34	2.4.4.	Outputs (Urine Output, faeces, Vomit)		X		
35	2.4.5.	Renal Replacement Therapy?		X		
36	2.4.6.	Invasive Ventilation?		X		
37	2.4.7.	Spontaneous Ventilation?		X		
38	2.4.8.	Non-invasive Ventilation?		X		
39	2.4.9.	Neuropsychic levels?		X		
40	2.4.10.	Scale of Pain 1?		X		
41	2.4.11.	Scale of Pain 2?		X		
42	2.4.12.	Scale of delirium?		X		
43	2.4.13.	Sedation Scale?		X		
44	2.4.15.	Glasgow?		X		
Question			**PU**	**PEOU**	**BI**	**UB**
45	2.4.16.	Metabolic Control?		X		
46	2.4.17.	Others?		X		
47	2.4.18.	Positioning?		X		
48	2.4.19.	Quality of the record from the previous day?	X	X		
49	2.4.20.	Quality of the record from the current day?	X	X		

continued on following page

Table 4. Continued

		Question	PU	PEOU	BI	UB
50	2.4.21.	The Balance is done correctly?	X	X		
51	2.4.22.	Evaluation of Performance (speed)?	X	X	X	X
52	2.4.23.	Global Evaluation of the Diary?	X	X	X	X
-	2.5.	Evaluate the potential of each registration presented on the Procedures Panel:				
53	2.5.1.	Procedures registration of the patient?		X		
54	2.5.2.	Graphic Registration?		X		
55	2.5.3.	Global Evaluation of the Procedures?	X	X	X	X
-	2.6.	Evaluate the potential of each registration presented on the Analysis Panel:				
56	2.6.1.	Disposition of data?		X		
57	2.6.2.	It is easy to read?		X		
58	2.6.3.	Global Evaluation of Analysis?	X	X	X	X
-	2.7.	Evaluate the potential of each registration presented on the Orders Panel:				
59	2.7.1.	Performed exams Registration?		X		
60	2.7.2.	Registration of the requested exams?		X		
61	2.7.3.	Utility?	X			
62	2.7.4.	Quality of information?	X			
63	2.7.5.	Global evaluation of Orders?	X	X	X	X
-	2.8.	Evaluate the potential of each registration presented on the Intervention's panel:				
64	2.8.1.	Can facilitate obtaining information regarding the realized interventions?		X		
65	2.8.2.	Can facilitate obtaining information regarding the therapeutic attitudes?		X		
66	2.8.3.	Graphic aspect?		X		
67	2.8.4.	Registration of the work plan?		X		
-	2.8.5.	Two + Two?				
68	2.8.6.	Utility of TISS28?	X	X	X	X
69	2.8.7.	Graphic aspect of TISS28?	X	X	X	X
70	2.8.8.	Global Evaluation of TISS28	X	X	X	X
-	2.9.	Evaluate the potential of each registration presented on the Historic Panel:				
71	2.9.1.	Ease of consulting of patient's Historic?		X		
72	2.9.2.	Automatic creation of PDF?		X		
73	2.9.3.	Global Evaluation of Historic?	X	X	X	X
-	2.10.	Evaluate the potential of each registration presented on the Scores panel:				
74	2.10.1.	The records made automatically, present similar values relatively to the manuscripts ones?	X	X		
75	2.10.1.1.	Utility of SOFA CHART?	X	X	X	X
76	2.10.1.2.	Utility of GLASGOW CHART?	X	X	X	X
77	2.10.1.3.	Graphic aspect is intuitive?	X	X	X	X
78	2.10.1.4.	The graphics can help to a better understanding of the real patient's condition?	X	X	X	X

continued on following page

Table 4. Continued

		Question	PU	PEOU	BI	UB
79	2.10.2.	By using the automation registration of Scores it facilitates the registration of SAPS II?	X		X	X
80	2.10.2.1.	SAPS III?	X		X	X
81	2.10.2.2.	GLASGOW?	X		X	X
82	2.10.3.	Global Evaluation of Scores?	X	X	X	X
-	2.11.	Evaluate the potential of each registration presented on the Vital Signs Panel:				
83	2.11.1.	Utility of Information?	X	X	X	
84	2.11.1.1.	Utility of consulting information (hourly, daily, continuous)?	X	X	X	
85	2.11.1.2.	Graphic aspect?	X	X	X	
86	2.11.1.3.	MEWS	X	X	X	
87	2.11.2.	Adverse events – Utility of system?	X		X	X
88	2.11.2.1.	The early warning system for Adverse Events is useful?	X	X		X
89	2.11.2.2.	Graphic Aspect?		X		
90	2.11.3.	Global evaluation of the vital signs?	X	X	X	X
91	2.12.	It is advantageous to use this system in intensive care units?	X		X	X
-	2.13.	Positive aspects of the system INTCare?				
-	2.14.	Suggestions to mitigate the less positive aspects previously evaluated?				
-	2.15.	Suggestions to make the system more advantageous?				

Table 5. Supplementary Table: Level of experience in Information Technology

Question	Answer	% - Q1	% - Q2
How much time do you spend at the computer?	Less than 2 hours/day	7%	20%
	Between 2 to 4 hours/day	57%	80%
	More 4 hours/day	36%	0%
Type of User?	Full Autonomy	62%	80%
	Rarely need technical support	38%	10%
	Need regular technical support	0%	10%
Uses computer preferably for? (multiple)	Application of office (email, text processing, spread sheet)	62%	80%
	Handling/Consult administrative info	31%	20%
	Handling/Consult clinical info	77%	50%
	Handling/Consult management Info	8%	10%
Did you participate in the first round (Q1)?	YES	- -	40%
	NO	-	60%

Chapter 13
Wireless Heartrate Monitoring Along Prioritized Alert Notification Using Mobile Techniques

Rajasekaran Rajkumar
Vellore Institute of Technology, India

ABSTRACT

The increasing number of problems that need to be addressed in the hospital sector calls for innovation in this field. It brings us the need to find cost-effective and memory-efficient solutions to handle the vast data and sector it into essential information to operate on the patient. There used to be many systems to manage clinical records which are fixed at a place. It is quite complicated to get the information and make this data available at a patient's bedside. This leads to a considerable amount of wasted time in moving to those storage PCs and also the cost afforded is comparatively high. A computer system that controls and accomplishes all the data in the hospital database to provide effective healthcare is called hospital information system (HIS). The introduction of HIS made billing and inventor easier for the staff. This paper discusses diverse methods that improve the cost, demands of HIS, and provide techniques to function efficiently using wireless networks. Also, the paper gives a comparative study on different aspects such as cost, quality of service, transportation, and security. A new system is proposed by combining the wireless healthcare system along prioritized alert notification.

INTRODUCTION

A Computer system that controls and accomplishes all the data in the hospital database to provide effective health care is called hospital information system (HIS). These health care systems have been existing since 1960s and have developed over time with better facilities. When they were in early stages, those systems didn't provide solution faster when applied in real time, but now system provide solution faster and reliable. The introduction of HIS made billing and inventor easier for the staff. But, now all the

DOI: 10.4018/978-1-7998-2451-0.ch013

Copyright © 2020, IGI Global. Copying or distributing in print or electronic forms without written permission of IGI Global is prohibited.

Figure 1. Hospital Information System Modules

HOSPITAL INFORMATION SYSTEM MODULES		
CORE MODULE	**SUPPORTING MODULE**	**ENTERPRISE MODULE**
Patient Accounts	Blood Bank	Finance
Diagnostic Imaging	Elderly services	Human Resource
Radiology	General Services	
Oncology	Patient Services	
Ophthalmology	Purchasing & Supply	
Orthopaedics	Therapy	
Otolaryngology	Pharmacy	
Laboratory	Health & Safety	

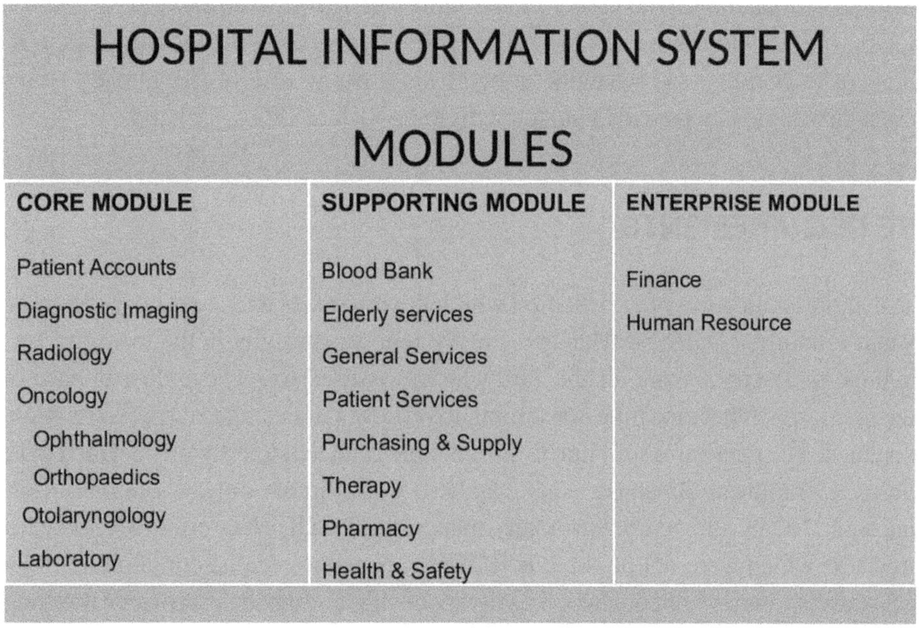

hospitals want to integrate the clinical, financial and other reports together to make the entire process a closed loop. This not only benefits the staff and patients to track the details but also make the discharge process also easier and faster.

Modern healthcare system requires integration of various departments which can be categorized as Core modules, supporting modules and Enterprise modules. Code Module includes Patient Accounts, Diagnostic Imaging, Radiology, Oncology, Ophthalmology, Orthopedics, Otolaryngology, etc. Supporting Modules includes Blood Bank, Elderly services, General Services, Patient Services, Purchasing & Supplies, Therapy, Pharmacy and Health & Safety. Enterprise management include Finance and Human Resources. These department needs to integrated to retrieve patient details easily during emergencies and discharge.

Earlier there used to be many systems which provide the facility for managing the clinical records which are fixed at a place. It is quite complicated to get the information and make this data available at patient's bed side. The attendants for the patient have to physically go to the location and manually enter that data into those PC's which can lead to redundancy, data misplacement and errors in recording the data. This leads to considerable amount of wastage of time in moving to those storage PCs and also the cost afforded is comparatively high. Now-a-days, almost all the European countries are already having local area network (LAN) and wide area network (WAN). This eliminates the conventional process of treatment for the patient.

When maintaining the clinical record, many other details should be continuously monitored like whether the hospital bills are clear as per the due date which is to be collected from the administration department and also the availability of all the essential drugs to be supplied for the patient should be checked in advance from the logistics department. All this patient data must be exchanged between doctor and nurse and always they should be synchronized accordingly.

This problem can be handled by having mobile computers which are connected to a central database through the wireless connection. The servers will be connected to the wired or wireless LAN with hospital systems. The appropriate alert messages can be triggered by the server if the drugs are out of stock or if the patient needs to be attended by the doctor at the hour. Many systems are already being developed using wireless technologies by provided personal digital assistant (PDA) in hand.

DATABASE REQUIREMENTS

A database is a digital collection of information which are organizes and stored in a secure way for easy accessibility and reliability. Database Management System was initially in the form of Flat files which contains one huge table comprising all the data which was used to retrieve data in case of concerns. When file size increased, it became time consuming to retrieve data using flat file, so relational database came into existence. The data were split into different tables and a hierarchy was defined to access them, this is known as Hierarchical Database. This Database was suitable only where one-to-one mapping is used. Relational DBMS allowed one-to-many mapping. NoSQL (Not only SQL) used information in unstructured text which were not possible is RDBMS, hence it became common in all industries. A NoSQL uses Datasets to arrive at conclusion easily. A healthcare database replaces the file system and paper documents. It follows OLTP database system (Online Transaction Processing Database) which is very convenient to retrieve data immediately. An OLTP is characterized by large number of transaction which included insertion, updation and deletion. It results in very fast retrieval of data of data by processing query and maintaining data integrity. The Electronic health record (EHR) is an ordinal version of patient's hospital records. EMR (Electronic Medical record is narrowed view of a patient's medical history whereas a EHR is a comprehensive record which includes primary information such as the personal details, patient's life-threatening allergy, lab results, medication records, etc. which is not only is for tracking/ monitoring data over time but also provides the following benefits:

- The data collected from the hospital can suggest an emergency treatment for an unconscious patient by knowing the medical record and his allergies.
- The patient can view his own record and his results from lab which can help him to take his medication outside hospital.
- Very useful for discharge process and follow-up process which makes the entire progression timesaving.
- Reduces the health care cost by avoiding repeated/ duplicate test since all the lab records are available hence providing an effective and cost-efficient process.

EXISTING SYSTEM

A Survey of E-Healthcare Information System Based on Android Application (Tupe & Kulkarni, 2015)

A device is used to sense optical/ electrical signals and take information such as temperature, BP, user defined data from a patient and converted into electrical data. Sensors is used to sense the data and are classified as active sensor and wearable sensor. The active sensor requires more power whereas the wearable sensor contains a small operating system. Hence, the wearable sensor is efficient and uses an embedded system to be attached along with it to connect with the other devices/ server. For this connection, A M2M gateway is used. This not only provides a medium to interact between devices but also establishes as secure communication so that the patient data are private. This paper proposes a system architecture which establishes such a network where user is authenticated and permitted to view/ send their data. The service-oriented architecture is used as it provides an enhanced healthcare management system by offering optimized data workflow on the medical experimental data. The data are processed before sending to server so as to maintain consistency. The data processing include cleaning, updating, converting, validating, sorting, summarizing, analyzing and reporting. It not only compares various algorithms with respect to throughput and delay but also the protocol used in the architecture.

WARD-IN-HAND Project (Ancona et al., 2000)

The network is a wireless LAN of sophisticated pen-based industrial terminals based on FSSH radio frequency communication at 2.4GHz with a communication bandwidth up to 2Mbs. They will connect to already existing wired LANs. Features of Ward-in-hand are:

- Achieving the maximum from the "hands-free" fault tolerance and security.
- Using the available hardware and software to cut down the cost and also be compatible with the existing hospital systems.
- It also provides the security and features for the authorized access into the patient record files.

Human Interface

To avoid the problems of using the conventional keyboards to type, this idea replaces the keyboard usage. It provides two modes of interaction:

- Pen-based
- Voice based

A Wireless Healthcare Service System for Elderly with Dementia (Lin et al., 2006)

The author proposes a system which does indoor, outdoor, emergency rescue and remote monitoring for dementia patients by locating the patient's position. The indoor system keeps a check on dementia patient and sends a notification to the neighborhoods. This uses a near field communication network whereas the outdoor monitoring uses a GSM network. The purpose of this paper is to integrate radio frequency identification (RFID) with GPS (global positioning system), Global system for mobile communication (GSM) and Global information system(GIS) to monitor and collect the status information from them. The architecture consists of a web server, a database and message controller server and a health GIS-server.

Indoor Monitoring

It makes a call to the call center automatically when the elder person leaves home alone without notice. This message will be immediately received by the patient's care takers.

Outdoor Monitoring

A pre-set outdoor area can be chosen, so that it constants checks if the patient is in that particular area. If the patient leaves the area, an alarm will be sent to the family through GSM network.

Emergency Rescue

The patient who is in emergency situation can signal the call Centre so that the geo position and profile details will be transmitted to the care takers. Remote monitoring: To get a single or periodic location report of the patient care takers can authenticate and use the system to track the patient.

The longitude and latitude co-ordinates of the patient received by the call center are converted to street map location using GPS and GIS parser and this information is combined with the personal profile information for a complete report. Each time a TIP (Tracing Information Packet) is generated and stored in the database. There will also be GPSlog, GISlog and Message log tables to store all up to date information of each segment of transmission process.

To monitor the patient constantly, sensors affixed to the body parts are used. To sense, process and transmit the sensor data use of RFID reader, a microprocessor and GSM communication module is beneficial. GSM satellite location module provides location information of the patient. The Short Message Controller receives the latest GPS data, H-GIS produces two GIS images with different resolutions to display appropriate GIS.

Emergency Response in Smartphone-Based Mobile Ad-Hoc Networks (Mitra & Poellabauer, 2012)

In this paper the author presents a framework Breathing Rate Monitoring (BREMON) which monitors the breathing activities of multiples patients in parallel from the accelerometer of their smart phones at a disaster site. It is placed on the chest to count BPM. Breaths per Minute (BPM) are sent over a multi hop MANET (mobile ad-hoc network). Any abnormal condition is reported to the smart phones of paramedics by making a pop up of the wave form of the recent breathing activities to decide on emergency of situation. BREMON uses Spontaneous Resource Sharing Infrastructure (SPIRIT) which allows to share the data as services within this infrastructure.

The process is done in three steps. They are sensing, computing of BPM and communicating the alert situation. The process of converting the accelerometer data into breathing rate is done in three steps. They are pre-processing, noise reduction and breathing rate. The force of gravity and other external factors influencing the reading are removed using the low pass filter and noise is smoothened. This data is transmitted over the window period of last 60 seconds.

At the point when a paramedic gadget (i.e., benefit looking for customer) in BREMON needs to find the patients as of now being observed (i.e., specialist co-ops) in its closeness, it communicates a Service Discovery Request (SDREQ) message with a related time-to-live (ttl) esteem. The SDREP messages over various bounces are totaled into a solitary SDREP message. Once the customer gets the SDREP message it chooses a specialist organization from the rundown of specialist co-ops in the SDREP message. Next, the customer sends a Service Access Request (SAREQ) message to the chose specialist organization. The asked for specialist co-op answers with a Service Access Reply (SSREP) message either permitting or declining the administration. On the off chance that the administration is without a doubt, then the specialist co-op sends intermittent Service Alive Messages (SAMSG) to the customer; these messages contain an overhaul the most recent BPM of the patient being observed. Utilization of Bluetooth makes it financially savvy than utilizing Wi-Fi or 3G or 4G systems.

SparkMed: A Framework for Dynamic Integration of Multimedia Medical Data into Distributed m-Health Systems (Constantinescu et al., 2012)

This paper proposes the SparkMed data integration framework for mobile healthcare which utilizes the LTE wireless technologies which has enhanced network capabilities, by enabling a wide range of heterogeneous medical software and uses peer-to-peer storage in multimedia cloud database systems. Through this it lets to transcode and access the multimedia data on any mobile device by moving the personal data in to the cloud by making it accessible. Remote users can view and also modify the data on cloud. SparkMed uses central server node based on reachability, network access time, and security/ or the storage capability.

This node is found by elimination procedure. Data synchronization is achieved by means of a priority-based synchronization system that propagates any data changes to central node, which interrupt dates the entire network of nodes.

Each non-central node registers data of interest (informed by the host software), Thenetworkthenensuresthateachnodeiskeptsynchronizedwithitsrespectivedat source(s) at all times. Conflict resolution is applied in case of incompatible changes.

A Secure Handshake Scheme with Symptoms-Matching for mHealthcare Social Network (Lu et al., 2011)

The objective is to develop securely and timely report patient's PHI to eHealth center for achieving better healthcare quality. sometimes, active patients can establish same symptom-based social relationship, and self-control and share their PHI to each other. It involves system setup, patient joining, patient same symptom based handshaking algorithms. This SSH scheme must ensure correctness, impersonator resistance and detector resistance that the patients who are trying to connect are genuinely trying for the right partner and the error detection must also be done properly to ensure there is no security breach of information.

Mobile Telemedicine System for Home Care and Patient Monitoring (Figueredo & Dias, 2004)

This system delivers a laid-back monitoring scheme to solve the health problems in out fast-paced world. Difficulties in searching for a hospital and travelling in traffic are the major problem that needed to be addressed. The telemedicine system for patient monitoring allows the device to collect the vital signal records, therapy and medication records and provide treatment for the patient. The Solution for telemedicine comprises a stable GSM or satellite communication which provides more flexibility in offering service. Since, a mobile phone has become a necessary product, it can be connected to electro medic devices to transfer the patient data. These data are transported through serial port using an RS232 Interface.

The architecture comprises of a server along with data storage which acquires the data through TCP/UDP. The electomedic device collect vital signals such as ECG, heart rate, Blood pressure, SPO2, respiration rate and temperature and sends to mobile phone through RS232 Interface. These signals are converted into packets and the sent to server through internet. Since the connectivity might become a problem, the communication protocol has to be defined in the module. In this paper, Agilent A3 patient monitor is used in implementation. JAVA MIDP (Mobile Information Device Profile) is used for simple user interface as it contains commands.

The data in the server needs to be retrieved and analyzed faster. Therefore, a distributed system was developed under JAVA technology. Their implementation provided options to visualize the list and export them if needed. The system's transmission rate was 0.6sec per packet for an ECG signal and 2sec for heartrate. The loss in the data signals were handled by Error correction method CRC resulting in a reliable transfer and retrieval of data. This project was aimed to be an alternative to elderly and handicapped patients to assist their health from a distance and also reduced the travelling cost and time.

Alerts in Mobile Healthcare Applications: Requirements and Pilot Study (Kafeza et al., 2004)

The hospital management workspace has become mobile due to irregular events such as rescheduling, crucial laboratory results and adverse drug events. Therefore, sending the appropriate message to the appropriate person in time needs to be taken care to avoid malfunctioning of the management. These messages are efficiently routed as ALERTS and are monitored to enhance the quality of service. The routing is systematically performed by correlating with medical events, availability of medical assistance and few other parameters. The urgent events are classified as Alert and acknowledgement is required for successful closure, else it triggers an additional notification to the respective patient/ parties. Existing methods include paging and notification in cellular phones but it's not efficient for future hospital management system. Technologies such as PDA (Personal Digital Assistance) and portable personal computers are becoming popular making the relationship between doctor and patient ubiquitous.

The methodology used in this paper provides a robust, cost and time efficient along with user friendly system to improve the communication between the doctors and between the doctor and patient outside the hospital. The implementation was divided into phases to provide an automated system. The first phase was to manage the alerts of the staff and monitor the alerts between them. The second phase was to integrate with the healthcare alert management system (HAMS) with the server in the hospital. The third phase is to communicate with other hospitals and suppliers to work efficiently. The HAMS consist of three parts, *the process and alert definition subsystem* is used to define the events and produce alerts accordingly. *The execution subsystem*s used for routing and monitoring of the alerts. *The Device subsystem* is used to represent a user environment that can show the alert messages. The medical emergency is further assessed depending on the severity of the event and the alert message are prioritized. Active alert table is maintained to keep track of unacknowledged messages and the priority of the unacknowledged alert messages is raised.

Even though the system provides flexibility and efficiency, it can be demanding if configured wrongly. An algorithm is needed to map the right person to send alert is nontrivial. Hence, the system has to be trained for all possible scenarios and further tuned to the requirements of different hospitals.

HCPP: Cryptography Based Secure EHR System for Patient Privacy and Emergency Healthcare (Sun et al., 2011)

In electronic health record (EHR) system, privacy is the major concern. The patients are willing to accept the record only if the data is protected and proper disclosure agreement is made resulting in high security, more efficient, less prone to errors and faster availability. This paper proposes an EHR system based on cryptographic constructions and existing wireless network infrastructure so as to provide protection of data.

The approach of this paper is based on healthcare system for patient privacy (HCPP) which satisfies few privacy regulations. A HCPP system contains the entities such as Patient, doctor, S-server, family, P-device and A-server. The patient is the user of the system with a device to store data whereas Doctor is the healthcare taker. The S-server stores the PHI of each patient in the hospital whereas the A-server is the trusted server which is run by the state government department. The P-device is the electronic device which the patient owns and has more capabilities such as cryptography, commutations, network access, etc. PHI is protected health information which contains the heath data of each individual. Usually, the HCPP has both PHI and de-identified information.

The device encrypts both PHI and de-identified information and store in server. The architecture is a LAN network which connects the device to the hospital and S-server interacts with the device through LAN network. The retrieval of data is of two types, PHI retrieval and MHI retrieval. PHI is used by the doctor to identify the patient id whereas the MHI is used in case of emergency. The MHI is collected and encrypted by the device and generates a key which is secure. The paper also takes about various security issues and attacks possible in HCPP system.

COMPARATIVE STUDY

All the methods proposed in various papers have their own advantages and disadvantages in terms of the feasibility and operational strategies. E-Healthcare Information System using android application needs no extra cost in terms of maintaining paper work for storing information or keeping track of it (Tupe & Kulkarni, 2015). It also minimizes error and flow of data in the system is optimized. Transportation of the patient is not needed for check-up and it is secured. Ward-In-Hand project has complex requirements and is not efficient in terms of cost and voice recognition is made easy for the users. This system is developed as an assistant to the hospital officials and so patients have to visit hospital to avail the services. There are no security measures taken in protecting the system from intrusion (Ancona et al., 2000). Wireless healthcare system needs communication cost and it is handy device. So, patient is remotely monitored by their dearer ones and also the corresponding physicians (Lin et al., 2006). Ad-hoc network for emergency response provides cost effective solution among wireless networks as it uses Bluetooth as mode of communication. It provides periodic notifications for the attenders in case of extreme conditions like calamities, or a disaster where large number of people need to be attended at the same time. There is no QoS as Bluetooth is unreliable (Mitra & Poellabauer, 2012). Multimedia

Table 1. Comparative study of various methods

PAPER	COST	QoS	Transposition	Security
E-Healthcare Information System using android application	No paperwork requirement	Reduced medical error and optimize dataflow	X	M2M gateway provide de data secure
Ward-In Hand project	Complex requirements	Voice- recognition on makes it easy for users.	✓	X
Wireless healthcare system	Communication cost	Handy device for dementia patients.	X	Secure monitor and report device
Ad-hoc network for emergency response	Cost effective as no Wi-Fi	Periodic notification are sent to attenders	X	X
Multimedia medical data integrated	Data on cloud so no	No QoS, future enhance	✓	All the data availa
Symptom matching secure handshake	-	Allows transparent to registered	X	✓
Telemedicine ne with RS232 Interface	reduce d	High	X	X
Alert notification with HAMS architecture	More efficient algorithms hm and device s for paging are need.	Provides high QoS by minimizi ng delay in alerts and monitori ng	✓	Stable securi ty
Cryptographic encryption uses LAN network	LAN network is needed	Efficient storage and retrieval of data	✓	Highly security

medical data integrated into distributive system stores data on cloud and also provides the access of medical images to all the devices in network acting as an assist for hospital systems (Constantinescu et al., 2012). Symptom-matching secure handshake method provides a social networking platform for the patients of a hospital to meet the patients of similar disease and build moral support and the application is secured by the algorithmic solution (Lu et al., 2011).

Telemedicine with RS-232 Interface reduces cost and quality of the system is high (Figueredo et al., 2004). Alert notification with HAMS architecture provides an efficient algorithm and devices for paging is needed. It provides high QoS by minimizing delay in rendering alerts. Patient must be a hospital admits to utilize this service. Necessary security measures are taken (Kafeza et al., 2004). Cryptographic encryption uses LAN network and provides efficient storage and retrieval mechanism. It uses cryptographic techniques to secure the data (Sun et al., 2011).

A comparison is show below with respect to Cost, Quality of Service, Transportation requirement and security of the Application as shown in Table 1.

PROPOSED METHODOLOGY

The Proposed Health care system contains patient, physician, SMS server, Patient App, Database server connected by wireless area network. The Azure Cloud database provides a secure and wide range access of health care information about the patient. NoSQL is used to extract data from the Database Server and connect with the Web Server and the GIS (geographic Information System). The Web server provides

Figure 2. Architecture diagram

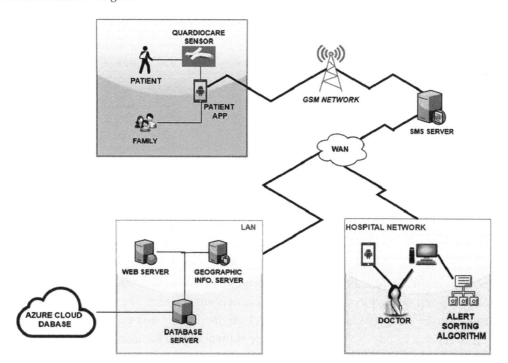

service for the users through the WAN network and responsible for integrating the information which will be converted into required format and sent to the user/ physician. The GIS is used in case of emergency situation to search the patient and efficiently acquire the location of the missing patient. It allows helps in finding the address of the patient by converting the GPS co-ordinates. Therefore, the patient movement will be recorded and will inform the patient and family in emergency situation as shown in Figure 2.

Patient and family are the users of the healthcare system where the patient health is tracked by the sensor attached through the wireless portable phone which has an installed Application to send the Protected Health Information details known as PHI.

The Patient Application is installed in electronic device such as smartphone, PDA or a secure wearable device. The device lets the family of the patient know the status of the patient and provides alert messages to the concerned persons of the patient in case of emergency based on the priority of the alert message and also it redirects the alert if the alert situation is not attended within a specific time period.

The ECG monitor used in the proposed model is DARDIOCARE which is a wireless wearable device. The device seamlessly fits the patient and provides accurate monitoring of the heart activity in daily basis. The data can be remotely accessed from the device and provides doctor/ physician accurate information. It not only measures heartrate but also body temperature, stress level, respiratory rate and tracks the activity of the patient as shown in Figure 3.

GSM network is used to notify the family members the movement of the patient while he is leaving home. It is also used for transmitting the emergency alert messages and to receive any commands as specified in the server.

The telecom short messaging service i.e. SMS server is used to control for handling the vast amount of data packets arrived at the server side through the GSM network from multiple devices.

Figure 3. QARDIOCARE sensor

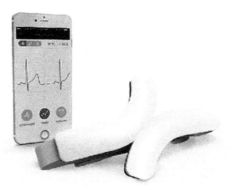

The LAN network is used for the local connection of the systems and the servers within the hospital to limit the information to the hospital management. While the WAN network is used for getting the remote data from mobile applications to store and update it in the database server as well as to get it checked and processed by the physician for future medical suggestions.

Web service server is for providing an online website facility for non-registered users. It can be accessed by an IP address by anyone without any prior authentication for using it.

GIS server uses the Global Positioning System to track the patient's location by converting the latitude and longitude co-ordinates into a geographical location and also adds additional information like the patient's profile like height, age, picture to generate missing report in emergency situations. It can also be used for providing transportation facilities to patients to the hospital for regular check-ups.

Cloud database is used for having backup of data on cloud and provide security for the server databases by restricting the access to them only for LAN devices. The data of server databases can be reflected in the cloud database regularly to protect data from theft or loss.

Microsoft Azure Cloud Database is used to build and maintain application and the algorithm runs on the cloud platform to provide service to the patient as well as the hospital staffs. The Microsoft Azure has maximum reliability with high data protection. The acquired data is taken from the Azure cloud and the data is processed by the sorting algorithm and once the patient is admitted the particular details of the patient is removed from the cloud. The data will be monitored continuously by the QardioCare sensor and stores the large amount of data in the Database. The actual reason of using cloud Database is to universally access the content and store large amount of ECG data for each patient.

Database server is used for storing and maintaining the information consistently in the database. Patient record, location details and status information of the patient are stored in various tables having interrelations between them.

The below Database is used for sorting algorithm to priorities the patient according thot he critical level Ci. Table 2 shows the database table for sorting algorithms.

Algorithm to assign critical value to the patient during emergency conditions: The critical category will be chosen by the patient / family during emergency cases and the respective value is calculated using the mean and Standard deviation.

Table 2. Database Table for Sorting Algorithm

Patient Id	Pi: Varchar
Critical level	Ci: Int
Admitted Status	Ai: Bool
Other Details	Di: Description

Alert sorting algorithm is used for ranking of the alerts from various devices who are in the emergency situations. Then these alerts are processed and served considering the urgency of the situation of that particular alert.

The algorithm checks for new alert in the background using New-Emergency function and appends the new emergency case to the set of alerts already present. The sorting algorithm

Priority_alert_Algorithmis called and pre-emitted the already running sorting algorithm similar PRE_EMPTION_PRIORITY_ALGORITHM used in Operating system for scheduling tasks. Initially the sorting algorithm will sort the Set of-Alerts with respect to the critical value and the action will be taken one by one until any other function pre-empt this function. For each alert in the sorted New-Alert, the staff availability is checked and if available then patient Pi with the critical level Ci is admitted and taken care. Else Divert () tries to find a staff in different hospital. If the patient is admitted, then Pi is removed from the Set-of-Alert and next patient is looped in the same procedure. This algorithm is used for providing a PRIORITY INVERSION method so that STARVING is avoided.

Async Prority_alert_algorithm(Set-of-Alert [ ] (Pi, Ci, Di, Ai)):
New-alert = {Pi,Ci, such that Ci is in decreasing order of alert as in formula
4.1}
For All Alerts:
// sorting with respect to the critical value
New-alert:= Sort (set-of-Alert [ ], Ci) {If Ci are equal then Consider Both}
// Looping alert to Request emergency action For (each alert in New-alert):
// Find the availability of staff
For (each Staff in Staff-in-hospital)
// If staff available then admit the patient
If (staff-availability = TRUE):
Schedule (alert (Si, Pi, Ci, Di, Ai)
Remove (Set-of-Alert [ ], Pi)
Else
// else check for other option
Flag = Divert(Pi, Ci, Hospital area)
If (Flag =TRUE && Ai:= TRUE):
Remove (Set-of-Alert [ ], Pi)
// Else increase the priority of alert
For(all other alerts):
Ci = Ci + 1
// If new alert comes

Async New-Emergency (New-alert (Pi, Ci, Di, Ai)): *// append the alert*
Add-new-alert (Set-of-Alert [ ], Pi, Ci, Di, Ai)
Prority_alert_algorithm(Set-of-Alert [ ])

CONCLUSION

As a result of the study performed among all the ideas, the ones proposed in "Wireless Healthcare Service System" (Lin et al., 2006) and "Alerts in Mobile Healthcare Applications: Requirements and Pilot Study" (Kafeza et al., 2004) are better solutions. The former one is better as it concentrates more on reducing transport expenses, constant monitoring and reporting services in case of missing patients while the latter is concentrating on handling the needs which are highly critical situations by prioritizing the alerts. On combining these two ideas a new system can be built which is a highly secured and which provides proper assistance to track the patient status and suggest medication through the application itself and also track the patient status. Introducing a Cloud Database throughout all the hospitals will helps in decision making by integrating the patient's information from multiple source. Other advantage of storing data in cloud is to provide security and use the information during discharge process. The proposed model provides a closed loop solution for emergency situation and informs the patient and their family in short span of time. The problem of eavesdropping might occur since the network is not secure and therefore the future work includes performing a cryptographic encryption using an Encryption server. This will concentrate more on maintaining confidentiality of the information which is available to the devices connected through LAN and help in providing proper assistant to track the patient status.

REFERENCES

Ancona, M., Dodero, G., Minuto, F., Guida, M., & Gianuzzi, V. (2000). Mobile computing in a hospital: the WARD-IN-HAND project. In *Proceedings of the 2000 ACM symposium on Applied computing* (vol. 2, pp. 554-556). ACM. 10.1145/338407.338419

Constantinescu, L., Kim, J., & Feng, D. (2012). SparkMed: A framework for dynamic integration of multimedia medical data into distributed m-health systems. *IEEE Transactions on Information Technology in Biomedicine*, *16*(1), 40–52. doi:10.1109/TITB.2011.2174064 PMID:22049371

Figueredo, M. V. M., & Dias, J. S. (2004, September). Mobile telemedicine system for home care and patient monitoring. In *Engineering in Medicine and Biology Society, 2004. IEMBS'04. 26th Annual International Conference of the IEEE* (Vol. 2, pp. 3387-3390). IEEE.

Honnegowda, L., Chan, S., & Lau, C. T. (2013). Embedded electronic smart card for financial and healthcare information transaction. *Journal of Advances in Computer Networks*, *1*(1), 57–60. doi:10.7763/JACN.2013.V1.12

Jung, S. J., & Chung, W. Y. (2013). Non-intrusive healthcare system in global machine-to-machine networks. *IEEE Sensors Journal*, *13*(12), 4824–4830. doi:10.1109/JSEN.2013.2275186

Jung, S. J., Myllylä, R., & Chung, W. Y. (2013). Wireless machine-to-machine healthcare solution using android mobile devices in global networks. *IEEE Sensors Journal, 13*(5), 1419–1424. doi:10.1109/JSEN.2012.2236013

Kafeza, E., Chiu, D. K., Cheung, S. C., & Kafeza, M. (2004). Alerts in mobile healthcare applications: Requirements and pilot study. *IEEE Transactions on Information Technology in Biomedicine, 8*(2), 173–181. doi:10.1109/TITB.2004.828888 PMID:15217262

Köpcke, F., & Prokosch, H. U. (2014). Employing computers for the recruitment into clinical trials: A comprehensive systematic review. *Journal of Medical Internet Research, 16*(7), e161. doi:10.2196/jmir.3446 PMID:24985568

Lin, C. C., Chiu, M. J., Hsiao, C. C., Lee, R. G., & Tsai, Y. S. (2006). Wireless health care service system for elderly with dementia. *IEEE Transactions on Information Technology in Biomedicine, 10*(4), 696–704. doi:10.1109/TITB.2006.874196 PMID:17044403

Lu, R., Lin, X., Liang, X., & Shen, X. (2011). A secure handshake scheme with symptoms-matching for mhealthcare social network. *Mobile Networks and Applications, 16*(6), 683–694. doi:10.100711036-010-0274-2

Mitra, P., & Poellabauer, C. (2012, June). Emergency response in smartphone-based mobile ad-hoc networks. In *Communications (ICC), 2012 IEEE International Conference on* (pp. 6091-6095). IEEE.

Poba-Nzaou, P., Marsan, J., Paré, G., & Raymond, L. (2014, January). Governance of Open Source Electronic Health Record Projects: A Successful Case of a Hybrid Model. In *System Sciences (HICSS), 2014 47th Hawaii International Conference on* (pp. 2798-2807). IEEE.

Sun, J., Zhu, X., Zhang, C., & Fang, Y. (2011, June). HCPP: Cryptography based secure EHR system for patient privacy and emergency healthcare. In *Distributed Computing Systems (ICDCS), 2011 31st International Conference on* (pp. 373-382). Academic Press.

Tang, B., Cao, H., Wu, Y., Jiang, M., & Xu, H. (2013). Recognizing clinical entities in hospital discharge summaries using Structural Support Vector Machines with word representation features. *BMC.*

Tupe & Kulkarni. (2015). A Survey of E-Healthcare Information System based on Android Application. *International Journal of Science and Research, 4*(1).

This research was previously published in the International Journal of Applied Research on Public Health Management (IJARPHM), 4(1); edited by Joseph Tan and Qiang (Shawn) Cheng; pages 35-46, copyright year 2019 by IGI Publishing (an imprint of IGI Global).

Chapter 14
Integrated Hospital Information System Architecture Design in Indonesia

Putu Wuri Handayani
Universitas Indonesia, Indonesia

Haya Rizqi Fajrina
Universitas Indonesia, Indonesia

Puspa Indahati Sandhyaduhita
Universitas Indonesia, Indonesia

Kasiyah M. Junus
Universitas Indonesia, Indonesia

Achmad Nizar Hidayanto
Universitas Indonesia, Indonesia

Indra Budi
Universitas Indonesia, Indonesia

Ave Adriana Pinem
Universitas Indonesia, Indonesia

Dumilah Ayuningtyas
Universitas Indonesia, Indonesia

ABSTRACT

Implementing Hospital Information System is an ultimately important practice that should be performed by hospitals in order to deliver accurate, timely, complete, and easily accessible data/information in an integrated manner. Given the specific characteristics of Indonesia, the objective of this research is to design an Information System Architecture as part of the Enterprise Architecture based on The Open Group Architecture Framework in order to support the Hospital Information System implementation in Indonesia. This research focuses on the hospitals basic processes, viz. the emergency processes, the inpatient processes and the outpatient processes. The integration aspect of the architecture should connect the hospitals with other related stakeholders. This research is a qualitative study by conducting interviews and observations in three government public hospitals, several directorate generals of the Indonesian Ministry of Health and a representative from the WHO. The result of this research is an integrated Information System Architecture model.

DOI: 10.4018/978-1-7998-2451-0.ch014

Copyright © 2020, IGI Global. Copying or distributing in print or electronic forms without written permission of IGI Global is prohibited.

INTRODUCTION

Hospitals as one of the public entities are expected to provide optimal services to the public and other stakeholders. To provide optimal services, information technology can be used, which has been acknowledged by the Directorate General of Health Development (*Direktorat Jenderal Bina Upaya Kesehatan*) of the Indonesian Ministry of Health by endorsing the use of information technology (IT), such as information systems, in the healthcare sector. The use of information technology in the healthcare sector is commonly known as e-health (Rawabdeh, 2007). The information system that is specifically designed for hospitals is widely known either as the Hospital Information System (HIS) or the Clinical Information System (CIS) (Petroudi & Giannakakis, 2011). According to Petroudi and Giannakakis' study, the Hospital Information System can provide solutions in producing effective and efficient operational processes in a hospital by integrating the entire process from the registration process to the payment process in conjunction with all of the required information.

The Hospital Information System is not only important for supporting operational processes in the hospitals but also important for the government, which is a stakeholder, because it can effectively and efficiently provide data of citizens' health information to enable the government to make decisions regarding healthcare facilities and healthcare programs to manage and finance healthcare facilities and medical research (World Health Organization, 2001). In addition, Law Number 14/2008 on the Public Information Disclosure, the President Regulation Number 12/2013 regarding Health Insurance, and the Minister of Health Regulation Number 1691/Menkes/Per/VIII/2011 regarding Hospital Patient Safety agree that hospitals should be able to provide accurate, timely, and complete health data/information that is easily accessible for the public and other relevant stakeholders. Thus, implementing the Hospital Information System is an important practice that should be performed by hospitals to not only produce effective and efficient operational processes but also to provide and deliver accurate, timely, complete, and easily accessible data/information in an integrated manner.

Pursuant to the Regulation of the Minister of Health Number 1144/Menkes/Per/VIII/2010 regarding the Organization and Working Procedure of the Ministry of Health, Article 106 states that the Directorate General of Health Development shall: (1) formulate and implement policies in the area of health development; (2) formulate norms, standards, procedures, and criteria in the area of health development; (3) provide technical guidance and evaluations in the area of health development; and (4) implement the administration of the Directorate General of Health Development. To date, although the Directorate General of Health Development acknowledges the importance of e-health, which includes the Hospital Information System, the Directorate General of Health Development has only issued one regulation (Kementrian Kesehatan RI, 2011), the Regulation of the Minister of Health Number 1171/MENKES/PER/VI/2011 on the Hospital Reporting System (HRS), which manages the reporting mechanisms and defines the types of reports that are required by the Ministry of Health from each hospital as the basis to determine health policies in Indonesia. In addition to the Directorate General of Health Development, the Indonesian Government has enacted Government Regulation Number 46/2014 concerning the Health Information System that defines the scope of health information as encompassing the health effort, health research and development, health funding, health workers, medical tools and equipment, health management and regulations, and community empowerment. Likewise, this regulation also lacks the standard procedures and guidelines in determining the business processes and data that are required to be exchanged between the hospitals and other relevant stakeholders. Therefore, despite the urgency to implement the Hospital Information System, the lack of regulations and the absence of standard procedures and guidelines contribute to the small number of public hospitals implementing the Hospital Information System. In addition, the lack of financial support also decreases the number (Health Metrics Network, 2008).

It can be inferred that the development of the procedures and guidelines for implementing the Hospital Information System in an integrated manner is very important to ensure the effective, efficient, and secure delivery of quality healthcare; however, the implementation of an integrated Hospital Information System in Indonesia poses a big challenge because Indonesia is a large archipelago in which the network and internet infrastructures are still not equally distributed throughout the country. These constraints limit hospitals to having loosely coupled integration architecture between hospitals and other related stakeholders, and a higher quality system is necessary to improve the quality and speed of healthcare work processes as well as to improve the availability and quality of data and information. Thus, it is expected that the rapid development of IT-related method/methodology can offer alternatives to these challenges. One of the best practices that is widely used in the industry is an approach called Enterprise Architecture, which can provide guidance for developing an integrated information system architecture (Niemi, 2006).

Enterprise Architecture (EA) can be defined as (1) a conceptual framework that depicts the primary components of an enterprise/organization and the relationship among these components and the environment and (2) the principles governing its design and evolution (Rood, 1994; IEEE, 2000). Enterprise Architecture Framework (EAF), such as TOGAF (The Open Group Architecture Framework), serves as an instrument that can be used as a guideline to design IT architecture and logic structure, to organize complex information, and to address IT/IS and business needs (Sajid & Ahsan, 2014). TOGAF defines the scope of applications of products and services that are in the domain of business and industry, technical infrastructure based on open system building blocks, including the definition of business process architecture, information system architecture, data architecture, and technology architecture. The phases of the enterprise architecture development method using TOGAF consist of a preliminary definition of frameworks and principles, architecture vision, business architecture, and information system architecture (McSweeney, 2000). A study conducted by Costetchi et al. (2014) shows that e-health enterprise system architecture provides a framework to support e-health in delivering coherent and interoperable e-health solutions that can form a true integrated e-health system aiming to deliver shared data and applications to healthcare participants. Therefore, it can be inferred that an enterprise architecture approach can be used as a frame of reference for designing information architecture in a planned, purposeful, and efficient manner.

Unfortunately, there are only a few studies related to enterprise architecture in the healthcare domain. Costetchi et al. (2014) designed an e-health framework that can be applied to meet both general and specific objectives called the Romania Healthcare Framework for Rare Diseases. The dimensions that are highlighted in the framework are the contextual level (strategy, objective, and goal), business architecture modeling, healthcare network, healthcare information system, technical/infrastructure architecture, data architecture, application architecture, technology/equipment architecture, and knowledge and educational/research/training. Thus, enriching the previous studies and considering the characteristics of Indonesia to develop an integrated Hospital Information System is needed to ensure an efficient integration of various systems from central to regional healthcare units. Furthermore, this architecture could also be implemented in other hospitals, especially in the developing countries that have similar characteristics to Indonesia.

Since an Enterprise Architecture Framework is deemed able to guide the development of an integrated architecture, the objective of this research is to design an Information System Architecture as part of the Enterprise Architecture based on TOGAF in order to support the Hospital Information System implementation in Indonesia. In the long term, it is expected that this Enterprise Architecture approach can improve the quality of hospital services and the provision of data to the Ministry of Health. Therefore, the scope of this research is defined as follows:

1. The focus is on basic hospital processes, such as emergency processes, inpatient processes, and outpatient processes, each of which include the registration, medical treatment, medical record management, billing, and payment process steps.
2. The integration aspect should connect the hospitals with the Ministry of Health, the provincial or the district/city Health Office, the National Population and Family Planning Board (*Badan Kependudukan dan Keluarga Berencana Nasional*/BKKBN), the Health Social Security Agency (*Badan Penyelenggara Jaminan Sosial/BPJS - Kesehatan*), international organizations, such as the World Health Organization (WHO), the manufacturers and suppliers of medical devices, and the public.
3. Designing the information system architecture in government public hospitals.

BACKGROUND

Hospital Information System (HIS)

The Hospital Information System (HIS), also often called the Clinical Information System (CIS), is a comprehensive, integrated information system designed to manage the administrative, financial, and clinical aspects of a hospital (Petroudi & Giannakakis, 2011). The aim of the Hospital Information System is to achieve the best possible process for patient care and administration by electronic data processing (Petroudi & Giannakakis, 2011). The Hospital Information System is an instance of the Health Information System (Haux, 2006). The Health Information System includes all health care systems involving patient care that must be integrated to generate consistent, valid, and correct data. To accommodate that objective, the Hospital Information System needs to provide services that can be used to exchange data with other health care systems.

It is common in a hospital environment that a number of systems are developed separately. To integrate entire business process in a hospital, Lu et al. (2005) designed the Enterprise Hospital Information System. The architecture was supposed to integrate three aspects in implementing the enterprise system: data integration, workflow integration and function integration. This enterprise system covered the Clinical Terminal, PACS (Picture Archiving and Communication System), Hospital Information System, and LIS (Laboratory Information System).

Indonesia has considered the Hospital Information System to be an important aspect in the health system. This is supported by Regulation Number 36/2009 issued by the Indonesian Minister of Health regarding Health. This regulation concerns health information system utilization and the integration across multiple sectors in healthcare. The Indonesian Health Information System Roadmap for the period from 2011-2014 (Pusat Data dan Informasi, 2012) states that one of the Ministry of Health's strategic plans is to effectuate the collection, the storage and the data dissemination system automatically through the utilization of information technology.

Though the benefits of a Hospital Information System have been emphasized, there is only a limited number of hospitals that have implemented the Hospital Information System (Bina Upaya Kesehatan, 2013). Although the Directorate of the Referral Health Effort (*Direktorat Bina Upaya Kesehatan Rujukan*) has launched a very basic package of the Hospital Information System, which is an open source Hospital Information System called SIMRS GOS (*Sistem Informasi Manajemen Rumah Sakit Generic Open Source*), hospitals still encounter obstacles in implementing the Hospital Information System. In addition, SIMRS GOS only implements very basic functions and does not have a clear and detailed architecture. The lack of funds, (IT) human resources, and an IT infrastructure are some elements that negatively influence hospital management decisions in implementing the Hospital Information System. Another issue that should be considered is the compatibility issue between the Hospital Information System and other existing systems and how these systems can be well-integrated.

The Open Group Architecture Framework (TOGAF)

According to Rood (1994), architecture is defined as a representation or model of components that build the system and the relationship of these components (Rood, 1994). Another definition of architecture is defined by ANSI/IEEE Std 1471-2000, as the "fundamental organization of a system, embodied in its components, their relationships to each other and the environment, and the principles governing its design and evolution" (IEEE, 2000, p.3). Based on these definitions, Enterprise Architecture (EA) can be defined as: (1) a conceptual framework that depicts the primary components of an enterprise/organization and the relationship among these components and the environment and (2) the principles governing its design and evolution (Rood, 1994; Winter & Fischer, 2007).

Enterprise Architecture is an architectural discipline that merges strategic business and IT objectives with opportunities for change and governs the resulting change initiatives (Jensen, Cline, & Owen, 2011). Enterprise Architecture is also a strategic planning tool and can be used as a reference architecture for modeling to develop a master plan that acts as an integrating force between aspects of (Dennis, 2010):

1. **Business Planning:** Including goals, visions, strategies and governance principles
2. **Business Operations:** Including clinical and business terms, organization structures, processes and data
3. **Automation:** Including application systems and databases
4. **The Business's Enabling Technological Infrastructure:** Including computers, operating systems and networks.

Enterprise Architecture goals can be divided into two categories: external and internal (Lange & Mendling, 2011). The external goal is related to fulfilling the regulatory requirements (Lange & Mendling, 2011). The internal goal is related to organizational goals, such as a business-IT alignment with the objective to align business with IT implementation, a cost reduction objective to reduce IT and business processes related to costs, standardization/consolidation that aims to simplify the architecture, management/governance with the objective to improve the decision making process, and agility with the objective to improve processes and IT flexibility. These goals would help organizations quickly respond to the change of environment and improve interoperability and integration (Lange & Mendling, 2011; National Institute of Health, 2011).

Enterprise Architecture Framework (EAF) is an instrument that can be used as a guideline to design IT architecture and logic structures, to organize complex information, and to address IT/IS and business needs, such as The Open Group Architecture Framework (TOGAF) (Sajid & Ahsan, 2014). TOGAF was introduced in 1995; it is based on the United States Department of Defense Technical Architecture Framework for Information Management (Sajid & Ahsan, 2014). TOGAF is an architectural framework that provides guidelines to design, evaluate, and build suitable architectures for enterprises/organizations. TOGAF includes the application of products and services that are in the domain of business and industry and the technical infrastructure based on open system building blocks, including the definition of business process architecture, application architecture, data architecture, and technology architecture. The phases of the Enterprise Architecture development method using the TOGAF framework consists of the preliminary definition of the framework and the principles, the architecture vision, the business architecture, and the information system architecture (McSweeney, 2000).

The preliminary definition of the framework and principles is a phase in which several aspects, such as the enterprise, the requirement for the architecture work, the architectural principles, the framework to be used, and the relationship between management frameworks are defined. The architecture vision phase is a phase in which a vision of capability and business value that will be delivered as a result of the proposed enterprise architecture is developed. It also defines the scope of the architecture, the key stakeholders, the business principles, the objectives, and the key business requirements. In the business architecture phase, the business architecture that represents the fundamentals of the organization based on the business strategy is built. The business architecture also defines the governance and the business processes of the organization. Two modeling methods that can be used to design business architecture are Unified Modeling Language (UML) and IDEF-0. During the information system architecture phase, the application and the data architecture are formed. The application architecture phase depicts the blueprint of each individual system needed by the organization based on their interactions and their relationships in the core business processes of the organization. The data architecture phase describes the logical and the physical data set structure and the data management resources (TOGAF 9.1, 2013).

Figure 1 describes a TOGAF content meta-model that could be used as a stand-alone framework for architecture within an enterprise. This content meta-model provides definitions of all types of building blocks that may exist within an architecture, showing how these building blocks can be described and related to one another (i.e., data entities held within applications and technologies implement those application) (TOGAF 9.1, 2013).

Indonesian Healthcare System

Access to health information will be effective and efficient if each stakeholder has implemented a Health Information System (Health IS), which has been considered by WHO to be one of the six major components of a health care system in a country (World Health Organization, 2011). Due to the development of the silo (computer-based) systems both within the Ministry of Health and almost in every health care facility (i.e., hospitals and clinics), the implementation of the Indonesian Health Information System still faces several obstacles, such as data redundancy and the inefficient use of resources in central and regional units (Pusat Data dan Informasi, 2012). Thus, a major challenge for the Ministry of Health, as explicitly stated in the Indonesia Health Information System Roadmap 2011-2014, is to

Figure 1. TOGAF Content Meta-model
(TOGAF 9.1, 2013)

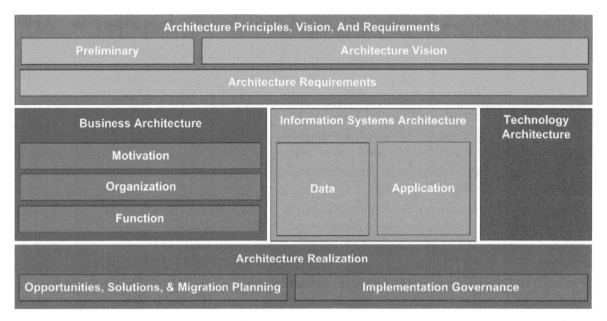

integrate different application components where integrity and different types of integration need to be achieved (Winter, et al., 2011). In order to solve these problems, the Ministry of Health has formulated a plan in the Indonesia Health Information System Roadmap 2011-2014 to build a National Health Data Repository that can accommodate all health data from all sources (i.e., the hospitals and the HSSA). In the future, this data repository is expected to be implemented in hospitals, province and city/district Health Offices, and other related stakeholders. In order to support that policy, which is also pursuant to the Regulation of the Minister of Health Number 82 Year 2013 regarding the Hospital Information System, every hospital in Indonesia must implement a Hospital Information System; however, most of the hospitals to date still do not have an appropriate plan to implement a Hospital Information System due to the lack of IT knowledge and awareness as well as funding issues. Therefore, the design of the Enterprise Architecture for a Hospital Information System is deemed to be urgently required.

The Indonesian Healthcare System involves several stakeholders who manage the flow of health information, health services, products, and funding. The key players in the Indonesian Healthcare System are the hospitals. Hospitals, as depicted in the Hospital Supply Chain (Figure 2), should be able to provide the Ministry of Health, the provincial or the district/city Health Office, the National Population and Family Planning Board (*Badan Kependudukan dan Keluarga Berencana Nasional*/BKKBN), the Health Social Security Agency (*Badan Penyelenggara Jaminan Sosial/BPJS - Kesehatan*), international organizations, such as the WHO, the manufacturers and suppliers of medical devices, and the public with health care information..

As shown in Figure 2, the flow of products, information, and funding from each party in the supply chain is affected by specified policies or regulations by the external parties. Related data/information about products and funding can be exchanged between the parties in the supply chain with external parties and vice versa. In the internal and upstream supply chain, the medical device procurement process is conducted by the integration between the suppliers and the manufacturers of the medical devices and

Figure 2. The Hospitals Supply Chain

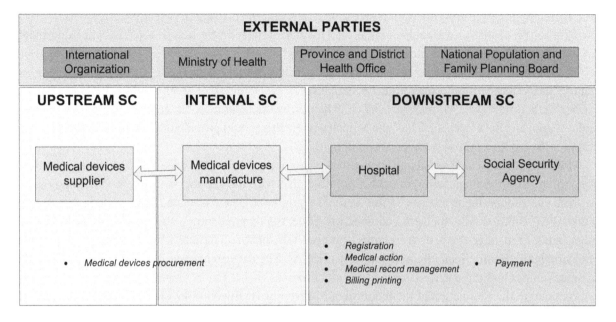

the hospital. The downstream supply chain focuses on the basic process steps, such as the registration, medical treatment, medical record management, and billing. The payment will be made by the social security agency. Figure 3 explains the detailed flow of information among the health care stakeholders mentioned in Figure 2.

The highest level of data exchange occurs between the WHO and the Ministry of Health and between the Ministry of Health and the BKKBN. The data exchange between the Ministry of Health and the WHO is conducted manually (requires paperwork). It involves the exchange of the groups of data which consists of diseases, environmental health, maternal and child health, health care facilities, health care, and the budget. The data exchange between the Ministry of Health and the BKKBN is specific to maternal and child health data.

The primary data exchange occurs between the hospitals and the Ministry of Health. The data is obtained by the Ministry of Health from all hospitals in Indonesia through the hospital reports submitted periodically by the hospitals. The hospitals' annual report submission is regulated by the Regulation of the Indonesian Ministry of Health Number 1171/MENKES/PER/VI/2011 regarding the Hospital Reporting System (HRS) (*Sistem Informasi Rumah Sakit* or *SIRS*), which requires hospitals to submit their annual reports to the Ministry of Health. The hospitals' annual reports are sent directly by the hospitals to the Ministry of Health via the Hospital Reporting System (HRS), a web-based application developed and managed by the Directorate of the Referral Health Effort (DRHE) of the Ministry of Health. The submission is performed by uploading the report file to the Hospital Reporting System website. The hospitals' annual reports include the profile data and the hospitals' performance. In addition to the Hospital Reporting System, the Directorate of the Referral Health Effort also develops and manages the Medical Equipment Procurement Application (MEPA) (*Aplikasi Pengadaan Alat Kesehatan*/ASPAK), a web-based application for submitting hospital data regarding the facilities, the infrastructures, and the medical equipment that are owned and managed by the hospitals. The submission is performed by uploading the data to the MEPA. For hospitals with IT infrastructure constraints, they can send the hardcopy of the data manually to the nearest district/city Health Office, and the district/city Health Office will forward the data to the Ministry of Health through the Hospital Reporting System or the Medical Equipment Procurement Application website.

In addition to the highest level data exchange and the primary data exchange, community groups require access to health information that is managed by the Ministry of Health, which includes data of the health facilities, diseases, maternal and child health, health insurance, budgeting, nutrition, medicine, and research and development. Thus, the Ministry of Health should provide information services for the community groups to provide the corresponding data.

Moreover, to achieve internal and upstream supply chain performance excellence, the hospitals must collaborate with the manufacturers (and if possible also with the suppliers) of the medical devices to perform the procurement process of the medical equipment. The associated data include the device name, the brand, the type, the serial number, the price, the manufacturers, and the distributors. On the other hand, to manage the patients' claims, the hospitals must collaborate with the healthcare providers, namely the Health Social Security Agency (HSSA). The data exchanged in this process include the patients' names and the diagnosis of the patients' illnesses.

Pursuant to the Regulation of the Indonesian Minister of Health Number 001/2012 regarding the Individual Health Care Referral System, the health facilities in Indonesia are divided into three categories:

1. **First Health Facilities:** Primary healthcare provided by doctors and dentists in a health center, health center care (*puskesmas/pusat kesehatan masyarakat*), integrated health service posts (*posyandu/ pos pelayanan terpadu*), private hospitals with general medical services (*rumah sakit pratama*), health center clinics, government and private clinics that provide general medical services, private practice doctors or dentists, and physician practices or family dentists located within the region or city
2. **Second Health Facilities:** Specialized health services performed by a specialist physician or dentist who uses knowledge and medical technology in a public or special district hospital
3. **Third Health Facilities:** A sub-specialized health service performed by a physician or dentist sub-specialists who use their knowledge of health and technology in a public hospital, specialized center, or national referral hospital

Pursuant to the Ministry of Health Regulation Number 340/Menkes/Per/III/2010 regarding Hospital Classification, the classification of hospitals is generally divided into public and specialized hospitals. Public hospitals are hospitals that are owned by the government as well as by private parties that provide health care services to all areas and for all types of diseases. Specialty hospitals are hospitals that are owned by the government as well as by private parties that provide health care in one specific area or for one particular type of disease based on disciplines, age groups, organs, or types of diseases. Public and specialty hospitals are spread throughout the province and districts/cities. According to the range of facilities and service capabilities, the public hospitals are classified into the A class, the B class, the C class, and the D class. Specialized hospitals are similarly ranked. The A class hospitals have a larger number of facilities and wider service capabilities than the B class hospitals, and so forth.

Based on the Regulation of the Minister of Health of the Republic of Indonesia Number 001 of 2012 and the regionalization of the area, the distribution of health care facilities is divided into:

Figure 3. The Health Services Integration

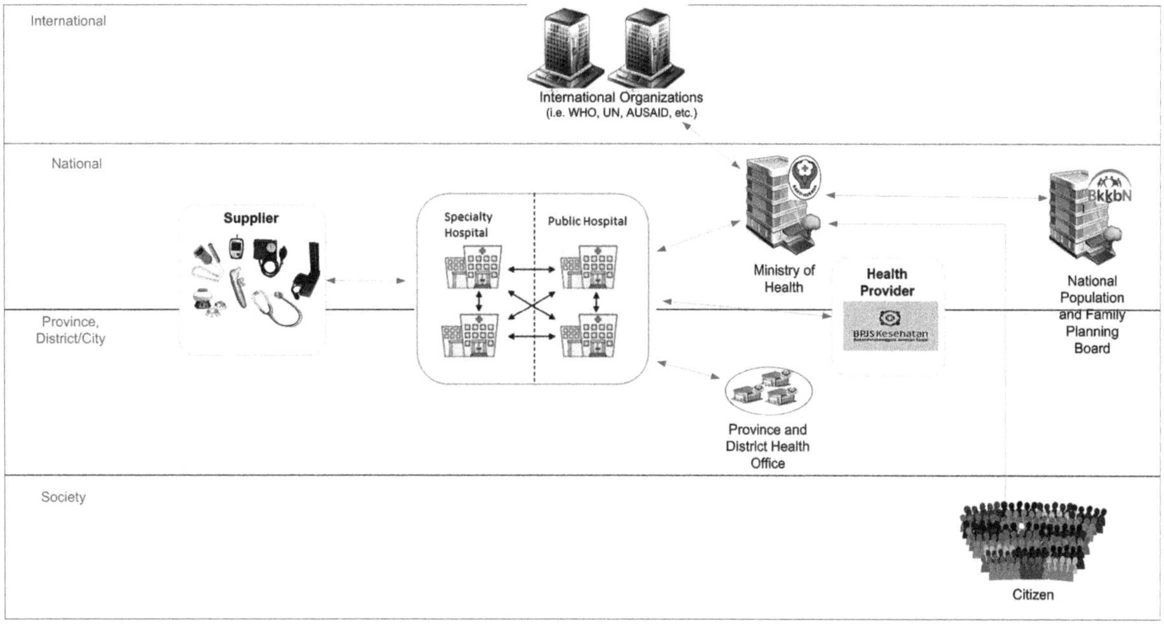

1. **The District Level:** Inpatient health centers, community health centers, mobile clinics
2. **The City Level:** Class C hospitals, class D hospitals, private hospitals with general medical services
3. **The Provincial Level:** Class A hospitals, class B hospitals, specialized Hospitals, national referral hospitals

The health care referral system is the provision of services that defines the delegation of tasks and responsibilities of health care services on a reciprocal basis. The referral system is required for patients covered by the National Health Insurance (NHI) (*Jaminan Kesehatan Nasional – JKN*) and registered for the Health Social Security Agency (HSSA) (*BPJS-Kesehatan*). The coverage includes the medical referral (based on the Regulation of the Indonesian Minister of Health Number 001/2012) defined as follows:

1. Consult patients for diagnostic purposes, treatment, operative measures, etc.
2. Deliver the materials (specimens) for a more complete laboratory examination
3. Bring more competent or specialized medical staff to improve the quality of medical care

The vertical referral is a referral between different health care levels from a lower level to the higher level or vice versa, while the horizontal referral is a referral for health services on the same level. The vertical referral and the horizontal referral is performed whenever the referrer cannot provide health care services according to the patients' needs because of the limited facilities, equipment, and/or medical staff. A vertical referral from a lower level to a higher one is normally done when patients require a specialist or sub-specialist for medical treatments. The refer-back process from a higher level health facility to a lower one can be performed when the following occurs (Regulation of the Indonesian Minister of Health Number 001/2012):

1. The patients' health problems can be treated by a lower level healthcare facility and its corresponding competency and authority
2. The competency and authority of the first or the second level of the healthcare facility can better handle the patients' needs than the higher ones
3. The patients' follow-up treatments can be handled by the lower level of the health facility as well as for reasons of convenience, efficiency, and long-term care
4. The higher level healthcare facility cannot provide health services that correspond to the patients' needs due to the limited facilities, infrastructure, equipment, and/or medical staff

Figure 4 describes the flow of the inter-hospital referral in accordance with the scope of this study. The referral process must obtain prior approval from patients and/or their families after the patients and/ or families receive an appropriate explanation from the hospital authority and health personnel, which includes the following information (Regulation of the Indonesian Minister of Health Number 001/2012):

1. Diagnosis and treatment and/or medical treatment necessary
2. Reason for referral and destination
3. Risks that can arise if a referral is not done
4. Referral transport
5. Risks or complications that may arise during the trip.

All of the information above is also included in the cover letter that contains the identity of the patient, the results of the examination (history, physical examination, and investigation), the working diagnosis, the therapy and/or the measures that have been provided, the purpose of the referral, and the name and signature of the medical staff who provided the services.

By having an integrated health data repository, as shown in Figure 5, the Ministry of Health can manage effective governance to make an efficient use of IT resources and budgets. This will help in achieving the Millennium Development Goals (MDGs) of the national health development: eliminating health services disparities and the barriers in accessing health services. In order to provide fast and mobile access to all related stakeholders, the Health Information System could be accessed through a smart phone, tablet, and the internet.

METHODOLOGY

We conducted the TOGAF phases to develop this research beginning with defining the architecture's needs and principles, the business process architecture, the application architecture, and the data architecture. During the preliminary phase, we interviewed hospital management of the inpatient, the outpatient, and the emergency services departments in three public hospitals to obtain information regarding their architecture needs, required principles, business processes, and information systems. The business processes mapping for the inpatient, outpatient, and emergency services was completed by reviewing the current operations performed by the hospitals' administration and then confirmed by the guidelines issued by the Directorate of the Referral Health Effort of the Ministry of Health. The interview results

Figure 4. The Referral Flow Process among Hospitals

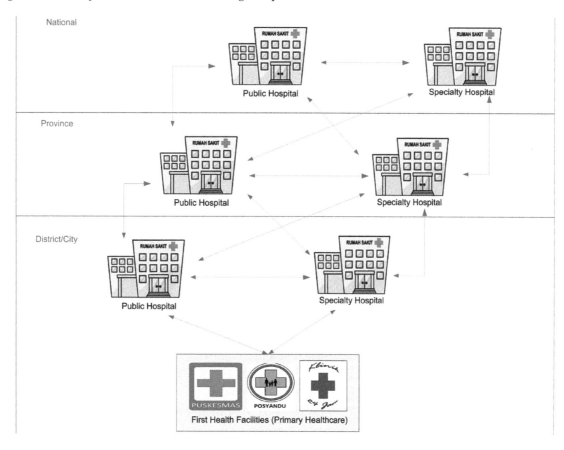

Figure 5. The Future Plan of the Enterprise Architecture Model of the Indonesian Health Information System

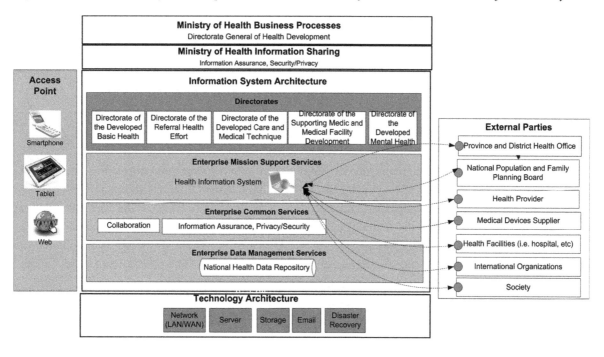

and our document analysis were then formulated in swim-lane flowcharts in order to depict the hospitals' basic business processes. Then, the data catalog and the main service class diagram were formulated based on those basic processes.

Regarding to the Indonesian Healthcare System, the artifacts yielded from this research are as follows:

1. **Architecture Principles, Vision, and Requirements Phase:** Hospitals' value chain, architecture principles, list of actors, business needs, problems and solutions
2. **Business Architecture Phase:** Hospitals basic business processes, use of case diagrams of the hospitals' basic services
3. **Information System Phase:** Data catalog, class diagrams for the hospitals' basic services

Data Collection Procedure

This research was a qualitative research study using in-depth interviews and case studies. The interviews were conducted from January to August of 2014 with eleven people from the management department of three public hospitals. The three public hospitals were chosen as case studies in this research because: (1) they had high scores for the national accreditation assessment, (2) they had partially implemented the Hospital Information System, and (3) they were public hospitals with several facilities and services. In addition, to understand the national and international health regulations and procedures, additional interviews were conducted with experts from the Directorate of the Referral Health Effort, the Directorate of the Supporting Medic and the Medical Facility Development (*Direktorat Bina Pelayanan Penunjang Medik dan Sarana Kesehatan*), the Center for Data and Information (*Pusat Data dan Informasi*) and a representative from the World Health Organization (WHO) in Indonesia.

Instruments

Interviews with all respondents included open-ended questions. The questions were related to the hospitals' business processes and organizational structures, current IT-related problems, existing information system, and their expectations for the Hospital Information System development.

RESULTS

Respondent Demographics

The respondents consisted of the management personnel from one government public hospital, i.e., the Head of the Health Information Management Installation, the Deputy Chief of Emergency Nursing, the Head of the Hospital Management Information System, and the Deputy Chief of the General Inpatient section A, and two government district public hospitals, i.e., the Deputy Director of Services, the Head of the Hospital Management Information System, two Heads of the Medical Record Sub Division, the Head of the Emergency Unit, and two Heads of the Inpatient Rooms. The respondents were selected due to their expertise and experience in hospital management and the hospital information system. In addition, to understand the national and international health regulations and procedures, the interview processes involved four experts from the Ministry of Health, i.e., one expert from the Directorate of the Referral Health Effort, two experts from the Directorate of Supporting Medic and Medical Facility Development, one expert from the Center for Data and Information, and one representative from the World Health Organization (WHO) in Indonesia.

Information System Architecture Design

Defining Architecture's Vision, Principles, and Needs

The business value chain analysis introduced by Michael Porter in 1985 is used to describe activities that an organization performs and links them to the organization's competitive position. According to Porter, activity is divided into primary and support activities (Porter, 1985). Primary activities are directly concerned the creation or delivery of a product or service. Each of these activities is linked and supported by support activities to improve an organization's effectiveness or efficiency. Primary activities can be grouped into the areas of logistics, operations, service, marketing, and sales. The main areas of support activities are related to procurement, technology development, human resource management, and infrastructure.

According to Porter's value chain, organization activity is divided into primary and support activities. The primary activities include the activities undertaken to provide high quality health care to the patients, which includes patient registration, medical care, medical care support (i.e., laboratory and radiology), medical records management, inventory management, payment, and customer service. These primary activities are supported by marketing, nutrition, finance, human resource management, waste management, pharmacy, information technology, and research and education. Moreover, to achieve excellent health services, the primary activities should be supported by the Hospital Information System. Figure 6 describes the hospital value chain.

Based on the interviews and observations conducted in one government public hospital and two government district public hospitals, it can be observed that the government public hospital and one of the government district public hospitals did not yet have an integrated Hospital Information System, but they did already have an IT unit and an IT manager as well as an adequate IT infrastructure and IT hu-

Figure 6. Hospital Value Chain

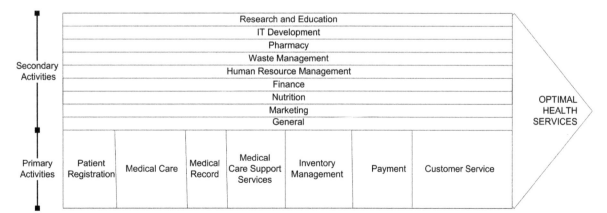

man resources. The other government district public hospital had implemented the Hospital Information System partially in the registration and billing modules but still did not have an IT unit, an IT manager, a sufficient IT infrastructure, or adequate IT human resources.

Based on the results of the interviews conducted in the hospitals regarding implementing the Hospital Information System, the business principles, the data principles, the application principles, and the technology principles required by the hospitals can be seen in Table 1.

Based on the identification of the hospitals' business activities from the interviews, the architecture principles and needs can be identified as the human actors and the basic business requirements required to implement the Hospital Information System. The basic business needs should be aligned primarily with the needs of the Ministry of Health as the national health policy maker. After mapping each actor to its business need, each problem is identified for each actor, and then each of the corresponding solutions is proposed to achieve the improvement target. Table 2 describes the mapping between the actors, the identification of business needs, the problems, and the proposed solutions.

Table 1. Defining Architecture Principles

Principle	Statement	Rationale	Implication
Business	5. Sustainability of excellent health care	Management can create policies for all major services to make the flow of information run smoothly, accurately, and in an integrated manner	If these policies have been formalized, the functions of each unit will work effectively and efficiently and will not interfere with the health services provided
	6. Service-oriented	The development of information technology-oriented architecture services can further facilitate the exchange of information between relevant stakeholders	Application developed and adapted to the business processes associated with it
	7. Comply with applicable laws	Organizational policies and business processes are executed following the rules and policies applicable	The management policy of the organization, data, and information technology must follow the rules of applicable law
	8. IT responsibility	The existence of IT managers in the organizational structure that is responsible for IT implementation activities	IT Unit is responsible for managing applications that support hospital business processes
Data	3. Data is an asset	The design of the data architecture must be able to see the data needs from the operator level to the management level	The existence of a data manager responsible for the availability of data
	4. Ease of data access	Authorization of data access rights for each user to respond quickly and maintain the data security	Information widely accessible, accurate and integrated
Application	3. Technology independence	Architecture development involving multiple platforms can prevent hospitals from depending on one particular party	Choosing a platform that can support interoperability
	4. Ease of use	Applications should be used easily by the user and involve users in the development of such applications	The design of user interface and displayed information provided by the application is easy to use and the information provided by the application is easily understood
Technology	2. Changes based on needs	Changes in IT should be done in response to hospital business needs	The need for IT planning that is aligned with future business planning

Table 2. Catalog of Actors, Business Needs, Problems, and Solutions

Actor	Basic Business Needs	Problem	Solution
Patient	Viewing patient medical record summary	Patient access to medical records is limited	Providing a Hospital Information System to facilitate patient access to medical records
Admission	Manage patients' data profile	Patient profile data scattered in several units often resulting in duplicate patient data	Providing a unified registration process along with an integrated Hospital Information System
Health workers	• Manage data relating to the clinical aspects of the order on each unit of measure (e.g. able to place an order for a package of measures or laboratory) • Can be integrated with other modules that are interconnected such as medical records, billing, support (lab, radiology)	Order clinical measures cannot be done in an integrated way	Providing an integrated Hospital Information System
Cashier	Manage patient billing data	Patient billing data is scattered in related medical units	Providing an integrated Hospital Information System
Hospital management and external parties (e.g. Ministry of Health, Province and District Health Offices, Health Providers, Medical Device Suppliers, hospitals)	Viewing hospital performance report	Hospital performance data is scattered in related medical units	Implement best practice processes and a Hospital Information System

Business Architecture

The government public hospital business processes begin when the patients complete registration in each unit of the targeted service. The patients who experience an emergency based on the results of the medical examination and need further treatment must register in advance at emergency registration; however, if it is not an emergency, the patient can be admitted in the outpatient registration section for further examination. If the patient is determined by medical personnel to require intensive care hospitalization, the patient must register with inpatient admissions subject to settling the payment process on an outpatient basis. Once the registration process is completed, the medical staff will perform the necessary medical treatment for patients throughout the subsequent medical action that will be recorded in the patients' medical records. If a patient is declared cured by medical personnel, then the patient will be provided with a bill according to the type of services provided. Billing is merged in one application for emergency room and inpatient services. In other cases, billing is printed separately. The payment process will be conducted in accordance with the billing documents received by the patient. If the patient is covered by both private and government insurers, then billing will be done by the hospital and vice versa. A patient who pays in person is required to pay in full either in cash or using a debit/credit card.

Currently, to support the business processes in government public hospitals (Figure **7**), there are three different applications where each application has functions to:

- Assist in the registration and management of billing for the inpatient and emergency department (Hospital Information System ER application)
- Assist in the registration and management of billing for the outpatient department (Hospital Information System ER application)
- Manage patient medical records (Hospital Information System OP application)

Based on Figure **7**, it can be seen that there are redundant processes carried out by more than one party and more applications involved in the current business processes in the department of central general state hospital. In addition, billing documents for all departments are still managed by IT unit.

On the other hand, one of the district general state hospitals had not implemented an integrated Hospital Information System and did not have an IT unit and adequate number of IT human resources as well as an adequate infrastructure. IT managers were in a sub-section of the Medical Records Department. The other district general state hospital had implemented an integrated Hospital Information System and had an IT unit in the finance department. In addition, these hospitals were supported by employees categorized as civil servants, regional honors (contract employee with a salary paid by the local government), and honor employees of the public service board (contract employee with a salary paid by the hospital).

According to the Head of Medical Records, there are still barriers in Hospital Information System implementation, such as lack of human resources in terms of both number and capacity (related workload) of the human resources for the use of a Hospital Information System. With the change of status as the Public Service Board in 2010 (PPID, 2013), according to the Deputy Speaker Services Director, the hospital must be able to independently obtain financing to support its operations, including paying salaries of honor employees of public service boards. Financial support from the local government is limited to the construction of facilities, such as buildings. In addition, as a referral hospital, the hospital may not refuse warranty patients, so the possibility of 'buddy' for inpatient cases to a higher class of service often cannot be avoided. Most patients who come to the government public hospitals are assurance patients. According to the way the payments are made by the patients, the patients served by this hospital are divided into cash and insurance patients (i.e., public and private social security, *Jaminan Kesehatan Masyarakat* [*Jamkesmas*] and *Jampersal* [extension of Jamkesmas], cooperation association with the company or factory and *Jamkesda*). Figure 8 shows the details of the basic business process services provided by government district public hospitals.

Government district public hospitals' basic services include emergency, outpatient, and inpatient services. As shown in Figure 8, the patients who come to the hospitals can receive these services. Patients who require emergency room services must first perform a triage examination to determine the severity of the patients' conditions. After that, the patients will receive medical treatment, and the patients must register as an emergency patient and are required to pay for administrative costs, physician services, and treatment. If the patients require medical personnel to undergo intensive treatment, the patients will complete inpatient registration.

Inpatient services require the patients to receive a room in accordance with the disease, gender, and economic circumstances of the patients. If a room is available, the patients are required to register for hospitalization. Medical treatment received by the patients will be recorded in the patients' medical record documents. If the patients are allowed to go home, they will then complete the payment, and the bill is printed. Outpatient services begin with patient registration. At the time of registration, the patients are required to pay for administrative costs, physician services, and medical treatment. After registering, the patients will receive medical treatment, and all medical treatments will be recorded in the patients'

Figure 7. Government Public Hospitals Basic Business Processes Flowchart

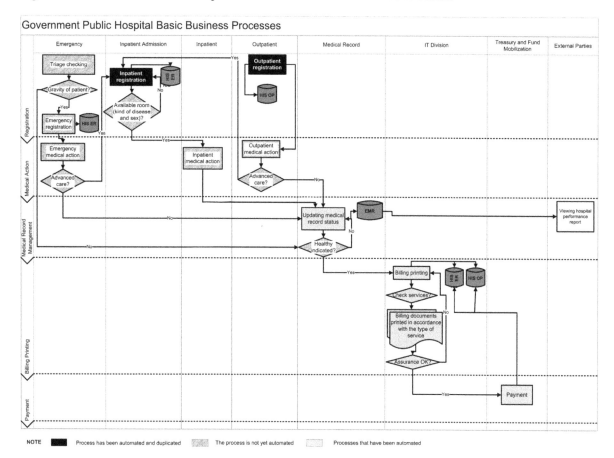

medical record documents. The information contained in the medical records is very important for hospital management to plan their healthcare facilities and services, conduct medical research, and to provide healthcare statistics to all required stakeholders. This designates medical record management as the center of integration between related units in the hospital. If the hospital is able to take care of a patient, the hospital should accept this patient for treatment; otherwise, this hospital should refer the patient to other hospitals, as stated in Figure 8.

Figure 7 and Figure 8 show that the hospitals' generic processes begin with the registration process performed in an integrated manner for the inpatient, the outpatient, and the emergency unit (Figure 9). There is only one registration process for the three basic services. Once the registration process is completed, the medical personnel will conduct the medical action/treatment according to the type and level of severity of the patient's condition. Then, all flow of activities performed by the medical personnel will be recorded automatically in the medical records of the patients. After the patient is declared healthy and discharged by the medical personnel, the billing process (printing) can be performed, and, subsequently, the payment process can be completed by the patient.

From a business standpoint, the registration process should be able to accommodate the three basic services. The same should hold for the billing process. Therefore, at the implementation level, it is possible that a bill for more than one service can be printed on one single billing document. In addition, the roles

Figure 8. Government District Public Hospitals' Basic Business Processes Flowchart

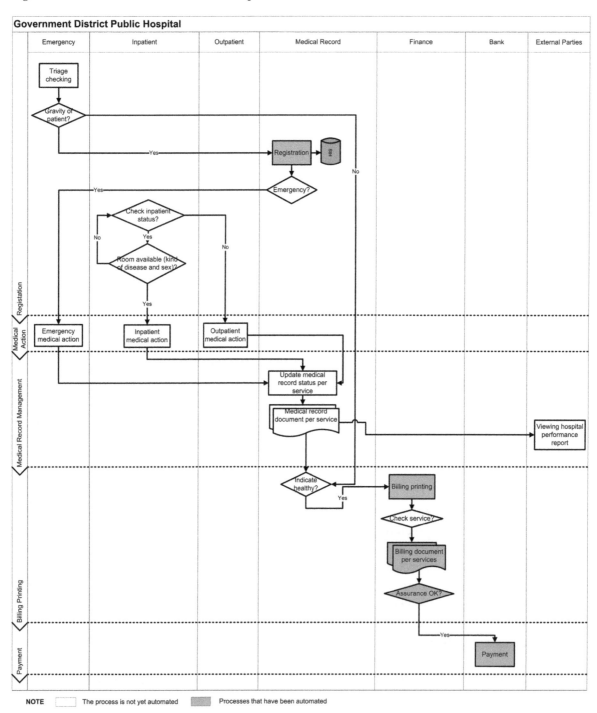

Figure 9. Government Public Hospital Basic Services' Business Processes

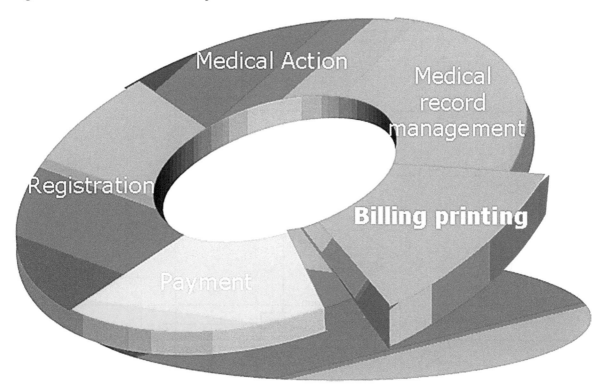

and responsibilities to manage the billing document should not be managed by the IT unit but should be managed by the finance unit performed by cashier and supported by the application. Therefore, this study proposes a generic business process flow as an end-to-end service to patients, as described in Figure 10.

A future business architecture formulated using a use case diagram can show the relationships between actors and the associated modules in the Hospital Information System (Figure 11). The data in the Hospital Information System can be processed, preferably automatically, to produce periodic reports for the Ministry of Health via the Hospital Reporting System. Reports that are required to be submitted through the reporting application are as follows (Bina Upaya Kesehatan, 2011):

1. Hospital profile data
2. Hospital health workers
3. Hospital service activities recapitulation data
4. Disease/morbidity inpatients compilation data
5. Disease/morbidity outpatients compilation data.

Both the Ministry of Health and hospitals require the same data that can be provided by processes run by the hospitals. The medical record function may issue a summary of data related to the hospitals service activities and a compilation of diseases/morbidity for inpatients and outpatients. Details of data that should be prepared and automated by the hospitals can be seen in Table 3. Then, by analyzing and summarizing the medical record data, the external parties can access the hospitals' performance reports.

Figure 10. Proposed Government Public Hospitals' Basic Business Processes Flowchart

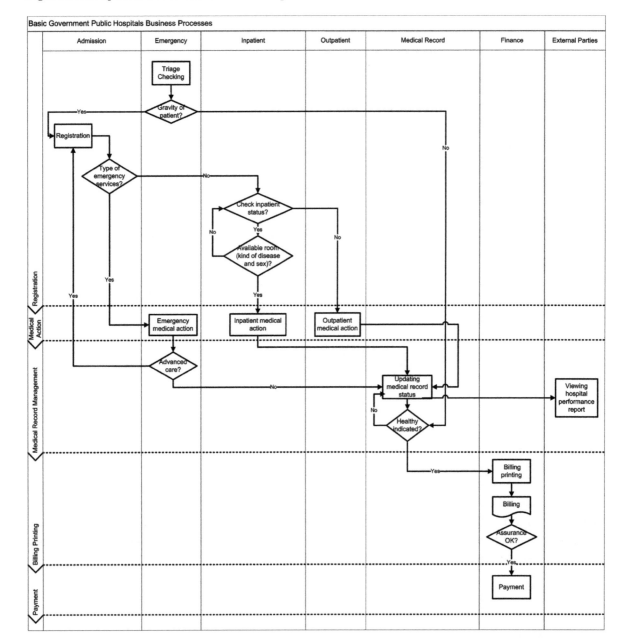

Information System Architecture

Information system architecture can be designed by defining the data architecture and the application architecture with the required modules of the Hospital Information System to support the hospitals' operations services. Data architecture defines various types and sources of data needed to support the business process needs of the hospitals, the Ministry of Health, and the patients. As shown in Figure 9, each process requires several data in order to complete the hospital business processes (Table 3). The

Figure 11. Government Public Hospital Basic Services' Use Case Diagram

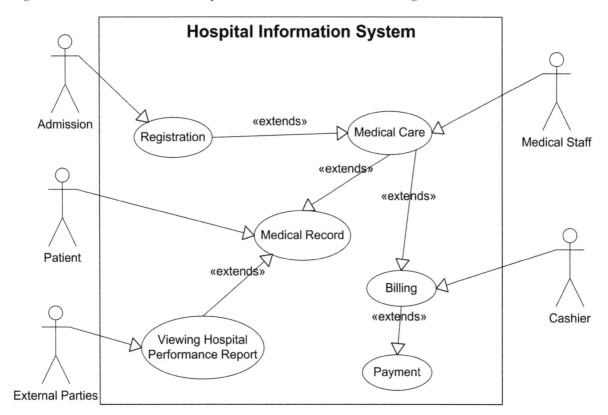

data are maintained by the corresponding business functions, such as admissions or registration staff, medical staff, and billing staff. The registration staff require data such as type of hospital, emergency department facility, facility per polyclinic, facility per room, disease type, patient profile, and health workers in order to generate reports of the number of patient visits for the hospital and to view the patient profile data and the summary of patient visits for certain hospitals in several periods, which is needed by the Ministry of Health. Next, the medical staff (in this case the steward of health data is the medical record staff) needs personal patient data, medical records, medical actions per emergency room, and medical actions per inpatient rooms in order to provide reports of the overall summary of patient medical records to identify the indicators of the hospitals' services, the activities of each unit of services, and the state of the inpatient morbidity/road, which is required by the hospitals and the Ministry of Health. The finance (billing) staff manages patient and billing data in order to view the summary of the billing statistics (including the payment methods) required by the hospitals and the Ministry of Health.

The health master data (e.g., patient, health workers, and disease types) as well as transaction data (e.g., billing and medical record) should be easily accessible by the emergency, the inpatient and the outpatient medical staff. The emergency, inpatient, and outpatient staff operate their facilities and administer medical actions that are conducted in their units. The data required by each major service units can be seen in Figure 12. The data sharing mechanism is conducted by defining the scope of common or shared data/information in the enterprise level and in the unit level. Sharing data can be easily done when there is a single repository accessible, e.g., through web services.

Finally, in order to describe the connectivity between data entities, a class diagram will be used (Figure 13). Figure 13 shows that patient data should be linked with medical activity data along with the facilities and the related health personnel. The data will be aggregated into a patient medical record entity. Some hospitals still separate the patients' medical records for emergency, inpatient, and outpatient activities. The billing entity will take the information from patients' medical records.

In accordance with the hospital's basic business processes that require a particular end-to-end process, the registration, the medical action, the medical record management, the billing, and the payment process, hospitals are required to implement Hospital Information System modules that at least consist of:

- **Registration Module:** Supports the integrated registration, scheduling, and queuing process for inpatient, outpatient, and emergency room departments
- **Order Communication System (OCS) Module:** Assists medical staff in performing medical procedures that need to be performed according to the disease suffered by the patient. This module involves the medical record module and other supporting modules, such as laboratory and radiology.
- **Medical Records Module:** Manages patient medical records (patient identification and numbering, patient's diagnose and procedure)
- **Billing Module:** Supports the process of calculating and printing the bill (billing) and payments (payment) made by the patient
- **Emergency, Inpatient and Outpatient Unit Module:** Support the activities in the emergency, inpatient, and outpatient medical departments

Table 3. Government Public Hospital Basic Services' Data Catalog

Process	Required Data Entity	By the Use of		
		Hospital	**Patient**	**Ministry of Health**
Registration	• Type of hospital • Emergency department facility • Facility per polyclinic • Facility per room • Disease type • Patient • Health workers	View the number of patient visits for each unit of service as well as a comparison of new and old patients	Managing the patient profile data	View the number of patient visits for each unit of service as well as a comparison of new and old patients
Medical Records	• Patient • Medical Records • Medical actions per emergency rooms • Medical action per inpatient rooms	Overall summary of patient medical record data can be processed to see indicators of hospital services, the activities of each unit of service, state of inpatient morbidity / road	Viewing medical record summary	Overall summary of patient medical record data can be processed to see indicators of hospital services, the activities of each unit of service, state of inpatient morbidity / road
Billing	• Patient • Billing	Overall summary of data can be processed to see billing statistics and payment methods of patients	Looking at the data transactions made while undergoing treatment	Overall summary of data can be processed to see billing statistics and payment methods of patients

Figure 12. Primary Data for Government Public Hospitals' Basic Services

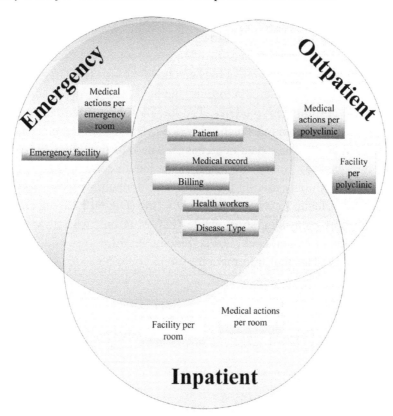

Figure 13. Government Public Hospital Basic Services' Class Diagram

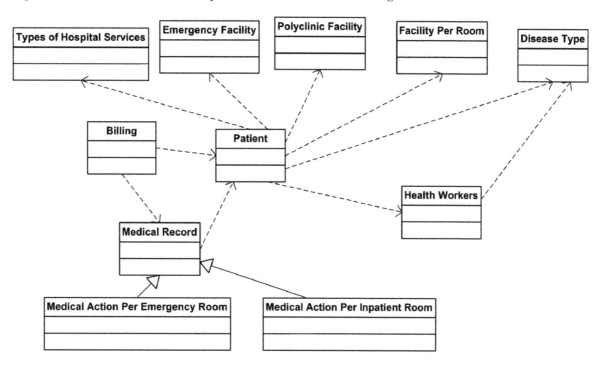

These modules are the core modules to support other hospital activities, making it easier for hospital management and staff to obtain and provide integrated and accurate data/information. Moreover, the best results could be achieved if the modules could also be integrated with other hospital modules and/or applications and health devices. Figure 14 depicts the integrated hospital information system architecture.

As shown in Figure 14, the integration point between hospitals and the external parties is located in the central integration modules, which are the billing, medical records, order communication system, referrals, and research and development modules. The integration between hospitals and the external parties can be performed using technologies such as service-oriented architecture, enterprise application integration technologies, and electronic data interchange. The information system architecture should also be supported by a technology architecture, such as the health communication standard (i.e. HL7, DICOM, CCOW), that is commonly used in the health care domain, network, server, storage, email, and disaster recovery. HL7 (Health Level Seven) and DICOM (Digital Imaging and Communications in Medicine) mainly support data integration, while CCOW (Clinical Context Object Workgroup) enables contextual integration (Winter, et al., 2011). Finally, in order to provide broad and fast access to all related stakeholders, the Hospital Information System could be accessed through smart phones, tablets, and the internet.

Figure 14. Government Public Hospital Information System Architecture

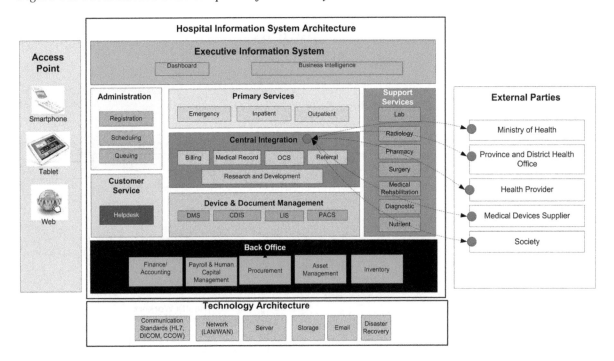

IMPLICATIONS

In order to implement an integrated hospital information system architecture, hospitals should assess their current business processes and applications. Based on existing processes and application assessments, hospitals could map their existing processes and applications using Figure 14. This research shows that hospitals have basic processes from the administration to the payment process in the emergency, inpatient, and outpatient units, so hospitals could adopt the information system architecture in Figure 14 for administration, primary services, and central integration modules. Other modules could be implemented according to the needs and characteristics of the hospital. Finally, in order to successfully implement this architecture, hospitals should be able to integrate the Hospital Information System with other related stakeholders (e.g., health care providers, medical device suppliers, and Ministry of Health).

In addition, based on the study by Handayani et al. (2014) and our analysis, the recommendations for the Ministry of Health are as follows:

1. The Ministry of Health needs to formulate IT governance policies for the hospitals so that the hospitals can define the position of the IT unit as well as the position of IT management and IT staff, including their career paths. This policy is required so that the hospital IT management can be well-integrated as part of the complete hospital management and can provide accountable support for the hospital operations.

2. The Ministry of Health needs to create a data dictionary (adjusted to the needs of health indicators and data/information for each unit in the Ministry of Health) and a standardized data exchange format that can support all platforms/technology to process the necessary data exchange between hospitals and the Ministry of Health. This is essential in order to support the integration of national e-health.

3. The Ministry of Health needs to compose an enterprise architecture guideline for Hospital Information System implementation, especially to help hospitals with limited IT budgets.

4. The Ministry of Health needs to create relevant assessment points for Hospital Information System implementations. This can be done by adding Hospital Information System implementation to the hospital accreditation criteria or by making regulations stating that hospitals that wish to join *BPJS - Kesehatan* programs (Health Social Security Agency) are required to implement a Hospital Information System.

5. The current Hospital Reporting System (*Sistem Informasi Rumah Sakit- SIRS)* has not yet implemented the validation and verification function. This function is required to improve the quality of data. The standard validation and verification procedure should be set in advance by the Ministry of Health to guide the process of validation and verification.

In principle, this hospital information system architecture could also be implemented in other hospitals in other developing countries with similar characteristics as Indonesia. In order to implement this architecture, there are several points that should be considered for adaptation. The architecture principle (Table 1) and the catalog of actors, business needs, problems, and solutions (Table 2) are relatively general, so it can be directly reused. If there is an additional constraint specific to the local context, e.g., in some countries, patient privacy is explicitly and strictly regulated, the principles and catalog can be easily extended to accommodate the issue. Second, since the business processes in this architecture are based on the referral system in Indonesia, specific referral systems should be examined and adjustments should be made regarding the health process (in the business architecture), the information flows, and the health data catalog (in the information system architecture, e.g., Table 3) within the architecture to formulize the appropriate business and information system architecture.

FUTURE RESEARCH DIRECTIONS

In order to design a complete enterprise architecture, future research should be conducted to define the information technology layers and to develop a hospital data dictionary. Other research that should be conducted in the future should focus on identifying the non-technical issues to increase awareness of their biggest impacts on the success of IT projects.

Theoretical Significance

Enterprise Architecture is one of the best practices that is currently widely used by the organization as a guideline to design IT architecture and logic structure, to organize complex information, and to address IT/IS and business needs (Sajid & Ahsan, 2014). TOGAF could be utilized to describe the organizational enterprise architecture because it provides guidelines to design, evaluate, and build the suitable architecture for an enterprise/organization. Until now, most healthcare organizations have not been aware and thus have not utilized enterprise architecture for their IT planning purposes.

This study shows that enterprise architecture, especially TOGAF, which provides quite extensive references, can be partially adopted to provide guidance for developing integrated information technology architecture to support hospitals' basic activities, namely the emergency unit, the inpatient unit, and the outpatient unit activities. The following steps and its corresponding artifacts of TOGAF utilized in this study are as follows: (1) Defining Architecture Principles, Vision, and Requirements (artifacts: architecture principle and value chain); (2) Defining Business Architecture (artifacts: catalog of actors, business needs, problems, and solutions); and (3) Defining Information Systems Architecture (artifacts: flowcharts, use case diagrams, data catalogs, information system architecture).

CONCLUSION

Hospitals are a public entity and therefore should provide optimal services to patients and other related stakeholders. Thus, hospitals should be encouraged to define their Information Technology (IT) standards and policies and subsequently implement health applications (e.g., Hospital Information System). One of the best practices that is widely used in the industry is Enterprise Architecture. Enterprise Architecture can provide guidance for developing integrated information system architecture, especially to support hospitals' basic activities from patient registration to the payment process. In order to develop a suitable enterprise architecture, hospitals should follow several required architecture principles related to business (i.e., sustainability of excellent health care, service-oriented environment, compliance with applicable laws, and IT responsibility), data (i.e., data as an asset and ease of data access), application (i.e., technology independence and ease of use), and technology (i.e., changes based on needs). The responding actors involved in the Hospital Information System are (1) the admission staff, which is responsible for the registration process; (2) the patients who wish to view a summary of their medical records; (3) the medical staff, which manages the patients' records; (4) the cashiers, who manage billing transactions; and (5) hospital management and external parties (i.e., health providers and the public) who wish to view hospital performance reports. Finally, to make hospital operations run efficiently and effectively, hospitals should at least implement the following IT application modules: registration, an order communication system, medical records, and payment.

ACKNOWLEDGMENT

We express our gratitude to the Directorate General of Higher Education for the *Program Penelitian Unggulan Perguruan Tinggi* (PUPT) Grant No. 1025/H2.R12/HKP.05.00/2014 and Universitas Indonesia for the continuous support particularly for the Directorate of Research and Community Engagement. Moreover, we would like to gratefully acknowledge the insightful contribution from Dr. R. Noviane Chasny, a Health Management Information Officer of the World Health Organization (WHO) Country Office for Indonesia.

REFERENCES

Bina Upaya Kesehatan Kementerian Kesehatan, R. I. (2011, November 8). *Juknis Sistem Informasi Rumah Sakit (SIRS) 2011*. Retrieved from www.buk.depkes.go.id

Bina Upaya Kesehatan Kementerian Kesehatan, R. I. (2013). *Ditjen BUK Sosialisasikan SIMRS Generik Open Source*. Retrieved from http://buk.depkes.go.id/index.php?option=com_content&view=article&id=376:ditjen-buk-sosialisasikan-simrs-generik-open-source&catid=1:latest-news

Costetchi, N., Danila, C., & Stanescu, A. M. (2014). Enterprise System Architecture to Sustain Cross-Domain e-Healthcare Applications. In Enterprise Interoperability VI (pp. 271-281). Springer International Publishing. doi:10.1007/978-3-319-04948-9_23

Dennis, S. (2010). IS World, 2003. *Journal of International Technology*.

Handayani, P. W., Hidayanto, A. N., Sandhyaduhita, P. I., Pinem, A. A., Fajrina, H. R., & Trisnanty, I. A. K. (2014). Critical Success Factors in Implementing Hospital Information System in Indonesia: Case Study Public Hospitals. In *Proceedings of the International Conference for Diversity, Technology and Innovation for Operational Competitiveness* (TIIM). Academic Press.

Haux, R. (2006). Health information systems- past, present, future. *International Journal of Medical Informatics*, 75(3-4), 268–281. doi:10.1016/j.ijmedinf.2005.08.002 PMID:16169771

Health Metrics Network. (2008). Retrieved from http://www.who.int/healthmetrics/library/countries/HMN_KEN_Assess_Final_2008_06_en.pdf

IEEE. (2000). *IEEE Recommended Practice for Architectural Description of Software Intensive Systems*. IEEE Std 1471- 2000.

Jensen, C. T., Cline, O., & Owen, M. (2011, March). *Combining Business Process Management and Enterprise Architecture for Better Business Outcomes.* IBM Redbook.

Kabupaten Bogor, P. P. I. D. (2013). *Profil RSUD Cibinong.* Retrieved from Pejabat Pengelola Informasi dan Dokumentasi (PPID) Kabupaten Bogor: http://ppid.bogorkab.go.id/?site=27

Kementrian Kesehatan, R. I. (2011, November 10). *Pertemuan Koordinasi Teknis IT Dalam Rangka E-Health.* Retrieved from http://buk.depkes.go.id/index.php?option=com_content&view=article&id=224:pertemuan-koordinasi-teknis-it-dalam-rangka-e-health

Lange, M., & Mendling, J. (2011). An Experts' Perspective on Enterprise Architecture Goals, Framework Adoption and Benefit Assessment. *15th IEEE International Enterprise Distributed Object Computing Conference Workshops (EDOCW).* Helsinki: IEEE.

Lu, X., Duan, H., Li, H., Zhao, C., & An, J. (2005). The Architecture of Enterprise Hospital Information. *Proceeding of the 2005 IEEE Engineering in Medicine and Biology 27th Annual Conference,* (pp. 6957-6960). IEEE.

McSweeney, A. (2000). *Enterprise Architecture and TOGAF.* The Open Group Architecture Framework.

National Institutes of Health. (2011, November 8). *Benefits of Enterprise Architecture.* Retrieved from https://enterprisearchitecture.nih.gov/Pages/BenefitsEnterpriseArchitecture.aspx

Niemi, E. (2006). Enterprise Architecture Benefits: Perceptions from Literature and Practice. *Proceedings of the 7th IBIMA Conference Internet & Information Systems in the Digital Age.* IBIMA.

Petroudi, D., & Giannakakis, N. (2011). New Technologies in Hospital Information System. In Clinical Technologies: Concepts, Methodologies, Tools and Applications, (pp. 2029-2034). IGI Global. doi:10.4018/978-1-60960-561-2.ch801

Porter, M. E. (1985). *Competitive advantage: creating and sustaining competitive performance.* New York: The Free Press.

Pusat Data dan Informasi Kementerian Kesehatan RI. (2012). *Roadmap Sistem Informasi Kesehatan tahun 2011-2014.* Jakarta: Kemenkes RI.

Rawabdeh, A. A. A. (2007). An E-health Trend Plan for the Jordanian Health Care System. *International Journal of Health Care Quality Assurance, 20*(6), 516–531. doi:10.1108/09526860710819459 PMID:18030969

Rood, M. A. (1994). Enterprise Architecture: Definition, Content, and Utility. *Proceedings of the IEEE Third Workshop on Enabling Technologies: Infrastructure for Collaborative Enterprises,* (pp. 106-111). IEEE.

Sajid, M., & Ahsan, K. (2014). Enterprise Architecture for Healthcare Organizations. *World Applied Sciences Journal, 30*(10), 1330–1333.

TOGAF 9.1. (2013). Retrieved from http://pubs.opengroup.org/architecture/togaf9-doc/arch/index.html

Winter, A., Haux, R., Ammenwerth, E., Brigl, B., Hellrung, N., & Jahn, F. (2011). *Health Information System Architectures and Strategies*. London: Springer-Verlag London Limited. doi:10.1007/978-1-84996-441-8

Winter, R., & Fischer, R. (2007). Essential Layers, Artifacts, and Dependencies of Enterprise Architecture. *Journal of Enterprise Architecture*, 1-12.

World Health Organization. (2001). *Medical Records Manual A Guide for Developing Countries*. World Health Organization.

World Health Organization. (2011, November 8). *Key Components of a Well-Functioning Health System*. Retrieved from http://www.who.int/healthsystems/EN_HSSkeycomponents.pdf

This research was previously published in Maximizing Healthcare Delivery and Management through Technology Integration edited by Arthur Tatnall and Tiko Iyamu; pages 207-236, copyright year 2016 by Medical Information Science Reference (an imprint of IGI Global).

Chapter 15
Design of a Hospital Interactive Wayfinding System:
Designing for Malaysian Users

Ashok Sivaji
MIMOS Berhad, Malaysia

Hizbullah Kampo Radjo
MIMOS Berhad, Malaysia

Mohd-Faizal Amin
MIMOS Berhad, Malaysia

Mohd Azrin Hafizie Abu Hashim
MIMOS Berhad, Malaysia

ABSTRACT

United Nations reported the importance of wayfindng as part of providing sustainable and beneficial accessibility to the public in built environment such as a hospital. Despite this, the survey conducted in this study found that current wayfinding system in hospitals does not meet the requirements of the Malaysian demography which is multilingual and multicultural. Furthermore, the various literacy levels in this country make the design more challenging. The objective of this study is to design, develop and test a hospital interactive wayfinding system (HIWS) that is targeted towards the West Malaysian population. Using the established symbols that has been validated by other studies and from the survey feedback obtained, the HIWS was designed and developed and tested with 24 Malaysian users using the lab based user experience testing. Although the results seems promising whereby 83% of users liked the system, the qualitative feedback revealed various improvements to the system, that would be valuable to the design and development team to improve HIWS.

DOI: 10.4018/978-1-7998-2451-0.ch015

Copyright © 2020, IGI Global. Copying or distributing in print or electronic forms without written permission of IGI Global is prohibited.

INTRODUCTION

Wayfinding system is a method for users to find ways to their desired destination that is not based merely on signage. It is a complex system that includes environment and behavioral aspect enabling users to interpret and endure their surroundings to get to their destination without long thoughts. The growth of population, trend and the expansion of technology precipitate the development of effective communication to fulfil the needs of people with various levels of literacy, memorizing ability and social culture. This requires a universal system that can easily be understood by various levels of age, literacy, language, culture and gender. Human's high demand and level of persona had created a need of optimal user experience (UX), a crucial factor in the development of a highly effective Interactive Wayfinding System (IWS). International standards such as ISO 21542:2011 ("ISO 21542:2011 Building construction -- Accessibility and usability of the built environment," 2011) specifies a range of requirement and recommendation for signage and wayfinding for internal and external environment. A United Nations report by (Rapley, 2013) has also emphasized the importance of wayfinding as part of providing sustainable and beneficial accessibility to global public in built environment, transport systems and in information and communication technologies (ICT). Wayfinding has become important for both outdoor and indoor building environments. For instance, in the design of shopping malls, various color themes has been used to indicate various areas to ease wayfinding in the shopping mall. Study (Ashok Sivaji, Downe, Mazlan, Soo, & Abdullah, 2011) found that when it comes to the design of shop layout, some shopping mall owners pay attention to the Gestalt principle of similarity(Soegaard, 2010), which indeed assist the consumer's in wayfinding. This is achieved by advocating similar design concepts in terms of shop label and color scheme which helps the consumer to form and associate with the shopping theme (whether shopping for souvenirs or clothes, or food) within the shopping mall.

According to (Mollerup, 2009), there are few reason why people have difficulty in finding their way around the hospital. Firstly, hospitals accommodate large real estate and complicated built environments. Secondly, the rapid nature of change and development in hospital environment to meet the changing needs of the demography. Thirdly, the usage of medical terminology for signage that is not familiar to visitor and/or patients. In the design of The Royal Children's Hospital in Melbourne, Australia designers and architects (Whittle, 2009) have created design inspired by nature that stimulates and engages children mentally and socially. For instance, it was shown in (Whittle, 2009) that dappled colors helps wayfinding. Additionally, views up and out of the street provide simple and strong wayfinding cues with consistent connection to external landmarks. Wayfinding has widely been used for inpatient and staffs to ease their way around when under stressful conditions (Sansom & Brooks, 2012). A good wayfinding system can be installed in hospitals to benefit patrons as it promotes 'healing' by enabling patrons to be in control of an environment to find healing. The key factor is to reduce stress, anxiety and fear, which are common feelings that undermine the body's ability to heal (Arthur & Passini, 1992).

The objective of this chapter is to firstly understand the requirement and challenges faced in a government hospital in Malaysia. To achieve this objective, a survey was conducted among the patients and visitors to a hospital. Based on the feedback, the second objective is to design a prototype IWS system and the third objective is to validate the design based on some established UX methods.

The scope of this chapter is only for the specialist clinics of a hospital. Hence the requirement gathering was confined to Malaysians ranging from three major ethnics, which are Malay, Chinese and Indians (including Punjabis) who do not suffer from visual impairment. This study was confined to Peninsular or West Malaysian population; hence it does not involve other Bumiputra who are mainly settled in East Malaysia.

BACKGROUND

Wayfinding was initially intended for outdoor environment. An urban planner Kevin Lynch in his influential book, The Image of the City, penned the term wayfinding. Lynch claimed that wayfinding is about forming mental images of our environmental surrounding based on sensation and memory (Lynch, 1960). He used the concept of image ability to evaluate city form and to recommend principles for city design. Romedi Passini, environmental psychologist and also an architect prolonged Lynch's theory to signage, architectural spaces, and other graphic communications. Passini made the first empirical study of wayfinding process, in his doctoral dissertation in man-environment relation (Arthur & Passini, 1992). As the era evolves, wayfinding has become important for indoor such as shopping malls, hospitals (Mollerup, 2009; Sansom & Brooks, 2012; Whittle, 2009). The usage of signage as a form of wayfinding in hospital has been studied by (Basri & Sulaiman, 2013). It was found that ergonomically, the height of the signage does not meet the directional purpose of the staffs and visitors. Hence, this study proposes the use a wayfinding information system, which could be used as a mobile application. The similarity of this proposal to that of the hospital information system (Ismail et al., 2010) is that it is a software based system. The difference however is that while (Ismail et al., 2010) compared and contrasted the various systems in Serdang, Selayang and UKM Medical Center, those system were targeted towards managing and administrating the financial and clinical aspects such as digital records of patients to improve decision making by care provider; the system discussed in this chapter is more for facilitating wayfinding for patients and visitor in a large real estate such as the various medical centers in Malaysia. It is imperative for medical center to have a vision to become a center of excellence through the integration of healthcare, smart partnership and service satisfaction rendered. With the mission of providing the best and professional service from the heart with the use of advanced and sophisticated technology, the medical center could easily serve a large population from various walks of life.

Figure 1. List of services offered by typical medical center

Medical	Surgery	Woman & Children
Anesthesiology Department	Cardiothoracic Surgery	Pediatrics Department
Dermatology Department	Ophthalmology/Eye Institute	Obstetrics & Gynecology Department
Gastroenterology & Hematology Department	Plastic/Reconstructive Surgery Department	Pediatrics: Critical Care
Geriatrics & Gerontology Department	Surgical Oncology Department	
Infectious Diseases Division	Vascular and Endovascular Surgery Department	
Nephrology Department	Cardiac Surgery Department	
Neurology Department	Oral and Maxillofacial Surgery Department	
Radiology Department	Orthopedics Department	
Rheumatology Department	Vascular Surgery Department	
Pathology Department	Gastrointestinal Surgery Department	
Allergy and Immunology Department	Department of Neurosurgery	
Urology Department		

Figure 1 shows the list of services offered by a typical medical Center. In Malaysia, it is common for medical centers that provide this array of services built with the purpose of serving about half a million population from surroundings areas and spans hundreds of square meters of total area. With the range of services provided across many departments within the large area to a large population, this study proposes a wayfinding user interface (UI) for a hospital or medical Center known as Hospital Interactive Wayfinding System (HIWS). When it comes to the design of a system, the waterfall model could be used in the software development cycle, which comprises of requirement gathering, workflow prototyping, users interface design, code development and testing.

DESIGN, DEVELOPMENT, AND TESTING OF HOSPITAL INTERACTIVE WAYFINDING SYSTEM (HIWS)

Literature Review

This section reviews the various literature and issues involving designing a wayfinding system for a multilingual and multicultural population with various levels of literacy. It also reviews related works and policies in developed nations to tackle some of the challenges associate with conventional way finding systems

Wayfinding System in a Multilingual and Multicultural Society

Wayfinding strategies should communicate effectively to the broadest group possible, including people with a wide range of sensory, language, intellectual abilities, ages, social and cultural backgrounds (Arthur & Passini, 1992). It is necessary and intuitive process enabling users to perceive and organize their environment. Nevertheless, the investment in wayfinding systems is the least devoted, compared to other categories of planning. The process is dynamic and it is more than generating a static mental map of an area claimed by Arthur and Passini. They postulated that wayfinders are a sequential process of decision-making navigating their journeys. Design consistency in signage technology is an important aspect of guidance and wayfinding systems because it enables users to identify the forms of the particular systems. Wayfinding is about effective communication, and relies on a succession of communication clues delivered through our sensory system of visual. One such cue is a signage, which facilitate users to identify the signs and enable them to navigate their ways.

Malaysian comprise of a multilingual and multicultural society. According to the Department of Statistics, with population strength of 28.1 million in 2009 at annual growth rate of 1.8%, the literacy rate in the country is at 97.3% in 2010; whereby literacy rate is defined by the attendance in school, but not necessarily completion. Among the Malaysian citizens however, from the 21.5 million who attended a formal schooling system, only 70% of the citizens have completed up to secondary school which is equivalent to SPM or GCE 'O' Levels. The remaining 17% have completed either a Pre-University certificate (equivalent to STPM or GCE 'A' Levels) or Certificate, Diploma, Degree or Postgraduate (*Educational and Social Characteristics of the Population 2010*, 2014) from a polytechnic or university. In 2010, the ethnic composition of Malaysia comprise of Malays (54.5%), Other Bumiputra (12.8%), Chinese (24.5%), Indian (7.3%) and Others (0.9%). ("Intercensal Mid-Year Population Estimates Malaysia and States," 2014).

The multi-linguism in Malaysia has been intensified with colonialism, immigration and nation's language policy (Brown & Asmar, 2006). The national language policy has emphasized both Malay and English in education, social and professional lives of Malaysian, (Brown & Asmar, 2006). In terms of language, the official language of Malaysia is Bahasa Malaysia (Malay), with English as the second language. Although, the country contains speakers of 137 living languages, it is common for Malaysian to speak Manglish, which is a colloquial form of English with heavy Malay, Chinese, and Tamil influences ("myGovernment - The Government of Malaysia's Official Portal," n.d.). Hence, it is common for education to take place within a multilingual environment. With this also comes the challenges to policy makers in many areas such as in the road and building signages, which should cater for a multilingual population (Brown & Romaine, 2006).

Wayfinding System in Hospitals

Issues such as low literacy rate and language standardization for a multi-lingual population remain a challenge in the design of a wayfinding system. The situation becomes more crucial in a hospital environment as the lack of understanding of language could create health risk to the citizens. Additionally, in the medical industry, there is the extra burden of medical terminologies on top of language barrier. This also creates productivity loss to the medical practitioners and administrative staffs who get queried on how to get to a particular destination or specialist clinic. The literacy and multilingual issues have also surfaced in the United States, whereby the 2000 census reported that 4.13% of the population could neither speak English well or at all, which created a burden to the health care industry. This lead to the establishment of the national program, known as Hablamos Juntos, or "We speak together", with the aim to promote adoption of graphical symbols in health care facilities. The target audience for this program are the public, with low literacy and with limited English proficiency (Berger & Juntos, 2005).

From the first phase of testing the Universal Symbol in Health Care (USHC), it was found that symbols can be more effective than text based signage in assisting patient and visitors in finding their way around the health care facility. As a result of further comprehensive research, design, testing at various sites with multilingual diverse group of users and redesign for consistency, a comprehensive 50 symbol set was designed as shown in Figure 2. The successes of the effectiveness of these symbols were attributed to the user experience (UX) analysis.

In another study, (Rooke, Tzortzopoulos, Koskela, & Rooke, 2009) found that it is possible to embed other forms of knowledge in hospital signage such as prominent landmarks and colors as cue. This study believes that strategically placing prominent landmarks or cues could minimize stress, confusion and frustration during the wayfinding in complex environment such as large hospital areas with many services and facilities as shown in Figure 1. Another study proposed the use of a Thorough Life Management to ensure the sustainability of a wayfinding system for all stages of the product life-cycle (Rooke, Koskela, & Tzortzopoulos, 2010). In a more recent report by (Foley, 2012), in an attempt to improve communication with the changing needs of the diverse community culturally and linguistically, a new wayfinding system will be designed incorporating aspects of culture and arts. This project which is to take place at the Western Sydney Local Health District will mainly target those with low medical and English literacy skills. The sustainability of these projects are promising and in line with Australia's National Art and Health Framework(*Meeting of Cultural Ministers - National Arts and Health Framework*, 2014),which includes efforts in improving wayfinding system in hospital.

Figure 2. Universal symbol in health care
Adopted from (Berger & Juntos, 2005).

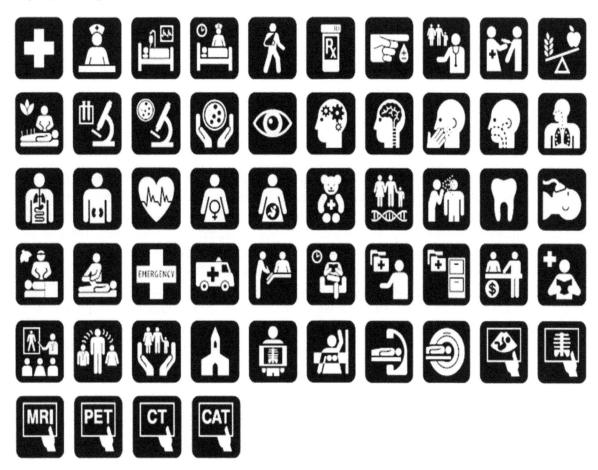

The Design, Development, and Testing of HIWS

Winston W. Royce has defined waterfall model in 1970 (www.princeton.edu). It is a sequential design process, which the progress is seen as flowing steadily downwards like a waterfall. The flow will go through the phases of requirement analysis, design process, implementation of the system, verification and maintenance. The method is widely used for software project in defining research process for the system

User Requirement Elicitation

Before the design and development efforts take place, it is important to understand the requirement of the user. The practice of user centered analysis (UCA), user centered design (UCD) and testing begins with the user requirement elicitation. The first step is to correctly identify the users or stakeholder for the HIWS. The targeted users of the HIWS are the Malaysian patients and visitors who use the services of the medical center. As proposed by (Cheng & Atlee, 2007), since requirement gathering is a challenging activity, it is proposed that a partnership be established between researcher with practitioners such as software system designers, developers, testers during the user requirement elicitation.

User Research: Survey Design and Interview

In a report compiled by the User Experience (UX) Professionals Association (Sherman, 2009), UX professional from 34 countries comprising of UX practitioners, usability professionals, user researchers, UCD practitioner, interface designer, UX Manager / Director, Information Architect from the US, UK, Canada, Spain and Australia, it was found that the UX techniques most often used included

1. User research such as interviews and surveys (75%);
2. Heuristic/expert review (74%);
3. Interface/interaction design (70%).

As proposed by (Cheng & Atlee, 2007), in this study, the partnership was established by having set up a team comprising of a user experience (UX) researcher, user interface designer, interaction designer, programmer and tester. Another proposal by the (Cheng & Atlee, 2007) is that researchers need to think beyond the current requirement engineering and software engineering knowledge and capabilities and include collaborators from other discipline. This is where the UX researcher who has knowledge and experience in user centered analysis, design and testing could fit in. Based on the common practice in developed countries and the benefits of user research, the team visited the hospital and interviewed the subjects and recorded the feedback using a survey (Gray & Malins, 2004; Sherman, 2009; Ashok Sivaji & Soo, 2013). In total, one hundred successful samples were gathered. The survey was divided into four (4) sections to gauge the levels of perception, understanding and familiarization from the patients and visitors to the specialist clinics within the medical center:

Section A: Demography.

This section comprises of 7questions and is targeted towards understanding the demography such as the gender, age range, ethnicity, nationality and spoken language. Knowing the demography provides some insight into the possibility of developing a system that is preferred by mobile or smartphone users or even users for those who are internet savvy. The Internet User Survey 2012 from MCMC ("Internet User Survey 2012," 2012) shows that the top 3 locations respondents of internet access are from home (63.1%), workplace (34.8%) and on-the-go (24.3%). The same survey found that Malaysian use multiple devices to access the internet. From here, it is clear that Malaysian would expect optimal user experience regardless of which device or location the internet being accessed. The purpose of asking the ethnicity, spoken language and literacy level is to confirm the various challenges that could impact them and whether a visual based system could be the solution to uncover the problems faced. The reason for asking the statistics on the visit frequency is to understand their behavioral change with respect to the frequency of visits.

Section B: Level of perception towards the medical center's specialist clinics signage system.

The purpose of these questions is to gauge the effectiveness level of the existing wayfinding system. It comprise of question to understand the suitability of the typography, readability and consistency used in the existing system. The questions set are also aimed at gauging the level of awareness of the respondent in the usage of color codes and the user opinion and ratings on the signage used currently at the medical center.

Section C: Level of understanding on the medical terminology.

Section C measures the level of hospital patrons' knowledge of the medical terminologies used to categorize the various departments as shown in Figure 1. In total 16 medical terminologies are shown with textual and visual signage as shown in Table 2 respectively. Indirectly this is to measure their preference level in using textual signage with and without visual cue.

Section D: Level of aestheticizing, cognitive and familiarization of ICT gadgets.

Section D measures whether the hospital patrons' prefer a two dimensional or a three dimensional representation. It also measure their familiarization with ICT gadgets such as smartphone, laptop or tablets

Problem Statement Derived from Outcome of User Research

From the respondents of the survey, 56% comprise of patients while the remaining 44% accompanied the patients to the specialist clinic. Among them 27% are visiting the clinics for the first time, while the majority (73%) of respondents make regular visits. The breakdown of the frequency of visits to the clinic is shown in Table 1. To understand further whether the users are familiar with ICT, when asked only 67% or two thirds of the responded answered 'Yes' to being familiar with computers, smartphones and tablet users. This is an important finding as it reveals that one third of the respondents are not really ready for a mobile apps based system, commonly found in a smartphone or tablet.

To understand further, how respondents feel about the current signage, two questions were asked. The first question attempts to understand how helpful were the current signage used in the hospital. The results revealed that 28% agree (19% agree, 9% strongly agree) that the signage were helpful, 12% were unsure while the majority of 60% disagree (45% disagree, 15% strongly disagree) that the existing signage were helpful in guiding the patients or visitors to the specialist clinic (First graph in Table 2). When it came to the rating of the existing signage system of the hospital, 22% found it to be good (9% very good, 13% good), 24% unsure while a majority of 54% found the system bad (37% bad, 17% very bad) (Second graph in Table 2). The respondents also provided some qualitative feedbacks to support their responses during the survey. The next section summarizes both the literatures and qualitative feedback.

Previous studies have found that there is a common misunderstanding between medical terminologies used by health care providers (HCP) and patients. Study by (Lerner, Jehle, Janicke, & Moscati, 2000) found that HCP need to be clear and conscious with the medical terminologies and vocabulary used especially when communicating with the young, urban and poorly educated. Another study proposes

Table 1. Frequency of visits to the specialist clinic

Number of Visit	1st	2nd – 3rd	4th – 5th	6th – 7th	> 8th
Number of Respondents	27	32	23	10	8

the use of nursing informatics in assessing patient's terms for health-related matters, which could involve a multi-disciplinary efforts including linguist, medical librarian, nurses and patients from varying culture, ethnic background and education levels (Zielstorff, 2003). Based on the qualitative feedback obtained from the survey respondents, it was found that more than half of the respondents (63%) are not familiar with the medical terminology such as Cardiology, Ophthalmology, Oral Surgery, Orthopedic and Nephrology. Unfortunately, these terminologies are currently used in the signages across the medical center and even in the service offered by a typical medical center as shown in Figure 1. When an alternative is provided to the respondent, it was interesting to note that more than half the respondents or 57% responded positively to being able to now understand the medical terminology / classification of various departments. The preliminary findings are similar to that reported by the Hablamos Juntos program (Berger & Juntos, 2005) whereby

- Comparing the respondent's demography in Table 1, it could be seen that, most respondents to the medical center found that the existing signage system is not helpful and not effective in guiding them to the specialist clinics. As shown in the first graph of Table 2, 45% of respondents disagreed and a further 15% strongly disagree that the current signage was helpful. As such the ratings on the existing signage system was more skewed towards being 'Not Sure'(24%) or 'Bad'(37%) or Very Bad (17%), as shown in the second graph in Table 2. This was seen on respondents who were not only on the first time visit but also for regular patients as shown in Table 1. Furthermore, when asked on how they rate the current signage in the medical center, it was found that in total 54% of respondents provide negative ratings.
- In terms of familiarity of medical terminologies used to label the specialist clinic, there is a significant increase from 24% (third graph in Table 2) to 57% (fourth graph in Table 2) in terms of usage of Universal Symbol in Health Care (USHC) as a visual aid to textual signage. At the same time, there is also a significant drop from 63% (third graph in Table 2) to 34% (fourth graph in Table 2) in terms of respondent not being familiar when the USHC is used as an aid as a visual signage.

User Centered Analysis

Based on the survey respondents, it was found that most of public hospital patron is from middle income group, pensioners and government servants accompanying their children or parents. They prefer public hospital because it cost much less than the private hospital. Based on observation, it is the trend that most public hospital patron age 40 below do have Internet gadget (smartphone, tablet or laptop). Less of age 50 and above have Internet gadget. Based on the analysis from the survey and observation conducted, it was found that a visual and web based interactive wayfinding system is feasible. At this point, the risk or limitation of this study is foreseen. As shown in fourth graph in Table 2, even the visual based icons are used, 33% respondents were not familiar and 10% are not sure when the medical terminology is guided with icons. The adoption of appropriate UX, design and psychology principle as described in the next section could minimize this risk.

Table 2. Finding from preliminary study

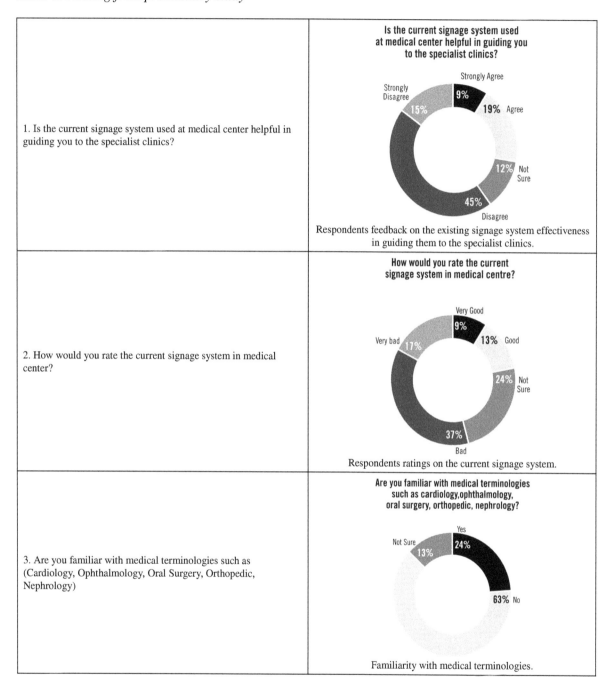

1. Is the current signage system used at medical center helpful in guiding you to the specialist clinics?	**Is the current signage system used at medical center helpful in guiding you to the specialist clinics?** Strongly Agree 9%, Agree 19%, Not Sure 12%, Disagree 45%, Strongly Disagree 15%. Respondents feedback on the existing signage system effectiveness in guiding them to the specialist clinics.
2. How would you rate the current signage system in medical center?	**How would you rate the current signage system in medical centre?** Very Good 9%, Good 13%, Not Sure 24%, Bad 37%, Very bad 17%. Respondents ratings on the current signage system.
3. Are you familiar with medical terminologies such as (Cardiology, Ophthalmology, Oral Surgery, Orthopedic, Nephrology)	**Are you familiar with medical terminologies such as cardiology, ophthalmology, oral surgery, orthopedic, nephrology?** Yes 24%, No 63%, Not Sure 13%. Familiarity with medical terminologies.

continued on following page

Table 2. Continued

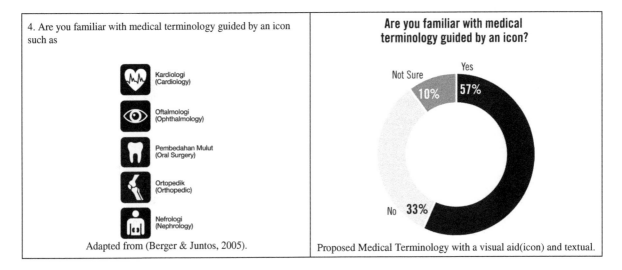

| 4. Are you familiar with medical terminology guided by an icon such as

 Kardiologi (Cardiology)
 Oftalmologi (Ophthalmology)
 Pembedahan Mulut (Oral Surgery)
 Ortopedik (Orthopedic)
 Nefrologi (Nephrology)

 Adapted from (Berger & Juntos, 2005). | **Are you familiar with medical terminology guided by an icon?**

 Not Sure 10% — Yes 57% — No 33%

 Proposed Medical Terminology with a visual aid(icon) and textual. |

Designing the User Interface

Visual communication is communication with visual aids. It is a conveyance of ideas and information that relies on vision presented with two-dimensional images. It relies both on eyes that function and on a brain that interprets all sensory information received. According to (Lester, 2013), an active curious mind remembers and uses visual messages in thoughtful and innovative ways. Visual communication is very effective by implementing UX elements. In an e-Commerce study by (Ashok Sivaji, Downe, et al., 2011), UX elements such as social presence, emotional, trust, word of mouth are found enhance UX on top of fundamental psychology principle such as Gestalt Theory and Fitt's Law. A great UX will excite user to do what they want to do, passionate and engage with it. According to another study by (Garrett, 2010), UX elements comprise of the following:

- Surface Plane,
- Skeleton Plane,
- Structure Plane,
- Scope Plane,
- Strategy Plane.

For this chapter, this GUI design is based on Garret's UX elements.

Surface Plane

In developing a comprehensive and usable IWS, various disciplines must be considered and carefully thought for the Surface Plane that is the GUI. There are three components of good GUI design. The components are aesthetic design, information design and interface design. Aesthetic design is more about appropriately designing a user interface. Information designs is about preparing the information about the medical center IWS in the best possible way for users (patient, visitor) to efficiently and effectively digests and comprehend information. Interface design is the makeup of how users can interact

Table 3. Respondents rating of the current typography

Type of Answers	Very Good	Good	Not Sure	Bad	Very Bad
Typography application	32	39	17	12	0
Readability	18	74	8	0	0

with medical center IWS. Good interface design is about making the experience of using the IWS easy, intuitive and effective. This includes icons, color, typography, animation and sound. Icons used for IWS function as buttons, which load the following page that shows the direction of patrons' desired specialist clinics. The icons is based on Hablamos Juntos (Berger & Juntos, 2005), which could be a viable and an effective communication tool, particularly for a country with low literacy and limited English proficiency. For a Malaysian context, the icons could be usable and adequate for hospital patrons with limited medical terminology proficiency and speak multi languages.

Typography is part of IWS. During the survey conducted to analyze the effectiveness of typography used in current wayfinding system at the medical center, it was found that the current typography used was applicable and has good readability as shown in Table 3. With these findings, the current typography which is 'Sans Serif' font was decided to be used as part of the design of the newly proposed wayfinding system.

Storyboards

Storyboards are graphic organizers form of illustration in sequence for the purpose pre-visualizing of a HIWS. The main page shows the IWS title with design elements animation on the background as an attraction element. The rest of the pages show presentation of the desired direction to specialist clinics. Table 4 shows the storyboard for the main page, oral surgery page and pediatrics page. It reflects a typical scenario of how the hospital visitor would carry out activities that would lead them to achieving their goals. In this case, a scenario could be

- A patient visiting one specialist to consult for oral surgery
- Followed by bringing his/her child to the pediatrics clinic

Skeleton Plane

The skeleton of the user interface includes the placement of buttons, illustrations and text. The skeleton is designed to optimize the composition of these elements for the best effect and efficiency so that user remembers what is desired and find it when required. Buttons are place at the bottom of the page to cater for left and right-handed patrons. If the buttons are on the left side of the page, right-handed patrons might not be comfortable using it and vice versa. The title of the IWS and hospital logo on the main page is prominently at the center of the page to make it noticeable, as shown in Figure 3. For the rest of the pages, the title for every location is displayed with prominent text at the top of the pages to make it noticeable for the patrons. The animated of the floor plan is at the center of the page as shown in Figure 4, making it a focal point for patron to focus in finding their way to their desired specialist clinics.

Table 4. Storyboarding

No.	Descriptive Text
Main Page (Refer to Figure 6)	
1	Text indicates the guide to specialist clinics with hospital logo displayed on light blue frame. Icons represent the specialist clinics with text of medical terminology function as buttons at the bottom of the main frame.
2	Animated design elements loops on the background.
Oral Surgery Page (Refer to Figure 7)	
1	Oral surgery button changed to light green (colour code for oral surgery for the respective hospital) when touched.
2	The light blue frame horizontally compress to the top of the main frame as the text of specialist clinics indicator disappears while the text of door number and floor level for oral surgery gradually appears on it. The visual of the floor plane horizontally compress and floor outline vertically compress appear below the light blue frame.
3	The visual of the floor plane horizontally decompress and floor outline vertically decompress below the light blue frame.
4	The floor plane and floor outline form to an isometric view below the light blue frame. Corresponding indicator of oral surgery gradually appear with respect the colour code of the department within the hospital while the registration counter gradually appear and moves down from the top indicating the location of the clinic. Human icon and *'Anda di sini'* indicator gradually appear.
5	Human icon moves to the registration counter where the location is and the indicator *'Destinasi anda'* gradually appears. The human icon animation will loop for 60 seconds. This page will automatically go back the main page if it is idle more than 60 seconds. The whole animation of this page will repeat if oral surgery button is touched.
Paediatrics Page (Refer to Figure 8)	
1	Paediatrics button changed to light brown (colour code for paediatrics for the respective hospital) when touched.
2	The light blue frame horizontally compress to the top of the main frame as the text of specialist clinics indicator disappears while the text of door number and floor level for paediatrics gradually appears on it. The visual of the floor plane horizontally compress and floor outline vertically compress appear below the light blue frame.
3	The visual of the floor plane horizontally decompress and floor outline vertically decompress below the light blue frame.
4	The floor plane and floor outline form to an isometric view below the light blue frame. Indicator of paediatrics gradually appears with respect to the department's colour code while the registration counter gradually appears and moves down from the top indicating the location of the clinic. Human icon and 'Anda di sini' indicator gradually appear.
5	Human icon moves to the registration counter where the location is and the indicator 'Destinasi anda' gradually appears. The human icon animation will loop for 60 seconds. This page will automatically go back the main page if it is idle more than 60 seconds. The whole animation of this page will repeat if paediatrics button is touched.

Structure Plane

The skeleton is a concrete expression of the more abstract structure of the site. The skeleton might define the placement of the interface elements on the page; the structure would define how users arrive at the desired page and where they could go when they finish. The skeleton might define the arrangement of navigational items allowing the users to browse what they desire. This is shown in the flow chart as shown below in Figure 5.

Scope Plane

The features and functions of HIWS define by structure to fit together, which composed the scope of IWS. HIWS offer a feature that enables users to play the same page again by touching the same button. Users can also go to another page without going back to the main page. If the page is left idle for more than 60 seconds it will automatically go back to the main page.

Figure 3. Skeleton showing placement of specialist clinics

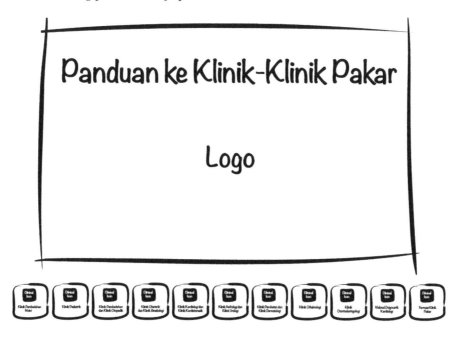

Figure 4. Skeleton showing placement of specialist clinics with animated 2D floor plan

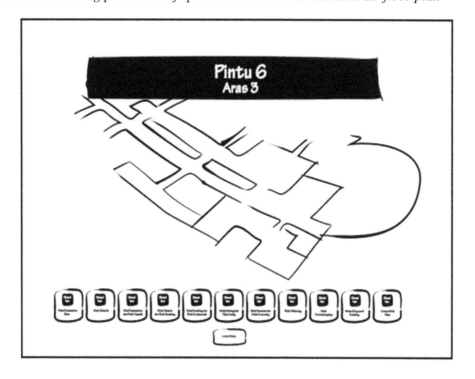

Figure 5. Flow chart showing navigation items

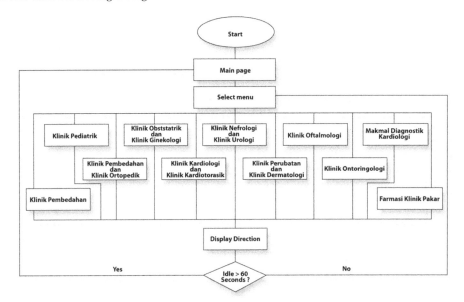

Strategy Plane

The icons that are used to represent the medical terminology enable patrons easily identify the specialist clinic. With a User Centric research in gathering requirement and identifying the problem faced by the patron, an appropriate design and development strategy is devised based on the Malaysian demography.

Development of the HIWS

The system is developed using Hype 2.0.1, which is a tool to develop web site prototype. All the images and design elements were developed using Adobe Illustrator CS6 and converted to Portable Network Graphics (PNG) files with Adobe Photoshop CS6. All the medical terminology used in a hospital could be applied in the GUI to enable patrons to associate the current signage system with HIWS.

Image Development

All images in the GUI design of HIWS were developed using Adobe Illustrator. Based on the location of the specialist clinics, whether within the same floor or multi-floor, the images could be designed. For the HIWS, the images of two levelled floor was designed which encompasses the floor plans that included the specialist clinics within the medical center, the specialist clinics indicators, the medical icons and the human icon that is animated in Hype. Due the Adobe Illustrator CS6 vector format, the images need to be converted as raster format files that enable them to be imported into Hype 2.0.1. All the images developed with Adobe Illustrator CS6 were converted to PNG.

GUI Development

The GUI for HIWS was developed using Hype 2.0.1. Each of the interfaces for the specialist clinics in HIWS was constructed in one scene.

Figure 6. Sequence of images and animated design element in the main page

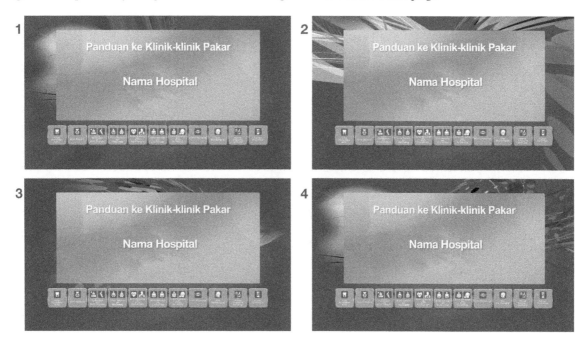

The animations and actions of the GUI were developed in the scene frame with three different layers of timeline for all specialist clinics pages. Each layers consist of the animation of the specialist clinics floor plan, the human icon animation which show the direction to the specialist clinics desired and the automatic revert to main page when the GUI of the specialist clinics are left idle for more than sixty seconds. Figure 6, 7 and 8 shows the GUI for the Main Page, Oral Surgery and Pediatrics.

The GUI is exported as HTML5 when completed. During the export process the HoSIWS.html file is developed with HTML script, Font script and JAVA script. The system compiled all the images together into a folder named HoSIWS.hyperesource. The files and the folder is compiled together in one folder to enable it to be displayed using a web browser. The HIWS will be displayed when HoSIWS.html file is clicked and the system will link all the images gathered in HoSIWS.hyperesource.

User Experience Testing

According to (Sherman, 2009), among the commonly used evaluation and/or testing techniques include

- Heuristic or expert review (Chrimes, Kitos, Kushniruk, & Mann, 2014; Ashok Sivaji, Abdullah, & Downe, 2011);
- Informal usability testing (Ashok Sivaji et al., 2014);
- Lab based user experience testing (Ashok Sivaji, Abdullah, Downe, & Ahmad, 2013).

This study involves performing lab based usability testing using eye tracking which is less prevalent. One of the reason for this is the cost of ownership of an eye tracker system is high as compared to other techniques which do not rely on using an eye tracker (Rapley, 2013; A. Sivaji & Soo, 2012). However, there

Figure 7. Sequence of images and animation for oral surgery specialist clinic

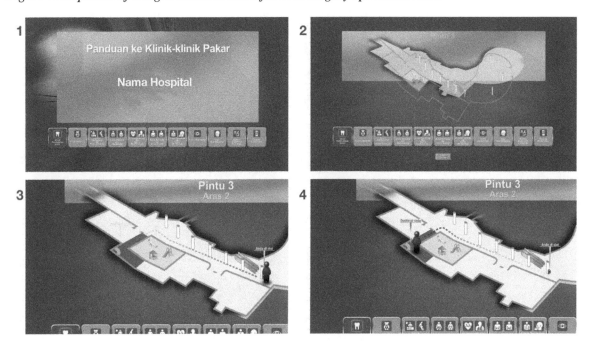

are some advantages in using an eye tracker. Firstly, since the target audience for this study are Malaysian and previous study have found that they suffer from high power distance, there are high tendencies for users to hold back their feedback during the usability testing (Hofstede, 2010; Ashok Sivaji & Ahmad, 2014). Additionally, studies have shown that eye tracking is able to capture visual cues represented in heat map and gaze plots. When incorporated with Retrospective Think Aloud, the eye tracking analysis is beneficial in uncovering insights from respondent's verbal and non-verbal feedback (Bojko, 2006; Goh et al., 2013; Jacob & Karn, 2003; Olmsted-Hawala, Holland, & Quach, 2014; Rashid, Soo, Sivaji, Naeni, & Bahri, 2013; Ashok Sivaji & Ahmad, 2014).

The user experience test (UET) gives a direct input on how real users use the system. It measures the usability or ease of use with the application of aesthetic design, information design and interface design. The test involves carefully creating a scenario of realistic situation, wherein the person perform a list of task using HIWS being tested while observers watch and take notes. The objective is to observe how people function in a realistic manner. With this, the system designer and developer can directly see the problems faced by users or whether the system meets their requirements.

Some of the metrics measured during the UET include

- The degree of the system meeting the requirements that were elicited in the previous section during the user research
- System effectiveness in ensuring user is able to complete the task
- System efficiency in ensuring the user is able to complete the task effectively and also in a shortest time as possible

Figure 8. Sequence of images and animation for pediatric clinic

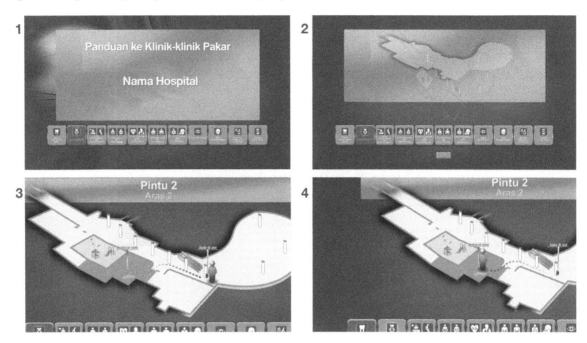

The testing was conducted in an independent Software Testing laboratory that has been accredited by the Department of Standards Malaysia. MIMOS Software Testing Laboratory is the first organization in Malaysia to be recognized with the International Standard ISO/IEC 17025:2005 in Software Testing in December 2013. This accreditation, under the Laboratory Accreditation Scheme of Malaysia (SAMM), demonstrates technical competence for a defined scope and the operation of a laboratory quality management system. The accreditation scope covers Functional, Performance, Security and Usability testing ("Accolades & Accreditations," 2013, "Standards Malaysia Recognises MIMOS As The First Malaysian Lab To Receive MS ISO/IEC Accreditation Certificate For Software Testing," 2014). Under the scope of usability testing, user experience test was conducted in a lab that has been featured in the Global Usability Studies(Yeo et al., 2011)

User Recruitment

To facilitate the user recruitment and test setup, a UX research and testing tool known as Mi-UXLab 1.0 (formerly known as URANUS) was used (A. Sivaji & Soo, 2012). Previous UX research in e-Commerce (Goh et al., 2013; Tzuaan & Sivaji, 2014) and industrial ergonomics (Ashok Sivaji, Shopian, Nor, Chuan, & Bahri, 2013) has shown how using such an automated tool could improve UX research data gathering productivity and accuracy. Since the Hospital Interactive Wayfinding System (HIWS) is designed for users of various walks of life, the targeted audience recruited was from various levels of income and literacy level, who represent the Malaysian ethnic group which is Chinese, Indians and Malays.

As shown in the Literacy Column of Table 5, the category of literacy is based on High, Medium and Low. High literacy comprise of users who have completed up to minimum of tertiary education such as an undergraduate, postgraduate or professional degree, while medium tertiary comprise of users who have completed up to a diploma level and those who are below a diploma level of education will fall under the low category level. In this study, a total of 24 subjects were recruited equally based on low (8 users), medium (8 users) and high (8 users) literacy level respectively (First graph in Table 5). These subjects comprise of various age groups to reflect the visitors and / or patients who visit the hospital, as shown in the age group column of Table 5 (Second graph in Table 5). The users comprise demography

Table 5. Demography for user experience test

No	Demography		Frequency	Analysis
	Literacy (Highest Qualification (Multi-Literacy))			
1	Low	Anything below Diploma	8	**Multi-literacy level** Low 34% High 33% Medium 33% Literacy levels of subjects for user experience test.
	Medium	Minimum Pre-U or Diploma Studies	8	
	High	Minimum Degree (Undergraduate)	8	
	Age Group			
2	Range	21-30	10	**Age distributioin** Age 21-30 **10** Age 31-40 **5** Age 41-50 **7** Age 51-60 **2** Age distribution for user experience test.
		31-40	5	
		41-50	7	
		51-60	2	
	Types of Device/Computer Literacy (Yes/No)			
3	Device	Laptop/Yes	18	**Device used** Desktop 20% Handphone 17% Laptop 25% Smartphone 30% Tablet 8% Multiple device experience.
		Smartphone Android/Yes	15	
		Desktop/Yes	14	
		Hand phone/No	12	
		Smartphone(IOS)/Yes	5	
		Tablet(Android)/Yes	4	
		Tablet(IOS)/Yes	2	
		Smartphone Blackberry/Yes	1	

of Malaysian from the midrange to the lower income group such as of students, technician, engineers, drivers, security guard and administrative assistant.

In terms of usage of technology or computer literacy, the majority of users are familiar with the smartphone (30%), laptop (25%), desktop 20% and hand phone (17%). Table 6 shows that 21 out of 24 or 88% of users are familiar with multiple devices which correspond to the internet usage survey by ("Internet User Survey 2012," 2012). This is despite the users having various levels of literacy and comprising of various age groups. A small portion of users (2 out of 24) are only familiar with basic handphone. These users have close to no experience in using neither the internet nor the computer. A handful of users ranging from 8% are familiar with tablet (Third graph in Table 5).

The gathering of the demography data was successfully done using the Mi-UXLab survey module. This survey module was previously used to also conduct employee 360 degrees self-assessment surveys, health awareness survey and also attendance tracking. The Mi-UXLab survey enables survey data to be

Table 6. Multiple device experience

User No.	Desktop	Hand-Phone	Laptop	Tablet		Smart-Phone		
				Android	(IOS)	Android	Blackberry	(IOS)
1	NO	YES	YES	NO	NO	NO	NO	YES
2	YES	NO	YES	NO	NO	YES	NO	NO
3	YES	NO	YES	NO	NO	YES	NO	NO
4	YES	NO	YES	NO	NO	YES	YES	NO
5	YES	NO	YES	NO	NO	YES	NO	NO
6	NO	NO	YES	NO	NO	YES	NO	NO
7	YES	YES	YES	NO	NO	NO	NO	NO
8	YES	NO	YES	NO	NO	YES	NO	NO
9	YES	YES	NO	NO	NO	NO	NO	NO
10	YES	YES	YES	YES	YES	YES	NO	YES
11	NO	NO	YES	NO	NO	NO	NO	YES
12	YES	YES	YES	NO	NO	YES	NO	NO
13	YES	NO	YES	YES	NO	YES	NO	YES
14	NO	YES	NO	NO	NO	NO	NO	NO
15	NO	NO	NO	NO	NO	YES	NO	NO
16	YES	NO	YES	YES	NO	YES	NO	NO
17	YES	YES	YES	NO	NO	NO	NO	NO
18	YES	YES	YES	NO	YES	NO	NO	YES
19	NO	YES	NO	NO	NO	NO	NO	NO
20	NO	NO	NO	NO	NO	YES	NO	NO
21	NO	YES	NO	NO	NO	YES	NO	NO
22	NO	YES	YES	NO	NO	NO	NO	NO
23	NO	NO	YES	YES	NO	YES	NO	NO
24	YES	YES	YES	NO	NO	YES	NO	NO

collected for open ended questions, multiple choice questions, matrix questions, ranking questions and Likert scale questions.

Test Setup and Scenario Based Testing

After completing the user recruitment, the usability analyst would schedule the appropriate timing for the users to take the test. Test is conducted with one user at a time, with the assistance of a moderator. Before the test starts, a briefing was conducted and user was required to sign a consent form on their agreement in participating with the test and the results could be used for the improvement of HIWS while their identity being anonymous.

Although, the users spoke multiple languages such as Cantonese, English, Malay, Mandarin and Tamil, the common language spoken is English and Malay. Hence the moderation was conducted in Manglish, which is a combination of English and Malay.

The various tasks to be performed are updated in Mi-UXLab, which will interact with the eye tracker (Tobii Studio and T60) to prompt the various scenarios, questions and user interface. The test comprise of the following scenario to resemble what happens in a hospital environment:

Task 1: You will have to visit the hospital for oral surgery in order to receive some treatment.
Task 2: After the treatment, proceed to the pharmacy to collect medications.
Task 3: Review each and every icon and let us know what you think each icon means.

1. Post Task Questionnaire (Close Ended):
   a. The way finding system is able to help me find the specialist clinic.
   b. The way finding system is easy to use.
   c. The symbols or icons used helps you to find the specialist clinic.
   d. Do you like the way finding system?

The similar scenarios are repeated for the various specialist clinics such as Cardiology, Cardiothoracic, Medical and Dermatology, Non-invasive Cardiology Laboratory Ophthalmology, Oral Surgery, Orthopedic and Nephrology, Obstetrics and Gynecology, Otorhinolaryngology, Urology, and Specialist Clinic Pharmacy.

Test Results for Task 1

While performing the first scenario, on the effectiveness of the users being able to identify the specialist clinic, it was found that 79% of the respondents were successful in their first attempt in locating the clinic, as shown in Figure 9. The remaining 21% could not identify the specialist clinic in the first go. These 5 respondents could not identify the icons used for the following specialist clinic:

- Ear Specialist;
- Heart diagnosis;
- Pregnancy related illness;
- Kidney related diseases;
- Fever related illness;

Figure 9. Success rate in first attempt for locating specialist clinic

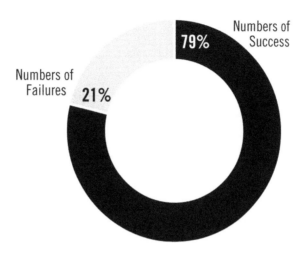

**Success rate in first attempt
in identifying specialist clinic**

These five respondents were given a second chance to identify the clinic and 2 out of 5 of them were successful in identifying the pregnancy and kidney related illness icons. The remaining 3 respondents could still not identify the appropriate clinic in the second attempt. These comprise of users 17 to 21. The reasons given for their choice are described in Table 7.

Figure 10 shows the time taken for all users. In terms of time taken for performing the task, in average users took about 55 seconds to perform the task. User 14 took only 16 seconds to correctly identify the dermatology clinic while user 7 took as long as 146 seconds to correctly identify the same clinic. Although user 14 identified the correct clinic in the fastest time, the user felt the icon used is not relevant. Refer to Table 7 for more qualitative feedback.

Feedback Capture after Task for Task 1

After completion of Task 1, Mi-UXLab system would automatically prompt the users to feedback their experience while performing the tasks. Table 7 summarizes their feedback.

Eye Tracking Analysis for Task 1

Based on the eye tracking data, it could be seen that users mostly fixate at the relevant areas of interest when tasked to visit a specialist clinic. As shown in Table 8, the darker spots on the heat map shows areas of high interest from other areas fixated by the users.

Test Results for Task 2

While performing the second scenario, on the effectiveness of the users being able to identify the pharmacy, it was found that 92% of the respondents were successful in their first attempt in locating the pharmacy, as shown in Figure 11. The remaining 8% could not identify in the first go but were successful in the second attempt.

Table 7. Qualitative feedback from users while performing Task 1

User No.	Feedback: How Well You Found the System Responding to Your Choice?
1	Confuse icon "Klinik Perubatan dan Klinik Dermalogi" dengan "Klinik Oftalmologi" sebab icon "Klinik Perubatan dan Klinik Dermatologi" tunjuk sakit tekak juga seperti icon "Klinik Oftalmologi".
2	N/A
3	N/A
4	N/A
5	N/A
6	N/A
7	N/A
8	N/A
9	N/A
10	Direction need to be showed. Since there is playground near to pediatrik clinic, I find that it is child clinic as well the teddy bear icon. I don't know the term pediatrik and others as well. I have not came across the term during my studies.
11	The 2 icon of Klinik Nefrologi dan Klinik Urologi represent kidney specialist.
12	The icon represent mouth problem so I assume it is to treat sore throat.
13	I have no idea whether the term and icon is relevant. I click on It based on eye icon. I don't know my current position.
14	The icon of Klinik Dermatologi is not relevant and I don't know what it is.
15	The term used Klinik Nefrologi dan Neurologi not understandable.
16	I know the dermatologi related to skin problem but I am not sure right now. The icon of dermatologi looks like pimples problem.
17	I chose this icon because the icon shows that it is ear ache. I don't understand the word Klinik dermatologi. I am not sure whether the icon and the terms are relevant or not.
18	I chose it because it should be the general treatment. I don't know what the icon of pharmacy is.
19	I chose it because it shows heart.
20	I chose it because it shows pregnant women In the icon.
21	Because there is icon/ picture representation.
22	There is icon/ picture representation.
23	Ear is usually associate with throat and eye.
24	There is an icon representing kidney

Figure 10. Time taken to perform Task 1

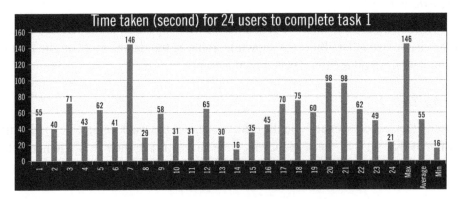

Table 8. Heat map generated from eye tracking analysis for Task 1

User	Scenario 1	Heatmap
1	Klinik Pediatrik	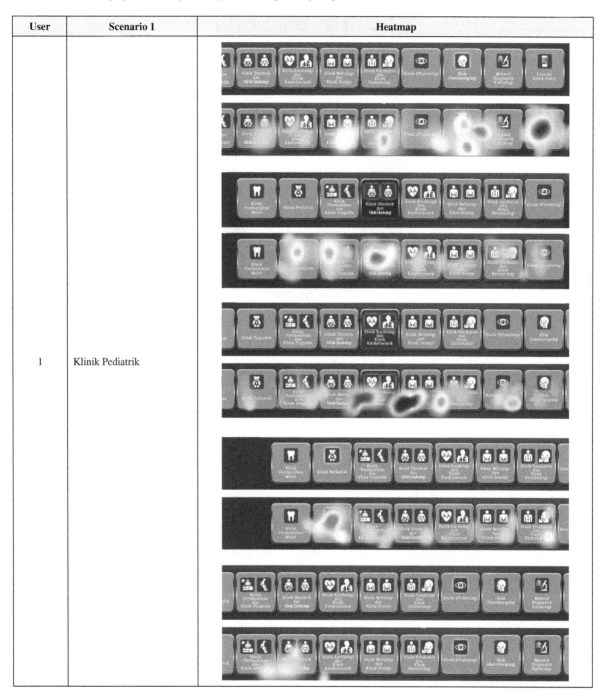

Figure 12 shows the time taken by the users to perform Task 2. The maximum amount of time was taken by user 7, being 118 seconds while the fastest time taken is only 5 seconds by user 24. While user 7 was only successful in the second attempt, user 5 could identify the correct pharmacy icon in the first attempt. The average time task for Task 2 35.55 seconds, which is 19.5 seconds faster than for Task 1.

Figure 11. Success rate in first attempt for locating pharmacy

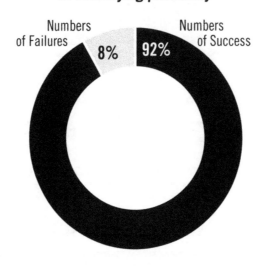

Figure 12. Time taken to perform Task 2

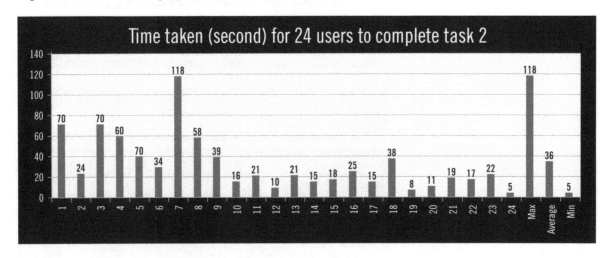

Feedback Capture after Task for Task 2

Similar to Task 1, Mi-UXLab will prompt for user feedback at the completion of the Task 2. This is summarized in Table 9.

Test Results for Task 3

After performing Task 1 and 2, it was found that although many users could complete the task, as shown in Figure 9 and 11, the FCAT shows that they were not really satisfied with the icons used. Taking into account this feedback, from user 10 onwards, a new task was included that is to gather feedback on each and every icons from the users. Table 10 shows the results for the review of various icons by each user.

Table 9. Qualitative feedback from users while performing Task 2

User No.	Feedback: How Well You Found the System Responding to Your Choice?
1	Not suitable icon for "Farmasi Klinik Pakar". Selalunya icon farmasi ada gambar macam tumbuk guna lesung.
2	N/A
3	N/A
4	N/A
5	N/A
6	N/A
7	N/A
8	N/A
9	N/A
10	I can find clinic easily.
11	The icon not relevant to pharmacy. I don't know what icon represented by Farmasi Klinik Pakar
12	The icon represent pharmacy.
13	I have no idea what the icon represent.
14	The icon of pharmacy looks like garbage bin. It is better to show pills.
15	The icon is not relevant to pharmacy and I also don't know what is general icon for pharmacy as well.
16	The Farmasi Klinik pakar not relevant with the icon and the icon should be something like pill.
17	I chose it because it is written pharmacy.
18	I chose it because, other options look too specific to certain treatment whereas this Farmasi Klinik Pakar looks like for general purpose or treatment.
19	I chose the icon because it is written pharmacy. I don't know what is the icon or picture is and it should be represented with some pills.
20	I chose it because of the Pharmacy term which I know. I don't know what the icon for.
21	Understand the term Farmasi but not relevant to the icon.
22	I chose it because of the Pharmacy term which I know. Not sure what the icon for.
23	I chose it because of the Pharmacy term which I know. Not sure what the icon for.
24	Understand Farmasi but doesn't understand the icon used.

Post Task Questionnaire

After the completion of all tasks, three sets of post task questions were used while rated by a 5 Point Likert scale as shown in Figure 13, 14 and 15. Figure 13 shows that 8% and 58% of users strongly agree and agree that the way findings system is able to help them find the specialist clinic, while the remaining 21% and 13% were unsure and disagreed that the system was helpful. From here, it could be summarized that 66% of users agree that the system is helpful while the remaining are either unsure or disagree that the system is useful.

As shown in Figure 14, 17% and 67% of users strongly agree and agree that the way finding system is easy to use, while the remaining 16% disagree that the system is easy. In summary, 84% of users found the system easy to use and 83% of users like to use the system as shown in Figure 14 and 16.

Table 10. Qualitative feedback from users while performing Task 3

User No.	Review Each and Every Icon and Let Us Know What You Think Each Icon Means
1	N/A
2	N/A
3	N/A
4	N/A
5	N/A
6	N/A
7	N/A
8	N/A
9	N/A
10	Not sure the icon for Klinik Geneologi is for men or women. I see the klink perubatan icon which is the doctor picture as general specialist. When I look at the klinik dermatologi picture it represent teeth ache specialist. Not sure what is Klinik Otorinolaringologi specialise in. The pharmacy icon is not relevant to pharmacy term and i have no idea what is that icon is.
11	The term Klinik Pembedahan Mulut not relevant to the icon. Klinik pediatrik term and the icon are relevant. Klinik Pembedahan dan Klinik Otopedik term and icon are relevant. Klinik Obsterik dan Klinik Ginekologi term and icon not relvant and I don't know the icon is what as well. Klinik Perubatan dan Klinik Dermatologi icon represent they are specialist in pimples. I dont know what is Klinik Otorinolaringologi.
12	Icon of Klinik Pembedahan Mulut not relevant to the term used. Klinik dermatologi icon is not relevant as it show teeth ache. Klinik Otorinolaringologi don't know what is the term is.
13	I don't know what is the Klinik Pediatrik term meaning. Klinik pembedahan icon looks like someone massaging. Klinik dermatologi looks like specialise in mouth symptom. I don't know what is the term Klinik oftalmologi meaning. I seriosly don't have any idea what is Klinik Otorinolaringologi. The makmal diagnostik looks relevant something like diagnostik but the term kardiologi makes me confuse.
14	The term Klinik Pembedahan Mulut not relevant to the icon. The icon of Klinik pembedahan mulut need to be changed. Klinik pediatrik term and the icon teddy bear are not suitable.I don't know what is the term Klinik Karidoterasik is. I don't have any idea what is Klinik Otorinolaringologi. Makmal diagnostik kardiologi is specialise in MRI and so on.
15	I don't know what is Klinik Dermatologi specialise in and the icon is not relevant. I don't understand what is the meaning of Klinik Oftalmologi. I don't understand what is the meaning of Klinik Otorinolaringologi. Don't know what is Makmal Diagnostik Kardiologi specialise in but I know its for diagnosis. The terminology used for all the icon is basic but it is just we depend on the pciture or icon.
16	The term Klinik Pembedahan Mulut not related to the icon as it shows teeth instead of mouth. The Klinik Pediatrik term shows me that it is child specialise whereby the icon or picture not at all. I don't know what is Klinik Otopedik. But when look at the picture it looks like they are bone specialise. I dont know what Klinik Otorinolaringologi specialise in but i think it should be mouth ache. Makmal Diagnostik Kardiologi more like R&D stuff. The terminology very hard to understand especially for village people.
17	The term Klinik Pembedahan Mulut not related to the icon as it shows teeth instead of mouth. Suppose it should show mouth icon. I don't know what is Klinik Pediatrik. I don't know what is makmal diagnostik kardiologi is for. Basically, I don't understand most of the terminology.
18	The term Klinik Pembedahan Mulut and icon not relevant and the term should be some sort of dental name. Klinik Pembedahan icon looks like someone massaging. They need to separate the Klinik Perubatan and Klinik Dermatologi into different options as there is huge distinction in their treatment specialisation. The dermatologi icon looks like someone slappig on the face. I dont know what is the term Klinik Otorinolaringologi is. Makmal Diagnostik kardiologi is maybe specialise in heart or fitness.
19	I don't know what is Klinik Otorinolaringologi is for as well the icon. I don't know what Makmal Diagnostik Kardiologi specialise in.
20	The term Klinik Pembedahan Mulut not related to the icon. Because mouth and teeth are different. I don't understand the term Klinik Otopedik. I don't know what is the icon that represented for Klinik Dermatologi. Makmal Diagnostik kardiologi is for any kind of research.
21	The term Klinik Pembedahan Mulut not related to the icon. Thinks that Klinik Dermatologi represents toothache.
22	The term Klinik Pembedahan Mulut not relevant to the icon. No obvious distinction between the two icon for Kilinik Neufrologi dan Klinik Urologi (2 icon seems to represent kidney). Icon for dermatologi seems to be representing clinic for tooth. Doesn't seems to understand some of the terminologies used. Makmal Diagnostik kardiologi seems to represent a lab.
23	The icon for Klinik Pembedahan Mulut is relevant to the icon used. Don't know the term for Urologi. Not sure of the term Klinik Perubatan dan Dermatologi
24	The icon for Klinik Pembedahan Mulut is relevant to the icon used. Thinks that icon for dermatologi represent mouth problems. Icon for Kilnik Otorinolaringologi seems to represent clinic for breathing problem(pernafasan).

Figure 13. The way finding system is able to help me find the specialist clinic

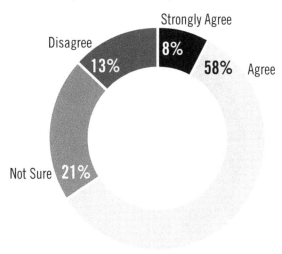

Figure 14. The way finding system is easy to use

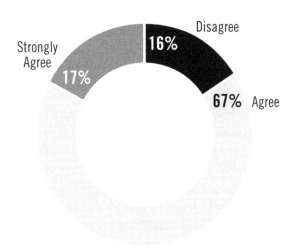

The symbols or icons used comprise of the entire system. Figure 15 shows that 17% and 41% strongly agree and agree to the statement that the symbols or icons used could help them find the specialist clinic, which is an overall 58% agreement on the symbol and icon design, which was based on the studies conducted in the US by Hablamos Juntos (Berger & Juntos, 2005).

Based on the qualitative feedback obtained and shown in Table 7, 9 and 10, which is based from a Malaysian demography, further improvement in terms of design and development could take place

Figure 15. The symbols or icons used helps you find the specialist clinic

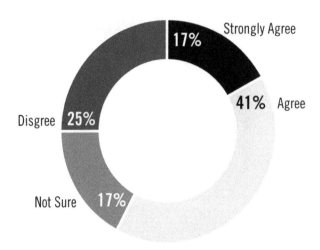

The symbols or icons used helps you find the specialist clinic

Table 11. Qualitative feedback from users while performing Task 3

Method	How Much Do You Agree that the Symbols or Icons Used Help You Find the Specialist Clinic?		
	Agree	Disagree	Neutral
Survey (Fourth graph in Table 2)	57%	34%	9%
User Experience Test (Figure 15)	58%	25%	17%

to the improvement of the effectiveness, helpfulness, ease of use and suitability of the HIWS system. When the finding from the user experience test (Figure 15) is compared to the survey conducted, it is not a surprise that the symbols do not appeal to the some of the respondents as shown in Table 11. One of the reasons for this is that the symbol used as a basis is based on the demography in the United States (US), instead from Malaysia. Both survey and user experience test users came to a similar agreement on the suitability of the symbols used, which is 57% and 58% respectively. However in terms of level of disagreement, there are lower levels of disagreements during the User Experience Test.

The pie chart in Figure 16 shows that 83% of the users like the HIWS. The reasons as provided by the users include:

- It enables estimation of a location.
- It enables direction to specific clinic.
- The like the icon, colors used and animation.
- Its simple and easily understandable.
- User friendly.
- Easy to find destination and location to clinic.

Figure 16. Do you like the way finding system?

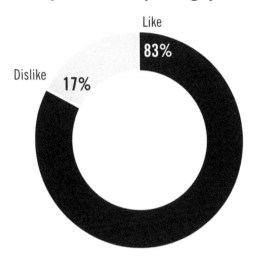

Do you like the way finding system

- Overall, it's easy to use and required less effort (no. of click).
- User friendly, good and nice interface, clear icon and picture.
- The logo is easy to understand with textual description.
- Interactive system is helpful to users.
- It makes convenient to locate direction to the specialist clinic.

However 17% of the users dislikes the system, the reason provided include

- Although overall the system looks good, it needs improvement in terms of usage of attractive colors and icons and more interesting interaction elements.
- There is no guiding arrows to clearly navigate the users to the targeted location.
- Unsuitable terminologies used.
- System is not user friendly, icons used do not correspond well to the terminology used for the specialist clinic.
- The design of the icon or pictures are not user friendly.
- Do not understand the application of the system.

FUTURE RESEARCH DIRECTIONS

This project is meant for the single kiosk use, which is recommended to be place near the escalator in the specialist clinics. There is a prospect to integrate the HIWS with the Total Hospital Information System (THIS) in the future. By having a data based system the kiosk can be place at many location for the use of the whole hospital. If this wayfinding system is uploaded to a website, QR code can be implemented for smartphone users. In this way patron do not have to go to the kiosk if they forgot the direction midway to their desired specialist clinics. Besides serving as interactive wayfinding system, online registration maybe made via this system without going to the registration counter. This will reduce waiting time, which currently occurs at the hospital. Patron can even search for their desired direction prior to visiting the specialist clinics. This will reduce much stress experienced by the patrons. Indirectly it could assist our government concern of inadequate integrated planning of health information system.

Some of the limitations of this study include:

1. The study does not represent entire Malaysian population and is only confined to West Malaysia, since the location of testing was conducted in Kuala Lumpur and it was difficult to find subjects from East Malaysia. Having excluded the diverse ethnic group such as from:
   a. Sabah and W.P. Labuan:
      i. Kadazan/Dusun,
      ii. Bajau,
      iii. Murut,
      iv. Other Bumiputra.
   b. Sarawak:
      i. Iban,
      ii. Bidayuh,
      iii. Melanau,
      iv. Other Bumiputra.
      who comprise of up to 13%, this study was designed to focus on the 87% of the population. It is recommended to perform similar studies take into account their feedback.
2. The sample size used for the testing is not sufficient and should be increased once the next iteration of design and development is completed based on the current feedback.

CONCLUSION

In conclusion, the study has met all its intended objectives. From the survey conducted, the first objective of understanding the Malaysian requirement and challenges faced in a government hospital has been gathered. From this, it could be seen that the majority of users found that the signage used with visual aid increased the familiarity with the specialist clinics. Based on design guidelines, the various icons and suitable fonts were used to design the system. This is followed by development of a web based interactive system. The final objective of validating the system was achieved by conducting a lab based user experience test to determine the effectiveness and time taken by the respondents in using the HIWS. In general, it could be seen that the system developed has met the requirements of majority of users. On the positive note, 79% of users were successful in their first attempt to find the specialist clinic with an average time taken of 55.05 seconds, which is less than a minute. This is also supported by the heatmap generated from the eye tracker as shown in Table 8. The success rate for finding the pharmacy was even higher at 92% with an average time taken of 35.55 seconds. In addition to this, 66% of users agree that the system is helpful in finding the specialist clinic and 86% reported that the system is easy to use. However, when it came to the appropriateness of symbols used, the number was lower whereby only 58% agreed that it was helpful, although in overall 83% like the way finding system. Based on the qualitative feedback obtained and Figure 15, significant localization efforts needs to be placed on redesigning the symbols and icons used which will boost the acceptance rate in the helpfulness of HIWS.

REFERENCES

Accolades & Accreditations. (2013). *MIMOS Berhad*. Retrieved August 04, 2014, from http://www. mimos.my/corporate/accolades-accreditations/

Arthur, P., & Passini, R. (1992). Wayfinding: people, signs, and architecture. McGraw-Hill, Incorporated.

Basri, A. Q., & Sulaiman, R. (2013). Ergonomics Study Of Public Hospital Signage. In *Advanced Engineering Forum* (Vol. 10, pp. 263–271). Trans Tech Publ. doi:10.4028/www.scientific.net/AEF.10.26310.4028/ www.scientific.net/AEF.10.263

Berger, C., & Juntos, H. (2005). Universal Symbols in Health Care Workbook: Executive Summary: Best Practices for Sign Systems. Hablamos Juntos.

Bojko, A. (2006). Using Eye Tracking to Compare Web Page Designs: A Case Study. Journal of Usability Studies, 1, 112–120. Retrieved from http://www.upassoc.org/upa_publications/jus/2006_may/ bojko_eye_tracking.html?pagewanted=all

Brown, K., & Asmar, H. O. (2006). Malaysia: Language Situation. In Encyclopedia of Language & Linguistics (pp. 462–464). doi:10.1016/B0-08-044854-2/01695-3

Brown, K., & Romaine, S. (2006). Language Policy in Multilingual Educational Contexts. In Encyclopedia of Language (pp. 584–596). Linguistics; 10.1016/B0-08-044854-2/00646-5

Cheng, B. H. C., & Atlee, J. M. (2007). Research Directions in Requirements Engineering. Future of Software Engineering, 2007. FOSE, 07. doi:10.1109/FOSE.2007.17

Chrimes, D., Kitos, N. R., Kushniruk, A., & Mann, D. M. (2014). Usability testing of Avoiding Diabetes Thru Action Plan Targeting (ADAPT) decision support for integrating care-based counseling of pre-diabetes in an electronic health record. International Journal of Medical Informatics, 83(9), 636–647. doi:10.1016/j.ijmedinf.2014.05.002 PubMed doi:10.1016/j.ijmedinf.2014.05.002 PMID:24981988

Educational and Social Characteristics of the Population 2010. (2014). *Department of Statistics Malaysia*. Retrieved from http://www.statistics.gov.my/portal/download_Population/files/census2010/education/5. Tables.pdf

Foley, M. (2012). NSW HEALTH Annual Report 2011 – 12. NSW Ministry of Health. Retrieved from http://www.health.nsw.gov.au/publications/Publications/annual_report12/HealthAR_2012.pdf

Garrett, J. J. (2010). Elements of User Experience, The: User-Centered Design for the Web and Beyond. Pearson Education. Pearson Education.

Goh, K. N., Chen, Y. Y., Lai, F. W., Daud, S. C., Sivaji, A., & Soo, S. T. (2013). A comparison of usability testing methods for an e-commerce website: A case study on a Malaysia online gift shop. In *Proceedings of the 2013 10th International Conference on Information Technology: New Generations, ITNG 2013* (pp. 143–150). IEEE. doi:10.1109/ITNG.2013.12910.1109/ITNG.2013.129

Gray, C., & Malins, J. (2004). Visualizing research. *A Guide to the Research*.

Hofstede, G. (2010). Geert hofstede. National Cultural Dimensions.

Intercensal Mid-Year Population Estimates Malaysia and States. (2014). *Department of Statistics Malaysia*, 7. Retrieved from http://www.statistics.gov.my/portal/download_Population/files/Anggaran_Penduduk_Pertengahan_Tahun_Antara_Banci2001_2009.pdf

Internet User Survey 2012. (2012). *Malaysian Communications and Multimedia Commision*. Retrieved from http://www.skmm.gov.my/Resources/Statistics/Internet-users-survey.aspx

Ismail, A., Jamil, A. T., Rahman, A. F. A., Madihah, J., Bakar, A., & Saad, N. M. (2010). The Implementation of Hospital Information System (HIS) in Tertiary Hospitals in Malaysia: A Qualitative Study. Malaysian Journal of Public Health Medicine, 10(2), 16–24.

ISO 21542:2011 Building construction -- Accessibility and usability of the built environment. (2011). *ISO (International Organization for Standardization)*. Retrieved from http://www.iso.org/iso/catalogue_detail?csnumber=50498

Jacob, R. J. K., & Karn, K. S. (2003). Eye tracking in human-computer interaction and usability research: Ready to deliver the promises. Mind, 2(3), 4.

Lerner, E. B., Jehle, D. V., Janicke, D. M., & Moscati, R. M. (2000). Medical communication: Do our patients understand? The American Journal of Emergency Medicine, 18(7), 764–766. doi:10.1053/ajem.2000.18040 PubMed doi:10.1053/ajem.2000.18040 PMID:11103725

Lester, P. (2013). Visual communication: Images with messages. Cenage Learning. Cengage Learning.

Lynch, K. (1960). The image of the city (Vol. 11). MIT Press.

Meeting of Cultural Ministers - National Arts and Health Framework. (2014). Council of Australian Governments Standing Council on Health (SCoH) including the Australian Health Workforce Ministerial Council (AHWMC). Retrieved from http://www.ahmac.gov.au/cms_documents/National Arts and Health Framework.pdf

Mollerup, P. (2009). Wayshowing in hospital. Australasian Medical Journal, 1(10), 112–114. doi:10.4066/AMJ.2009.85

myGovernment - The Government of Malaysia's Official Portal. (n.d.). Malaysian Administrative Modernisation and Management Planning Unit (MAMPU). Retrieved July 31, 2014, from https://www.malaysia.gov.my/en/about-malaysia?subCatId=3208956&type=2&categoryId=3208945

Olmsted-Hawala, E., Holland, T., & Quach, V. (2014). Eye Tracking in User Experience Design. Elsevier; doi:10.1016/B978-0-12-408138-3.00003-0 doi:10.1016/B978-0-12-408138-3.00003-0

Rapley, C. E. (2013). *Accessibility and Development: environmental accessibility and its implications for inclusive, sustainable and equitable development for all*. Department of Economic and Social Affairs, United Nations.

Rashid, S., Soo, S., Sivaji, A., Naeni, H. S., & Bahri, S. (2013). Preliminary Usability Testing with Eye Tracking and FCAT Analysis on Occupational Safety and Health Websites. Procedia: Social and Behavioral Sciences, 97, 737–744. doi:10.1016/j.sbspro.2013.10.295 doi:10.1016/j.sbspro.2013.10.295

Rooke, C. N., Koskela, L. J., & Tzortzopoulos, P. (2010). Achieving a lean wayfinding system in complex hospital environments: Design and through-life management. In *Proceedings of the 18th Annual Conference of the International Group for Lean Construction* (pp. 233–242). National Building Research Institute, Technion-Israel Institute of Technology.

Rooke, C. N., Tzortzopoulos, P., Koskela, L. J., & Rooke, J. A. (2009). Wayfinding: embedding knowledge in hospital environments. In HaCIRIC (pp. 158–167). London, UK: Imperial College Business School.

Sansom, M., & Brooks, E. (2012). WorldHealthDesign-Architecture-Culture-Technology. International Academy of Design and Health.

Sherman, P. (2009). *UPA 2009 Salary Survey. User Experience Professionals Association*. Retrieved from http://usabilityprofessionals.org/usability_resources/surveys/SalarySurveys.html

Sivaji, A., & Ahmad, W. F. W. (2014). Benefits of Complementing Eye-Tracking Analysis with Think-Aloud Protocol in a Multilingual Country with High Power Distance. In Current Trends in Eye Tracking Research (pp. 267–278). Springer. doi:10.1007/978-3-319-02868-2_21 doi:10.1007/978-3-319-02868-2_21

Sivaji, A., & Soo, S. (2012). Website user experience (UX) testing tool development using Open Source Software (OSS). *2012 Southeast Asian Network of Ergonomics Societies Conference (SEANES)*. doi:10.1109/SEANES.2012.6299576

Sivaji, A., & Soo, S. (2013). Understanding, Enhancing and Automating HCI Work Practices: Malaysian Case Studies. Procedia: Social and Behavioral Sciences, 97, 656–665. doi:10.1016/j.sbspro.2013.10.285 doi:10.1016/j.sbspro.2013.10.285

Sivaji, A., Abdollah, N., Soo, S., Chuan, N.-K., Nor, Z. M., Rasidi, S.-H., & Yoong, S.-W. (2014). Measuring Public Value UX based on ISO/IEC 25010 Quality Attributes. In *3rd International Conference on User Science and Engineering 2014 (i-USEr 2014)*. IEEEXplore. doi:10.1109/IUSER.2014.700267710.1109/IUSER.2014.7002677

Sivaji, A., Abdullah, A., & Downe, A. G. (2011). Usability testing methodology: Effectiveness of heuristic evaluation in E-government website development. In *Proceedings - AMS 2011: Asia Modelling Symposium 2011 - 5th Asia International Conference on Mathematical Modelling and Computer Simulation* (pp. 68–72). IEEE.

Sivaji, A., Abdullah, M. R., Downe, A. G., & Ahmad, W. F. W. (2013). Hybrid usability methodology: Integrating heuristic evaluation with laboratory testing across the software development lifecycle. In *Proceedings of the 2013 10th International Conference on Information Technology: New Generations, ITNG 2013,* (pp. 375–383). IEEE. doi:10.1109/ITNG.2013.6010.1109/ITNG.2013.60

Sivaji, A., Downe, A. G., Mazlan, M. F., Soo, S. T., & Abdullah, A. (2011). Importance of incorporating fundamental usability with social & trust elements for e-commerce website. In *ICBEIA 2011 - 2011 International Conference on Business, Engineering and Industrial Applications,* (pp. 221–226). Retrieved from http://ieeexplore.ieee.org/stamp/stamp.jsp?tp=&arnumber=5994248&isnumber=5994212

Sivaji, A., Shopian, S., Nor, Z. M., Chuan, N.-K., & Bahri, S. (2013). Lighting does Matter: Preliminary Assessment on Office Workers. Procedia: Social and Behavioral Sciences, 97, 638–647. doi:10.1016/j.sbspro.2013.10.283 doi:10.1016/j.sbspro.2013.10.283

Soegaard, M. (2010). Gestalt principles of form perception. *Interaction-Design. Org*, 8.

Standards Malaysia Recognises MIMOS As The First Malaysian Lab To Receive MS ISO/IEC Accreditation Certificate For Software Testing. (2014). BERNAMA. Retrieved August 04, 2014, from http://www.bernama.com/bernama/v7/newsindex.php?id=1011837

Tzuaan, S. S., & Sivaji, A. (2014). Measuring Malaysian M-Commerce User Behaviour. *Computer and Information Sciences (ICCOINS), 2014 International Conference*. IEEE.

Whittle, K. (2009). *The Nature of Healing. International Academy of Design and Health*. Retrieved July 29, 2014, from http://www.designandhealth.com/events/singapore-congress-kristen-whittle.aspx

Yeo, A. W., Chiu, P.-C., Lim, T.-Y., Tan, P.-P., Lim, T., & Hussein, I. (2011). Usability in Malaysia. In Global usability (pp. 211–222). Springer. doi:10.1007/978-0-85729-304-6_12 doi:10.1007/978-0-85729-304-6_12

Zielstorff, R. D. (2003). Controlled vocabularies for consumer health. Journal of Biomedical Informatics, 36(4-5), 326–333. doi:10.1016/j.jbi.2003.09.015 PubMed doi:10.1016/j.jbi.2003.09.015 PMID:14643728

KEY TERMS AND DEFINITIONS

Hablamos Juntos: A project funded by the Robert Wood Johnson Foundation, and administered by the UCSF Fresno Center for Medical Education & Research, a major educational and clinical branch of the UCSF School of Medicine. Targeted towards the Latino population, it is aimed at improved patient and medical care provider communication.

Mi-UXLab: Formerly known as URANUS, it is a software designed by MIMOS User Experience Lab to facilitate user experience testing, heuristic evaluation, survey and Kansei engineering. It has been used in user experience research, design and testing projects in various domains and purposes such as e-Government, e and m-Commerce, industrial ergonomics, Human Resource Information System, Cloud Computing, Mobile Testing and Cultural UX.

SAMM (Skim Akreditasi Makmal Malaysia): A National Laboratory Accreditation Scheme set up by the Malaysian Government on August 15th 1990 managed by the Department of Standards Malaysia. SAMM accredits almost every testing facility and technology such as software testing. A SAMM endorsed test report gives confidence that the test was done in accordance with the stated specification, test or calibration method and correct test environment.

Universal Symbol in Health Care (USHC): A universal symbol comprising of 50 symbols that was found to be more effective than text based signage in assisting patient and visitors in finding their way around the health care facility.

User Experience (UX) Professionals Association: An international association devoted to assisting new and established professionals in the user experience disciplines.

User Experience (UX): Designing the User Experience comprise of User Centered Analysis, User Centered Design, Development and Testing. It is a well-established method commonly referred to in the field of Human Computer Interaction (HCI) under the Association of Computing and Machinery (ACM) classification.

Wayfinding System: A method for users to find ways to their desired destination that is not based merely on signage. It is a complex system that includes environment and behavioral aspect enabling users to interpret and endure their surroundings to get to their destination without long thoughts.

This research was previously published in Critical Socio-Technical Issues Surrounding Mobile Computing edited by Murni Mahmud, Norshidah Mohamed, Teddy Mantoro, and Media Ayu; pages 88-123, copyright year 2016 by Information Science Reference (an imprint of IGI Global).

Section 3
Management and Operations

Chapter 16
Managing Emergency Units Applying Queueing Theory

Salvador Hernández-González
Instituto Tecnologico de Celaya, Mexico

Manuel Dario Hernández-Ripalda
Instituto Tecnologico de Celaya, Mexico

Anakaren González-Pérez
Instituto Tecnologico de Celaya, Mexico

Moises Tapia-Esquivias
Instituto Tecnologico de Celaya, Mexico

Alicia Luna-González
Instituto Tecnologico de Celaya, Mexico

ABSTRACT

Today managers of health systems must manage the resources at their disposal to ensure that service quality is adequate, this leads at the same time making decisions to ensure that these resources are managed efficiently and effectively. The decision process in healthcare systems is not trivial given the complexity of these systems. The application of tools (like queueing theory) for decision making in hospital systems is an area of opportunity because of the increasing financial pressure and the growing demand for care. This document shows how queueing theory can be applied for analyzing the performance of an Emergency Unit under different capacity scenarios. The analysis shows that increasing the number of servers required to maintain constant congestion(emphasis on efficiency)is more expensive than adding servers to maintain constant the probability that a patient has to wait (emphasis on quality and efficiency). The paper ends with recommendations for future research.

DOI: 10.4018/978-1-7998-2451-0.ch016

Copyright © 2020, IGI Global. Copying or distributing in print or electronic forms without written permission of IGI Global is prohibited.

INTRODUCTION

Administration of Health Systems and Hospitals

Hospital systems administrators are responsible for managing resources at their disposal, in order to provide quality service to patients and beneficiaries.

Hospital systems were used to operate without major limitations regarding the available resources, since it was essential to preserve the integrity of the patient, also administration was supported to a greater extent by trial and error, therefore, the application of tools from different areas, as Operations Research have been (at least until recently) ignored; but today health institutions, especially government institutions suffer from increasing financial pressure from governments, which require that assigned resources are managed effectively and efficiently.

While this applies to all hospitals in the world, it is in the countries known as emerging economies such as Mexico, where the effects of lack of tools to support the decision process have a greater impact. As others, Health systems are not easy to analyze and problems are challenging.

For example: Mexico is among the few OECD countries that have not yet achieved universal or near universal coverage of health insurance. Also, the public share of health care financing in México has increased to 50% in 2012, but it is one of the lowest across the OECD members (the average is 72%) (OECD 2005, OECD 2014), in other words, around half of all health spending is paid by Mexican patients.

Expenditure cuts to the health systems are common and result in the zero generation of vacancies for new doctors and nurses, shortages of medicines, materials and equipment; however it continues increasing demand service. According to OECD statistics, in Mexico the number of doctors per capita raised in the past years moving from 1.6 per 1000 population in 2002 to 2.2 per 1000 population in 2012, which it is just above Korea (2.1), Chile(1.7) and Turkey(1.7). The 34 members of the OECD average 3.2 (OECD, 2014).

It should be noted that one of the priorities of governments should be to ensure greater coverage of health services, ensuring that the workforce (doctors, nurses) have the necessary skills and resources to carry out their tasks.

The question arises about what managers should do before making a decision. According to Litvak, Long, Arroye and Jarillo (2000) the following question is proposed: How much can be cut in spending of a health system without affecting the quality of service?

In Health systems timely access has been identified as one of the key elements of healthcare quality (Green 2005). What kind of tools can be applied to measure the time a patient spends waiting in a queue to receive attention? How many doctors are needed to guarantee a reasonable waiting time and generate the perception of a good quality in the service? How much a "good" policy cost?

This chapter shows a set of relationships derived from queuing theory which are (among many others) very useful for decision-making and enable an administrator to evaluate different decisions and also their impact on the quality of service provided to patients and so to answer questions as the previous paragraph. We present an application example of the emergency system of a public hospital in Mexico where it is necessary to calculate the number of doctors required to satisfy the demand of service and ensuring the quality of service, the costs of different alternatives and the robustness to face scenarios of increased demand.

Table 1. Emergency classification

Priority	Features	Estimated Waiting Time
1	Imminent risk of death.	immediate attention
2	Uncontrolled bleeding, chest pain accompanied by low pressure, loss of consciousness, multiple traumas with or without fracture.	< 60 minutes
3	Patient with respiratory stability, with vomiting or evacuation of blood, seizures, abdominal pain, fever greater than 38 °C / 100.4 °F (children under 3 months), wounds requiring stitches.	< 120 minutes
4	Patient with respiratory stability without reaching symptoms in Priority 3	Up to 4 hours of waiting

Emergency Department in Hospital Systems

The Emergency Department at hospitals is the service area with the highest demand of patients, each patient has his respective degree of urgency; however all patients, independent of the degree of urgency, require speed and quality of care (Table 1).

The perception of the quality of service provided by the hospital through their doctors and nurses depends largely on the care provided by emergency department. Today it is recognized that the attention of real and perceived emergencies in a hospital is a problem that must be addressed, appropriate care in the emergency department reduce the effects of trauma in the population, temporary sequels, permanent and secondary to these (Arellano & Martinez, 2012). For example, in México the measured average waiting time is 26 minutes for a consultation in a primary care clinic and 18 minutes after arrival for emergency services (OECD 2005).

Service Discipline in the Emergency Department

The mechanism usually consists of the patient's arrival at the window, for information, once it has provided information to the patient, it is channeled to the "Triage" (the French word for classification), the patient is evaluated by a medical and vital signs are recorded, the result of the evaluation classifies the patient, assigning a priority level of care (Reyes & Grimaldi, 2012).

In this sense, so that the different areas of health systems in general provide better services to the amount of available resources, administration officials need tools to plan, prioritize and make informed decisions (Green, 2005).

BACKGROUND

The patient care process in an emergency department, have been modeled by different conceptual models such as the input-throughput-output model, the Fields chaos model, the ED Cardiac Analogy Model, formula-based equations, regression modeling, queuing theory–based models and discrete-event (or process) simulation models.

To select which model to use should be considered the problem to be faced. The queuing model is particularly useful for measuring the impact of a change in the parameters of the care process.

The queuing model expresses the model of patient care in the form of equations, these equations to measure average values of the emergency system such as the time spent in the system while waiting to be served, number of patients in the system, number of patients waiting to be served, and the number of patients who leave without being served. All these measurements are defined universally and accurately.

The models developed in queuing theory consider situations such as: different patterns of arrival, arrivals either individually or in groups, with different probability distributions, service times with different probability distributions, service configurations in the form of networks with different stages, different service disciplines.

Queueing models provide estimated measures as could be the steady state of a queuing system under different considerations in the arrival time, service time, service disciplines, different network configurations of servers, and restrictions on system capabilities. These descriptions in a steady state are defined unambiguously in a mature scientific discipline, with useful and fruitful applications in telecommunications and production areas to name a few.

It is worth mention that queueing models are not used to forecast demand, especially in the short term. Equations from queueing theory were not built for that purpose. On the other hand, allow a quantitative description that occurs by changing the system configuration. Changes in a system, for example, can be: change service discipline, giving priority to certain patients; increase or decrease the number of servers they serve; configure networks with different trajectories, for patients with different services.

The waiting line models (or alternatively queueing models), they are not used to optimize, directly, the configuration of a system according to some criterion. Queueing models are used to estimate the consequences of the decisions on the system in service metrics that are of interest. Knowing these estimated effects, they can be used to better decide on the most appropriate change.

The waiting lines models are analyzed either with equations as computer simulation, this is according to the case presented. The equations of the waiting line models can be put into a spreadsheet, and allow rapid analysis of various system conditions.

For example, Panayiotopoulos and Vassilacopoulos in 1984 article, describes an emergency department system with the following characteristics: (1) general independent interarrival distribution, (2) general service-time distribution, (3) limited waiting room, (4) patient's priorities increase up to a certain number, (5) time-dependent number of servers (doctors), (6) infinite patient population, (7) each server meets the system only once within a certain period of time, while the total number of the available servers is known. The model was analyzed by computer simulation. The following is a review of the most recent literature related to the application of different approaches used to analysis of health care systems, including queueing theory.

Queuing theory–based models are applied in Au (2009),to model the bypass of ambulances due to the lack of beds in ED, Cochran and Roche (2009) develop a spreadsheet used as a tool for managers to follow the flow of patients in real-time, Huang (1995) develop a model to analyze the capacity of ED, Mayhew and Smith (2008) apply queueing models to analyze completion times in Accident and emergency departments, Panayiotopoulos and Vassilacopoulos(1984) apply queueing models to study parameters as arrivals distribution, service distributions, level of urgency ann capacity in the waiting room, Siddharthan, Jones and Johnson (1996) study how delay time increases due to the presence of non-emergency patients, Green, Soares, Giglio and Green (2006) apply queueing models to analyze and optimize the timely care of patients, Stout and Tawney (2005) develop a spreadsheet to support the management of an ED, Broyles and Cochran (2007) constructs a non-linear regression to estimate adjust the abandonments of patients without care, Roche, Cochran and Fulton (2007) details the use of queuing networks to model patient flow in an extreme 'fast-track' ED design.

In Bruin, Van Rossum, Visser and Koole (2007) queuing theory is applied to analyze the flow of patients in a cardiology unit, in order to identify system bottlenecks and the effect of the variation demand in the time spent in the system (cycle time).

Erdmann, Boessenkool Hogewoning and Does (2012) show how a Lean approach to reducing work in process of a public hospital is used. Process control is using a CONWIP system.

Tan, Tan and Lau (2013) propose the implementation of a dynamic queuing model for the emergency department, particularly in a hospital in Singapore, the model incorporates a strategy to prioritize patients dynamically.

Lin, Patrick and Labeau (2013) use queuing models focusing on patient flow and limited capacity in the waiting line, i.e., incorporated into the model the phenomenon of blocking. The model is implemented for the analysis of patient flow in the emergency department and intensive care unit.

Dogan and Unutulmaz (2014) propose the Value Stream Map to build a model of flow of patients in a care unit for recovery, and then an analysis of various decisions with simulation is performed.

From the review of the literature we conclude:

1. Queuing theory models allow the analysis of the effect of demand, the distribution of service times, level of urgency, bed capacity, abandonment of patients without care and to identify the bottleneck.
2. It is noted that spreadsheets provide a means to access and apply queuing models in managing hospital systems.
3. It is not common the economic analysis of the proposed solutions (e.g. the cost of adding more doctors).

Other Approaches

In the next section we present different approaches to the analysis of healthcare systems:

- **Input-Throughput-Output Model:** Asplin, Magid, Solberg, Lurie and Camargo (2003).
- **Fields Chaos Model:** Fields (2003).
- **ED Cardiac Analogy Model:** Richardson, Ardagh and Gee (2005).
- **Formula -Based Equations:** Bernstein, Verghese, Leung, Lunney and Perez (2003), Epstein and Tian (2006), Hoot and Aronsky (2006), Reeder and Garrison (2001).
- **Regression Modeling:** Weiss, Derlet, Arndahl, Ernst, Richards, Fernández-Frackelton, Schwab, Stair, Vicellio, Levy, Brautigan, Johnson and Nick (2004), Weiss, Ernst, Derlet, King, Bair and Nick, (2005), Batal, Tench, McMillian, Adams and Mehler (2001).
- **Time-Series Analysis:** Jones, Thomas, Evans, Welch, Haug and Snow (2008), Milner (1988), Milner (1997), Champion, Kinsman, Lee, Masman, May, Mills, Taylor, Thomas and Williams (2007), Tanberg and Qualls (1994), Schweigler, Desmond, McCarthy, Bukowski, Ionides and Younger (2009).
- Puente, Priore, Pine and Fountain (2002) used fuzzy logic and simulation to analyze the emergency department of a hospital, it should be noted that the paper does not mention if taken into account the priorities emergency care.

- **Discrete-Event (or Process) Simulation Models:** Connelly and Bair (2004), Zilm (2004), Khare, Powell, Reinhardt and Lucenti (2009), Coats and Michalis (2001), Hung, Whitehouse, O'Neill, Gray and Kissoon (2007), Garcia, Rivera, Centeno and, DeCario (1995), van Oostrum, Van Houdenhoven, Vrielink, et al., 2008), Chin and Fleisher (1998), Ohboshi, Masui, Kambayashi and Takahashi (1998) and Levin, Dittus, Aronsky, et al. (2008).

Software

The application of queuing models is greatly facilitated through the use of software available for analysis and estimation. Given the complexity of the equations, it is convenient to have a tool that speeds up the calculations and allows doctors the access to these tools. In this sense spreadsheets allow managers to build templates that facilitate the calculation and construction of graphs to analyze queuing systems. Through search engines managers nowadays can find spreadsheet files that can be used immediately. There are only two spreadsheet based tools developed to health systems:

The page Improving Patient Flow contains several downloadable spreadsheets files developed for decision analysis in health care systems (Steyn, 2015).

Consolidated Clinic Planning Model (CCPM) is a spreadsheet-based model designed to organize, aggregate and analyze mass dispensing of vaccines and clinic operations (University of Maryland, 2015).

Nowadays managers also can find basic programs for educational purposes to systems formed by modules that perform very difficult tasks.

In the web site http://www2.uwindsor.ca/~hlynka/qsoft.html there is a list of software to queuing models, with over 70 references and links. The list was compiled by Dr. Myron Hlynka of the University of Windsor (Last updated: June 10, 2014). Examples of software that can be found in the list are:

The Queue Network Analyzer (QNA) developed by Bell Laboratories to calculate properties of queueing networks (Whitt, 1983).

WinPepsy-QNS developed by the Erlangen Research Group on Analytical Modelling of Dept. of Computer Science 4 (Distributed Systems and Operating Systems) (Bolch, Greiner, de Meer, Trivedi, 2006).

Again it is interesting to note the lack of software dedicated to healthcare systems in the aforementioned web page.

QUEUING THEORY

Queues are part of daily life. The phenomenon of waiting for a service is present in any field: banks, supermarkets, cinemas, fast food restaurants, etc. The phenomenon of waiting can not be avoided, but it can be controlled; the waiting time in line or queue is a factor to be taken into account to measure the quality of service and to measure the efficiency of its operation (Taha 2011, Hillier & Lieberman 2010).

The study queuing systems involves the quantification metrics such as the number of customers in the queue, how long a customer stays formed (cycle time) and the average use of the site, the operation also generates a cost that has two elements: the cost of operation of the station and the cost of waiting.

It should be mentioned there is a set of equations to calculate these metrics, as well as to obtain a balance between the cost of service and cost for waiting. These formulas have the advantage for understanding the relationships between each of the elements of a system unlike other analysis approaches that often resemble black boxes (Hopp & Spearman, 2008).

Figure 1. Queueing system

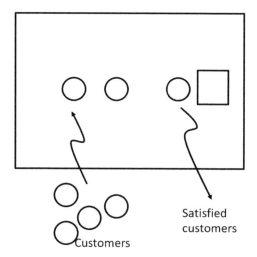

The basic process of operation is as follows (Figure 1): Customers requiring service, arriving at λ customers per unit time (demand). Customers who enter the system and in accordance with the discipline are served by the server, if it is empty or the clients are incorporated into a queue to wait their turn.

At one point, a customer is selected from the queue and is attended by a server (e.g. a doctor) which provides the service at a rate of μ customers per unit of time; as mentioned above the customer is served according to the discipline of the queue, the most common (for example in manufacturing systems) is to attend the first to arrive (First-in-First-Out discipline or FIFO), although in hospital systems the predominant attention policy is based on the level of priority or urgent attention. Later the service is performed to the customer needs through a service mechanism, and finally the customer leaves the system.

To adequately describe a system queuing performance measures are used. They are briefly described below.

Performance Measures of Queuing Systems

Administrators need a way to measure the quality of service, as well as to study the effect of changing system conditions. The following is a list of some performance measures applied to queueing systems (Hall, 1991).

For Customers

- **Cycle Time in the System:** Is the period that the client remains in the system, including the time remaining in the queue plus the service time (CTs).
- **Cycle Time in the Queue:** It is the time that the client remains in the queue waiting to be served (CTq).
- **Service Time ($1/\mu$):** period to receive the service. A shorter wait is better than a longer wait.
- **Waiting Cost:** waiting time will be more costly for some customer than other: the cost for a patient that waits in an Emergency Unit is infinite.

- **Proportion of Completed on Time:** If a customer is not server by a deadline, a penalty is incurred: The customer leaves the queue and complains for a poor service.

For Servers

- **System Congestion:** Indicating fraction of capacity utilization of the system and it is given by the relationship $\rho = \dfrac{\lambda}{\mu}$. It is assumed that the capacity of attention of the server is greater than the demand, that is, $\rho < 1$.
- **Number of Customers in the System:** It is also known as work in process (WIP). The number of customers in the queue plus being served L.
- **Number of Customers in the Queue:** The symbol is usually Lq.
- **System Throughput:** The long run number of customers passing through the system. The symbol is *th*.

Characterizing Demand and Service Time

The first step in the analysis of queuing systems is to determine the demand and capacity of the stations (service time), then it must be determined the type of distribution that explains the behavior of both variables. In queuing theory there are analytical models that assume that the process arrival and service distributions are exponential, however it is necessary perform a goodness of fit test to check how probability function fits the data (Hall, 1991).

Kendall Notation

There is a notational shorthand due to Kendall for characterizing queueing models. This notation appears in queueing theory books and present very useful information about the system assumptions (Curry & Feldman, 2009) (Table 2). The Kendall notation is a list of characters separated by diagonal lines "/" where:

- **First Element:** The inter-arrival time distribution between customers (the demand of service).
- **Second Element:** The service time distribution.
- **Third Element:** The number of servers and is an integer number.
- **Fourth Element:** The maximum number of customers allowed in the system at one time and is an integer number.
- **Fifth Element:** The optional and specifies the queueing discipline.

The general form of Kendall notation is:

```
arrival process / Service time process / Number of servers / Maximum possible
allowed in the system / Queue discipline
```

Table 2. Queueing symbols for the Kendall notation

Symbol	Definition
M	Exponential (Markovian system) inter-arrival or service time
D	Discrete inter-arrival or service time
W	Weibull type inter-arrival or service time
G	General inter-arrival or service time
1, 2, 3, ...	Number of servers, capacity, integer
FIFO	First-In-First-Out discipline
LIFO	Last-In-Fisrst-Out discipline

Exponential Distribution

A nonnegative variable X is said to have an exponential distribution function with parameter $\lambda > 0$ if the probability density function is:

$$f_X(x) = \begin{cases} \lambda e^{-\lambda x} & x \geq 0 \\ 0 & \text{other case} \end{cases} \tag{1}$$

The expected value and the variance are as follows:

$$E[X] = \frac{1}{\lambda} \tag{2}$$

$$V[X] = \frac{1}{\lambda^2} \tag{3}$$

An important property of the exponential distribution is that it contains no memory. As a result of this lack of memory, is that if the number of events within an interval of time are according to a Poisson random variable, then the time between events is exponential (Taylor & Karlin 1998). The exponential distribution is applied in probabilistic modelling like queueing theory, random failures, call centers, and reliability.

Calculating Properties: Equations

Consider a queueing system that has been operating over a long time and have reached an appropriate steady state. The fundamental equation that relates the demand, the cycle time and the number of customers in the system is as follows:

$$L = \lambda \times CT \tag{4}$$

Table 3. Properties and equations of M/M/1 queueing systems

Number of customers in the queue	$L_q = \dfrac{\rho^2}{(1-\rho)}$	(5)
Number of customers in the system	$L = L_q + \dfrac{\lambda}{\mu}$	(6)
Cycle time in the system	$CT = \dfrac{1}{\mu - \lambda}$	(7)
Probability that the system is empty	$P_0 = 1 - \rho$	(8)

This equation is known as Little's Law: if demand λ is known, and is known the average number of customers in the system L. Then you can calculate the cycle time CT or residence time of a customer in: the period between their arrivals until their departure after completion of service. The validity of equation (4) does not rest on the details on of any particular model, but depends only upon long run mass flow balance relations (Taylor & Karlin 1998).

M / M / 1 Queue

It is the simplest type of structure. Assuming that the time between arrivals of customers are distributed exponentially and in addition, the service also follows a distribution of exponential type, then known as

Figure 2. Average number of customers in the system for an M/M/1 queue

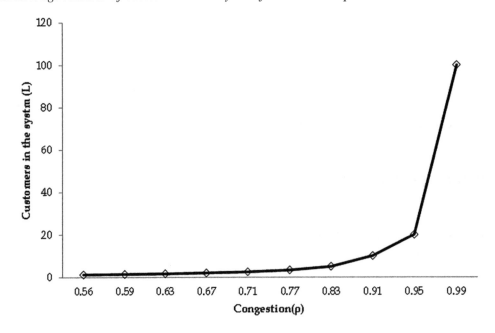

M / M / 1 system (arrivals Markov type or Poisson, service time service Markov or exponential and one server). If discipline is first come first serve, the properties can be calculated with formulas of Table 3.

Figure 2 shows the relationship between the average number of customers in the system (L) and the queue congestion (ρ). As can be seen, L is an increasing function of ρ. For low values of ρ, L increases slowly and then, as ρ gets closer to 1, L increases rapidly, and growing to infinite limit as $\rho \rightarrow 1$. There is a misconception of some managers who think that keeping the server busy most of the time maximizes the server productivity. But the reality is that this policy eventually is at the cost of extreme delays (more people in the queue, more waiting time to be attended), at the same time, as $\rho \rightarrow 1$, the probability of find the server empty tends to zero and, on the field, the chaos in the waiting area is evident. It should be noted too that the waiting time in the queue is a measure of the quality of service provided to customers (Figure 3).

In systems such as hospitals, patients arrive with the expectation of being served immediately; any delay in the attention is interpreted as a poor quality of service and severe management problems.

M / M / c Queue

Examples of M / M / c are banks, stores, or cinemas. In the case of both arrivals and service times are exponentially distributed, it is known as M / M / c system. If discipline is first come first serve then the properties are calculated using the formulas of Table 4.

Systems with Service Priorities

As mentioned above, in health systems it is common to use a discipline-based care priorities and degree of urgency of the patient. To calculate the properties in this kind of service, it is necessary to take into

Figure 3. Probability the server is empty

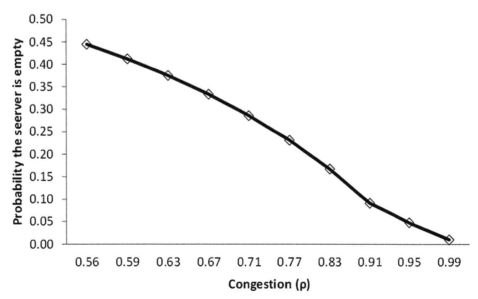

Table 4. Properties and equations of M/M/c queueing systems

Number of customers in the queue	$$L_q = \frac{P_0 \left(\lambda/\mu\right)^c \rho}{c!\left(1-\rho\right)^2}$$	(9)
Cycle time in the queue	$$CT_q = \frac{L_q}{\lambda}$$	(10)
Cycle time in the system	$$CT = CT_q + \frac{1}{\mu}$$	(11)
Probability that the system is empty	$$P_0 = \left[\sum_{n=0}^{c-1}\left[\frac{\left(\lambda/\mu\right)^n}{n!} + \frac{\left(\lambda/\mu\right)^c}{c!}\left(\frac{1}{1-\lambda/(c\mu)}\right)\right]\right]^{-1}$$	(12)
congestion in the system	$$\frac{\lambda}{c\mu}$$	(13)

Table 5. Equations for properties in queues with priorities

Cycle time in the system	$$CT = \frac{1}{A B_{k-1} B_k} + \frac{1}{\mu_k}$$ Where:	(14a)
	$$A = c!\frac{c\mu - \lambda}{\left(\lambda/\mu\right)^c}\sum_{j=0}^{c-1}\frac{\left(\lambda/\mu\right)^c}{j!} + c\mu$$	(14b)
	$$B_0 = 1$$	(14c)
	$$B_k = 1 - \frac{\sum_{i=1}^{k}\lambda_i}{c\mu}$$	(14d)
Total demand of service	$$\lambda = \sum_{i=1}^{N}\lambda_k$$	(15)
Number of customers of priority k	$$L_k = \lambda_k CT_k$$	(16)

Where the subscript $k = 1,2, \dots$ indicates the class or priority level of the client or patient. Equations assume non preemptive priorities.

account the significance or weight of the patient. For this case, the properties are calculated with the equations of Table 5.

Selecting the Number of Servers

Within the management and control of a system of waiting lines, frequently it is desired determine the number of necessary servers to provide a service. It should take into account that adding servers:

1. Service quality is improved.
2. Operating costs of the system are increased.

Therefore to solve the problem correctly it involves balancing quality of service against the costs of the operation.

According to Gross (2008), the following approaches are proposed to assess the desirability of increasing the number of servers:

*   "A" policy: Select the number of servers required to maintain constant congestion (emphasis on quality of service).
*   "B" policy: Select the number of servers required maintaining constant efficiency and quality of service simultaneously, for example, the basis is the probability that a patient has to wait (emphasis on quality and efficiency).

Analysis of Serial Systems

In a pure serial system, the customers out of one stage and enter to next stage to receive another service. The departures from each stage are the inflows into the next stage as illustrated in Figure 4. This system is a serial one where for each stage i, i=1, 2, 3, ..., n are specified the service time and the number of servers ($E[T_{S,i}], c_i$) (Curry & Feldman, 2009). If each stage satisfies the assumption of exponential inter-arrival times and service times, then it can be considered as a serial M/M/c queue system and the equations (9 – 13) can be applied independently to each stage to obtain their properties.

Figure 4. Pure serial system

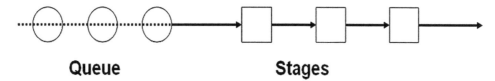

Queue   **Stages**

Table 6. Area data

Demand	Triage Service Time	Doctors Service Time (c=3)
11 patients / 60 minutes	4.17 minutes	20.91 minutes

CASE STUDY: ANALYSIS OF AN EMERGENCY UNIT

To illustrate the process of analysis and selection of servers and the differences between these approaches to increase the number of servers, data from emergency department of a public hospital will be used. In this case we know that the system works with the following operating conditions according to the data reported by Rodríguez, González, Hernández and Hernández (2016) and resumed in Table 6.

The area of "Triage" has a demand (average arrival rate) of 11 patients/hour. Once admitted, a nurse takes vital signs, and evaluates the patient with a series of questions about symptoms and other signs it presents. On this basis the level of urgency of the patient is determined. Patients rated, leaving the "triage" and sent to the section of specialists, where they are attended by level of urgency.

Under these conditions authors determined that the "Triage" has the capacity to meet current demand. However in the area of medical specialists, it is observed that the congestion is$\rho=1.25$, i.e., the demand is greater than the capacity of attention: the area works chaotically and the number of patients grows without limit, causing complaints from upset patients, because of their waiting time for attention (Rodríguez, González, Hernández & Hernández, 2016).

METHODOLOGY

Since demand is a variable outside the control of administrators, so they want to improve service in the area. While it is clearly necessary to increase the number of doctors, it is necessary to analyze what criteria is better to make these changes and how they would impact the perception of attention. The fundamental questions are:

- How to improve patient flow?
- How to reduce the feeling of waiting for a patient?
- How to improve the patient's perception of the service?

"A" Policy

For example, suppose you want to maintain a congestion of 75% both in the area of "triage" as in the area of medical attention (servers) (Figure 5).

Applying the queueing theory equations, the results show that the "Triage" satisfies the current demand using a single server, if demand increases, then it will be necessary to add a second server to the area. However, in the doctor's area the situation is different: with the base demand at least 5 doctors (2 additional doctors to currently working 3) are required. If demand increases 10% then at least 6 doctors (Figure 6) are required.

Figure 5. System congestion versus number of patients for different demand scenarios: "Triage" area

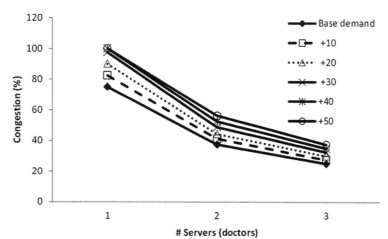

Figure 6. System congestion versus number of patients for different demand scenarios: Doctors area

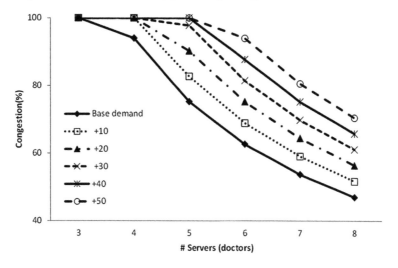

"B" Policy

Suppose it is desired a probability ≤ 0.75 that a patient must wait for treatment at the "Triage", with the current demand it will not be necessary to increase the number of servers. But if demand increases 10%, it will be necessary to add a server, and this can be kept to a 50% increase in demand (Figure 7).

In doctor's area, the results indicate that at least 5 doctors are needed for the base demand, and no change is necessary even to an increase in demand of 20%. If demand increases to 30% it is necessary to increase servers to 6 doctors (Figure 8).

Figure 7. Prob. of waiting versus number of servers for different demand scenarios: "Triage" area

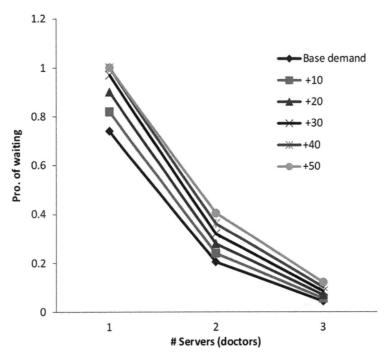

Figure 8. Prob. of waiting versus number of servers for different demand scenarios: Doctor's area

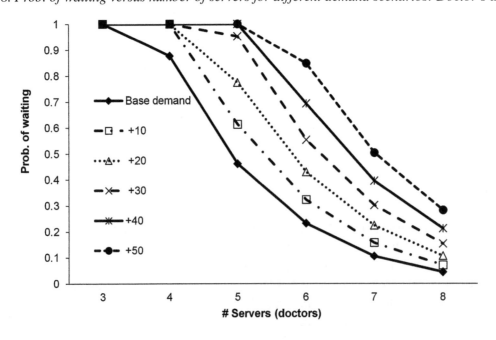

Properties: Cycle Time and Work in Process

To evaluate the performance of the system with both policies, we calculated cycle time and the number of patients in the system for each strategy ("Triage": Equations 5 – 8; Doctors: Equations 9 – 12).

In the case of "Triage" it shows that the cycle time for both policies is about 5 minutes, except for the last case the demand scenario, where the cycle time is 6 minutes as can be seen in Table 7.

Table 8 shows the cycle times for each demand scenario in the doctor's area, with the number of doctors required to meet the target congestion.

For example the base demand requires at least 6 doctors, the cycle times are 0.99, 1.37, 1.79 and 3.44 minutes for each level of urgency. If demand increases by 10%, then cycle times are 1.40, 2.03, 2.75, and 6 minutes.

With regard to control the probability of waiting for service, it is appreciated that for the current demand, 5 doctors are required, and the cycle times are 2.51, 3.80, 5.36 and 14.31 minutes for each level of urgency, if demand increased 10%, cycle times change to 3.38, 5.39, 8.04 and 29.22 minutes respectively (Table 9).

When comparing cycle times, it is clear that the policy of congestion control, resulting in less cycle time than the policy of controlling the probability of waiting for service. However, further analysis shows that the investment is higher because they must incorporate double resources (3 additional doctors) to meet the target and current demand. This is not always possible, especially for public health institutions, which often suffer of lack of the financial resources needed to meet capacity requirements.

By comparison, the policy based on the probability of waiting for service shows that cycle times are greater, however this policy is more robust to increased demand. This is most apparent for high-demand scenarios.

To complement this part, in the next section an economic analysis of both strategies is performed.

Table 7. Cycle time in triage (minutes)

Servers	Base Demand	10%	+20%	+30%	+40%	+50%
1	16.67	23.81	41.65	165	∞	∞
2	4.85	5.02	5.22	5.46	5.75	6
3	4.25	4.27	4.3	4.34	4.38	4.43

Table 8. Cycle time for the "A" strategy (minutes)

Level of Urgency	Base Demand	+10%	+20%	+30%	+40%	+50%
1	0.99	1.40	0.81	1.13	0.68	0.92
2	1.37	2.03	1.15	1.64	0.97	1.35
3	1.79	2.75	1.51	2.23	1.28	1.85
4	3.44	6.11	3.01	5.08	2.64	4.28
Number of doctors	6	6	7	7	8	8

Table 9. Cycle time for the "B" strategy (minutes)

Level of urgency	Base demand	+10%	+20%	+30%	+40%	+50%
1	2.51	3.38	1.91	2.53	3.25	1.96
2	3.80	5.39	2.89	3.99	5.37	3.08
3	5.36	8.04	4.08	5.90	8.35	4.52
4	14.31	29.22	10.90	20.17	41.21	14.83
Number of doctors	5	5	6	6	6	7

Economic Analysis

So far it has observed:

1. "A" strategy obtains shorter cycle time; however, this policy is more sensitive to changes in demand.
2. "B" strategy implies higher cycle times but this policy is robust to changes in demand.

This section ends making an economic analysis of two strategies, in this case the doctors area because has the highest congestion; compared with other areas (window, *triage*) (Rodríguez, González, Hernández and Hernández, 2016).

We will compare the cost of policies A and B; we assume that a doctor earns about $ 15,000 pesos/month ($ 1,000 USD / month) (El informador, 2010). We did not take into account the costs of waiting, because in this case it is not feasible monetarily to quantify death of a patient due to a very high waiting time for treatment. The equation cost is as follows:

Figure 9. Costs of both strategies

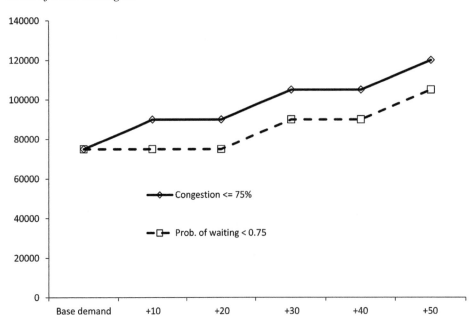

$$\text{TotalCost} = \text{Earn} \times \text{\#Doctors} \tag{17}$$

Figure 9 shows the cost of each strategy, which was obtained by applying the equation (17). The results show that from the point of view of cost, using the combined strategy (B) a lower cost is obtained compared to the pure strategy (A) of system efficiency (Gross, 2008), as mentioned above, this is because in the combined approach, increasing servers to meet the target is slower, directly impacting the cost.

CONCLUSION

Today managers of health systems must manage the resources at their disposal to ensure that service quality is adequate, this leads at the same time making decisions to ensure that these resources are managed efficiently and effectively.

The decision is not trivial given the complexity of these systems. This makes it necessary to apply tools for assessing the impact of a decision on measures of system performance.

The review of the literature shows that managers are more interested in the application of tools to support decision -making in health systems and hospitals.

Among the set of tools that can be applied to management performance measures are equations and relations from queueing theory. Spreadsheets provide a means to access and apply queuing models in managing hospital systems. It is not common the economic analysis of the proposed solutions (e.g. the cost of adding more doctors).

This chapter shows an application example of the application of queueing models with priorities to the analysis of an emergency department of a public hospital in Mexico.

Service demand is greater than the capacity of attention and therefore is necessary to determine how many doctors are needed to provide the service. The study was conducted comparing two approaches:

A. Select the number of servers required to maintain constant congestion (emphasis on quality of service).
B. Select the number of servers required to maintain constant efficiency and service quality simultaneously, for example, taken as the base the probability that a patient has to wait (emphasis on quality and efficiency).

In both cases, the response time is within the standards required for the emergency department. However, in the "A" strategy it is obtained as a result, a shorter response time to the patient but is very sensitive to increase in demand. On the other hand, with the "B" strategy, an outcome with longer patient stays was obtained but ensures a better quality of service (ensures a probability of care) and is less sensitive to demand.

Finally the economic analysis showed that strategy "B" is cheaper.

FUTURE RESEARCH

The queuing theory can be applied to model various problems within hospital systems. Here are some examples:

The supply of medicines and supplies of a hospital can be modeled through a queuing network where each stage (warehouse, factory, warehouse) is a system where the entity (purchase order, batch, emergency vehicle) must form a row before being served. If one takes into account the service costs, waiting cost and flow cost, then you can think of an optimization model that allows to determine the operating conditions that minimize the cost of the entire supply chain network.

In emergency situations such as natural disasters or chemical emergency response time of first aid is vital to address these eventualities. It should be noted that vehicles must pass through saturated streets, where there may be long lines to move from one point to another.

In controlling patient flow, it is important to quantify the cycle time within the system and in each individual stage in the hospital. Similarly, in situations where the demand for care is growing continuously and it is necessary to determine the necessary personnel (doctors, nurses, etc.) to increase capacity.

Applying the equations of queuing theory, managers can get the measures used to evaluate the performance of a health system. One of the benefits of this approach is that in the future, the Health ministers can standardize the measurement methods and results between different hospitals can be compared each other to evaluate the performance.

REFERENCES

Arellano, N., & Martínez, M. G. (2012). Satisfacción de los usuarios de Urgencias basada en la sistematización del Servicio. Hospital General Dolores Hidalgo; Guanajuato, México. *Archivos de Medicina de Urgencia de México, 4*(1), 13–19.

Arroyave, G., & Jarillo, E. (2000). *Costos Hospitalarios: costo del día-paciente. Memorias del VII Congreso Internacional de Costos. León, España*. Retrieved 10/june/2015 from: http://www.intercostos. org/documentos/Trabajo243.pdf

Asplin, B. R., Magid, D. J., Rhodes, K. V., Solberg, L. I., Lurie, N., & Camargo, C. A. Jr. (2003). A conceptual model of emergency department crowding. *Annals of Emergency Medicine, 42*(2), 173–180. doi:10.1067/mem.2003.302 PMID:12883504

Au, L., Byrnes, G. B., Bain, C. A., Fackrell, M., Brand, C., Campbell, D. A., & Taylor, P. G. (2009). Predicting overflow in an emergency department. *IMA Journal of Management Mathematics, 20*(1), 39–49. doi:10.1093/imaman/dpn007

Batal, H., Tench, J., McMillian, S., Adams, J., & Mehler, P. S. (2001). Predicting patient visits to an urgent care clinic using calendar variables. *Academic Emergency Medicine, 8*(1), 48–53. doi:10.1111/j.1553-2712.2001.tb00550.x PMID:11136148

Bernstein, S. L., Verghese, V., Leung, W., Lunney, A. T., & Perez, I. (2003). Development and validation of a new index to measure emergency department crowding. *Academic Emergency Medicine, 10*(9), 938–942. doi:10.1111/j.1553-2712.2003.tb00647.x PMID:12957975

Bolch, G., Greiner, S., de Meer, H., & Trivedi, K. S. (2006). *Queueing networks and Markov chains* (2nd ed.). New York: Wiley Interscience. doi:10.1002/0471791571

Broyles, R., & Cochran, J. (2007) Estimating business loss to a hospital emergency department from patient reneging by queueing-based regression. *Proceeding of Industrial Engineering Research Conference*.

Champion, R., Kinsman, L. D., Lee, G. A., Masman, G. A., Mills, T. M., Taylor, M. D., ... Williams, R. J. (2007). Forecasting emergency department presentations. *Australian Health Review*, *31*(1), 83–90. doi:10.1071/AH070083 PMID:17266491

Chin, L., & Fleisher, G. (1998). Planning model of resource utilization in an academic pediatric emergency department. *Pediatric Emergency Care*, *14*(1), 4–9. doi:10.1097/00006565-199802000-00002 PMID:9516622

Coats, T. J., & Michalis, S. (2001). Mathematical modeling of patient flow through an accident and emergency department. *Emergency Medicine Journal*, *18*(3), 190–192. doi:10.1136/emj.18.3.190 PMID:11354210

Cochran, J. K., & Roche, K. T. (2009). A multi-class queueing network analysis methodology for improving hospital emergency department performance. *Computers & Operations Research*, *36*(5), 1497–1512. doi:10.1016/j.cor.2008.02.004

Connelly, L. G., & Bair, A. E. (2004). Discrete event simulation of emergency department activity: A platform for system-level operations research. *Academic Emergency Medicine*, *11*(11), 1177–1185. doi:10.1111/j.1553-2712.2004.tb00702.x PMID:15528582

Curry, G. L., & Feldman, R. M. (2009). *Manufacturing systems modeling and analysis* (2nd ed.). New York: Springer.

de Bruin, A. M., van Rossum, A. C., Visser, M. C., & Koole, G. M. (2007). Modeling the emergency cardiac in-patient flow: An application of queuing theory. *Health Care Management Science*, *10*(2), 125–137. doi:10.100710729-007-9009-8 PMID:17608054

Doğan, N. O., & Unutulmaz, O. (2014). *Lean production in healthcare: a simulation-based value stream mapping in the physical therapy and rehabilitation department of a public hospital*. Total Quality Management & Business Excellence. doi:10.1080/14783363.2014.945312

El Informador. (2010). *Las 10 profesiones mejor pagadas de México*. Retrieved 28/06/2015 from http://www.informador.com.mx/economia/2010/252791/6/las-10-profesiones-mejor-pagadas-de-mexico.htm

Epstein, S. K., & Tian, L. (2006). Development of an emergency department work score to predict ambulance diversion. *Academic Emergency Medicine*, *13*(4), 421–426. doi:10.1111/j.1553-2712.2006.tb00320.x PMID:16581932

Erdmann, T. P., Boessenkool, H., Hogewoning, L., & Does, R. (2012). Quality Quandaries: Reducing Work in Process at an Emergency Assistance Center. *Quality Engineering*, *25*(1), 78–84. doi:10.1080/08982112.2012.731929

Erlangen Research Group. (2015). *WinPepsy software*. Retrieved 28/06/2015 from http://www4.cs.fau.de/Research/ana/Projekte/

Fields, W. W. (2003). Calculus, chaos, and other models of emergency department crowding. *Annals of Emergency Medicine*, *42*(2), 181–184. doi:10.1067/mem.2003.347 PMID:12883505

Garcia, M. L., Rivera, C., Centeno, M., & DeCario, N. (1995) Reducing time in emergency room via a fast track. *Winter Simulation Conference Proceedings*. 10.1109/WSC.1995.478898

Green, L. V., Soares, J., Giglio, J. F., & Green, R. A. (2006). Using queueing theory to increase the effectiveness of emergency department provider staffing. *Academic Emergency Medicine*, *13*(1), 61–68. doi:10.1111/j.1553-2712.2006.tb00985.x PMID:16365329

Green, L. (2005). *Capacity planning and management in hospitals. In M. L. Brandeau, F. Sainfort, & W. P. Pierskalla (Eds.), Operations Research and Healthcare* (pp. 15–43). New York: Kluwer Academic Publishers.

Gross, D., Shortle, J. F., Thompson, J. M., & Harris, C. M. (2008). *Fundamentals of queueing theory*. Wiley. doi:10.1002/9781118625651

Hall, R. W. (1991). *Queueing methods for manufacturing and services*. Prentice Hall.

Hillier, F. S., & Lieberman, G. J. (2005). *Introduction to operations research* (8th ed.). Boston: McGraw-Hill.

Hlynka, M. (2014). *List of Queueing Theory Software*. Retrieved 28/06/2015 from http://web2.uwindsor.ca/math/hlynka/qsoft.html

Hoot, N., & Aronsky, D. (2006) An early warning system for overcrowding in the emergency department. *AMIA Annual Symposium Proceedings*.

Hopp, W. J., & Spearman, M. L. (2008) Factory Physics (3rd ed.). Long Grove: Waveland Press Inc.

Huang, X. (1995). A planning model for requirement of emergency beds. *IMA Journal of Mathematics Applied in Medicine and Biology*, *12*(3-4), 345–353. doi:10.1093/imammb/12.3-4.345 PMID:8919569

Hung, G. R., Whitehouse, S. R., O'Neill, C., Gray, A. P., & Kissoon, N. (2007). Computer modeling of patient flow in a pediatric emergency department using discrete event simulation. *Pediatric Emergency Care*, *23*(1), 5–10. doi:10.1097/PEC.0b013e31802c611e PMID:17228213

Jones, S. S., Thomas, A., Evans, R. S., Welch, S. J., Haug, P. J., & Snow, G. L. (2008). Forecasting daily patient volumes in the emergency department. *Academic Emergency Medicine*, *15*(2), 159–167. doi:10.1111/j.1553-2712.2007.00032.x PMID:18275446

Khare, R. K., Powell, E. S., Reinhardt, G., & Lucenti, M. (2009). Adding more beds to the emergency department or reducing admitted patient boarding times: Which has a more significant influence on emergency department congestion? *Annals of Emergency Medicine*, *53*(5), 575–585. doi:10.1016/j.annemergmed.2008.07.009 PMID:18783852

Levin, S. R., Dittus, R., Aronsky, D., Weinger, M. B., Han, H., Boord, J., & France, D. (2008). Optimizing cardiology capacity to reduce emergency department boarding: A systems engineering approach. *American Heart Journal*, *156*(6), 1202–1219. doi:10.1016/j.ahj.2008.07.007 PMID:19033021

Lin, D., Patrick, J., & Labeau, F. (2013). Estimating the waiting time of multi-priority emergency patients with downstream blocking. *Health Care Management Science*, *17*, 1–12. PMID:23690253

Litvak, E., & Long, M. (2000). Cost and Quality Under Managed Care: Irreconcilable Differences? *The American Journal of Managed Care*, *6*, 305–312. PMID:10977431

Mayhew, L., & Smith, D. (2008). Using queueing theory to analyse the government's 4-H completion time target in accident and emergency departments. *Health Care Management Science*, *11*(1), 11–21. doi:10.100710729-007-9033-8 PMID:18390164

Milner, P. C. (1988). Forecasting the demand on accident and emergency departments in health districts in the Trent region. *Statistics in Medicine*, *7*(10), 1061–1072. doi:10.1002im.4780071007 PMID:3206002

Milner, P. C. (1997). Ten-year follow-up of ARIMA forecasts of attendances at accident and emergency departments in the Trent region. *Statistics in Medicine*, *16*(18), 2117–2125. doi:10.1002/(SICI)1097-0258(19970930)16:18<2117::AID-SIM649>3.0.CO;2-E PMID:9308136

Ohboshi, N., Masui, H., Kambayashi, Y., & Takahashi, T. (1998). A study of medical emergency workflow. *Computer Methods and Programs in Biomedicine*, *55*(3), 177–190. doi:10.1016/S0169-2607(97)00063-1 PMID:9617517

OECD. (2005). *OECD Reviews of Health Systems*. Retrieved 23/09/2015 from http://www.borderhealth.org/files/res_839.pdf

OECD. (2014). *OECD Health Statistics 2014. How does Mexico compare?* Retrieved 23/09/2015 from http://www.oecd.org/els/health-systems/Briefing-Note-MEXICO-2014.pdf

Panayiotopoulos, J. C., & Vassilacopoulos, G. (1984). Simulating hospital emergency departments queueing systems: (G/G/m(t)):(IHFF/N/Inf.). *European Journal of Operational Research*, *18*(2), 250–258. doi:10.1016/0377-2217(84)90191-7

Puente, J., Priore, P., Pino, R., & de la Fuente, D. (2002). La Gestión de Colas en un Servicio de Urgencias Hospitalario. Un Enfoque Borroso. II Conferencia de Ingeniería de Organización.

Reeder, T. J., & Garrison, H. G. (2009). When the safety net is unsafe: Real-time assessment of the overcrowded emergency department. *Academic Emergency Medicine*, *8*(11), 1070–1104. doi:10.1111/j.1553-2712.2001.tb01117.x PMID:11691670

Reyes, A. G., & Grimaldi, B. (2012). *Triage en la sala de urgencias*. Retrieved 08/05/2015 from: http://salud.tamaulipas.gob.mx/wp-content/uploads/2012/03/triagedeurgencias.pdf

Richardson, S. K., Ardagh, M., & Gee, P. (2005). Emergency department overcrowding: The Emergency Department Cardiac Analogy Model (EDCAM). *Accident and Emergency Nursing*, *13*(1), 18–23. doi:10.1016/j.aaen.2004.10.010 PMID:15649683

Roche, K. T., Cochran, J. K., & Fulton, I. A. (2007) Improving patient safety by maximizing fast-track benefits in the emergency department–a queueing network approach. *Industrial Engineering Research Conference Proceedings*.

Rodríguez, G. R., González, A., Hernández, S., & Hernández, M. D. (2016, forthcoming). *Análisis del servicio del área de Urgencias aplicando teoría de líneas de espera*. Revista Contaduria y Administración.

Schweigler, L. M., Desmond, J. S., McCarthy, M. L., Bukowski, K. J., Ionides, E. L., & Younger, J. G. (2009). Forecasting models of emergency department crowding. *Academic Emergency Medicine*, *16*(4), 301–308. doi:10.1111/j.1553-2712.2009.00356.x PMID:19210488

Siddharthan, K., Jones, W. J., & Johnson, J. A. (1996). A priority queueing model to reduce waiting times in emergency care. *International Journal of Health Care Quality Assurance*, *9*(5), 10–16. doi:10.1108/09526869610124993 PMID:10162117

Steyn, R. (2015). *Improving Patient Flow software*. Retrieved 28/06/2015 from http://www.steyn.org.uk/

Stout, W. A., & Tawney, B. (2005). An Excel forecasting model to aid in decision making that effects hospital bed-resource utilization-hospital capability to admit emergency room patients. *Systems Information Engineering Design Symposium Proceeding*. 10.1109/SIEDS.2005.193261

West, R. (2001). Objective standards for the emergency services: Emergency admission to hospital. *Journal of the Royal Society of Medicine*, *94*, 4–8. PMID:11383429

Tan, K. W., Tan, W. H., & Lau, H. C. (2013). Improving patient length-of-stay in emergency department through dynamic resource allocation policies. *Proceedings of 2012 IEEE International Conference on Automation Science and Engineering (CASE)*. 10.1109/CoASE.2013.6653988

Tanberg, D., & Qualls, C. (1994). Time series forecasts of emergency department patient volume, length of stay, and acuity. *Annals of Emergency Medicine*, *23*(2), 299–306. doi:10.1016/S0196-0644(94)70044-3 PMID:8304612

Taylor, H. M., & Karlin, S. (1994). *Introduction to stochastic modeling* (4th ed.). Academic Press.

University of Maryland. (2015). *Consolidated Clinic Planning Model*. Retrieved 28/06/2015 from http://www.isr.umd.edu/Labs/CIM/projects/clinic/ccpm.html

van Oostrum, J. M., van Houdenhoven, M., Vrielink, M. M., Klein, J., Hans, E. W., Kimek, M., ... Kazemier, G. (2008). A simulation model for determining the optimal size of emergency teams on call in the operating room at night. *Anesthesia and Analgesia*, *107*(5), 1655–1662. doi:10.1213/ane.0b013e318184e919 PMID:18931229

Whitt, B. (1983). The queueing network analyzer. *The Bell System Technical Journal*, *62*(9), 2779–2815. doi:10.1002/j.1538-7305.1983.tb03204.x

Weiss, S. J., Derlet, R., Arndahl, J., Ernst, A. A., Fernández-Frackelton, M., Schwab, R., ... Nick, T. G. (2004). Estimating the degree of emergency department overcrowding in academic medical centers: Results of the national ED overcrowding study (NEDOCS). *Academic Emergency Medicine*, *11*(1), 38–50. doi:10.1111/j.1553-2712.2004.tb01369.x PMID:14709427

Weiss, S. J., Ernst, A. A., Derlet, R., King, R., Bair, A., & Nick, T. G. (2005). Relationship between the national ED overcrowding scale and the number of patients who leave without being seen in an academic ED. *The American Journal of Emergency Medicine*, *23*(3), 288–294. doi:10.1016/j.ajem.2005.02.034 PMID:15915399

Zilm, F. (2004). Estimating emergency service treatment bed needs. *The Journal of Ambulatory Care Management*, *27*(3), 215–223. doi:10.1097/00004479-200407000-00005 PMID:15287211

KEY TERMS AND DEFINITIONS

Customer: Entity requiring or requesting service (person, piece, part).

Cycle Time: Time spent by a customer from entering the system until it is removed.

Healthcare System Management: Set of techniques and tools applied to the effective and efficient management of resources in health systems, hospital systems and in general all those dedicated to the diagnosis, treatment and cure of diseases of persons.

Hospital: A facility where sick customers are cared for to provide diagnosis and treatment.

Patient Flow: Movement of customers in a hospital through each stage of care treatment.

Queueing Theory: It is the study of the phenomenon of waiting to be served, trying to predict the time in the system as well as the average number of customers.

Service Cost: Resource cost per patient treated.

Triage: A classification system used by doctors of Emergency Units for the selection and classification of patients based on the priorities of care, favoring the possibility of survival, according to the therapeutic needs and available resources.

Waiting Cost: The cost incurred by each client to expect formed to be addressed. In the case of hospital systems this cost is infinite.

Work in Process: Number of customers waiting to be served.

This research was previously published in the Handbook of Research on Managerial Strategies for Achieving Optimal Performance in Industrial Processes edited by Giner Alor-Hernández, Cuauhtémoc Sánchez-Ramírez, and Jorge Luis García-Alcaraz; pages 469-493, copyright year 2016 by Business Science Reference (an imprint of IGI Global).

Chapter 17
A Simulation Model for Resource Balancing in Healthcare Systems

Arzu Eren Şenaras
Uludag University, Turkey

Hayrettin Kemal Sezen
Uludag University, Turkey

ABSTRACT

This study aims to analyze resource effectiveness through developed model. Changing different number of resources and testing their response, appropriate number of resources can be identified as a basis of resource balancing through what-if analysis. The simulation model for emergency department is developed by Arena package program. The patient waiting times are reduced by the tested scenarios. Health care system is very expensive sector and related costs are very high. To raise service quality, number of doctor and nurse are increased but system target is provided by increased number of register clerk. Testing different scenarios, effective policy can be designed using developed simulation model. This chapter provides the readers to evaluate healthcare system using discrete event simulation. The developed model could be evaluated as a base for new implementations in other hospitals and clinics.

INTRODUCTION

The growing costs of healthcare are a major concern for healthcare providers. As healthcare organizations move towards the goals of reducing costs, optimizing patient experience, and improving health of populations; operations research tools are becoming more important. These tools provide the ability to assess trade-offs between resource utilization, quality of service, and operating costs (Lal and Roh, 2013).

The Emergency Department (ED) is the service within hospitals responsible for providing care to life threatening and other emergency cases over 24 hours daily, 7 days a week. Therefore, such departments are highly frequented by patients and this frequency is continuously increasing (Weng et al. 2011, Saghafian et al. 2012, Ghanes et al. 2014).

DOI: 10.4018/978-1-7998-2451-0.ch017

Copyright © 2020, IGI Global. Copying or distributing in print or electronic forms without written permission of IGI Global is prohibited.

Emergency Departments (ED) are one of the most complex parts of hospitals to manage, and yet a major entry point for patients. It deals with patients without an appointment and with a wide range of illnesses. Even if most patients arriving to an ED leave the hospital after having seen a physician at the ED, a significant part of them need to be hospitalized. In many hospitals, finding available beds for unscheduled patients is extremely complicated. Even if all patients arriving at the ED do not require the same level of care, many hospitals proceed with the following policy: accept any patient until no bed is available. However, more sophisticated policies, including bed booking strategies and dynamic decisions, can lead to significant improvement of overall hospital performance (Prodel et al., 2014).

Discrete event simulation (DES) is one of the most commonly used operations research tool in healthcare. Its unique ability to account for high levels of complexity and variability that exist in the real world, along with animation capability makes it easier to illustrate and gain buy-in from physicians and other clinical providers compared to other black-box mathematical models offered by operations research. However, DES also has some limitations. In scenarios where there is a large number of stochastic input decision variables and there is little information about the structure of output function using simulation modeling by itself can be tedious and complicated. In such cases, optimization via simulation can help to maximize or minimize measures of the performance by evaluating the system using discrete event simulation (Banks et al, 2004).

DES models for healthcare facilities commonly focus on improving wait time, patient flow and management of capacity (Hamrock et al. 2014; Jacobsen et al. 2006). Although DES is adept at modeling the complex queuing structure for patients in healthcare environments, transition process variation driven by organizational and human factors is more difficult to capture mathematically. For example, analyses of patient location data used to construct DES models may find that patients are consistently waiting for servers (e.g., beds, imaging suites, clinicians) at time-points despite their availability. In the DES, queued patients would efficiently shift to open servers. However in clinical practice, transition process factors such as inefficient communication, lack of awareness of server availability, complex administrative guidelines, interruptions, and cumbersome documentation create further delays (Shi et al. 2015; Armony et al. 2010). These delays are not inherent to queuing nor well understood from time-stamped patient flow data alone. To fully capture the dynamics of healthcare facilities or any flow-based socio-technical system, transition process variability should be understood.

Not accounting for these processes can lead to results that severely under-estimate waiting. Moreover, DES wait time distributions may be difficult to validate against the observed healthcare system. To achieve sufficient validation, the model developer may be motivated to input additive time intervals to patients at transition points that are drawn from a distribution representing the difference between the current model and observed waits (Shi et al. 2015). A more in-depth approach, borrowed from lean methods, may motivate the model developer to map out the transition process and measure or elicit expert estimates of time distributions for each component; independent value of this investigation exists (Kang et al. 2014; Simon and Canacari 2012).

The aim of this paper is to develop methods to identify efficient hospitalization admission control policies for the emergency department patients.

LITERATURE REVIEW

It is impossible and impractical to have a whole hospital DES model that includes everything in a hospital: all models are simplifications (Pidd, 2003). An appropriate level of abstraction and scope must be chosen when attempting whole hospital simulation. The literature has very few examples of such studies. Surprisingly, though, Fetter and Thompson (1965) is a very early example of DES that reports a whole hospital simulation, with a special interest in maternity processes. The aim of this work was to give a decision support tool to hospital administrations to predict the consequences of design changes and alternative policies. They created three models of hospital subsystems: (1) maternity suite, (2) a surgical pavilion, and (3) an outpatient clinic. The maternity model was used to analyze patient load and bed occupancy (Gunal & Pidd, 2010: 46). Recent examples of application of this method in healthcare include study of Sundaramoorthi (2010), where this technique was used to plan nurse resource allocation to patients based on workload needs. Ahmed (2009) used simulation based optimization to design a decision support tool to determine the optimal number of doctors and other staff to maximize the number of patients seen. Ferrand et al. (2010) have compared two distinct resource-allocation policies to handle the flow of scheduled elective surgeries and unpredictable emergency surgeries. The flexible policy is the historical way of assigning patients to operating rooms. Under the flexible policy, emergency surgeries access any operating room and have priority over electives. The new policy provides the surgeon with more focus as the operating rooms are divided into two subsets and patients access the subset of rooms that corresponds to their type, either elective or emergency. Roberts (2011), recognizes that in healthcare it is often difficult to define a single performance characteristic. Especially in healthcare further investigation is often needed to understand how a change in the process leads to downstream impact. Hence simulation is considered an ideal technique to be used. Zhang (2012) applied this integrated approach to determine the staffing requirements of a long term care facility. Tan et al. (2013) presented an integrated framework for dynamic queue management from both demand and supply perspectives. Their experimental analysis showed that the demand-side strategies work seamlessly with both static and dynamic strategies of the supply-side. Likewise, supply-side strategies are performing well with each demand-side strategies. In addition, the dynamic staffing (supply of doctors) can adapt to demand surges or cut cost when demand is reduced. The integrated framework allows healthcare decision makers to play a role in achieving the desired service quality and select from a list of possible strategies that suit the operation needs of the ED. Ghanes et al (2014), proposed a Discrete Event Simulation (DES) model for an emergency department (ED). The model was developed in close collaboration with the French hospital Saint Camille, and is validated using real data. The objective of this model is to help ED managers better understand the behavior of the system and to improve the ED operations performance. Using DES in Arena software, they have built a realistic ED model taking into account all common structural and functional characteristics of at least French EDs. Their experiments focused on human staffing levels and provided useful insights to decision makers.

Espinoza et al. (2014) studied the impact of the model's ability to predict ER performance with a limited amount of input information, such that what-if questions may be asked to guide decision making. Towards this end, two input data scenarios are compared to a case of perfect information. One scenario considers only patient arrival times and the other assumes additional knowledge of patient care pathways. Although both generate similar performance measures, the case with least information yields a slightly worse estimate of patient care pathway composition. This project studies two different cases of real-time data obtained from an ER patient workflow, each representing less or more information useful to feed a discrete event simulation model of an emergency room. Moon et al. (2015) introduces EMSSim that is an agent-based simulation of emergency medical services during disasters. We developed EMSSim to encompass the disaster victims' pass-ways from their rescues to their definitive care. This modeling scope resulted that our model delivers the detailed geographical and medical modeling which are often modeled separately. This is an effort to fill the gap between the prehospital delivery and the in-hospital care over the disaster period. They specified the model with a variant of the dynamic DEVS formalism so that the complex models could be better understood and utilized by others. Also, we suggest a modeling approach to create a profile with mathematical modeling on the victims' survival rates, which would enable our models to simulate the effectiveness of the treatments by the responders. Finally, they provide a case study of virtual experiments that analyzes the sensitivity of rescue performances by varying the disaster response resources. Frank et al (2015) have compared two different configurations in two different geriatric hospitals. The integrated care scenario (Saint-Etienne hospital) means that Short Stay and Rehabilitative Care are both in the same department and separated scenario (Clermont-Ferrand hospital) means that both services are located in different departments. They used Discrete Event Simulation to evaluate both scenarios and a design of experiment to study the impact of the bed ratio in SS and RC. The model uses a data collection (one year of hospitalization) from the Saint-Etienne Hospital. Performance indicators are occupancy rates, admissions (admitted or refused), number of waiting patient, total LOS and total transfer time. Then a cost analysis considering the French hospital funding system was performed. The most interesting configuration is the one with integrated care. Lal et al (2015) discussed the methodology and applications of simulation based optimization, highlighting advantages, challenges and opportunities of using this method in healthcare. They summarized the needs of simulation based optimization in healthcare. They also introduce the key concepts and practical implications of using simulation based optimization to help the users identify the need and model the problems appropriately. Levin and Garifullin (2015) describe a novel method to integrate regression models for survival data in DES capable of quantifying the drivers of transition processes to estimate wait time. These methods are illustrated by example within a large hospital DES. Pepino et al. (2015) proposed a prototype simulation of a hospital ward which permits the study of the workload and task distribution among nursing and auxiliary personnel. In our study, we took both X a generic ward in a complex healthcare structure and a case study of a hospital immunology department as reference models. Both analyses were carried out together with a team of expert head nurses and following a specific simulation model developed in the Simul8 environment, which allowed the calculation of patient assistance timing as well as the efficiency of personnel use depending on the patient autonomy.

DISCRETE EVENT SIMULATION

We will define simulation as the process of designing a model of a real system and conducting experiments with this model for the purpose of understanding the behavior of the system and /or evaluating various strategies for the operation of the system. Thus it is critical that the model be designed in such a way that the model behavior mimics the response behavior of the real system to events that take place over time. The term's model and system are key components of our definition of simulation. By a model we mean a representation of a group of objects or ideas in some form other than that of the entity itself. By a system we mean a group or collection of interrelated elements that cooperate to accomplish some stated objective. One of the real strengths of simulation is the fact that we can simulate systems that already exist as well as those that are capable of being brought into existence, i.e. those in the preliminary or planning stage of development (Shannon, 1998: 7).

Simulation is one of the most powerful analysis tools available to those responsible for the design and operation of complex process or systems. In an increasingly competitive world, simulation has become a very powerful tool for the planning, design, and control of systems (Pegden, 1990).

We consider simulation to include both the construction of the model and the experimental use of the model for studying a problem. Thus, we can think of simulation modeling as an experimental and applied methodology, which seeks to (Shannon, 1998: 7):

- Describe the behavior of a system.
- Use the model to predict future behavior, i.e. the effects that will be produced by changes in the system or in its method of operation.

The majority of modern computer simulation tools implement a paradigm, called discrete-event simulation (DES). This paradigm is so general and powerful that it provides an implementation framework for most simulation languages, regardless of the user worldview supported by them (Altiok & Melamed, 2007: 11).

Discrete event systems simulation is the modeling of systems in which the state variable changes only at a discrete set of points in time (Banks et al, 2005: 13). In a discrete model, though, change can occur only at separated points in time, such as a manufacturing system with parts arriving and leaving at specific times, machines going down and coming back up at specific times, and breaks for workers (Kelton & Sadowski, 2004: 9).

The simulation event list is a means of keeping track of the different things that occur during a simulation run (Law & Kelton, 2000). Anything that occurs during the simulation run that can affect the state of the system is defined as an event. Typical events in a simple simulation include entity arrivals to the queue, the beginning of service times for entities, and the ending of service times for entities. These events change the state of the system because they can increase or decrease the number of entities in the system or queue or change the state of the resources between idle and busy. The event list is controlled by advances in the simulation clock. In our basic simulation model, the simulation clock advances in discrete jumps to each event on the event list. This type of model is called a discrete event simulation (Chung, 2004: 10).

A Discrete Event Simulation simulator executes the following algorithm (Altiok and Melamed, 2007: 12):

1. Set the simulation clock to an initial time (usually 0), and then generate one or more initial events and schedule them.
2. If the event list is empty, terminate the simulation run. Otherwise, find the most imminent event and unlink it from the event list.
3. Advance the simulation clock to the time of the most imminent event, and execute it (the event may stop the simulation).
4. Loop back to Step 2.

Although discrete event simulation could conceptually be done by hand calculations, the amount of data that must be stored and manipulated for most real-world systems dictates that discrete event simulations need to be done on a digital computer (Law & Kelton, 2000: 6).

Steps in Simulation Study

The essence or purpose of simulation modeling is to help the ultimate decision-maker solve a problem. Therefore, to learn to be a good simulation modeler, you must merge good problem solving techniques with good software engineering practice (Shannon, 1998: 9).

The steps in simulation study are as follows (Banks et al, 2005: 14-18; Shannon, 1998:9):

- **Problem Formulation:** Clearly defining the goals of the study so that we know the purpose, i.e. why are we studying this problem and what questions do we hope to answer? Every study should begin with a statement of the problem. If the statement is provided by the policymakers, or those that have the problem, the analyst must ensure that the problem being described is clearly understood. If a problem statement is being developed by the analyst, it is important that the policymakers understand and agree with the formulation.
- **Setting of Objectives and Overall Project Plan:** The objectives indicate the questions to be answered by simulation. At this point, a determination should be made concerning whether simulation is the appropriate methodology for the problem as formulated and objectives as stated.
- **Model Conceptualization:** The art of modeling is enhanced by an ability to abstract the essential features of a problem, to select and modify basic assumptions that characterize the system, and then to enrich and elaborate the model until a useful approximation results.
- **Data Collection:** There is a constant interplay between the construction of the model and the collection of the needed input data (Shannon, 1975). As the complexity of the model changes, the required data elements can also change. Also, since data collection takes such a large portion of the total time required to perform a simulation, it is necessary to begin it as possible, usually together with the early stages of model building.
- **Model Translation:** Most real-world systems result in models that require a great deal of information storage and cumputation, so the model be entered into a computer-recognizable format. We use the term "program" even though it is possible to accomplish the desired result in many instances with little or no actual coding.
- **Verified:** Verification pertains to the computer program prepared for the simulation model. Is the computer program performing properly? With complex models, it is difficult, if not impossible, to translate a model successfully in its entirety without a good deal of debugging; if the input parameters and logical structure of the model are correctly represented in the computer, verification has been completed.
- **Validated:** Validation usually is achieved through the calibration of the model, an iterative process of comparing the model against actual system behavior and using the discrepancies between the two, and the insight gained, to improve the model. This process is repeated until model accuracy is judged acceptable.
- **Experimental Design:** The alternatives that are to be simulated must be determined.
- **Production Runs and Analysis:** Production runs, and their subsequent analysis, are used to estimate measures of performance for the system designs that are being simulated.

- **More Runs:** Given the analysis of runs that have been completed, the analyst determines whether additional runs are needed and what design those additional experiments should follow.
- **Documentation and Reporting:** There are two types of documentation: program and progress. Program documentation is necessary for numerous reasons. If the program is going to be used again by the same or different analyst, it could be necessary to understand how the program operates. Musselman (1998) discuss progress reports that provide the important, written history of a simulation project. Project reports give a chronology of work done and decision made.
- **Implementation:** The success of the implementation phase depends on how well the previous 11 steps. It is also contingent upon how thoroughly the analyst has involved the ultimate model user during the entire simulation process.

Advantages and Disadvantages of Simulation

Simulation is a widely used and increasingly popular method for studying complex systems. Some possible advantages of simulation that may account for its widespread appeal are the following (Law and Kelton, 2000: 91-92):

- Most complex, real-world systems with stochastic elements cannot be accurately described by a mathematical model that can be evaluated analytically. Thus, a simulation is often the only type of investigation possible.
- Simulation allows us to estimate the performance of an existing system under some projected set of operating conditions.
- Alternative proposed system designs can be compared via simulation to see which best meets a specified requirement.
- In a simulation we can maintain much better control over experimental conditions than would generally be possible when experimenting with the system itself.
- Simulation allows us to study a system with a long time frame.

Simulation is not without its drawbacks. Some disadvantages are as follows:

- Each run of stochastic simulation model produces only estimates of a model's true characteristics for a particular set of input parameters. Thus, several independent runs of the model will probably be required for each set of input parameters to be studied. For this reason, simulation models are generally not as good at optimization as they are at comparing a fixed number of specified alternative system designs. On the other hand, an analytic model, if appropriate, can often easily produce the exact true characteristics of that model for a variety of sets of input parameters. Thus, if a "valid" analytic model is available or can easily be developed, it will generally be preferable to a simulation model.
- Simulation models are often expensive and time-consuming to develop.
- The large volume of numbers produced by a simulation study or the persuasive impact of a realistic animation often creates a tendency to place greater confidence in a study's results than is justified. If a model is not a "valid" representation of a system under study, the simulation results, no matter how impressive they appear, will provide little useful information about the actual system.

A Simulation Concept

Although there are several different types of simulation methodologies, we will limit our concerns to a stochastic, discrete, process oriented approach. In such an approach, we model a particular system by studying the flow of entities that move through that system. Entities can be customers, job orders, particular parts, information packets, etc. An entity can be any object that enters the system, moves through a series of processes, and then leaves the system. These entities can have individual characteristics which we will call attributes. An attribute is associated with the specific, individual entity. Attributes might be such things as name, priority, due date, required CPU time, ailment, account number etc. As the entity flows through the system, it will be processed by a series of resources. Resources are anything that the entity needs in order to be processed. For example, resources might be workers, material handling equipment, special tools, a hospital bed, access to the CPU, a machine, waiting or storage space, etc. Resources may be fixed in one location (e.g. a heavy machine, bank teller, hospital bed) or moving about the system (e.g. a forklift, repairman, doctor). A simulation model is therefore a computer program which represents the logic of the system as entities with attributes arrive, join queues to await the assignment of required resources, are processed by the resources, released and exit the system. In addition to the logic of how an entity flows through the system, the computer program keeps track of and advances time, as well as keeping track of resource utilization, time spent in queues, time in the system (processing time), and other desired statistics. Much of what happens in the system is probabilistic or stochastic in nature. For example the time between arrivals, the time for a resource to process the entity, the time to travel from one part of the system to another and whether a part passes inspection or not, are usually all random variables. It is these types of data for input to the model that are difficult to obtain (Shannon, 1998: 8).

Components and Organization of a Discrete Event Simulation

The following components will be found in most discrete event simulation models using the next event time advance approach programmed in a general purpose language (Law and Kelton, 2000):

- **System State:** The collection of state variables necessary to describe the system at a particular time.
- **Simulation Clock:** A variable giving the current value of simulated time.
- **Event List:** A list containing the next time when each type of event will occur.
- **Statistical Counters:** Variables used for storing statistical information about system performance.
- **Initialization Routine:** A subprogram to initialize the simulation model at time 0.
- **Timing Routine:** A subprogram that determines the next event from the event list and then advances the simulation clock to the time when that event is to occur.
- **Event Routine:** A subprogram that updates the system state when a particular type of event occurs (there is one event routine for each event type).
- **Library Routines:** A set of subprograms used to generate random observations from probability distributions that were determined as part of the simulation model.

- **Report Generator:** A subprogram that computes estimates (from the statistical counters) of the desired measures of performance and produces a report when the simulation ends.
- **Main Program:** A subprogram that invokes the timing routine to determine the next event and then transfers control to the corresponding event routine to update the system state appropriately. The main program may also check for termination and invoke the report generator when the simulation is over.

Areas of Application

The applications of simulation are vast. The Winter Simulation Conference (WSC) is an excellent way to learn more about the latest in simulation applications and theory. Some presentations, by area, from a recent WSC are listed next (Banks et al, 2005; Sezen and Günal, 2009):

- Manufacturing Applications
- Semiconductor Manufacturing
- Construction Engineering and Project Management
- Military Applications
- Logistics, Supply Chain, and Distribution Applications
- Transportation Modes and Traffic
- Business Process Simulation
- Health Care

CASE STUDY

In this study, an investigated emergency department is found in a second stage public hospital in Turkey. To begin our study, all patients who come to hospital are entity and our resources are doctors, nurses, and lab technicians, registration clerks and X ray technicians.

The hospital that is investigated in this study is located in a town. Its population is 157000. In this town there is only one state hospital. Apart from this state hospital, the town has two private hospitals.

Problem Description

To begin simulation study, conceptual understanding of the system must be done. When a patient arrives to emergency department, if there is a life-threatening condition, she/he is accepted to resuscitated zone without registration. If there isn't a life-threatening condition; registration of patient must be done. Pendant registration patient is classified as red or green and patient priority change according to this classification. When a patient is red, first nurse accepts patient and she realizes her first controls and medical examination is done by a doctor. After medical examination doctor asks patient to go to the lab or X-ray area, or ask nurse to apply a cure to patient. If patient's classification is green, than his priority is less then the patient whose classification is red; patient wait for a doctor and after doctor examination nurse can apply a cure according to the doctor decision or he can go to the lab or he can leave system.

If a patient goes to the lab or X-ray room, he/she waits in the queue. Patient waits also given her/his results. Then he/she returns to the examination room and doctor decides which cure nurse applies. After treatment patient passes observations room. In observation room, patient's keeping is done by nurses. When observation time is up, patient waits for doctor for last examination and then patient goes to the registration office and then leave system.

Simulation Model

Based on gathered data simulation model is built. System includes many stochastic variables such as arrivals time and service time. Some assumptions and simplification must be made. First in emergence department there is no appointment rule. Patient can arrive to emergency department through ambulance or by his own. Service time is in general triangular or normal. Based on gathered data arrivals time are fitted to exponential distribution with parameter 7.2 minutes. Patient with life threating condition is the %3,2 of patient. Service time for these patients is triangle with parameter 10, 20, 30. In fact after first intervention patient leaves system to enter intensive care department. Patients without life threating condition pass registration stage. Registration time is fitted to normal distribution with mean 3,2 and standard deviation 1,3. In registration, %23 of the patient are classified as red, the rest is green. For patient in red class, nurse service time is fitted to normal distribution with mean 3,2 and standard deviation is 0,5; doctor service time is fitted to triangular (4.2, 5.7, 9.1). %40 of this part of patient goes to lab and the rest wait for nurse to treat. Nurse service time is fitted to triangular (3.5, 7.5, 9.7) and patient passes to observation room. For patients in green class, their priority in queue is second. Their examination is realized by a doctor. Doctor service time is fitted to normal distribution with mean 7.3 mn and std is 2,5 mn. %40 of patients in green class leave system; %20 go to the lab and the rest wait for nurse to treat. Test and diagnosis part consists of Lab and X ray .X ray service time is fitted to normal (2.5, 0.8) and lab service time is fitted to normal distribution with parameter(10.1, 3.2) after lab operation ;we assume that patient must wait 15mn for test results. When patient takes results, patient returns to examination room to show his test results to doctor. Doctor's service time is fitted to triangular distribution (3.1, 7.2, 8.6). At the end of doctor examination, doctor decides either let patient to leave or send patient to observation room. In observation room, a nurse visits patient every 15 minutes and before patient leaves the observation rooms, a doctor gives approval. Doctor service time is fitted to triangular (1.8, 3.5, 5.6). To leave system, patient must visit registration office and registers clerk service time is fitted to normal distribution with parameter mean 5,2 minute and standard deviation is 2,1.

Simulation model was developed by Arena package program. The following commands are used in developed simulation model: Create, Assign, Branch, Seize, Release, Route, Delay, Station, Queue and Dispose.

Simulation Results

Simulation model runs for 1000 minutes and 100 minutes is assumed to warm up period. To initialize our system we begin with all resources with 1 capacity. Table 1 shows the number of resources for scenario 1.

Simulation model's results show that 118 patients came to the emergency service and 75 patients leave system during simulation. Table 2 shows the utilization rates of resources for scenario 1.

Table 1. Number of Resources for Scenario 1

Resource Name	Number of Resources
Doctor	1
Register Clerk	1
Nurse	1
X-ray technician	1
Lab.Tech	1

Table 2. Utilization rate for Scenario 1

Resource Name	Utilization
Doctor	% 94,96
Register Clerk	% 81,95
Nurse	% 89,70
X-ray technician	% 2,00
Lab. Tech	% 6,32

The Average number of patients waiting for doctor in green class for first examination is 8,5 . Then number of doctor is increased. Number of resources, utilization rate and number of patients that leave system are shown below. Table 3 shows the utilization rates of resources for scenario 2. 87 patient leave the system.

87 patients leave the system. Number of patients who wait for nurse in observation room is 5,23 in average and at the end of simulation 23 patients wait for nurse in this room. So number of nurses is increased. Table 4 shows the utilization rates of resources for scenario 3.

83 patients leave system. Number of nurse is increased one in scenario 3. Therefore utilization rate of nurse decreased to (1,15/2) 57,5. Number of doctor is increased to 3 in Scenario 4. Table 5 shows the utilization rates of resources for scenario 4.

89 patients leave system. Number of doctors is increased one in scenario 4. Therefore utilization rate of doctor is decreased to (1,15/3) 35. Table 6 shows the utilization rates of resources for scenario 5.

Table 3. Utilization rate for Scenario 2

Resource Name	Number of Resources	Utilization
Doctor	2	1,10
Register Clerk	1	0,89
Nurse	1	0,94
X-ray technician	1	0,01
Lab.Tech	1	0,07

Table 4. Utilization rate for Scenario 3

Resource Name	Number of Resources	Utilization
Doctor	2	1,21
Register Clerk	1	0,86
Nurse	2	1,15
X-ray technician	1	0,01
Lab.Tech	1	0,04

Table 5. Utilization rate for Scenario 4

Resource Name	Number of Resources	Utilization
Doctor	3	1,15
Register Clerk	1	0,88
Nurse	2	1,02
X-ray technician	1	0,03
Lab.Tech	1	0,05

Table 6. Utilization rate for Scenario 5

Resource Name	Number of Resources	Utilization
Doctor	3	1,23
Register Clerk	1	0,90
Nurse	3	0,99
X-ray techniciantechnician	1	0,01
Lab.Tech	1	0,05

85 patients leave system. Number of nurse is increased one in scenario 5. Therefore utilization rate of doctor is decreased to (0,99/3) 33. Table 7 shows the utilization rates of resources for scenario 6. Number of nurses is increased one in scenario 6.

88 patients leave system. Table 8 shows the utilization rates of resources for scenario 7. Number of doctors is increased one in scenario 7.

86 patients leave system. Number of nurse is increased one in scenario 8. Table 9 shows the utilization rates of resources for scenario 8.

86 patients leave system. Number of nurse is increased one in scenario 9. Table 10 shows the utilization rates of resources for scenario 9.

86 patients leave system. Number of doctor is increased one in scenario 10. Table 11 shows the utilization rates of resources for scenario 10.

111 patients leave system. Number of register clerks is increased one in scenario 11. Table 12 shows the utilization rates of resources for scenario 11.

113 patients leave system. Number of doctors is decreased to three in scenario 12. Table 13 shows the utilization rates of resources for scenario 12.

114 patients leave system. Number of nurse is decreased to four in scenario 13. Table 14 shows the utilization rates of resources for scenario 13.

As a result of scenario 13; utilization rate of doctor is (1,3/3) %43, utilization rate of register clerk is %52,5, utilization rate of nurse is (1,15/4) %28,7, utilization rate of x-ray technician is %2, utilization rate of lab.tech is % 9.

Table 7. Utilization rate for Scenario 6

Resource Name	Number of Resources	Utilization
Doctor	3	1,19
Register Clerk	1	0,89
Nurse	4	1,13
X-ray techniciantechnician	1	0,02
Lab.Tech	1	0,03

Table 8. Utilization rate for Scenario 7

Resource Name	Number of Resources	Utilization
Doctor	4	1,19
Register Clerk	1	0,88
Nurse	4	1,10
X-ray technician	1	0,01
Lab.Tech	1	0,04

Table 9. Utilization rate for Scenario 8

Resource Name	Number of Resources	Utilization
Doctor	5	1,14
Register Clerk	1	0,88
Nurse	4	1,01
X-ray technician	1	0,01
Lab.Tech	1	0,04

Table 10. Utilization rate for Scenario 9

Resource Name	Number of Resources	Utilization
Doctor	5	1,14
Register Clerk	1	0,88
Nurse	5	1,01
X-ray technician	1	0,01
Lab.Tech	1	0,04

Table 11. Utilization rate for Scenario 10

Resource Name	Number of Resources	Utilization
Doctor	6	1,18
Register Clerk	1	0,88
Nurse	5	1,05
X-ray technician	1	0,02
Lab.Tech	1	0,03

Table 12. Utilization rate for Scenario 11

Resource Name	Number of Resources	Utilization
Doctor	6	1,22
Register Clerk	2	1,01
Nurse	5	1,06
X-ray technician	1	0,01
Lab.Tech	1	0,07

Table 13. Utilization rate for Scenario 12

Resource Name	Number of Resources	Utilization
Doctor	3	1,28
Register Clerk	2	1,03
Nurse	5	1,09
X-ray technician	1	0,03
Lab.Tech	1	0,07

Table 14. Utilization rate for Scenario 13

Resource Name	Number of Resources	Utilization
Doctor	3	1,30
Register Clerk	2	1,05
Nurse	4	1,15
X-ray technician	1	0,02
Lab.Tech	1	0,09

CONCLUSION

The simulation model for emergency department is developed by Arena package program. The patient waiting times are reduced by the tested scenarios. This chapter provides the readers to evaluate healthcare systems using discrete event simulation. The developed model could be evaluated as a base for new implementations in other hospitals and clinics.

From scenario 1 to scenario 10, number of doctors and nurses are increased but service quality and number of patients does not increase. At scenario 11, number of register clerks is increased to 2 and service quality and number of patient who leave system rise. On the other hand utilization of X-ray technician and lab tech is very low. If it is possible, for 2 responsibilities using same staff will increase effectiveness of the system.

Health care system is very expensive sector and related costs are very high. To raise service quality, number of doctors and nurses are increased but system target is provided by increased number of register clerk. Testing different scenarios, effective policy can be designed using developed simulation model.

REFERENCES

Alessandro, P., Adriano, T., Annunziata, M., & Oscar, T. (2015). A Simulation Model For Analyzing The Nurse Workload In A University Hospital Ward. *Proceedings of the 2015 Winter Simulation Conference.*

Altiok, T., & Melamed, B. (2007). Simulation Modeling and Analysis with Arena. Academic Press.

Armony, M., Shlomo, I., Mandelbaum, A., Marmor, Y., Tseytlin, Y., & Yom-Tov, G. (2010). *On Patient Flow in Hospitals: A Data-Based Queuing-Science Perspective.* Working paper. New York University.

Banks, J., Carson, J. S., Nelson, B. L., & Nicol, D. M. (2004). *Discrete-Event System Simulation* (4th ed.). Upper Saddle River, NJ: Prentice-Hall, Inc.

Camila, E., Francisco, R., Jimena, P., & Daniel, B. (2014). Real-Time Simulation As A Way To Improve Daily Operations In An Emergency Room. *Proceedings of the 2014 Winter Simulation Conference.*

Chung, C. A. (2004). *Simulation Modeling Handbook A Practical Approach.* CRC Press.

Fetter, R. B., & Thompson, J. D. (1965). The Simulation Of Hospital Systems. *Opns Res, 13*(5), 689–711. doi:10.1287/opre.13.5.689

Garifullin. (2015). *Simulating Wait Time In Healthcare: Accounting For Transition Process Variability Using Survival Analyses.* Academic Press.

Günal, M., & Pidd, M. (2010). Discrete event simulation for Performance Modelling in Health care: A review of the Literature. *Journal of Simulation, 4*(1), 42–51. doi:10.1057/jos.2009.25

Hamrock, E., Paige, K., Parks, J., Scheulen, J., & Levin, S. (2012). Discrete Event Simulation for Healthcare Organizations: A Tool for Decision Making. *Journal of Healthcare Management, 58*(2), 110–124. PMID:23650696

Il-Chul, M., Won, B. J., Junseok, L., Doyun, K., Hyunrok, L., Taesik, L., ... Woon, K. G. (2015). EMS-SIM: Emergency Medical Service Simulator With Geographic And Medical Details. *Proceedings of the 2015 Winter Simulation Conference.*

Jacobsen, S., Hall, S., & Swisher, J. (2006). Discrete-Event Simulation of Health Care Systems. In R. Hall (Ed.), *Patient Flow: Reducing Delay in Healthcare Delivery* (pp. 211–252). Springer. doi:10.1007/978-0-387-33636-7_8

Kang, H., Nembhard, H., Rafferty, C., & DeFlitch, C. (2014). Patient Flow In The Emergency Department: A Classification And Analysis Of Admission Process Policies. *Annals of Emergency Medicine, 64*(4), 335–342. doi:10.1016/j.annemergmed.2014.04.011 PMID:24875896

Karim, G., Oualid, J., Zied, J., Mathias, W., Romain, H., Valérie, T., & Ger, K. (2014). A Comprehensive Simulation Modeling Of An Emergency Department: A Case Study For Simulation Optimization Of Staffing Levels. *Proceedings of the 2014 Winter Simulation Conference.*

Kelton, W. D., Sadowski, R. P., & Sadowski, D. A. (2004). *Simulation with Arena.* McGraw Hill.

Lal Mohan, T., & Roh, T. (2013). Simulation in Healthcare. In J. A. Larson (Ed.), *A Book Management Engineering: A Guide to Best Practices for Industrial Engineering in Health Care* (1st ed.). Taylor and Francis Group.

Law, A. M. (2007). *Simulation Modeling and Analysis* (4th ed.). McGraw Hill.

Law, A. M., & Kelton, W. D. (2000). *Simulation Modeling and Analysis* (3rd ed.). New York: McGraw-Hill, Inc.

Martin, P., Vincent, A., & Xiaolan, X. (2014). Hospitalization Admission Control Of Emergency Patients Using Markovian Decision Processes And Discrete Event Simulation. *Proceedings of the 2014 Winter Simulation Conference.*

Mohan, L. T., Thomas, R., & Todd, H. (2015). Simulation Based Optimization: Applications In Healthcare. *Proceedings of the 2015 Winter Simulation Conference.*

Pegden, C. D. (1990). *Introduction to Simulation Using SIMAN.* McGraw-Hill, Inc.

Pidd, M. (2003). *Tools for Thinking: Modelling in Management Science* (2nd ed.). Chichester, UK: Wiley.

Roberts, S. D. (2011). Tutorial on the Simulation of Healthcare Systems. In *Proceedings of the 2011 Winter Simulation Conference.* Piscataway, NJ: Institute of Electrical and Electronics Engineers, Inc. 10.1109/WSC.2011.6147860

Saghafian, S., Hopp, W. J., Van Oyen, M. P., Desmond, J. S., & Kronick, S. L. (2012). Patient Streaming as a Mechanism for Improving Responsiveness in Emergency Departments. *Operations Research, 60*(5), 1080–1097. doi:10.1287/opre.1120.1096

Sezen, H. K., & Günal, M. M. (2009). *Yöneylem Araştırmasında Benzetim.* Bursa: Ekin Yayınevi.

Shannon, R. E. (1975). *Systems Simulation: The Art and Science.* Prentice-Hall.

Shannon, R. E. (1998). Introduction To The Art And Science Of Simulation. *Proceedings of the 1998 Winter Simulation Conference.* 10.1109/WSC.1998.744892

Shi, P., Chou, M., Dai, J., Ding, D., & Sim, J. (2015). Models and Insights for Hospital Inpatient Operations: Time Dependent ED Boarding Time. *Management Science, 24,* 13–14.

Simon, R., & Canacari, E. (2012). A Practical Guide to Applying Lean Tools and Management Principles to Health Care Improvement Projects. *Association of Perioperative Registered Nurses Journal, 95*(1), 85–100. doi:10.1016/j.aorn.2011.05.021 PMID:22201573

Thomas, F., Regis, G., Vincent, A., Xiaolan, X., & Emilie, A. (2015). Performance Evaluation Of An Integrated Care For Geriatric Departments Using Discrete-Event Simulation. *Proceedings of the 2015 Winter Simulation Conference.*

Way, T. K., Lau, H. C., & Lee, F. C. Y. (2013). Improving Patient Length-Of-Stay In Emergency Department Through Dynamic Queue Management. *Proceedings of the 2013 Winter Simulation Conference.*

Weng, S.-J., Cheng, B.-C., Kwong, S. T., Wang, L.-M., & Chang, C.-Y. (2011). Simulation Optimization for Emergency Department Resources Allocation. In *Proceedings of the 2011 Winter Simulation Conference.* Piscataway, NJ: Institute of Electrical and Electronics Engineers. 10.1109/WSC.2011.6147845

Yann, F., Michael, M., & Uday, R. (2010). Comparing Two Operating Room Allocation Policies For Elective And Emergency Surgeries. *Proceedings of the 2010 Winter Simulation Conference.*

KEY TERMS AND DEFINITIONS

Computer Simulation: Reproducing the behavior of a system using a mathematical model.

Discrete Event Simulation: DES is the modeling of systems in which the state variable changes only at a discrete set of points in time.

Discrete Model: Change can occur only at separated points in time.

Event List: A list containing the next time when each type of event will occur.

Simulation Clock: A variable giving the current value of simulated time.

Validation: Validation usually is achieved through the calibration of the model, an iterative process of comparing the model against actual system behavior and using the discrepancies between the two, and the insight gained, to improve the model. This process is repeated until model accuracy is judged acceptable.

Verification: Verification pertains to the computer program prepared for the simulation model. Is the computer program performing properly? With complex models, it is difficult, if not impossible; to translate a model successfully in its entirety without a good deal of debugging; if the input parameters and logical structure of the model are correctly represented in the computer, verification has been completed.

This research was previously published in the Handbook of Research on Data Science for Effective Healthcare Practice and Administration edited by Bijan Raahemi, Amir Albadvi, Behrouz H. Far, and Elham Akhond Zadeh Noughabi; pages 78-93, copyright year 2017 by Medical Information Science Reference (an imprint of IGI Global).

Chapter 18
Surgery Operations Modeling and Scheduling in Healthcare Systems

Fatah Chetouane
Université de Moncton, Canada

Eman Ibraheem
Université de Moncton, Canada

ABSTRACT

Surgery operations scheduling is a complex task due to operation duration uncertainties and resource sharing and availabilities in healthcare processes. In current health care systems it is important to minimize staff idle time and maintain a high utilization rate for surgery facilities. In the present study a nonlinear mathematical model for surgery scheduling is described, and an approximated linear model is deduced based on a set of assumptions. The linear model is solved using heuristic approach. The objective is to maximize the utilization of operating rooms and the surgery staff. Computational results show that our model improved the surgery schedule and the resources utilization. Our model also showed the potential of adding cases to the schedule due to minimizing the completion time of the schedule.

1. INTRODUCTION

Providing efficient healthcare services to patients are gaining an increasing attention over the past few years. Recent budgetary restrictions, prescribed by politics, due to economic changes, led public hospitals to seek and implement methodologies and techniques at their managerial and operational levels, to achieve efficient resource usage, without compromising the quality of their service, risking patient endangerment, or causing additional costs (patient waiting and resources usage costs). Emergency department and surgery department got to be the most critical subsystems in any hospital, due to their role in fulfilling emergent needs. Surgery departments service both urgent and elective surgery procedures, and are linked to referrals from physicians outside the hospital, and/or from other department within,

DOI: 10.4018/978-1-7998-2451-0.ch018

Copyright © 2020, IGI Global. Copying or distributing in print or electronic forms without written permission of IGI Global is prohibited.

such as the emergency department. The Surgery department is the hospital most expensive center (Health Care Financial Management Association.2005), and due to his linkage to other hospital services (intensive care, preoperative care, post anesthesia care, surgery admission, and recovery units), its impacts the performance of the hospital as whole. To provide an idea of surgery department cost distributions, based on data from statistics Canada collected for the period 2007-2008, the New Brunswick regional health authority expenditures averaged: staff wages (70%), medical and surgical supplies (13%), drugs and medicines (7%), equipment and miscellaneous (10%). When putting these expenditure figures in contrast with the increasing demand in surgery procedures inflicted on the same New Brunswick regional health authority (16% increase over the period from 2005 to 2008), seeking continuous improvement of the operating theatre management becomes critical to ensure quality healthcare delivery for all patients, by keeping a cost-effective, and a flexible scheduling of all surgery demands.

In the same line of thought, this study is aimed, in a first stage, toward the development of a general mathematical programming model (nonlinear) for elective surgery planning and scheduling. During modeling, surgeries are assumed to be of uncertain durations, also operating room, and surgeon preferences are taking into consideration. The two goal of increasing operating room utilization, and reducing surgeon idle times are combined in a single objective formulation. In the second stage of this study, a linear program is extracted from the general model and solved using a simple heuristic approach. Several feasible schedules (no optimal) can be obtained easily using the linear model, providing a flexibility in the decision making process.

The reminder of this chapter starts with a brief background on recent studies on modelling and scheduling of surgery procedures, followed by a mathematical description of the constraints involved in the surgery planning and scheduling problem. The nonlinear model is then simplified to a linear mathematical program, and a heuristic procedure is presented to solve the simplified model. Based on a case study, some results are discussed, with conclusion and future possible extensions.

2. RECENT MATHEMATICAL STUDIES ON SURGERY SCHEDULING

As succinctly defined in (Burke & Riise, 2008), the surgery scheduling problem is to find the optimal allocation of surgeries to operating rooms and days, and their optimal sequence for each day. Objectives are typically tardiness costs (over time), hospitalization costs, intervention costs, operating room utilization, patient's waiting time, patient or personnel preferences, etc. This problem is solved on different time scales, ranging from month-scale admission planning to daily detailed surgery scheduling, using different objectives and constraints. The most common objective is to maximize operating rooms usage (Hans et al., 2008) and staff utilization (Denton et al., 2007). Contributions on surgery scheduling can be classified according to several standpoints and criteria such as: single operating room vs. multiple operating room scheduling; surgery scheduling (not considering sequencing), and vice-versa, or simultaneously sequencing and scheduling (which lead generally to a combinatorial stochastic optimization problem); considering uncertainty, considering costs; and also depending on techniques used to approach the problem whether by using simulation methods, or mathematical optimization methods. For few decades ago mathematical programming models and optimization techniques have frequently used for surgery scheduling (Denton et al. 2007), (Santibáñez et al. 2007), and (Jeroen et al. 2008). A good literature review of surgery scheduling is provided in (Cardoen, B. 2009) and (Cardoen, B. et al. 2010), where authors studied one hundred and twenty four papers on operating room planning and scheduling, and compared their used terminology and primary contributions using several indicators such as: time horizon, accounted uncertainties, analysis and solving methods, patient types, performance metrics (resources, time, quality of care, economic aspects), and decision delineation (discipline, surgeon, patient). The main outcome of their study is an enhanced way to classify existing contribution using the proposed indicators that helps researcher identify manuscripts according to specific research interests. An early, though extensively cited study is described in (Magerlein and Martin. 1978). This citation appears in many succeeding contributions in the field of surgical system scheduling. It provides a comparison of three common surgery scheduling approaches, namely: no blocked (open) booking, blocked booking, admissions scheduling and control system. The conducted comparison is made with regards to operating room performance metrics, service quality, and implementation drawbacks vs. benefits. Blocked and no blocked approaches outperformed admissions control system approach, with regards to the capacity planning stability aspect, while the control system approach outperformed on the managerial and operational flexibility aspect, due its advantage in testing several decision rules for surgery scheduling (first-come-first-serve, longest-cases-first, and shortest-cases-first). The authors discussed the real challenge in surgery scheduling due to the multiple type of uncertainty and imprecision affecting the process, especially surgery procedure durations. Most estimation of surgery durations are based on surgeons' estimates, operating room schedulers' estimates, or historical averages (or a combination of the three). It was advised that accurate estimates are key to achieving quality process analysis and improvements, since lower estimates will result in an overloaded schedule causing cancellations, overtime, and low employee morale, while higher estimates will result in idle times, misused capacity and increased patient waiting times. The variability in surgery durations can also be caused by the fluctuation in surgeon experience and skills. A study on this fluctuation for a two-surgeon team (a responsible and an assistant) is described in (Molina-Pariente, Fernandez-Viagas & Framinan, 2015). A mixed integer linear programming model is proposed for an open surgery scheduling case, with surgeon experience level as an explicit parameter in the model. In addition to uncertainties on surgery durations, uncertainty on downstream resource availabilities (capacity constraints of surgical intensive, and/or post anesthesia care units) are studied in (Min & Yih, 2010b). They formulated thee elective surgery scheduling problem as a stochastic optimization model minimizing patient and overtime costs. Other performance measures were also collected such as: average overtime, average utilization, total number of scheduled patients and cancellations. The solution approach was conducted using sample average approximation method implemented using ILOG, CPLEX software. When compared to a deterministic version of the problem (replacing random variable by their expected value parameters) the stochastic optimization model outperformed the deterministic version by more than 17% in cost reduction. This proves the importance of considering the uncertainties in the modeling and solving of surgery scheduling problems.

Erdogan & Denton (2011) discussed how the design and physical layout of the entire surgical process stages (preoperative, intraoperative and postoperative) complicates the scheduling problem. They based their study on the comparison between two surgical suite designs: one with separate intake and recovery areas; and another with common intake, and recovery areas. Among the complicating factors are duration uncertainties (operative, preoperative and postoperative), variability of patients to be scheduled on a given day (cancelations, no-shows, and emergency add-ons), resource availabilities, and interactions between specialties. Authors discussed the efficiency and limitation of queuing, simulation, mathematical and optimization approaches in addressing these complicating factors. In reference to the interaction between different surgery specialties and units, the joint operating room planning and advanced scheduling problem, where several specialties share a fixed number of operating rooms, and post-surgery beds was studied in (Aringhieri, Landa, Soriano, Tànfani, & Testi, 2015). Using linear programming models, authors exploited the inherent hierarchical interaction between two decision levels: the time block assignment level to surgical specialties, and the patient assignment level to these time blocks. The influence of preoperative preparation tasks, such as sterilization and setting of needed equipment, on the sequencing of elective surgery operations with deterministic durations was also investigated in (Zhao, & Li, 2014), where the surgery sequencing problem is solved using two different approaches: mixed integer nonlinear programming, and constraint programming. Better performance with regards to solution quality and sensitivity to setup tasks where obtained using the constraint programming approach. In (Xiang, Yin, & Lim, 2015) the studied surgery scheduling problem considers nurse schedule constraints (role, specialty, qualification and availability). A mathematical formulation is proposed, and solved using ant colony optimization approach. Despite the resulting complexity of integrating nurse constraints, the obtained results exhibit a shorter completion time, and a balanced resource allocations when compared to those obtained without considering nurse rostering constraints. The problem of scheduling surgical services in a multistage operating room department was also studied in (Saremi, Jula, ElMekkawy & Wang, 2013). Several patient types with stochastic service time and punctual arrivals are considered. Admission is schedule-based, and each patient type is served by a specific specialty (surgeon type). Resource (surgeon) availabilities are restricted by time window constraints. The application of simulation methods enhanced with mathematical programming models improved the appointment scheduling in terms of completion time. Surgeries allocation and sequencing problem for multiple operating rooms and multiple surgical team, was also studied in (Koksalmis, Hancerliogullari & Hancerliogullari, 2014) using a mathematical formulation to minimize the number of unscheduled surgical operations. Adopting an open scheduling strategy, (Bouguerra, Sauvey & Sauer, 2015) studied the case where operating rooms are considered specialized for a given day but multi-functional on the scheduling horizon. The model was solved using heuristic approach, with an objective to maximize operating rooms utilization and to minimize idle time between planned surgeries.

More surgical procedures are now being performed in outpatient procedure centers. These centers are increasingly appealing for their ability to handle specialty procedures in a more accommodating way to patient preferences. These facilities are subjected to similar challenges with regards to surgery booking under uncertainties. Indeed, the problem of optimizing surgical procedure scheduling, in the presence of uncertainty on patient attendance and surgery durations is studied in (Berg, Denton, Erdogan, Rohleder, & Huschka, 2014). A stochastic programming model formulation is used allowing to test exact and heuristic resolution methods. Their study shows that heuristic scheduling methods (easy-to-implement) are more suitable to use in one or both of these cases: overtime costs greater than patient waiting time costs, or procedure duration uncertainty and no-attendance rate for the procedure are directly related. In the same study, the efficiency of double booking, and late-day scheduling of patients with high no-attendance rate, or procedures with high duration variance, is attested to lower waiting, idling, and overtime costs. Generally surgery can be of an elective or emergency type (Encyclopedia of surgery, 2010). This classification is broad and indicates the two essential priority categories for surgery operations. Other classifications such as elective, emergent, urgent can be found in literature (Cardoen, B. et *al.* 2010). Unlike elective surgeries which can be planned off-line, emergency surgeries cannot be planned in advance and must be handled on-line (Yigal, G. et al. 1996). In order to deal with this uncertainty on a daily basis, and to safely handle priority patients, hospitals must reserve a portion of their resource capacity for emergency add-on cases (Guinet and Chaabane. 2003). Lamieri et al. (2008) proposed a stochastic model for operating rooms scheduling where both elective and emergency surgeries were taken into account. Random capacity for emergency surgeries was reserved and the problem was formulated as a stochastic integer model.

Service capacity must be controlled effectively to handle most daily planned elective surgeries, in addition to emergency patients in a cost efficient manner. In (Huh, Liu, & Truong. 2013) this management problem is modelled as a multi-resource allocation scheduling problem in a dynamic and non-stationary environment, where demand and resource availability is continually updated, and patient reneging/no-shows may occur inflicting an additional waiting cost. An overtime cost is also inflicted when elective surgeries exceed available capacity. Authors established patient waitlist equation, and formulated the problem as a Markov decision process, allowing several scheduling algorithms to find the optimal trade-off between over-planning and under-planning for emergency patients. Their study is inspired by optimal control and look-ahead optimization theory. Unlike the common two-priority categories (elective and urgent), Min & Yih (2010a) studied the elective surgery scheduling with several priority categories in a limited capacity surgical facility. Their scheduling policy seeks an optimal trade-off between overtime cost and surgery postponement cost. A stochastic dynamic programming model is formulated to address the problem. Numerical examples point out the importance of taking into account patient priority in the surgery scheduling problem, it also proves that the schedule efficiency doesn't rely only on the total number of patients in a waiting list, but also on the number of patients in each priority category.

3. SURGERY SCHEDULING MATHEMATICAL MODEL

In the following a mathematical model for elective surgery planning and scheduling is proposed to highlight resources constraints and variability of surgical procedure durations. In the following model surgery procedures are assigned to surgery teams according to their specialties. College of surgeons in most hospitals, have different surgery specialties, with at least, one team by specialty. In our model, all surgical procedures are considered confirmed and all resources (medical teams, operating rooms, and equipment) are available over the scheduling horizon. The following notation is used to designate model parameters and variables:

SH: surgery scheduling time horizon
NS: number of elective surgical operations confirmed for scheduling
NR: number of operating rooms considered in the scheduling process
NT: number of surgical teams involved in the schedule plan
i: index for surgical operations, $i \in \{1...NS\}$
j: index for operating rooms, $j \in \{1...NR\}$
k: index for surgical teams (not surgical specialties index), $k \in \{1...NT\}$

Here, the index of surgical team is not used to differentiate between surgical specialties: two different values of index k designate two separate teams, albeit they have the same specialty (neurology, dermatology, orthopedic, etc.). To represent an operating room assignment, binary decision variables X are used as follows:

X(i,j): Equals 1 if surgery (*i*) is assigned to room (*j*), and 0 otherwise, $i \in \{1...NS\}$; $j \in \{1...NR\}$.

To consider the inherent uncertainty on surgical operation (*i*) durations, let us introduce scheduled beginning and completion times, with duration parameters, as follows:

Tb(i,j): Scheduled beginning time of operation (*i*) in room (*j*), $i \in \{1...NS\}; j \in \{1...NR\}$
Te(i,j): Scheduled completion time of operation (*i*) in room (*j*), $i \in \{1...NS\}; j \in \{1...NR\}$
D(i): Randomly distributed duration for operation (*i*), $i \in \{1...NS\}$.

On operation surgery schedule, these variables and parameters are linked by the constraint:

$$Te(i,j) - Tb(i,j) \geq D(i) \bullet X(i,j) \tag{1}$$

In the general case, the duration parameter in constraint (1) is an unknown random variable, making not predictable the respect of this constraint in practice.

An operating room can be idle, active, or undergoing maintenance/cleaning. At the beginning of the scheduling horizon, all operating rooms are assumed to be idle, and ready for use. The cleaning/maintenance duration of an operating room is specific to the surgical room and to the type of surgery completed in it.

Even if cleaning durations can be contained within, relatively accurate, limits, they are assumed to be randomly distributed. Let $M(i, j)$ be the random setup-time duration for operating room (*j*), between the two successively scheduled surgeries (*i*) and (*i'*), $i \neq i' \in \{1...NS\}; j \in \{1...NR\}$. The operating room cleaning constraint is:

$$\min_{i'>i \in \{1,...NS\}} \left[Tb(i',j) - Te(i,j) \right] \geq M(i,j) \cdot X(i',j) \cdot X(i,j) \tag{2}$$

The total idling time $UR(j)$ for operating room (*j*), over the entire scheduling horizon *SH*, can be expressed as:

$$UR(j) = \sum_{i=1}^{NS} \left(\min_{i'>i \in \{1,...NS\}} \left[Tb(i',j) \cdot X(i',j) - Te(i,j) \cdot X(i,j) \right] - M(i,j) \cdot X(i,j) \right) \tag{3}$$

The function "min" designates the minimum function. For surgery team allocations, binary decision variables *Y* are used as follows:

Y(i, k): Equals 1 if surgery (*i*) is assigned to team (*k*), and 0 otherwise, $i \in \{1...NS\}; k \in \{1...NT\}$. If the beginning and completion times of operation (*i*) by surgical team (*k*) are denoted by $Sb(i, k)$ and $Se(i, k)$ respectively, then:

$$Se(i,k) - Sb(i,k) \geq D(i) \bullet Y(i,k) \tag{4}$$

Usually, when a surgical team (*k*) performs several surgical procedure over the scheduling horizon, it is required to take a break period $R(i, k)$ after completing surgery (*i*) and before starting the next scheduled surgery (*i'*). Such requirement is described by constraint (5).

$$\min_{i'>i\in\{1,...NS\}}\left[Sb(i',k)-Se(i,k)\right]\geq R(i,k)\cdot Y(i',k)\cdot Y(i,k) \tag{5}$$

The break period duration $R(i, k)$ is usually, proportional to the duration of the completed surgical procedure (other criteria can also be considered such as the time of the day the surgery is completed). In this study, the break period duration is assumed to be linearly proportional to the completed procedure duration. This is described by constraint (6), where $i\in\{1...NS\}$; $k\in\{1...NT\}$; a, b real positives.

$$R(i,k) = [a +b\bullet D(i)]\bullet Y(i,k) \tag{6}$$

In constraints (2), (3) and (5), variables $Tb(i,...)$, $Sb(i,...)$, must be ordered according to their surgical procedure indexes: if surgery (i) precedes surgery (i'), then $Tb(i,...)< Tb(i',...)$ and $Sb(i,...)<Sb(i',...)$. Binary variables are also related in a way that, if $X(i, j)=Y(i, k)$, then equalities: $Tb(i, j)=Sb(i, k)$ and $Te(i,j)=Se(i,k)$, must be both satisfied. Moreover, for each surgical procedure (i), $i\in\{1...NS\}$, the binary variables must respect constraint (7).

$$\sum_{j=1}^{NR}\sum_{k=1}^{NT}X(i,j)\cdot Y(i,k)=1 \tag{7}$$

Similarly to constraint (3), the total idling time $US(k)$ for surgical team (k), over the entire scheduling horizon SH, is expressed by constraint (8).

$$US(k) = \sum_{i=1}^{NS}\left(\min_{i'>i\in\{1,...NS\}}\left[Sb(i',k)\cdot Y(i',k)-Se(i,k)\cdot Y(i,k)\right]-R(i,k)\cdot Y(i,k)\right) \tag{8}$$

The completion date of all tasks associated with room (j) over the scheduling horizon (SH) is $CR(j)$, $j\in\{1...NR\}$. As expressed by constraint (9), this represents the sum of idle, busy, and cleaning period times for room (j).

$$CR(j) =UR(j)+\sum_{i=1}^{NS}\left[D(i)+ M(i,j)\right]\cdot X(i,j) \tag{9}$$

Likewise, the completion date of all tasks associated with surgical team (k) over the scheduling horizon (SH) is $CS(k)$, $k\in\{1...NT\}$. As expressed by constraint (10), this represents the sum of idle, busy, and break period times for team (k).

$$CS(k) = US(k) + \sum_{i=1}^{NS}\left[D(i) + R(i,k)\right]\cdot Y(i,k) \tag{10}$$

For optimizing both operating room and surgical team utilization, let α be the weight coefficient, assigned by management team, to the operating room utilization metric in the efficient operation of the system, and β the weight factor indicator for surgical team utilization metric. Based on constraints (3) and (8), these two objectives can be merged into the single objective constraint (11), with $\alpha+\beta=1$.

$$\min[\alpha \bullet \max[UR(j)] + \beta \bullet \max[US(k)]] \tag{11}$$

The function "max" designates the maximum function. Minimizing surgery completion times is equivalent to minimizing constraint (11) for all defined indexes, $i \in \{1...NS\}$; $j \in \{1...NR\}$; $k \in \{1...NT\}$ over the scheduling horizon (*SH*), subject to constraints (1), (2), (4), (5), (6), (7) presented above, and to the constraints (12) to (16) below.

$$\alpha + \beta = 1 \tag{12}$$

$$CR(j) \leq SH \tag{13}$$

$$CS(k) \leq SH \tag{14}$$

$$D(i) \cong N(\mu_d, \sigma_d) \tag{15}$$

$$M(i,j) \cong N(\mu_m, \sigma_m) \tag{16}$$

In constraint (12), parameters α and β give the model the flexibility to prioritize optimizing operating rooms usage over surgical team and vice versa. A value $\alpha = 0$ means the goal is to maximize surgical staff usage, while $\beta = 0$ means the goal is to maximize operating room usage. Constraints (15) and (16), describe the normally distributed procedure and room maintenance. The model described above is nonlinear, since it involves products of variables in constraint (7), and nonlinear functions (minimum) in constraints (2), (3), (5) and (8). In the next section, based on the nonlinear model, an approximated linear program is deduced, and a heuristic is defined as a solving method.

4. LINEAR PROGRAMMING MODEL

In the following, few simplifying assumptions are introduced to transform the nonlinear model, presented in the previous section, to a linear form that can be solved using linear programming method. Let us assume that a room cleaning duration depends only to the type of surgery performed, and not on room designs or equipment. Thus, constraint (16) is replaced by constraint (17).

$$M(i) \cong N(\mu_m, \sigma_m) \tag{17}$$

When break period durations $R(i, k)$ are independent from surgical teams, and depend only on performed surgical procedures, constraint (6) is replaced by constraint (18).

$$R(i) = [a + b \bullet D(i)] \tag{18}$$

Assuming that all surgical procedures are indexed based on their order in their assigned resource (room, surgical team) queues constraints (1), (2), (3), (5), (8), (9) and (10), respectively, can be replaced by constraints (19), (20), (21), (22), (23), (24), and (25) correspondingly.

$$Te(i,j) - Tb(i,j) \geq D(i) \tag{19}$$

$$Tb(i+1,j) - Te(i,j) \geq M(i) \tag{20}$$

$$UR(j) = \sum_{i=1}^{NS} [Tb(i+1,j) - Te(i,j) - M(i)] \cdot X(i,j) \tag{21}$$

$$Sb(i+1,k) - Se(i,k) \geq R(i) \tag{22}$$

$$US(k) = \sum_{i=1}^{NS} \left[Sb(i+1,k) - Se(i,k) - R(i) \right] \cdot Y(i,k) \tag{23}$$

$$CR(j) = UR(j) + \sum_{i=1}^{NS} \left[D(i) + M(i) \right] \cdot X(i,j) \tag{24}$$

$$CS(k) = US(k) + \sum_{i=1}^{NS} \left[D(i) + R(i) \right] \cdot Y(i,k) \tag{25}$$

Consequently, the linear program is formulated as minimizing objective (11) subject to constraints (7), (12), (13), (14), (15), (17), and all constraints from (18) to (25).

Many approaches were used in the literature to solve linear program based model for surgery scheduling problem. A branch and price approach is used in (Fei, Chu, Meskens, & Artiba, 2008). The algorithm is based on a column generation approach, where each column represents a schedule for one operating room generated by solving a sub problem of the single operating room case. In (Santibáñez, Begen, & Atkins, 2007), the emphasis is on scheduling surgical blocks considering different surgical specialties. In (Fei, Meskens, & Chu, 2010), the scheduling problem is modeled as two-stage hybrid flow-shop problem and solved using hybrid genetic algorithm. The linear program described above, is solved using a heuristic that is described in the next section.

5. PROPOSED HEURISTIC SOLUTION APPROACH

The solution approach is based on surgery selection rules, programmed using computer codes and spreadsheets (*Microsoft Visual basic, Microsoft Excel*). The selection rules are: *surgical procedure with shortest duration first, surgical procedure with longest duration first, random selection of a surgical procedure*. Schedules obtained using these rules are compared with regards to the objective function (11), and classified based on their resource utilization best score, corresponding to lowest *UR* and *US* value using constraints (21) and (23). For example for the surgical procedure with shortest duration first strategy, the algorithm proceeds iteratively by rearranging the initial list of surgical procedures by increasing durations. The next phase is to update all surgeon and room data to match the produced list. A schedule is computed by screening the ordered list (top-to-bottom) and assigning the earliest start time for a surgical procedure based on its resource availability information. If a resource is not available (room and/or surgical team), the surgery is labeled as unscheduled, and the algorithm move to the next surgical procedure in the list. Two subroutines are used to update surgical team, and room availabilities. These subroutines are constantly accessed and updated by the scheduling algorithm using the scheduling constraints. All durations are entered using mean value and variance using a spreadsheet (*Microsoft Excel*). The schedule computing program is depicted in Figure 1.

Once all surgeries are scheduled according to one strategy (priority rule), the program on Figure 1 restarts again by selecting another strategy. All schedules found using the three strategies are evaluated with regards to the objective function (11). Although, using priority rules does not find an optimal schedule, the proposed program is flexible, and easy to use and to improve by incorporating other scheduling strategies.

Figure 1. Surgery scheduling algorithm flow chart

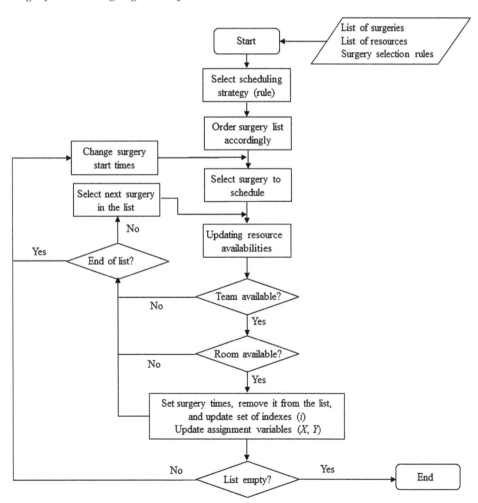

6. ILLUSTRATIVE EXAMPLE

A Canadian public hospital for a town of more than 120,000 people is considered in this example. The increase in surgical demands, results in a longer waiting time to access care. Figure 2 provides a classification of surgical procedures, by wait time, during a six month observation period. Such information is useful for planning elective surgery scheduling. More than 34% of patients waited 3 months to access care, while 22% waited a year or more. The waiting time is expected to increase, while resource are less and less available. In this example, operating room booking clerks are responsible for scheduling patient surgeries, and entering patient information into the hospital computerized system, so a surgical waitlist can be generated. Approximately, 400 new patients are added to the waiting list every month. A schedule is produced every week, and scheduled patients are notified on the surgery date and on the required preoperative tests and diagnosis. The increase in surgical demands with limited resources require the need to improve resources utilization and procedure scheduling.

Analyses were conducted for 10 operating rooms shared between 12 surgery teams. Due to the lack of data, surgery procedure durations were considered deterministic. Parameters α and β give are equally set to 0.5, which means that the same importance where given to surgery team and operating room utilizations. To study the effect of time horizon (SH) on surgery schedule, a week schedule (5 working days) is determined using two approaches: daily scheduling, where the algorithm is applied on a one-day surgery list; and weekly scheduling, where the algorithm is applied on a one-week surgery list.

7. RESULTS AND DISCUSSION

The make span is defined as the maximum time duration between the start of the first surgery to the completion of the last one in the list (daily or weekly). A comparison between the daily, weekly and actual schedule (used in the hospital) with regards to the make span (in minutes) is provided, for each week day in Table 1.

Figure 2. Classification of performed elective surgeries by wait time, from January to June 2010 (Source: Statistics Canada)

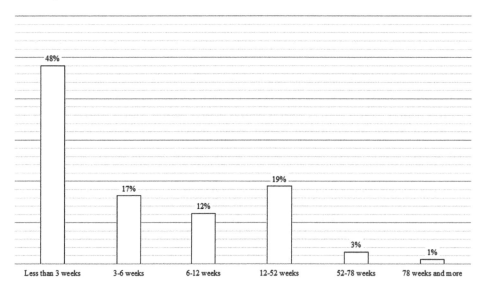

Table 1. Make span (in minutes) and number of scheduled surgeries (NSS)

Day	Actual schedule		Daily based scheduling		Weekly based scheduling	
	NSS	Make span	*NSS*	Make span	*NSS*	Make span
Day 1	31	520	31	480	33	480
Day 2	25	520	25	520	28	470
Day 3	25	480	25	440	30	480
Day 4	28	500	28	460	30	470
Day 5	38	600	38	520	26	480
Total	147	2620	147	2420	147	2380

From Table 1, the heuristic did improve surgery scheduling when compared to the actual schedule, and the make span is reduced. However, the improvement did vary according to the scheduling criteria (weekly vs. daily). The total make span over a week using daily based scheduling is 2420 min, and 2380 min when using weekly based scheduling. The same remark applies for each week day, where the make span varied between 470 min and 480 min for weekly schedule and between 440 min to 520 min for daily schedule. Reducing the make span means better resources utilization, and offers flexibility to integrate add on cases into the off-line schedule with reduced over time cost. Also, a bigger number of scheduled surgeries (*NSS*) reduces patient access waiting time to healthcare services. The proposed schedule strategies (daily and weekly) led towards better operating room utilization of and shorter idling periods, when compared with the schedule in use at the hospital. Parameters α and β allow managers to prioritize infrastructure or human resources according to their availability and cost.

8. CONCLUSION

In this study a mathematical model for elective surgery scheduling is proposed. The objective of the model is to improve resource utilizations. After linearization, the proposed model is transformed to a linear mathematical program that is solved using heuristic approach. The program computes different surgery schedules using a set of priority rules using surgery duration length as criteria, or random selection criteria. The program is tested on an illustrative example, and the obtained results show that the scheduling approach improved resource utilizations. In future research, simulation will be used to test the robustness of the proposed approach using random distribution for surgical procedure and room maintenance times. A key strength of simulation is the ability to model the behavior of a system as it develops over time and will allow significant exploration of multiple options. Like this study, most of studies focused on maximizing resource utilizations using mathematical programming models. With the perspective of using discrete event simulation approach, our future focus is toward the dynamic scheduling of add-on cases, by conducting experimentation with different algorithms and discrete event models as initiated in the study by (Dexter, Macario, & Traub, 1999).

REFERENCES

Aringhieri, R., Landa, P., Soriano, P., Tànfani, E., & Testi, A. (2015). A two level metaheuristic for the operating room scheduling and assignment problem. *Computers & Operations Research, 54*, 21–34. doi:10.1016/j.cor.2014.08.014

Berg, B. P., Denton, B. T., Erdogan, S. A., Rohleder, T., & Huschka, T. (2014). Optimal booking and scheduling in outpatient procedure centers. *Computers & Operations Research, 50*, 24–37. doi:10.1016/j.cor.2014.04.007

Bouguerra, A., Sauvey, C., & Sauer, N. (2015, May). *Mathematical model for maximizing operating rooms utilization.* Paper presented at the 15th IFAC/IEEE/IFIP/IFORS Symposium on Information Control Problems in Manufacturing INCOM'2015, Ottawa, Canada. 10.1016/j.ifacol.2015.06.068

Burke, E. K., & Riise, A. (2008, August). *Surgery Allocation and Scheduling.* Paper presented at the 7th International Conference on the Practice and Theory of Automated Timetabling, Montreal, Canada.

Cardoen, B., Demeulemeester, E., & Beliën, J. (2009). Operating room planning and scheduling: A literature review. *European Journal of Operational Research, 1016*(10), 14–25.

Cardoen, B., Demeulemeester, E., & Beliën, J. (2010). Operating room planning and scheduling: A literature review. *European Journal of Operational Research, 201*(3), 921–932. doi:10.1016/j.ejor.2009.04.011

Denton, B., Viapiano, J., & Vogl, A. (2007). Optimization of surgery sequencing and scheduling decisions under uncertainty. *Health Care Management Science, 10*(1), 13–24. doi:10.100710729-006-9005-4 PMID:17323652

Dexter, F. (1999). An operation room scheduling strategy to maximize the use of operation rooms. *Anesthesia and Analgesia, 89*(1), 7–20. PMID:10389771

Dexter, F., Macario, A., & Traub, R. D. (1999). Which algorithm for scheduling add-on elective cases maximizes operating room utilization? Use of bin packing algorithms and fuzzy constraints in operating room management. *Anesthesiology, 91*(5), 1491–1500. doi:10.1097/00000542-199911000-00043 PMID:10551602

Erdogan, S. A., & Denton, B. T. (2011). Surgery planning and scheduling. In J. J. Cochran, L. A. Cox, P. Keskinocak, J. Kharoufeh, & J. C. Smith (Eds.), *Wiley Encyclopedia of Operations Research and Management Science.* doi:10.1002/9780470400531.eorms0861

Fei, H., Chu, C., Meskens, N., & Artiba, A. (2008). Solving surgical cases assignment problem by a branch-and-price approach. *International Journal of Production Economics, 112*(1), pp. 96-108.

Fei, H., Meskens, N., & Chu, C. (2010). A planning and scheduling problem for an operating theatre using an open scheduling strategy. *Computers & Industrial Engineering, 58*(2), 221–230. doi:10.1016/j.cie.2009.02.012

Gerchak, Y., Gupta, D., & Henig, M. (1996). Reservation planning for elective surgery under uncertain demand for emergency surgery. *Management Science, 42*(3), 321–334. doi:10.1287/mnsc.42.3.321

Guinet, A., & Chaabane, S. (2003). Operating theatre planning. *International Journal of Production Economics*, *85*(1), 69–81. doi:10.1016/S0925-5273(03)00087-2

Hans, E. W., Wullink, G., Van Houdenhoven, M., & Kazemier, G. (2008). Robust surgery loading. *European Journal of Operational Research*, *185*(3), 1038–1050. doi:10.1016/j.ejor.2006.08.022

Health Care Financial Management Association. (2005). *Achieving operating room efficiency through process integration*. Technical Report, US National Library of Medicine, National Institutes of Health. *PubMed*, *57*(3), 113–119.

Huh, W. T., Liu, N., & Truong, V. A. (2013). Multi-resource allocation scheduling in dynamic environments. *Manufacturing & Service Operations Management*, *15*(2), 280–291. doi:10.1287/msom.1120.0415

Koksalmis, E., Hancerliogullari, K. O., & Hancerliogullari, G. (2014, May). *How to schedule surgical operations into operating rooms? An application in Turkey*. Paper presented at the IIE Industrial and Systems Engineering Research Conference, Montreal, Canada.

Lamiri, M., Xie, X., Dolgui, A., & Grimaud, F. (2008). A stochastic model for operating room planning with elective and emergency demand for surgery. *European Journal of Operational Research*, *185*(3), 1026–1037. doi:10.1016/j.ejor.2006.02.057

Magerlein, J. M., & Martin, J. B. (1978). Surgical demand scheduling: A review. *Health Services Research*, *13*, 418–433. PMID:367987

Min, D., & Yih, Y. (2010a). An elective surgery scheduling problem considering patient priority. *Computers & Operations Research*, *37*(6), 1091–1099. doi:10.1016/j.cor.2009.09.016

Min, D., & Yih, Y. (2010b). Scheduling elective surgery under uncertainty and downstream capacity constraints. *European Journal of Operational Research*, *206*(3), 642–652. doi:10.1016/j.ejor.2010.03.014

Molina-Pariente, J. M., Fernandez-Viagas, V., & Framinan, J. M. (2015). Integrated operating room planning and scheduling problem with assistant surgeon dependent surgery durations. *Computers & Industrial Engineering*, *82*, 8–20. doi:10.1016/j.cie.2015.01.006

Santibáñez, P., Begen, M., & Atkins, D. (2007). Surgical block scheduling in a system of hospitals: An application to resource and wait list management in a British Columbia health authority. *Health Care Management Science*, *10*(3), 269–282. doi:10.100710729-007-9019-6 PMID:17695137

Saremi, A., Jula, P., ElMekkawy, T., & Wang, G. G. (2013). Appointment scheduling of outpatient surgical services in a multistage operating room department. *International Journal of Production Economics*, *141*(2), 646–658. doi:10.1016/j.ijpe.2012.10.004

Sciomachen, A., Tànfani, E., & Testi, A. (2005). Simulation models for optimal schedules of operating theatres. *International Journal of Simulation*, *6*, 26–34.

Tyler, D. C., Pasquariello, C. A., & Chen, C. H. (2003). Determining Optimum Operating Room Utilization. *Anesthesia and Analgesia*, *96*(4), 1114–1121. doi:10.1213/01.ANE.0000050561.41552.A6 PMID:12651670

Van Houdenhoven, M., Van Oostrum, J. M., Hans, E. W., Wullink, G., & Kazemier, G. (2007). Improving operating room efficiency by applying bin-packing and portfolio techniques to surgical case scheduling. *Anesthesia and Analgesia, 105*(3), 707–714. doi:10.1213/01.ane.0000277492.90805.0f PMID:17717228

Van Oostrum, J. M., Van Houdenhoven, M., Hurink, J. L., Hans, E. W., Wullink, G., & Kazemier, G. (2008). A master surgical scheduling approach for cyclic scheduling in operating room departments. *OR-Spektrum, 30*(2), 355–374. doi:10.100700291-006-0068-x

Wullink, G., Van Houdenhoven, M., Hans, E. W., Van Oostrum, J. M., Van der Lans, M., & Kazemier, G. (2007). Closing emergency operating rooms improves efficiency. *Journal of Medical Systems, 31*(6), 543–546. doi:10.100710916-007-9096-6 PMID:18041289

Xiang, W., Yin, J., & Lim, G. (2015). A short-term operating room surgery scheduling problem integrating multiple nurses' roster constraints. *Artificial Intelligence in Medicine, 63*(2), 91–106. doi:10.1016/j.artmed.2014.12.005 PMID:25563674

Zhao, Z., & Li, X. (2014). Scheduling elective surgeries with sequence-dependent setup times to multiple operating rooms using constraint programming. *Operations Research for Health Care, 3*(3), 160–167. doi:10.1016/j.orhc.2014.05.003

This research was previously published in Effective Methods for Modern Healthcare Service Quality and Evaluation edited by Panagiotis Manolitzas, Evangelos Grigoroudis, Nikolaos Matsatsinis, and Denis Yannacopoulos; pages 90-108, copyright year 2016 by Medical Information Science Reference (an imprint of IGI Global).

Chapter 19
Application of Fuzzy Soft Set in Patients' Prioritization

Samira Abbagholizadeh Rahimi
Université Laval, Canada

ABSTRACT

Based on studies, access to healthcare services and long waiting time is one of the main issues in many countries including Canada and United States. Healthcare organizations can't increase their limited resources nor treat all patients simultaneously. Then, patients' access to these services should be prioritized in a way that best uses the scarce resources and insures patients' safety. Prioritization is essential and inevitable not only because of resource shortage, which have not been improved during years, but also because it is a crucial issue that could contribute to the capability and stability of the healthcare systems, and most importantly to patients' safety. On the other hand, inappropriate prioritization of patients waiting for treatment, could affect directly on inefficiencies in healthcare delivery, quality of care, and most importantly on patients' safety and their quality of life and satisfaction. Inspired by these facts, in this chapter the importance of patients' prioritization and using fuzzy logic in this area will be discussed, and a novel hybrid framework using fuzzy soft sets for patients' prioritization will be proposed. The proposed framework may have a significant impact on patients' safety, and on both medical community and the public's faith in justice and equity.

INTRODUCTION

Medical knowledge and clinical practices are always associated with considerable amounts of uncertainty and about everything in medicine is inevitably vague (Sadegh-Zadeh, 2012). Many complicated problems like patients' prioritization problem involves such uncertainties. Despite this issue's importance, (to the best of our knowledge) no valid tool has been proposed in the literature to prioritize patients for medical treatment considering these uncertainties, and associated risks all together. To this end, this chapter will give useful impulses to face these major challenges in patients' prioritization, by developing a novel integrated framework which covers the current drawbacks and will provide theoretical solutions for them. This chapter focuses on uncertainties in clinicians' decisions and involving associated risks that

DOI: 10.4018/978-1-7998-2451-0.ch019

Copyright © 2020, IGI Global. Copying or distributing in print or electronic forms without written permission of IGI Global is prohibited.

could threaten patients while they are waiting for treatment, and proposes a novel integrated framework to deal with these crucial issues.

This problem, cannot be solved using classical mathematic methods. There are several well-known theories (such as theory of probability, theory of fuzzy sets, theory of vague sets, theory of interval mathematics, and etc.) to describe uncertainty, but all of these theories have their inherit difficulties as Molodtsov (1999) mentioned in his paper. The reason for these difficulties is, possibly, the inadequacy of the parameterization tool of the theories (Celik & Yamak, 2013). To overcome these difficulties, Molodtsov initiated the concept of soft sets as a new mathematical tool for dealing with uncertainties (Molodtsov, 1999). This so-called soft set theory seems to be free from the difficulties affecting the existing methods (Maji et al., 2003).

Maji et al. (2001) defined various operators for soft set theory. and in 2010, Ali & Shabir (2010) made some improvements of the introduced operations by Maji et al. Fundamental properties of soft sets has been defined by Aktas and Cagman (2007). They combined the soft set theory and group theory to defined soft groups. Some new operation were studied in Ali & Shabir (2010), Ali et al. (2009), and Feng and Li (2013). They gave the new concept of the soft product in soft set theory and discussed generalized decision making schemes, and many other researchers such as Li (2014), Li and& Ren(2015), and Yu and Li (2014) have studied soft set theory in different aspects.

Recently, research works on soft sets in different industries are very active and progressing rapidly. Applications of fuzzy soft set theory in many disciplines and real life situations have been studied by many researchers but, its application in healthcare industry is in its infancy stages. To the best of our knowledge this is the first time in literature that such novel integrated framework is introduced for patients' prioritization. This chapter focuses on developing an interdisciplinary, systematic and innovative prioritization framework which is inspired by Celik and Yamak (2013) work on medical diagnosis. The proposed framework considers uncertainty, multiple criteria, risks and their inherent interactions to prioritize patients' access to healthcare services. In this chapter, Analytical Network Process (ANP) is used to find relative importance weights of criteria and risks considering their possible interactions. Then, by using the notion of a fuzzy soft set together with arithmetic operations on fuzzy number, authors introduce how fuzzy soft set technology could be used for patients' prioritization.

The rest of the chapter is organized as follows. In the next two sections prioritization of patients' access to healthcare services, the related literature review and shortcomings are discussed in details. Basics of Fuzzy soft set theory are explained briefly after. Then the proposed framework is discussed. To illustrate the application and effectiveness of the proposed framework, a numerical example in surgery ward is illustrated. In order to demonstrate robustness of the proposed method, sensitivity analysis under various criteria/risks-weight-change scenarios is performed and the results are discussed. Finally, the proposed framework is compared with some of well-known Multi Criteria Decision Making (MCDM) methods in the comparison section to show its benefits and advantages. This chapter concludes with a summary of the chapter, a discussion on the major contribution of this framework and future directions.

PRIORITIZING PATIENTS ACCESS TO HEALTHCARE SERVICES

Patients in the Organization for Economic Co-operation and Development (OECD) countries (including United States and Canada) continue to wait too long to receive medically necessary treatment. Waiting times' situation not only have not been improved during years till 2016, but also they have gotten slightly worse (Barua, 2015). One of the main reasons for long waiting times is imbalance between demand and availability of scarce resources in healthcare organizations. Clinicians can't treat all patients simultaneously. Due to high costs, managers can't increase number of their limited resources either. Then, patients' access to these services should be prioritized in a way that best uses existence scarce resources, and insure patients' safety.

However, prioritization may not be the only option responding to limited resources in health care, but it may be one of the best options in identification of high risk patients and increasing safety of patients' waiting for treatment. There are other alternative like increasing efficiency or the overall amount spent for health care, and rationing by delay. But, rationing implicitly goes along with problems in principle (Nagel & Lauerer, 2016), and is not sufficiently narrowing the gap that occurs between demand and supply (Williams et al., 2012). Rationing regularly refers to actual withholding of health services, while prioritization describes a systematic and comprehensive approach to analyze what is more and what is less important. It leads to a ranking order (Meyer & Raspe, 2012) and a precise selection of patients' for treatment. Prioritization in healthcare domain is preferable approach over implicit approaches like rationing when tight budgets force clinicians to make allocation decisions (Nagel & Lauerer, 2016). Prioritization helps to allocate scare resources fairly and transparently (Nagel & Lauerer, 2016).

Currently, in healthcare systems after patients are referred to treatment, their situation is examined. If patients have non-life threatening condition, they will be enrolled on a first-come, first serve basis (Abbasgholizadeh Rahimi et al., 2016). But if their conditions are life-threatening they will be registered two or three emergency groups/priority levels. Higher priority-patients will be selected for service prior to those with a lower priority, regardless of when they are placed on the list (Barua, 2015). In the literature review, the comprehensive explanation of the different developed/used prioritization tools will be explained in details.

Inappropriate prioritization of patients waiting for treatment, affect directly on inefficiencies in health care delivery, quality of care, and most importantly on patients' medical conditions. Reports regarding the harms related to long waiting times and inappropriate prioritization of patients on waiting list are increasing. These harms include:

- Poorer medical results from care and decreased quality of life,
- Reduction in effectiveness of treatment (Day, 2013),
- Increased pain, and risk of adverse events (Barua & Esmail, 2013),
- Mortality (Prentice & Pizer, 2007), and so more.

An appropriate patients' prioritization can play an important role in diminishing these undesirable outcomes. Besides, it can have significant impact on both medical community and public's faith in justice and equity.

An excellent prioritization in health system requires not only good recognition of the system, expertise to analyze and understand the information (related to patients, clinicians and other resources) but also to consider and organize that information regularly in a way to make an adequate decision and to promote a collaboration among key stakeholders (e.g. managers, clinicians, patients).

There are different major challenging aspects in prioritization of patients' access to healthcare services as (Abbasgholizadeh Rahimi et al., 2016):

- How to involve confronting trade-offs between multiple, often conflicting, factors?
- How can groups of clinicians' opinions be simultaneously involved in the decision making procedure?
- How can patients and their families be involved in the decisions?
- What are the main criteria for prioritizing patients?
- What are the risks that could threaten patients on waiting list?
- How important are selected risks and criteria compared to each other?
- How can we handle uncertainties in clinicians' decisions in the procedure be handled?
- How dynamic nature of the health system could be considered in prioritization of patients?

Currently, access to healthcare services are not prioritized in a way that best uses limited resources and to ensure a transparent, equal and accurate rank of patients on waiting lists. There is no reliable and comprehensive method of assessing the relative priority of patients on waiting lists, and some researchers (Peacock et al., 2009;Domènech et al., 2013;Abbasgholizadeh Rahimi et al., 2014, 2016; Mullen, 2003; Russell et al., 2003; Abbasgholizadeh Rahimi & Jamshidi, 2014; Comas et al., 2008) in their studies stressed the need for an interdisciplinary and collaborative research to explore systematic and precise prioritization framework. Although some prioritization approaches have been developed for this aim but, they have several major shortcomings (Abbasgholizadeh Rahimi et al., 2016). following, we will discuss on how patients are prioritized currently and what are their main shortcomings.

LITERATURE REVIEW

The earliest publications on 'priorities in medicine' are from England (Butterfield, 1968; Godber, 1970) and Denmark (Pornak & Raspe, 2015), Norway was the first country worldwide that considered prioritization on a national level (Raspe, 2016).

Patients' prioritization is a complex decision making process and according to Hadorn (2000), "the normative basis for prioritization is that patients with more urgent conditions should receive services ahead of those with less urgent conditions, and patients with approximately the same degree of urgency should wait about the same length of time". Broadly, patients' priority can be defined by the position of patient in the waiting queue (leading to e.g., first-come, first-served (FCFS)), patient specific characteristics or the contribution to an objective function or to a combination of factors (Riet & Demeulemeester, 2015).

Some authors (Davis & Johnson, 1998; Fordyce & Phillips, 1970; Hadorn, 2000; Lack et al., 2000), (Domènech et al., 2013; Mariotti et al., 2014; Dowseya et al., 2014; Montoya et al., 2014) proposed various prioritization scoring systems to assist health professionals to make better decisions in determining which patient receive treatment sooner than others. A scoring system or points system consists of a method for deciding patients' relative priorities for treatment. In this type of prioritization system, a weighted set of criteria is proposed and each patient is assessed with respect to every criterion. The sum of all the values gives a "total score" for each patient, which is used to rank patients between them.

Pioneer scoring systems introduced in 1990s were criticized for being arbitrary and resulting in significant numbers of patients being mistakenly denied treatment (sometimes with fatal consequences). However, scoring systems have been proposed and are largely in use in:

- Italy,
- Sweden,
- New Zealand,
- United Kingdom,
- Norway,
- Germany,
- Canada and other OECD countries.

For instance, currently used scoring tools in Canada are in the following five main clinical areas:

- i.e. Cataract surgery,
- General surgery procedures,
- Hip and knee replacement,
- Magnetic resonance imaging scanning,
- Children's mental health.

Prioritization formulae were also developed (mostly by considering specific criteria like waiting time or emergency) with the aim of reducing waiting times and improving access of patients to healthcare services, Mullen (2003) gave a complete review of developed prioritization formulas. A summary of Mullen's review is shown in Table 1.

Naylor et al. (1993) suggested to assign to each patient, at referral's moment, a priority code based on an Urgency Rating Scale (URS). Prioritization based on other considerations has also been proposed for situations where the risk of death is low (Hadorn, 2000). In Dolan and Cookson's (2000) work the different principles of priority-setting decision makings have been focused qualitatively (e.g. need, equity and fairness principles). Nagel and Lauerer (2016) comprehensively discussed the different prioritization factors in their book and MacCormick et al. (2003) thoroughly discussed the different prioritization factors and their weighing, in a review study on patients' prioritization systems.

The prioritization has been rarely evaluated and considered within scheduling problem for surgical patients as well. However, in Testi et al. (2008) and Valente et al. (2009), the subset of patients to be operated on among the patients on waiting list and their order of admission (based on the prioritization system) was introduced which were based on both the waiting time of the patient since its referral and its urgency status. Valente et al. (2009) developed a model to prioritize access to elective surgery on the basis of clinical urgency and waiting time. While, Testi et al. (2008) in their research emphasized the importance of using both urgency related groups (URGs) and scoring system for scheduling patients' admissions in an explicit and transparent way, and a similar approach was also used in Min and Yih (2010) . Most recently, in 2015, Addis et al. considered the problem of selecting a set of patients among a given waiting list of elective patients and assigning them to a set of available operating room blocks. In their study, each patient was prioritized by a recommended maximum waiting time.

In emergency departments (EDs) upon their arrival to the ED, patients have a triage interview, then the triage nurse prioritizes them to three or five clinically distinct levels based on their vital signs, present illnesses and past medical history. The contemporary Emergency Severity Index (ESI) triage system sorts patients into five clinically distinct levels in EDs. ESI level 1 or level 2 are assigned to the most acutely-ill patients, and ESI levels 3, 4, and 5 are assigned to the lowest acutely-ill patients. There are several serious limitation of using the ESI triage sorting system in EDs; physicians and nurses in current triage

Table 1. Developed prioritization formulae

Description	Proposed Prioritization Formula	Description
(Luckman et al., 1969)	$P = S^a \, DT^{w^b}$	where P= priority score; S =social factor (1–3);D= disability factor (1–3); w=deterioration factor(1–3); T = time on waiting list(weeks); a and b are constants.
(Fordyce & Phillips, 1970),	$AI=(aS)(bD)(T)c^w$	where S =social factor; D =disability factor (1–5); w =urgency of condition (0–5); T=time on waiting list (weeks); a, b and c are constants.
(Phoenix, 1972)	$P = DT^{\sqrt{w}}$	Luckman J. (1969) proposed formula simplified to this one
(Eltringham & Clare, 1973)	$P=800(1 - e^{-kT})$	where P =patient's priority score; k = f(urgency);T =time on waiting list.
(Clare, 1973)	$P = \dfrac{c^w T}{\sqrt{L}}$	where P =priority score; L= expected length of stay; c =constant; w =urgency or deterioration factor; T= time on waiting list.
(Culyer & Cullis, 1976)	$P = \dfrac{c^w \left(T + 28\right)}{\sqrt{L}}$	
(Langham & Thorogood, 1996) ; (Soljak, 1997); (Hadorn & Holmes, 1997),	$P = \sum\limits_{i=1}^{5} S_i$	where P= priority score; S_i= score for ith clinical factor
(Dennett & Parry, 1998),	$P = \sum\limits_{i=1}^{3} A_i \cdot \sum\limits_{j=1}^{2} B_j$	where P= total priority score; A_i= score on ith element of the clinical severity criterion (i =1 suffering (physical or mental) (values 0, 3, 5 or 7);i = 2 disability (1, 3, 5 or 7); i = 3 clinical cost of delay (1, 3 or 6)); B_j=score on jth element of the capacity to benefit criterion (j = 1 degree of improvement anticipated; j = 2 likelihood of improvement).
(Seddon et al., 1999),	$P = E\sum\limits_{i=1}^{5} S_i$	where E =(100 – age)/30 if age > 70
(Lack et al., 2000)	$P = \sum\limits_{i=1}^{5} S_i . w_i + \left(\dfrac{5t}{m} - 1\right)^2$	where t = time already waited and m=waiting time of the longest waiter.

system are not able to determine how to proceed when they faced with the scenario of multiple same level patients in the waiting room (Tanabe et al, 2005; Andersson et al., 2006). And, the main challenge is how to prioritize patients and how to identify who should proceed first for the treatment (Andersson et al., 2006). Moreover, patient medical state might change while waiting for treatment, which means that decisions should change dynamically as well (Claudio & Okudan, 2010).

The use of the utility theory to prioritize ED patients assigned to the same acuity level was recently increased. In 2010, Claudio and Okudan illustrated the use of the multi-attribute utility theory (MAUT) in patient prioritization using a hypothetical example. They explained the choice of MAUT due to the inherent uncertainty in ED settings, and that MAUT accounts for uncertainty (Ashour & Kremer, 2016).

Ashour and Okudan (2010) also prioritized patients in ED using MAUT, and considering patient age, gender, pain level, and the assigned ESI. These factors were not considered in the ESI algorithm nor in Claudio and Kudan's study (Claudio & Okudan, 2010).

Argon and Ziya (2009) in their study assumed that each customer arrives with a signal that can be used as an indicator for his/her identity. They considered three different prioritization policies i.e., highest-signal-first (HSF) policy, two-class policy, first-come-first-served (FCFS) policy, and the generalized cμ (GE-cμ) policy. Then, they compared these policies based on waiting cost. Their study showed that when the waiting cost is linear with time, HSF policy outperformed any finite class priority policy otherwise the two-class policy and the FCFS policy performed better than the HSF policy (Ashour & Kremer, 2016). Even though Argon and Ziya (2009) have described techniques to choose the better signal, they did not develop a way to prioritize patients who visit the ED.

Ashour and Kremer (2016) most recently developed a dynamic prioritization tool for EDs. They applied group technology (GT) concept to the triage process to develop a dynamic grouping and prioritization (DGP) algorithm. They implemented discrete event simulation (DES) to investigate the impact of the DGP algorithm on the performance measures of the ED system. Their study demonstrated that DGP algorithm outperforms the ESI algorithm by shortening patients' average length of stay (LOS), average time to bed (TTB), time in emergency room, and lowering the percentage of tardy patients and their associated risk in the system (Ashour & Kremer, 2016). Patients' prioritization has been considered also in other types of medical activities such as:

- Organ Transplant (Cholongitas et al., 2010; Cholongitas & Burroughs, 2012; Lin & Harris, 2012; Lavee & Brock, 2012; Abbasgholizadeh Rahimi & Jamshidi, 2014; Ahlert & Kliemt, 2013; Al-Ebbinia et al., 2016),
- Trauma (Fieldsa et al., 2013), (Andersson et al., 2006), and in
- Cardiothoracic ICU (Yang et al., 2013).

Despite all these efforts, some important points are still overlooked and major shortcomings in current prioritization systems need to be improved (Peacock et al., 2009; Domènech et al., 2013; Abbasgholizadeh Rahimi et al., 2014; Mullen, 2003; Russell et al., 2003). These shortcomings are explicitly stated in the following:

1. Current prioritization tools cannot ensure that the ranking results are robust to face uncertainty. Uncertainties are inherent to most of real-life decision making processes and particularly in medicine, where the lack of information, as well as its imprecision and conflicting nature are common facts (Noseworthy et al., 2003; Abbasgholizadeh Rahimi et al., 2016).
2. Associated risks that could threaten patients' health during the waiting time have been overlooked. In all patient-related procedures, presents' risks are associated with severe effects and unavoidable consequences which increase along with the waiting time. By considering these risks in the prioritization procedure, decision makers could make sure that patients with the highest risks (e.g. the risk of injury, stroke, disability or even death) will be selected first (Abbasgholizadeh Rahimi et al., 2016).
3. Lack of group decision making is another shortcoming of current prioritization tools which cause biased and inaccurate prioritization of patients (Abbasgholizadeh Rahimi et al., 2016). For instance, in surgery wards medical staff may have different priorities or concerns that could conflict with

surgeons' ones. But, at the end, surgeon is the only one who prioritizes patients based on his/her opinion. This may cause bias in the prioritization procedure, and dissatisfaction of other medical staff as well. To benefit from all surgery team members' knowledge and experience in prioritization procedure, other team member's assessments should be considered. Albeit, in order to have an accurate prioritization, the surgery team members should have different weights.

4. Possible interrelationships among criteria have been overlooked (Abbasgholizadeh Rahimi et al., 2016). Real life situations usually confirm possible interrelationships among decision criteria that can influence the final results. However, this issue rarely has been considered in patients' prioritization procedures up to date.

5. Dynamic behavior of system has rarely been considered. Practically, waiting lists are dynamic, new patients arrive and others quit continuously. Moreover, patients' condition evolve in time. Therefore, any prioritization procedure must take into account this dynamic behavior of the system in order to adequately support decision makers (Abbasgholizadeh Rahimi et al., 2016).

6. Last but not least, there is no systematic and comprehensive framework for patients' prioritization on waiting list.

Based upon the increasing number of demand for healthcare services and mentioned shortcomings of existing prioritization systems, there is need for a quantitative and qualitative approach that dynamically identifies and assesses the patients' priority and considers uncertainties and risks. The approach should improve the capability of prioritization systems to make differentiations among mix of patients, while lowering the cognitive stress and load on medical staff, which resulted from the dynamic nature of prioritization process and the complex environment of healthcare organizations, and aiding them to make better decisions. Methodology part of the chapter focuses on our developed methodologies to deal with some of the mentioned shortcomings in prioritization systems.

FUZZY SOFT SETS

In this section, authors give some known and useful definitions and notations regarding a soft set and a fuzzy soft set. The definitions and notions in this part may be found in references (Molodtsov, 1999; Celik & Yamak, 2013; Maji et al., 2003; De et al., 2001; Chetia & Das, 2010; Sanchez, 1979). Let U be an initial universal set and E be a set of parameters. The power set of U is denoted by P(U) and A is a subset of E.

Definition 1: A pair (F, A) is called a soft set over U, where F is a mapping given by F: A→P (U) (Molodtsov, 1999; Ali et al., 2009).

Definition 2: A fuzzy subset μ of U is defined as a map from U to [0, 1]. The family of all fuzzy subsets of U is denoted by F (U). Let $\mu, \nu \in$ F (U) and x $\in$ U. Then the union and intersection of μ and ν are defined in the following way (Zadeh, 1965):

$$(\mu \vee \nu)(x) = \mu(x) \vee \nu(x),$$

$$(\mu \wedge \nu)(x) = \mu(x) \wedge \nu(x),$$

$\mu \le \nu$ if and only if $\mu(x) \le \nu(x)$ for all x $\in$ U.

Definition 3: Let U be a common universe, E be a set of parameters and A $\subseteq$ E. Then a pair (F, A) is called a fuzzy soft set over U, where F is a mapping given by F: A$\rightarrow$F (U) (Maji et al., 2003).

Definition 4: For two fuzzy soft sets (F, A) and (G, B) over a common universe U, we say that (F, A) is a fuzzy soft subset of (G, B) if: (i) A $\subseteq$ B, (ii) F (a) $\le$ G (a) for all a $\in$ A. In this case, we write (F, A) $\subseteq$ (G, B) [26].

Proposition: Let (F, A) and (G, B) be two fuzzy soft sets over a common universe U, (Maji et al., 2001; Ali & Shabir, 2010) Then:

1. (F, A) $\cup$ (F, A) = (F, A),
2. (F, A) $\cap$ (F, A) = (F, A),
3. $\left(\left(F,\ A \right) \cup \left(G,\ B \right) \right)^{c} = (F,A)^{\circ} \cap (G,B)^{\circ}$,
4. $\left(\left(F,\ A \right) \cap \left(G,\ B \right) \right)^{c} = (F,A)^{\circ} \cup (G,B)^{\circ}$,
5. $\left(\left(F,\ A \right) \vee \left(G,\ B \right) \right)^{c} = (F,A)^{\circ} \wedge (G,B)^{\circ}$,
6. $\left(\left(F,\ A \right) \wedge \left(G,\ B \right) \right)^{c} = (F,A)^{\circ} \vee (G,B)^{\circ}$.

Definition 5:

1. A fuzzy subset μ on the universe of discourse $\mathbb{R}$ (the set of all real numbers) is convex if and only if for a, b $\in$ U μ (αa + βb) $\ge \mu$(a) $\wedge \mu$(b), where $\alpha + \beta = 1$ (Maji et al., 2003; Kaufmann & Gupta, 1991).
2. A fuzzy subset μ on the universe of discourse U is called a normal fuzzy subset if there exist $a_i \in U$ such that $\mu(a_i) = 1$ (Maji et al., 2003; Kaufmann & Gupta, 1991).
3. A fuzzy number is a fuzzy subset defined on the universe of discourse $\mathbb{R}$ which is both convex and normal. For more information on fuzzy numbers readers could refer to (Li, 2014; Li & Ren, 2015; Li & Liu, 2015).

Fuzzy number can take various forms such as Triangular Fuzzy Number (TFN), Trapezoidal Fuzzy Number, and Gaussian Fuzzy Number. TFN is the most popular form due to its simple membership function which is represented by three parameters as (a, b, c). The parameters a, b, and c denote the smallest possible value, the most promising value, and the largest possible value of the fuzzy number, respectively. And the membership function is defined as below (Maji et al., 2003; Kaufmann & Gupta, 1991).

$$\mu\left(u\right) = \begin{cases} 0 & if\ u < a, \\ \dfrac{u - a}{b - a} & if\ a \le u \le b, \\ \dfrac{c - u}{c - b} & if\ b \le u \le c, \\ 0 & if\ \ u \ge c\ . \end{cases}$$

If the membership function μ (u) is piecewise linear, then μ is said to be a trapezoidal fuzzy number. Now let μ and β be two triangular fuzzy numbers parameterized by the triplet $b_1 = (a_1,b_1,c_1)$ and $b_2 = (a_2,b_2,c_2)$ respectively.

Then addition and multiplication of μ and β are as below (Maji et al., 2003; Kaufmann & Gupta, 1991):

- $\mu \oplus \beta = \tilde{a}_2 \oplus \tilde{b}_2 = (a_1,a_2,a_3) \oplus (b_1, b_2, b_3) = (a_1+b_1, a_2+b_2, a_3+b_3)$
- $\mu \otimes \beta = \tilde{a}_2 \otimes \tilde{b}_2 = (a_1,a_2,a_3) \otimes (b_1, b_2, b_3) = (a_1 \times b_1, a_2 \times b_2, a_3 \times b_3)$

It is required to reduce a given fuzzy number into a single crisp representative value. This is called defuzzification operation. Then in the next step authors give the defuzzification method of a triangular fuzzy number. The defuzzification value t of a triangular fuzzy number (l, m, u) is equal to (Maji et al., 2003):

$$t = \frac{l + m + m + u}{4} \tag{1}$$

METHODOLOGY: FUZZY SOFT SET FOR PATIENTS' PRIORITIZATION

In Figure 1 an algorithm of our proposed framework for patients' prioritization using ANP and fuzzy arithmetic operations is presented. This approach focuses on shortcomings related to uncertainty, risks and interrelationship among criteria and risks in prioritizing patients' access to healthcare services.

Assume that there is a set of m patients, $P = \{p_1,p_2,p_3,...,p_m\}$, set of n criteria $C = \{c_1, c_2, c_3, ..., c_n\}$ (these criteria could be medical, social or other factors as explained in the previous chapter) related to a set of k risks $R = \{R_1, R_2, R_3, ..., R_k\}$. Authors apply fuzzy soft set theory to distinguish which patient's risks is high and is in priority to receive care and treatment considering uncertainty. For this, a fuzzy soft set (F, P) over C where F is a mapping $F: P \rightarrow F(C)$ is constructed.

This fuzzy soft set gives a relation matrix PC, called patient-criteria matrix, where the entries are fuzzy numbers $\tilde{p}$ parameterized by a triplet $(p - 1, p, p + 1)$. For instance, $\tilde{a}_{11}$ shows a fuzzy number for the first patient's situation considering first criterion. Then construct another fuzzy soft set (G, C) over R, where G is a mapping $G: C \rightarrow F(R)$. This fuzzy soft set gives a relation matrix CR, called criteria-risk matrix, where each element denotes the impact of the criteria for a certain risk. For instance, $\tilde{b}_{11}$ shows a fuzzy number for the first criterion's impact on first risk. These elements are also taken as triangular fuzzy numbers. Thus the general form of PC *matrix* is shown in Figure 1.

$$PC = \begin{array}{c} c_1\left(W_{C_1}\right) c_2\left(W_{C_2}\right) \cdots \cdots c_n\left(W_{C_n}\right) \\ \begin{bmatrix} \tilde{a}_{11} & \tilde{a}_{12} & \cdots & \cdots & \tilde{a}_{1n} \\ \tilde{a}_{21} & \tilde{a}_{22} & \cdots & \cdots & \vdots \\ \vdots & \vdots & \cdots & \cdots & \vdots \\ \vdots & \vdots & \cdots & \cdots & \vdots \\ \tilde{a}_{m1} & \tilde{a}_{m1} & \cdots & \cdots & \tilde{a}_{mn} \end{bmatrix} \end{array}$$

Figure 1. Systematic algorithm of proposed prioritization method

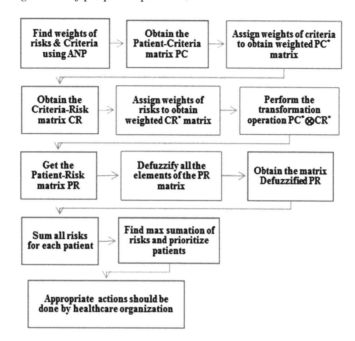

And the general form of *CR matrix* is:

$$CR = \begin{array}{c} \\ \\ c_1 \\ c_2 \\ \vdots \\ \vdots \\ c_n \end{array} \begin{array}{c} R_1\left(W_{R_1}\right) R_2\left(W_{R_2}\right) \ldots \ldots R_k\left(W_{R_n}\right) \\ \begin{bmatrix} \tilde{b}_{11} & \tilde{b}_{12} & \cdots & \cdots & \tilde{b}_{1k} \\ \tilde{b}_{21} & \tilde{b}_{22} & \cdots & \cdots & \tilde{b}_{2k} \\ \vdots & \vdots & \cdots & \cdots & \vdots \\ \vdots & \vdots & \cdots & \cdots & \vdots \\ \tilde{b}_{n1} & \tilde{b}_{n2} & \cdots & \cdots & \tilde{b}_{nk} \end{bmatrix} \end{array}$$

Since some risks have a higher impact than others, it's better to treat all risks uniquely. The risks that can cause the biggest losses, should have the biggest importance weights. It's the same for criteria, each criterion has a relative importance weight comparing to other criteria.

For finding each criterion's importance weight (i.e. W_C) and each risk's importance weight (i.e. W_R), medical experts should compare each risk to all other risks and also each criterion to all other criteria using a questionnaire which has been developed based on ANP method. The reason of using ANP technique in this framework is that, ANP enables us to consider all possible interrelationships among these criteria and risks. For further information on ANP approach please refer to Saaty & Özdemir (2005). Now each of k risk and n criterion have weights, which indicates risk's/criterion's importance in comparison to others.

The numbers inside parenthesis in PC and CR matrices are weights obtained using ANP methodology. In PC and CR matrices each criterion and each risk's weight should be multiplied in its related column to get the weighted PC and CR matrices which are shown by PC* and CR*. For instance, W_{C_1} (Weight of first criteria, C_1) should be multiplied in first column of CP matrix.

Now, after obtaining weighted PC (i.e. PC*) and weighted CR (i.e. CR*) matrices, the transformation operation PC*⊗CR* is performed, the Patient-Risk matrix (PR) would be as follows:

$$PR = \begin{array}{c} \\ p_1 \\ p_2 \\ \vdots \\ \vdots \\ p_m \end{array} \overset{\begin{array}{ccccc} R_1 & R_2 & \cdots & \cdots & R_k \end{array}}{\begin{bmatrix} \tilde{d}_{11} & \tilde{d}_{12} & \cdots & \cdots & \tilde{d}_{1k} \\ \tilde{d}_{21} & \tilde{d}_{22} & \cdots & \cdots & \tilde{d}_{2k} \\ \vdots & \vdots & \cdots & \cdots & \vdots \\ \vdots & \vdots & \cdots & \cdots & \vdots \\ \tilde{d}_{m1} & \tilde{d}_{m2} & \cdots & \cdots & \tilde{d}_{mk} \end{bmatrix}}$$

where:

$$\tilde{d}_{il} = \left(\sum_{j=1}^{n} (a_{ij} - 1).(b_{jl} - 1), \ \sum_{j=1}^{n} a_{ij}.b_{jl}, \ \sum_{j=1}^{n} (a_{ij} + 1).(b_{jl} + 1) \right) \tag{2}$$

Then, defuzzifying each element of the above matrix by equation (1), and the defuzzified Patient-Risk (PR) matrix would be as below:

$$\text{Defuzzified } PR = \begin{array}{c} \\ p_1 \\ p_2 \\ \vdots \\ \\ p_m \end{array} \overset{\begin{array}{ccccc} R_1 & R_2 & \cdots & \cdots & R_k \end{array}}{\begin{bmatrix} v_{11} & v_{12} & \cdots & \cdots & v_{1k} \\ v_{21} & v_{22} & \cdots & \cdots & v_{2k} \\ \vdots & \cdots & \cdots & \cdots & \vdots \\ \vdots & \cdots & \cdots & \cdots & \vdots \\ v_{m1} & v_{m2} & \cdots & \cdots & v_{mk} \end{bmatrix}}$$

Now to get the final prioritization, the summation of each row should be calculated $Sv_m = \sum_{j=1}^{k} v_{mj}$ for example for the first patient $Sv_1 = \sum_{j=1}^{k} v_{1j}$. Then the final matrix *sum* (which is the result of summation) would be:

$$Sum = \begin{array}{c} p_1 \\ p_2 \\ \vdots \\ p_m \end{array} \begin{bmatrix} Sv_1 \\ Sv_2 \\ \vdots \\ Sv_m \end{bmatrix}$$

In this matrix $Sv1$ is the priority number of the first patient and Sv_m is the priority number of mth Patient.

Now patients can be ranked based on their priority score. The patient with the largest overall priority number should be the one selected for treatment first. This proposed framework can be applied in different clinical settings. Fields such as organ transplant, surgery, cancer treatment or other critical care.

In numerical example, application of proposed framework will be explained for prioritizing surgical patients.

NUMERICAL EXAMPLE

In this section, to illustrate the proposed framework, a hypothetical numerical example is presented. Suppose that in a hospital's surgery ward, there are four surgical patients $\{p_1, p_2, p_3, p_4\}$ on waiting lists. Surgeons reached to consensus to consider three criteria $\{C_1, C_2, C_3\}$ to prioritize these patients. They also selected three risks of R1 (Risk of death), R2 (Risk of comorbidity), and R3 (Risk of infection) $\{R_1, R_2, R_3\}$ which may threaten patients' health if patients' treatment is delayed. Authors used ANP technique and medical experts' opinion to obtain each criterion's and each risk's relative importance weights.

The ANP approach four phases (Saaty & Özdemir, 2005) (Chung et al., 2005), and detailed explanation of ANP can be found in Saaty (Saaty & Özdemir, 2005):

Phase 1: *Construction of model and problem structuring*: In this step the problem should be stated clearly and decomposed into a rational system like a network.
Phase 2: *Pairwise comparisons and priority vectors:* In ANP, like (AHP) pairs of decision elements at each cluster are compared with respect to their importance towards their criteria. In addition, interdependencies among criteria of a cluster must also be examined in pairs. The relative importance values are determined with Saaty's scale.
Phase 3: *Formation of Super-matrix*: A super-matrix is a partitioned matrix, where each matrix part represents a relationship between two clusters in a system. The super-matrix concept is similar to the Markov chain process. To obtain global priorities in a system with interdependent influences, the local priority vectors should be entered in the appropriate columns of a matrix.
Phase 4: *Synthesizing the criteria/risks*: The priority weights of the criteria/risks can be found in the normalized super-matrix.

In this study we used Super Decisions software version number 2.0.8. (which implements ANP) to obtain the relative weights of the risks and criteria. For more details on process of obtaining relative weights of criteria/risks for patients' prioritization using AHP/ANP in real practice, please refer to (Abbasgholizadeh Rahimi et al., 2016; Abbasgholizadeh Rahimi & Jamshidi, 2014). The calculated weights are as followings:

Criteria's Weights = {0.08, 0.68, 0.24},

Risks' Weights = {0.79, 0.15, 0.06},

Suppose that surgeons assign following numbers to multiple criteria for each of four patients:

$F(p_1) = \{C_1/3, C_2/5, C_3/6\}$,

$F(p_2) = \{C_1/4, C_2/7, C_3/9\},$

$F(p_3) = \{C_1/5, C_2/8, C_3/2\},$

$F(p_4) = \{C_1/1, C_2/3, C_3/4\},$

Then the fuzzy soft set (F, P) is a parameterized family of all fuzzy sets over C and gives a collection of an approximate description of the Patient-Criteria in the hospital. This fuzzy soft set (F,P) represents the relation matrix Patient-Criteria (PC) and is:

$$PC = \begin{array}{c} \\ p_1 \\ p_2 \\ p_3 \\ p_4 \end{array} \begin{array}{ccc} C_1(0.79) & C_2(0.15) & C_3(0.06) \\ \begin{bmatrix} \tilde{3} & \tilde{5} & \tilde{6} \\ \tilde{4} & \tilde{7} & \tilde{9} \\ \tilde{5} & \tilde{8} & \tilde{2} \\ \tilde{1} & \tilde{3} & \tilde{4} \end{bmatrix} \end{array}$$

And the relation matrix of Criteria-Risk (CR) is as followings:

$$CR = \begin{array}{c} \\ c_1 \\ c_2 \\ c_3 \end{array} \begin{array}{ccc} R_1(0.79) & R_2(0.15) & R_3(0.06) \\ \begin{bmatrix} \tilde{4} & \tilde{2} & \tilde{3} \\ \tilde{6} & \tilde{5} & \tilde{7} \\ \tilde{9} & \tilde{8} & \tilde{1} \end{bmatrix} \end{array}$$

Then, after assigning weights to relative columns in PC and CR matrices, and performing the transformation operation PC*⊗CR* is performed and authors get the Patient-Risk matrix PR as:

$$PR = \begin{array}{c} \\ p_1 \\ p_2 \\ p_3 \\ p_4 \end{array} \begin{array}{ccc} R_1 & R_2 & R_3 \\ \begin{bmatrix} \widetilde{27.1} & \widetilde{4.3} & \widetilde{1.5} \\ \widetilde{38.9} & \widetilde{6.2} & \widetilde{2.1} \\ \widetilde{30.4} & \widetilde{4.7} & \widetilde{2.3} \\ \widetilde{16.7} & \widetilde{2.7} & \widetilde{0.9} \end{bmatrix} \end{array}.$$

where:

$\widetilde{27.1} = (18.7, \ 27.1, \ 37), \widetilde{4.3} = (2.9, \ 4.3, \ 6), \widetilde{1.5} = (0.99, \ 1.5, \ 2.2),$

$\widetilde{38.9} = (28.8, \ 38.9, \ 50.6), \widetilde{6.2} = (4.5, \ 6.2, \ 8.3), \widetilde{2.1} = (1.49, \ 2.1, \ 2.9),$

$$\widetilde{30.4} = (21.07,\ 30.4,\ 41.4),\ \widetilde{4.7} = (3.1,\ 4.7,\ 6.6),\ \widetilde{2.3} = (1.75,\ 2.3,\ 3.13),$$

$$\widetilde{16.7} = (9.9,\ 16.7,\ 25.1),\ \widetilde{2.7} = (1.57,\ 2.7,\ 4.1),\ \widetilde{0.9} = (0.48,\ 0.92,\ 1.48),$$

Above numbers are gained using equation (2). Now, after defuzzifying the above numbers using equation (1), the defuzzified PR will be as following:

$$\text{Defuzzified } PR = \begin{array}{c} \\ p_1 \\ p_2 \\ p_3 \\ p_4 \end{array} \begin{array}{ccc} R_1 & R_2 & R_3 \\ \left[\begin{array}{ccc} 19.5 & 40.25 & 15.45 \\ 28.1 & 58.25 & 21.45 \\ 17.5 & 33.75 & 22.35 \\ 11.9 & 25.25 & 8.85 \end{array} \right] \end{array}$$

After summation of each row what is obtained will be summation of risks for each patient. The final matrix *Sum* is:

$$\rightarrow Sum = \begin{array}{c} p_1 \\ p_2 \\ p_3 \\ p_4 \end{array} \left[\begin{array}{c} 33.5 \\ 47.8 \\ 38.1 \\ 20.8 \end{array} \right]$$

Considering the obtained priority scores in the *Sum* matrix, the second patient's (p_2) situation is more risky than others and this patient should be the first priority for surgery. Other patients' prioritization would be as following: $p_3 > p_1 > p_4$.

ROBUSTNESS ANALYSIS

The proposed framework is deemed robust if it obtains the same result under different (uncertain) operating conditions. Will the same patient be recommended for treatment if the criteria and risks' weights vary? This analysis is important to validate model's reliability. This is especially important for critical problems, where the margin of error could mean fewer life years saved for waiting patients. Figure 2 illustrates the sensitivity analysis results in multiple scenarios when the weight of the most important criterion (i.e. C_2) and the most important risk (i.e. R_1) varied by ±10% and ±20% of its original value. Scenarios 1-4 are related to criteria and scenarios 5-8 are related to risks.

From the experiments, authors can conclude that the proposed framework is robust under all eight scenarios, and the decision makers should be confident that patient 2 is the optimal choice, even though the derived criteria/risk's importance weights may be imperfect, and the probability of choosing the wrong patient for treatment is therefore almost zero.

Figure 2. Sensitivity analysis under eight different scenarios
For a more accurate representation of this figure, please see the electronic version.

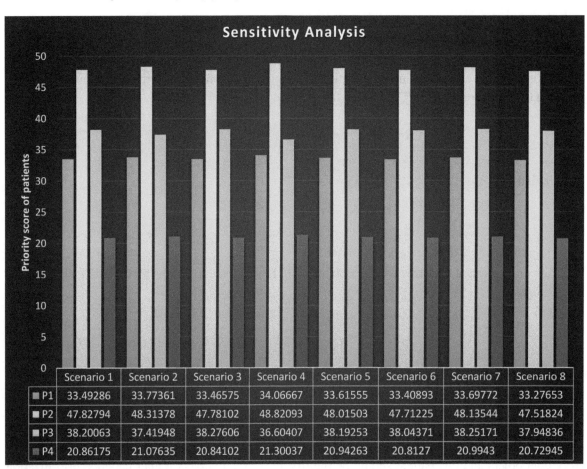

	Scenario 1	Scenario 2	Scenario 3	Scenario 4	Scenario 5	Scenario 6	Scenario 7	Scenario 8
■ P1	33.49286	33.77361	33.46575	34.06667	33.61555	33.40893	33.69772	33.27653
■ P2	47.82794	48.31378	47.78102	48.82093	48.01503	47.71225	48.13544	47.51824
■ P3	38.20063	37.41948	38.27606	36.60407	38.19253	38.04371	38.25171	37.94836
■ P4	20.86175	21.07635	20.84102	21.30037	20.94263	20.8127	20.9943	20.72945

COMPARISON

For illustrating the advantages and contributions of the proposed framework, Table 2 is provided. This table compares the proposed integrated method with four other well-known methods (namely: Analytic Hierarchy Process (AHP), Analytic Network Process (ANP), Technique for Order of Preference by Similarity to Ideal Solution (TOPSIS), and Data Envelopment Analysis (DEA)) from different perspectives.

In brief, none of the mentioned methods consider the associated uncertainties in patients' prioritization procedure except the proposed framework. Besides, in the proposed framework the authors involved the associated risks in the procedure as an important factor while this important issue has been overlooked in others. All of the methods including the proposed framework consider multiple criteria and we can assign importance weights for these criteria, but none of them except ANP and proposed framework considers the relationships among criteria. This framework can consider group of decision makers' opinion like other methods. From the time point of view, the required time for prioritizing patients in large scale in the proposed framework is less than others. This comparison has been done based on experts' opinion

Table 2. Comparison of the proposed framework with other we-known methods

	AHP	ANP	TOPSIS	DEA	Proposed Method
Consider uncertainty					✓
Involve associated risks					✓
Involve multiple criteria	✓	✓	✓	✓	✓
Involve group of Decision Makers (DMs)	✓	✓		✓	✓
Consider importance weight of each expert (based on their knowledge)	✓	✓			✓
Assign importance weights for criteria	✓	✓	✓	✓	✓
Consider dependency among criteria		✓			✓
Easiness of the procedure (simplicity)	✓		✓		✓
Time-efficiency in large scale					✓

however, for more precise comparison further studies in practice is required. This could be done by conducting a clinical studies, involving clinicians in the procedure, and implementing each methodology in practice and comparing the results and each of the mentioned aspects in different methodologies.

CONCLUSION

Access to healthcare services and long waiting time is one of the main issues in most of the countries including Canada and United States, and based on recent reports, this situation not only have not been improved during years till 2016, but also they have gotten slightly worse. Healthcare organizations can't increase their limited resources nor treat all patients simultaneously. Then, patients' access to these services should be prioritized in a way that best use the scarce resources and most importantly insure safety of patients who are waiting for treatment.

Prioritization is essential and inevitable not only because of resource shortage, which have not been improved during years, but also because it may be one of the best options in identification of high risk patients and increasing safety of patients' waiting for treatment. Prioritization is a crucial issue that will contribute to the capability and stability of the systems as well. This decision making under complex, uncertain and dynamic environments is not simple as ABC so in order to reduce the workload of clinicians and impact on waiting times for healthcare services, development of prioritization tools are necessary.

In this chapter, the authors proposed a novel integrated and easy to use framework which prioritizes a diverse mix of patients in waiting lists into an order of importance considering the following strengths and main features:

1. The importance of each criterion and each risk is computed, considering group of medical experts' opinions,
2. Associated uncertainties are handled,
3. Importance of each decision maker's opinion has been considered by assigning weights to their knowledge and experience to obtain more precise results,

4. Possible interrelationships among criteria and also among risks are considered, and
5. Various risks that threaten patients' safety have been considered as an important and distinguished factor.

This is an original and innovative framework and the above features, distinguish it from currently used methods. To exhibit the simplicity, and applicability of the proposed framework, in this chapter authors provided an example of surgical patients' prioritization. The proposed framework not only considers uncertainties and risks in determining patients' priorities, but also remains noticeably robust. Finally, the proposed method is compared with some of the well-known methods in the comparison section to show its main benefits. The results of this study may increase safety of patients' waiting for treatment, and could have a significant impact on both medical community and the public's faith in justice and equity.

Although the authors believe this study provides real value, there are areas for future enhancements. The main weakness of the proposed model is that patients were not involved in the prioritization procedure. Besides, dynamic nature of the healthcare system has not been considered in this study, involving these aspects could increase the validity and efficacy of the results. Another interesting future research in this regard would be to study whether the proposed framework yield a fruitful result in real practice in different clinical settings.

REFERENCES

Abbasgholizadeh Rahimi, S., & Jamshidi, A. (2014a). *Prioritization of Organ Transplant Patients using Analytic Network Process*. Montreal, Canada: Academic Press.

Abbasgholizadeh Rahimi, S., Jamshidi, A., Ruiz, A. & Ait-Kadi, D. (2014b). *Applied Methods in Prioritization of Patients in Surgery Waiting Lists*. Montreal, Canada: Academic Press.

Abbasgholizadeh Rahimi, S., Jamshidi, A., Ruiz, A., & Ait Kadi, D. (2016). A new dynamic integrated framework for surgical patients prioritization considering risks and uncertainties. *Decision Support Systems*, *88*, 112–120. doi:10.1016/j.dss.2016.06.003

Addis, B., Carello, G., Grosso, A., & Tanfani, E. (2015). *Operating room scheduling and rescheduling: a rolling horizon approach*. Flex Serv Manuf J.

Ahlert, M., & Kliemt, H. (2013). Problems of priority change in kidney allocation and beyond. *The European Journal of Health Economics*, *14*(3), 383–390. doi:10.100710198-012-0382-y PMID:22358456

Aktas, H., & Cagman, N. (2007). Soft sets and soft groups. *Inf Sci*, *177*(13), 2726–2735. doi:10.1016/j.ins.2006.12.008

Al-Ebbinia, L., Oztekin, A., & Chen, Y. (2016). FLAS: Fuzzy lung allocation system for US-based transplantations. *European Journal of Operational Research*, *248*(3), 1051–1065. doi:10.1016/j.ejor.2015.08.001

Ali, M., Feng, F., Liu, X., Min, W. K., & Shabir, M. (2009). On some new operations in soft set theory. *Computers & Mathematics with Applications (Oxford, England), 57*(9), 1547–1553. doi:10.1016/j. camwa.2008.11.009

Ali, M., & Shabir, M. (2010). Comments on De Morgan's law in fuzzy soft sets. *J. Fuzzy Math., 18*(3), 679–686.

Andersson, A., Omberg, M., & Svedlund, M. (2006). Triage in the emergency department—a qualitative study of the factors which nurses consider when making decisions. *Nursing in Critical Care, 11*(3), 136–145. doi:10.1111/j.1362-1017.2006.00162.x PMID:16719019

Argon, N., & Ziya, S. (2009). Priority Assignment Under Imperfect Information on Customer Type Identities. *Manuf Serv Oper Manag, 11*, 674–693.

Ashour, O., & Kremer, G. (2016). Dynamic patient grouping and prioritization: A new approach to emergency department flow improvement. *Health Care Management Science, 19*(2), 192–205. doi:10.100710729-014-9311-1 PMID:25487711

Ashour, O. & Okudan, G. (2010). *Patient sorting through emergency severity index and descriptive variables' utility.* Academic Press.

Barua, B. (2015). *Waiting Your Turn: Wait Times for Health Care in Canada, 2015 Report.* Fraser institute.

Barua, B., & Esmail, N. (2013). *Why are we waiting so long? Health care wait times nearly double over the past two decades to 18.2 weeks.* Fraser Institute.

Butterfield, W. (1968). *Priorities in medicine.* London: The Nuffield Provincial Hospitals Trust.

Celik, Y., & Yamak, S. (2013). Fuzzy soft set theory applied to medical diagnosis using fuzzy arithmetic operations. *Journal of Inequalities and Applications, 82*, 1–9.

Chetia, B., & Das, P. (2010). An application of interval valued fuzzy soft set in medical diagnosis. *Int. J. Contemp. Math. Sci., 5*(38), 1887–1894.

Cholongitas, E., & Burroughs, A. (2012). The evolution in the prioritization for liver transplantation. *Annals of Gastroenterology, 25*(1). PMID:24713804

Cholongitas, E., Germani, G., & Burroughs, A. K. (2010). Prioritization for liver transplantation. *Gastroenterology & Hepatology Nature Reviews, 7*(12), 659–668. doi:10.1038/nrgastro.2010.169 PMID:21045793

Chung, S., Lee, A., & Pearn, W. (2005). Analytic network process (ANP) approach for product mix Planning in semiconductor fabricator. *International Journal of Production Economics, 96*(1), 15–36. doi:10.1016/j.ijpe.2004.02.006

Clare, P. (1973). *Waiting Lists: Priority Formulae.* Birmingham, UK: Notes taken at a meeting of the Midlands Health Services Discussion Group.

Claudio, D., & Okudan, G. (2010). Utility function based patient prioritization in the emergency department. *European Journal of Industrial Engineering, 4*(1), 59–77. doi:10.1504/EJIE.2010.029570

Comas, M., Castells, X., Hoffmeister, L., Román, R., Cots, F., Mar, J., ... Espallargues, M. (2008). Discrete-Event Simulation Applied to Analysis of Waiting Lists. Evaluation of a Prioritization System for Cataract Surgery. *Value in Health*, *11*(7), 1203–1213. doi:10.1111/j.1524-4733.2008.00322.x PMID:18494754

Culyer, A., & Cullis, J. (1976). Some economics of hospital waiting lists in the NHS. *Journal of Social Policy*, *5*(3), 239–264. doi:10.1017/S0047279400004748

Davis, B., & Johnson, S. (1998). Real-time priority scoring system must be used for prioritisation on waiting lists. *British Medical Journal*. PMID:10373189

Day, B. (2013). *Reducing Wait Times for Health Care*. Fraser Institute.

De, S., Biswas, R., & Roy, A. (2001). An application of intuitionistic fuzzy sets in medical diagnosis. *Fuzzy Sets and Systems*, *117*(2), 209–213. doi:10.1016/S0165-0114(98)00235-8

Dennett, E., & Parry, B. (1998). Generic surgical priority criteria scoring system: The clinical reality. *The New Zealand Medical Journal*, *111*, 163–166. PMID:9612483

Dolan, P., & Cookson, R. (2000). A qualitative study of the extent to which health gain matters when choosing between groups of patients. *Health Policy (Amsterdam)*, *51*(1), 19–30. doi:10.1016/S0168-8510(99)00079-2 PMID:11010223

Domènech, M., Adam, P., Tebé, C., & Espallargues, M. (2013). Developing a universal tool for the prioritization of patients waiting for elective surgery. *Journal of Health Policy*, *113*(1-2), 118–126. doi:10.1016/j.healthpol.2013.07.006 PMID:23932414

Dowseya, M., Gunn, J., & Choong, P. (2014). Selecting those to refer for joint replacement: Who will likely benefit and who will not? *Best Practice & Research. Clinical Rheumatology*, *28*(1), 157–171. doi:10.1016/j.berh.2014.01.005 PMID:24792950

Eltringham, D., & Clare, P. (1973). *Waiting List Management by Computer*. OR Unit Regional Hospital Board.

Feng, F., & Li, Y. (2013). Soft subsets and soft product operations. *Inf Sci*, *232*, 44–57. doi:10.1016/j.ins.2013.01.001

Fieldsa, E., Okudana, G., & Ashour, O. (2013). Rank aggregation methods comparison: A case for triage prioritization. *Expert Systems with Applications*, *40*(4), 1305–1311. doi:10.1016/j.eswa.2012.08.060

Fordyce, A., & Phillips, R. (1970). Waiting list management by computer. *The Hospital*, *66*(9), 303–305.

Godber, G. (1970). Priorities in medicine. *The Journal of the Royal College of General Practitioners*, *20*, 313–322. PMID:5500451

Hadorn, D. (2000). Setting priorities for waiting lists: Defining our terms. *Canadian Medical Association Journal*, *163*(7), 857–860. PMID:11033717

Hadorn, D., & Holmes, A. (1997). The New Zealand priority criteria project Part 2: Coronary artery bypass graft surgery. *British Medical Journal*, *314*(7074), 135–138. doi:10.1136/bmj.314.7074.135 PMID:9006478

Kaufmann, A., & Gupta, M. (1991). Introduction to Fuzzy Arithmetic Theory & Applications. Van Nostrand.

Lack, A., Edwards, R., & Boland, A. (2000). Weights for waits: Lessons from Salisbury. *Journal of Health Services Research & Policy*, *5*(2), 83–88. PMID:10947552

Langham, S., & Thorogood, M. (1996). Waiting lists, Bypassing the time. *The Health Service Journal*, *106*(33). PMID:10156829

Lavee, J., & Brock, D. (2012). Prioritizing registered donors in organ allocation: An ethical appraisal of the Israeli organ transplant law. *Current Opinion in Critical Care*, *18*(6), 707–711. doi:10.1097/MCC.0b013e328357a2e2 PMID:22914426

Li, D.-F. (2014). *Decision and Game Theory in Management With Intuitionistic Fuzzy Sets*. Springer. doi:10.1007/978-3-642-40712-3

Li, D.-F., & Liu, J.-C. (2015). A parameterized non-linear programming approach to solve matrix games with payoffs of I-fuzzy numbers. *IEEE Transactions on Fuzzy Systems*, *23*(4), 885–896. doi:10.1109/TFUZZ.2014.2333065

Li, D.-F., & Ren, H.-P. (2015). Multi-attribute decision making method considering the amount and reliability of intuitionistic fuzzy information. *Journal of Intelligent & Fuzzy Systems*, *28*, 1877–1883.

Lin, C., & Harris, S. (2012). A Unified Framework for the Prioritization of Organ Transplant Patients: Analytic Hierarchy Process, Sensitivity and Multifactor Robustness Study. *Journal of Multi-Criteria Decision Analysis*, *20*(3-4), 157–172. doi:10.1002/mcda.1480

Luckman, J., Mackenzie, M., & Stringer, J. (1969). *Management Policies for Large Ward Units*. Coventry, UK: Institute for Operational Research.

MacCormick, A., Collecutt, W., & Parry, B. (2003). Prioritizing patients for elective surgery: A systematic review. *ANZ Journal of Surgery*, *73*(8), 633–642. doi:10.1046/j.1445-2197.2003.02605.x PMID:12887536

Maji, P., Biswas, R., & Roy, A. (2001). Fuzzy soft set. *J. Fuzzy Math.*, *9*(3), 677–692.

Maji, P., Biswas, R., & Roy, A. (2003). *Soft set theory*. Comp.&Math.Appl.

Mariotti, G., Siciliani, L., Rebba, V., Fellini, R., Gentilini, M., Benea, G., ... Liva, C. (2014). Waiting time prioritisation for specialist services in Italy: The homogeneous waiting time groups approach. *Health Policy (Amsterdam)*, *117*(1), 54–63. doi:10.1016/j.healthpol.2014.01.018 PMID:24576498

Meyer, T., & Raspe, H. (2012). Priority setting: Priorisierung: Was ist das und wie geht das? *Rehabilitation*, *51*(2), 73–80. doi:10.1055-0032-1306288 PMID:22570153

Min, D., & Yih, Y. (2010). An elective surgery scheduling problem considering patient priority. *Computers & Operations Research*, *37*(6), 1091–1099. doi:10.1016/j.cor.2009.09.016

Molodtsov, D. (1999). Soft set theory first results. *Computers & Mathematics with Applications (Oxford, England)*, *37*(4-5), 19–31. doi:10.1016/S0898-1221(99)00056-5

Montoya, S., González, M., López, S., & … . (2014). Study to Develop a Waiting List Prioritization Score for Varicose Vein Surgery. *Annals of Vascular Surgery, 28*(2), 306–312. doi:10.1016/j.avsg.2012.11.017 PMID:24084264

Mullen, P. (2003). Prioritizing waiting lists: How and why? *European Journal of Operational Research, 150*(1), 32–45. doi:10.1016/S0377-2217(02)00779-8

Nagel, E., & Lauerer, M. (2016). *Prioritization in Medicine An International Dialogue*. Springer International. doi:10.1007/978-3-319-21112-1

Nagel, E., & Lauerer, M. (2016). *Prioritization in Medicine: An International Dialogue*. Springer International Publishing. doi:10.1007/978-3-319-21112-1

Naylor, C. (1993). Waiting for coronary revascularization in Toronto: 2 years' experience with a regional referral office. *Canadian Medical Association Journal, 149*(7), 955–962. PMID:8402424

Noseworthy, T., McGurran, J., & Hadorn, D. C. (2003). Waiting for scheduled services in Canada: Development of priority-setting scoring systems. *Journal of Evaluation in Clinical Practice, 9*(1), 23–31. doi:10.1046/j.1365-2753.2003.00377.x PMID:12558699

Peacock, S., et al. (2009). Overcoming barriers to priority setting using interdisciplinary methods. *Health Policy, 92*(2-3), 124-32. doi:10.1016/j.healthpol.2009.02.006

Phoenix, C. J. (1972). *Waiting list management and admission scheduling*. Butterworth.

Pornak, S., & Raspe, H. (2015). Die dänische Debatte über Priorisierung und Posteriorisierung in der Medizin – Was gibt es Neues? *Gesundheitswesen (Bundesverband der Arzte des Offentlichen Gesundheitsdienstes (Germany)), 77*, 1–7.

Prentice, J., & Pizer, S. (2007). Delayed Access to Health Care and Mortality. *Health Services Research, 42*(2), 644–662. doi:10.1111/j.1475-6773.2006.00626.x PMID:17362211

Raspe, H. (2016). Prioritisation: (At Least) Two Normative. In *Prioritization in Medicine: An International Dialogue* (pp. 85–99). Springer International Publishing. doi:10.1007/978-3-319-21112-1_7

Riet, C., & Demeulemeester, E. (2015). Trade-offs in operating room planning for electives and emergencies: A review. *Operations Research for Health Care, 7*, 52–69. doi:10.1016/j.orhc.2015.05.005

Russell, C., Roberts, M., Williamson, T. G., McKercher, J., Jolly, S. E., & McNeil, J. (2003). Clinical categorization for elective surgery in Victoria. *ANZ Journal of Surgery, 73*(10), 839–842. doi:10.1046/j.1445-2197.2003.02797.x PMID:14525579

Saaty, T., & Özdemir, M. (2005). *The Encyclion: A Dictionary of Decisions with Dependence and Feedback based on the ANP*. RWS Publications.

Sadegh-Zadeh, K. (2012). *Handbook of analytic philosophy of medicine*. New York: Springer Dordrecht Heidelberg. doi:10.1007/978-94-007-2260-6

Sanchez, E. (1979). Inverse of fuzzy relations, application to possibility distributions and medical diagnosis. *Fuzzy Sets and Systems, 2*(1), 75–86. doi:10.1016/0165-0114(79)90017-4

Seddon, M., French, J. K., Amos, D. J., Ramanathan, K., McLaughlin, S. C., & White, H. D. (1999). Waiting times and prioritisation for coronary artery bypass survey in New Zealand. *Heart (British Cardiac Society), 81*(6), 586–592. doi:10.1136/hrt.81.6.586 PMID:10336915

Soljak, M. (1997). *The Use of Scoring Systems in the NHS: Cardiac Surgery in London. From Waiting Lists to Booking Systems HSMC*. University of Birmingham.

Tanabe, P., Travers, D., Gilboy, N., Rosenau, A., Sierzega, G., Rupp, V., ... Adams, J. G. (2005). Refining emergency severity index (ESI) triage criteria. *Academic Emergency Medicine, 12*(6), 497–501. doi:10.1111/j.1553-2712.2005.tb00888.x PMID:15930399

Testi, A., Tanfani, E., Valente, R., Ansaldo, G. L., & Torre, G. C. (2008). Prioritizing surgical waiting lists. *Journal of Evaluation in Clinical Practice, 14*(1), 59–64. doi:10.1111/j.1365-2753.2007.00794.x PMID:18211645

Valente, R., Testi, A., Tanfani, E., Fato, M., Porro, I., Santo, M., ... Ansaldo, G. (2009). A model to prioritize access to elective surgery on the basis of clinical urgency and waiting time. *BMC Health Services Research, 9*(1), 1. doi:10.1186/1472-6963-9-1 PMID:19118494

Williams, I., Robinson, S., & Dickinson, H. (2012). *Rationing in health care: the theory and practice of priority setting*. Bristol: The Policy Press.

Yang, M., Fry, M., & Raikhelkar, J. (2013). A Model to Create an Efficient and Equitable Admission Policy for Patients Arriving to the Cardiothoracic ICU. *The Clinical Investigator, 41*(2), 414–422. PMID:23263573

Yu, D.-J., & Li, D.-F. (2014). Dual hesitant fuzzy multi-criteria decision making and its application to teaching quality assessment. *Journal of Intelligent and Fuzzy Systems, 27*(4), 1679–1688.

Zadeh, L. (1965). Fuzzy sets. *Information and Control, 8*(3), 338–353. doi:10.1016/S0019-9958(65)90241-X

KEY TERMS AND DEFINITIONS

First-Come First-Served: A basic prioritization rule mentioning the first arrived client should be the first to receive the service.

Group Decision Making: Group decision making give an opportunity to group of experts and professionals to express their decisions and opinions and considers the values that each point of views as important.

Multi Criteria Decision Analysis: A valuable tool that could solve complex decision making problems, usually involve the problems that are characterized as a choice among alternatives.

Prioritization: Deciding which clients are perceived or measured important or significant and ranking them based on their importance or significance called prioritization.

Risks: A thing that may happen or be the cause of loss, injury, disease, or death.

Soft Set: In order to deal with uncertainty in a parametric manner, (in 1999) Molodtsov proposed a generalization of fuzzy set theory called Soft set theory.

The Organization for Economic Co-Operation and Development (OECD): OECD is a forum consisting of the governments of 34 democracies with market economies work with each other to promote economic growth, prosperity, and sustainable development.

Waiting List: A waiting list is a queue of clients who are assumed to need a service that is in short supply.

This research was previously published in Theoretical and Practical Advancements for Fuzzy System Integration edited by Deng-Feng Li; pages 221-244, copyright year 2017 by Information Science Reference (an imprint of IGI Global).

Chapter 20
Evaluation of the Length of Hospital Stay Through Artificial Neural Networks Based Systems

Vasco Abelha
University of Minho, Portugal

Fernando Marins
University of Minho, Portugal

Henrique Vicente
University of Evora, Portugal

ABSTRACT

The mentality of savings and eliminating any kind of outgoing costs is undermining our society and our way of living. Cutting funds from Education to Health is at best delaying the inevitable "Crash" that is foreshadowed. Regarding Health, a major concern, can be described as jeopardize the health of Patients – Reduce of the Length of Hospital. As we all know, Human Health is very sensitive and prune to drastic changes in short spaces of time. Factors like age, sex, their ambient context – house conditions, daily lives – should all be important when deciding how long a specific patient should remain safe in a hospital. In no way, ought this be decided by the economic politics. Logic Programming was used for knowledge representation and reasoning, letting the modeling of the universe of discourse in terms of defective data, information and knowledge. Artificial Neural Networks and Genetic Algorithms were used in order to evaluate and predict how long should a patient remain in the hospital in order to minimize the collateral damage of our government approaches, not forgetting the use of Degree of Confidence to demonstrate how feasible the assessment is.

DOI: 10.4018/978-1-7998-2451-0.ch020

Copyright © 2020, IGI Global. Copying or distributing in print or electronic forms without written permission of IGI Global is prohibited.

Figure 1. Variables relevant on the length of stay

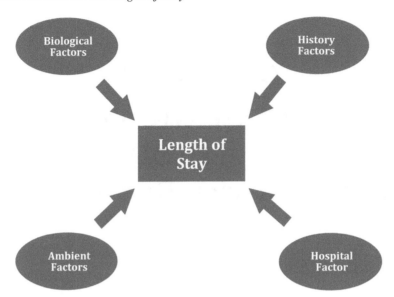

1. INTRODUCTION

Over the past few years, the dogma of reducing costs has grown rapidly. We are currently facing a worldwide economic crisis that is affecting every sector of our society. This leads to erroneous behaviors and actions by our leaders, when trying to delay and repeal the possibility of a foreshadowed economic crash. And how do they try to bypass the crash? Reduction of all costs. Sections such as Education, Health, Social Security, etcetera, are being forced to cut down the costs, to counterbalance the lack of funding by the government. In education, schools are closing down, teachers are fired or compelled to lecture more students and to work for more hours, culminating in a diminution of performance in the art of teaching and learning. The same can be applied to Health.

Nowadays, closing health facilities and laying off medical staff are some of the headlines of our lives, both doctors and patients are suffering the consequences of our leader's convictions in reducing costs. None is getting the respect they deserve. Health practitioners are, as well as teachers, enforced to practice extra hours, to reduce the duration of medical evaluations and, last but not the least, to priori-tize the health of the institution above the patient health, which ends up in minimizing the length of the patient's stay at the hospital.

Ethically, this view is unacceptable. Objectively, this is happening. In no circumstances, should a medical patient be seen as a number, as a monetary cost. The Hospital must be regarded only as a tool, a place to treat maladies, illness. A Patient's fate must not be decided by arithmetic, but by his health condition, his context, his past and present. These are the only decisive aspects to determine the duration of a sick person in the medical facility. And what is this context?

In the medical universe, the context can be referred as the life story of a patient. In order to make any type of medical judgment, a health professional has to consult all the information on the patient. This information comes from two sources:

- Patient
- Hospital

From the patient, we can obtain age, sex, comorbidities - physiological / morphological features - as well as data related to their daily lives. It is important to note that this information is subjective and may also not correspond to the truth, since we can never confirm the honesty of the patient. The ill-founded can induce the health professional in error through lies or due to memory problems.

The data relative to the Hospital includes all kinds of medical history of the patient: examinations, consultations, cultures and medical journals. It can be said that this information is objective and concrete, as these are obtained through medical procedures and exact methods.

We can see, based on the literature, that these information sources fit perfectly in the medical universe, specifically, SOAP note - (an acronym for subjective, objective, assessment, and plan) is a method of documentation employed by health care providers to write out notes in a patient's chart.

The aspects, previously enumerated, are more than necessary, as presented in a wide-range of literature or among experts, to do a risk assessment– Determine, with a certain Degree of Confidence, if a patient should stay in health care or not. Of course not all aspects have the same importance (Fry, 1993; Pritchard, 1981; World Health Organization [WHO], 1978). The most prominent aspects can be linked to Patient History, Comorbidity and Daily Context. To shed some light, the latter refers to the patient daily lives. If they have no conditions to be "set out in the open" – home hygienic conditions, no guidance - they ought to stay in the hospital, because, if not, they will most likely deteriorate their health and be routed once again to the hospital in a near future and even increase their cost to the hospital.

"It is better to do it right the first time and not having the past come back to bite". Nevertheless and in spite of these politics, this is exactly what happens most of the times. Patients tend to decrease their already short time span of admission in the hospital. The rest of aspects are easy to infer their relevance and why they should as well be taken into consideration. Such variables as *current treatments, exams and daily hospital diaries* have a correlation between them. Most of the time they share information or complement each other.

Thus and in order to easily apply and explain the concepts soon to be described. The aspects needed to determine the length of stay in a hospital were clustered in 4 groups displayed in *Figure 1*. All the data relative to the patient such as age, sex, and comorbidity are linked to the Biological Factors. Patient History refers to the detailed patient medical history. The information here comes from the sufferer, himself, or any past records that the health system has regarding his previous admissions. Ambient Factors is simply the context embracing the patient. Anything that surrounds him is, as well, important for determining the length of stay. Hospital Factor simply summarizes every exam, diagnosis he did at the hospital.

After a briefly description of the relevance and meaning of the values, one setback that arises is the incomplete information, noise and uncertainty. Sometimes we may not be completely certain of such information or we may not even have access to that specific data. Our investigation aims to speculate and estimate the necessary length of stay in a hospital of a certain patient, while reducing any mishap in their health. This is achieved by the use of logical programming based approach to knowledge representation and reasoning, complemented with a computational framework based on Artificial Neural Networks.

2. KNOWLEDGE REPRESENTATION AND REASONING

Many approaches for knowledge representation and reasoning have been proposed using the *Logic Programming* (*LP*) paradigm, namely in the area of Model Theory (Pereira, 2009; Neves, Machado, Analide, Abelha, & Brito, 2007; Neves, 1984) and Proof Theory (Halpern, 2005; Kovalerchuck & Resconi, 2010). We follow the proof theoretical approach and an extension to the *LP* language, to knowledge representation and reasoning. An *Extended Logic Program* – acronym E.L.P – is a finite set of clauses in the form:

$$p \leftarrow p_1, \ldots, p_n \text{ not } q_1, \ldots, q_m \tag{1}$$

$$?(p_1, \ldots, p_n, \text{ not } q_1, \ldots, q_m) \ (n, m \geq 0) \tag{2}$$

where *?* is a domain atom denoting falsity, the p_i, q_j, and p are classical ground literals, i.e., either positive atoms or atoms preceded by the classical negation sign ¬ (Kovalerchuck & Resconi, 2010). Under this representation formalism, every program is associated with a set of abducibles (Pereira & Anh, 2009; Neves, Machado, Analide, Abelha, & Brito, 2007; Neves, 1984) given here in the form of exceptions to the extensions of the predicates that make the program. Once again, LP emerged as an attractive formalism for knowledge representation and reasoning tasks, introducing an efficient search mechanism for problem solving.

Due to the growing need to offer user support in decision making processes some studies have been presented (Lucas, 2011; Machado, Abelha, Novais, João Neves, & José Neves, 2010), related to the qualitative models and qualitative reasoning in Database Theory and in Artificial Intelligence research. With respect to the problem of knowledge representation and reasoning in Logic Programming (LP), a measure of the *Quality-of-Information* (*QoI*) of such programs has been object of some work with promising results (Liu & Sun, 2007; Caldeira et al., 2010). The *QoI* with respect to the extension of a predicate *i* will be given by a truth-value in the interval [0,1], i.e., if the information is *known* (*positive*) or *false* (*negative*) the QoI for the extension of *predicate*$_i$ is 1. For situations where the information is unknown, the *QoI* is given by:

$$QoI_i = \lim_{n \to \infty} \frac{1}{n} = 0 (N \gg 0) \tag{3}$$

where *N* denotes the cardinality of the set of terms or clauses of the extension of *predicate*$_i$ that stand for the incompleteness under consideration. For situations where the extension of *predicate*$_i$ is unknown but can be taken from a set of values, the *QoI* is given by:

$$QoI_i = \frac{1}{Card} \tag{4}$$

where *Card* denotes the cardinality of the *abducibles* set for *i*, if the *abducibles* set is disjoint. If the *abducibles* set is not disjoint, the *QoI* is given by:

$$QoI_i = \frac{1}{C_1^{Card} + \ldots + C_{Card}^{Card}}$$ (5)

where C_{Card}^{Card} is a card-combination subset, with *Card* elements. The next element of the model to be considered is the relative importance that a predicate assigns to each of its attributes under observation, i.e., w_i^k, which stands for the relevance of attribute k in the extension of *predicate$_i$*. It is also assumed that the weights of all the attribute predicates are normalized, i.e.:

$$\sum_{1 \leq k \leq n} w_i^k = 1, \forall_i$$ (6)

where $\forall$ denotes the universal quantifier. It is now possible to define a predicate's scoring function $V_i(x)$ so that, for a value $x=(x_1,\ldots,x_n)$, defined in terms of the attributes of *predicate$_i$*, one may have:

$$V_i(x) = \sum_{1 \leq k \leq n} w_i^k \times \frac{QoI_i(x)}{n}$$ (7)

It is now possible to engender all the possible scenarios of the universe of discourse, according to the information given in the logic programs that endorse the information depicted in Figure 3, i.e., in terms of the extensions of the predicates *Biological Factors, Historical Factors, Hospital Factors and Ambient Factors*.

It is now feasible to rewrite the extensions of the predicates referred to above, in terms of a set of possible scenarios according to productions of the type:

$$predicate_i(X_1,\ldots,X_n) :: QoI$$ (8)

and evaluate the *Degree of Confidence* (*DoC*) given by $DoC = V_i(x_1,\ldots,x_n)/n$, which denotes one's confidence in a particular term of the extension of *predicate$_i$*. To be more general, let us suppose that the Universe of Discourse is described by the extension of the predicates:

$$a_1(\ldots), a_2(\ldots), \ldots, a_n(\ldots) \text{ where } (n \geq 0)$$ (9)

Therefore, for a given *scenario$_i$*, one may have (where $\perp$ denotes an argument value of the type unknown; the values of the others arguments stand for themselves):

$$
\begin{cases}
\neg a_1\left(x_1, y_1, k_1, z_1\right) \leftarrow not\ a_1\left(x_1, y_1, k_1, z_1\right) \\
a_1\left(27, [10,12], 15,\right) :: 0.5 \quad \underbrace{[25,30][10,12][3,25][0,5]}_{\text{atribute's domains for } x_1, y_1, k_1, z_1} \\
\neg a_2\left(x_2, y_2, k_2, z_2\right) \leftarrow not\ a_2\left(x_2, y_2, k_2, z_2\right) \\
a_2\left([33,42], 10, [10,12], \perp\right) :: 0.48 \quad \underbrace{[20,50][8,10][6,14][20,50]}_{\text{atribute's domains for } x_2, y_2, k_2, z_2}
\end{cases}
$$

$\Downarrow$ 1st interaction: transition to continuous intervals

$$
\begin{cases}
\neg a_1\left(x_1, y_1, k_1, z_1\right) \leftarrow not\ a_1\left(x_1, y_1, k_1, z_1\right) \\
a_1\left([27,27], [10,12], [15,15], [0,5]\right) :: 0.5 \quad \underbrace{[25,30][10,12][3,25][0,5]}_{\text{atribute's domains for } x_1, y_1, k_1, z_1} \\
\neg a_2\left(x_2, y_2, k_2, z_2\right) \leftarrow not\ a_2\left(x_2, y_2, k_2, z_2\right) \\
a_2\left([33,42], 10, [10,12], [20,50]\right) :: 0.48 \quad \underbrace{[20,50][8,10][6,14][20,50]}_{\text{atribute's domains for } x_2, y_2, k_2, z_2}
\end{cases}
$$

$\Downarrow$ 2nd interaction: normalization $\dfrac{Y - Y_{min}}{Y_{max} - Y_{max}}$

$$
\begin{cases}
\neg a_1\left(x_1, y_1, k_1, z_1\right) \leftarrow not\ a_1\left(x_1, y_1, k_1, z_1\right) \\
a_1\left(\left[\dfrac{27-25}{30-25}, \dfrac{27-25}{30-25}\right], \left[\dfrac{10-10}{12-10}, \dfrac{12-10}{12-10}\right], \left[\dfrac{15-3}{25-3}, \dfrac{15-3}{25-3}\right], \left[\dfrac{0-0}{5-0}, \dfrac{5-0}{5-0}\right]\right) \equiv \\
a_1\left([0.4,0.4], [0,1], [0.545,0.545], [0,1]\right) :: 0.5 \quad \underbrace{[0,1][0,1][0,1][0,1]}_{\text{atribute's domains for } x_1, y_1, k_1, z_1} \\
\neg a_2\left(x_2, y_2, k_2, z_2\right) \leftarrow not\ a_2\left(x_2, y_2, k_2, z_2\right) \\
a_2\left(\left[\dfrac{33-20}{50-20}, \dfrac{42-20}{50-20}\right], \left[\dfrac{10-8}{10-8}, \dfrac{10-10}{10-8}\right], \left[\dfrac{10-6}{14-6}, \dfrac{12-6}{14-6}\right], \left[\dfrac{20-20}{50-20}, \dfrac{50-20}{50-20}\right]\right) \equiv \\
a_2\left([0.433,0.733], [1,0], [0.5,0.75], [0,1]\right) :: 0.48 \quad \underbrace{[0,1][0,1][0,1][0,1]}_{\text{atribute's domains for } x_2, y_2, k_2, z_2}
\end{cases}
$$

The *Degree of Confidence* (*DoC*) is evaluated using the equation $DoC = \sqrt{1 - \Delta l^2}$, as it is illustrated in Figure 2. Here Δl stands for the length of the arguments' intervals, once normalized.

Below, one has the expected representation of the universe of discourse, where all the predicates' arguments are nominal. They speak for one's confidence that the unknown values of the arguments fit into the correspondent intervals referred to above.

Figure 2. Degree of Confidence evaluation

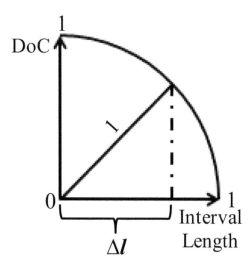

$$
\begin{cases}
\neg a_{1_{DoC}}\left(x_1, y_1, k_1, z_1\right) \leftarrow not\ a_{1_{DoC}}\left(x_1, y_1, k_1, z_1\right) \\
a_{1_{DoC}}\left(1, 0, 1, 0\right) :: 0.5 \quad \underbrace{\left[0.4, 0.4\right]\left[0, 1\right]\left[0.545, 0.545\right]\left[0, 1\right]}_{\text{atribute's domains for } x_1, y_1, k_1, z_1} \quad \underbrace{\left[0, 1\right]\left[0, 1\right]\left[0, 1\right]\left[0, 1\right]}_{\text{atribute's domains for } x_1, y_1, k_1, z_1} \\
\neg a_{2_{DoC}}\left(x_2, y_2, k_2, z_2\right) \leftarrow not\ a_{2_{DoC}}\left(x_2, y_2, k_2, z_2\right) \\
a_{2_{DoC}}\left(0.95, 0, 0.97, 0\right) :: 0.48 \quad \underbrace{\left[0.433, 0.733\right]\left[1, 0\right]\left[0.5, 0.75\right]\left[0, 1\right]}_{\text{atribute's domains for } x_2, y_2, k_2, z_2} \quad \underbrace{\left[0, 1\right]\left[0, 1\right]\left[0, 1\right]\left[0, 1\right]}_{\text{atribute's domains for } x_2, y_2, k_2, z_2}
\end{cases}
$$

3. A CASE STUDY

Therefore, and in order to exemplify the applicability of our model, we will look at the relational database model, since it provides a basic framework that fits into our expectations (Vicente et al., 2012), and is understood as the genesis of the LP approach to knowledge representation and reasoning.

Consider, for instance, and speaking hypothetically, where a relational database is given in terms of extends of the relations or predicates depicted in Figure 3, which stands for a situation where one has to interpret the various information and data about a Patient. Adding to this, there is the hypothesis of surfacing some incomplete data. For instance, in relation *Ambient Factors* the presence/absence of underlying problems for Case 1 is unknown, while in Case 2, it varies from 5 to 7. The Length of Stay Database (Figure 3) is populated according to the various results of the different columns:

- Biological Factors;
- Historical Factors;
- Hospital Factors;
- Ambient Factor.

Figure 3. A summary of the Relational Database model

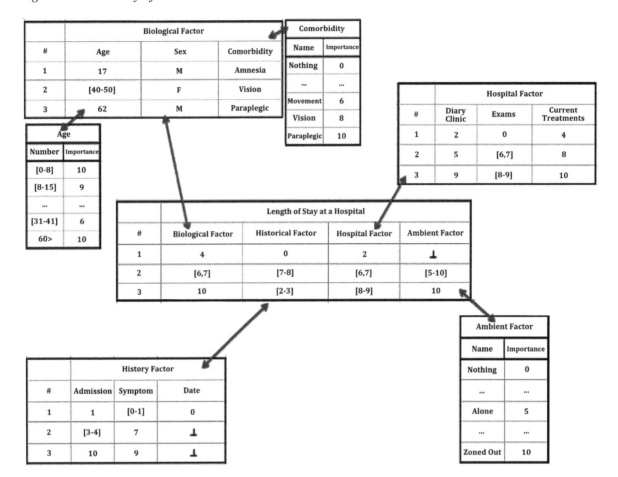

These are all the necessary variables to estimate the importance/risk of a patient remaining in Hospital Care, as well as their boundaries.

It should be reminded and noted that every single value is classified from level 0 to 10. The higher the level goes the more important it is. As seen in the Figure 3 every set has the equivalent result. Nevertheless, we must remark and not forget that these values, present on Figure 3 are merely example to aid on the explanation of the algorithm. These will and can be later calibrated by the medical staff for their needs.

Through this we can deduct and describe the extension of the length predicate as:

length: bio Factor, Hist.Factor, Hosp.Factor, Amb.Factor → {0,1}

where 0 (zero) and 1 (one) denote, respectively the aspect of *non need or need* of keeping them in health care. It is now possible to give the extension of the predicate length, in the form:

$$\{\neg length\left(Bio, Hist, Hosp, Amb\right) \leftarrow not\ length(Bio, Hist, Hosp, Amb)$$

$$length(\ \underbrace{4, 0, 2, \perp}_{\substack{\text{attribute's values} \\ [0,10][0,10][0,10][0,10] \\ \text{attribute's domains}}}\ ) :: 1 \quad length(\underbrace{[6,7], [7,8], \perp, [5,10]}_{\substack{\text{attribute's values} \\ [0,10][0,10][0,10][0,10] \\ \text{attribute's domains}}}) :: 1\}$$

In this program, the first clause denotes the closure of predicate *length*. The next clauses correspond to the four terms taken from the extension of the *length* relation. For example, the second clause corresponds to a female patient "2": a age uncertain, somewhere between 40 to 50 years with problems in her vision – blind. Analyzing Table Age with Comorbidity (both are filtered), we realize the values from 0-10 to her respective age can be between [6,7]. Assuming her age is between 40 and 50, it can belong to *level 6 [31,41] or level 5 [41,51] – interval should be [5,6]*. Comorbidity of vision corresponds to level 8. So doing an average of the respective values to her biological factors will give us a variable between [6,7]. We keep doing these kinds of operations for all the aspects that aren't unknown. If they are unknown we just assume the level can go from 1 to 10. To eliminate any doubt, Case 1, refers to a patient that should no longer remain in Health Care, while Case 2 is the opposite and ought to remain held for further examination and care. For further enlightenment, it is essential to explain that – in the Table History Factor – *Admission, Symptom* and *Date* is relative to the severity of his past status. Date is the number of times he has been in the hospital. The latter – admission and symptom – is referent to his health condition and how it evolved during the admission and posterior time on the medical facility.

Moving on, the next step is to transform all values into continuous intervals and then normalize the predicate to obtain the *Degree of Confidence* of the length predicate.

$$\{\neg length\left(Bio, Hist, Hosp, Amb\right) \leftarrow not\ length(Bio, Hist, Hosp, Amb)$$

$$length(\ \underbrace{[0.4, 0.4], [0,0], [0.2, 0.2], [0,1]}_{\substack{\text{attribute's values ranges once normalized} \\ [0,1][0,1][0,1][0,1] \\ \text{attribute's domains}}}\ ) :: 1$$

$$length(\ \underbrace{[0.6, 0.7], [0.7, 0.8], [0.1, 0.1], [0.5, 1]}_{\substack{\text{attribute's values ranges once normalized} \\ [0,1][0,1][0,1][0,1] \\ \text{attribute's domains}}}\ ) :: 1\}$$

The logic program referred to above, is now presented in the form:

$$\{\neg length(Bio, Hist, Hosp, Amb) \leftarrow not\ length(Bio, Hist, Hosp, Amb)$$

$$length_{DoC} \left(\underbrace{1,1,1,0}_{\text{attribute's confidence values}} \right) :: 1 \quad \underbrace{[0.4, 0.4], [0,0], [0.2, 0.2], [0,1]}_{\text{attribute's values ranges}}$$

$$\underbrace{[0,1][0,1][0,1][0,1]}_{\text{attribute's domains}} \quad length_{DoC} \left(\underbrace{0.99, 0.99, 1, 0}_{\text{attribute's confidence values}} \right) :: 1$$

$$\underbrace{[0.6, 0.7], [0.7, 0.8], [0.1, 0.1], [0,1]}_{\text{attribute's values ranges}} \quad \underbrace{[0,1][0,1][0,1][0,1]}_{\text{attribute's domains}} \}$$

where its terms make the training and test sets of the Artificial Neural Network given in Figure 4.

4. ARTIFICIAL NEURAL NETWORKS

Neves et al. (2010, 2012, 2013) demonstrated how Artificial Neural Networks (ANNs) could be successfully used to model data and capture complex relationships between inputs and outputs. ANNs simulate the structure of the human brain being populated by multiple layers of neurons. As an example, let us consider the case where one may have a situation in which a prolonged stay is needed, which is given in the form:

$$\{length\ attributes : (Bio, Hist, Hosp, Amb)$$

$$length \left(\underbrace{10, [2,3], [8,9], 10}_{\text{attribute's values}} \right) :: 1 \quad \underbrace{[0,10][0,10][0,10][0,10]}_{\text{attribute's domains}}$$

$\Downarrow$ 1st interaction: transition to continuous intervals

$$length \left(\underbrace{[10,10], [2,3], [8,9], [10,10]}_{\text{attribute's values ranges}} \right) :: 1 \quad \underbrace{[0,10][0,10][0,10][0,10]}_{\text{attribute's domains}}$$

$\Downarrow$ 2nd interaction: normalization $\dfrac{Y - Y_{min}}{Y_{max} - Y_{min}}$

$$length \left(\underbrace{[1,1], [0.2, 0.3], [0.8, 0.9], [1,1]}_{\text{attribute's values ranges once normalized}} \right) :: 1 \quad \underbrace{[0,1][0,1][0,1][0,1]}_{\text{attribute's domains}}$$

⇓ *DoC* calculation: $DoC = \sqrt{1 - \Delta l^2}$

$$length \left(\underbrace{1, 0.99, 0.99, 1}_{\text{attribute's confidence values}} \right) :: 1 \quad \underbrace{[1,1],[0.2,0.3],[0.8,0.9],[1,1]}_{\text{attribute's values ranges}} \quad \underbrace{[0,1][0,1][0,1][0,1]}_{\text{attribute's domains}} \}$$

In Figure 4 it is shown how the normalized values of the interval boundaries and their *DoC* values work as inputs to the ANN. The output translates the necessity of increasing the length of stay on a Hospital of a patient, and *DoC* the confidence that one has on such a happening.

5. CONCLUSION AND FUTURE WORK

To understand if the increase of the length of hospital stay is mandatory for the well being of the patient is a hard and complex task, which needs to consider many different conditions with intricate relations among them. These characteristics put this problem into the area of problems that may be tackled by AI based methodologies and techniques to problem solving. Despite that, little to no work has been done in that direction. This work presents the founding of a computational framework that uses powerful

Figure 4. A possible Artificial Neural Network Topology

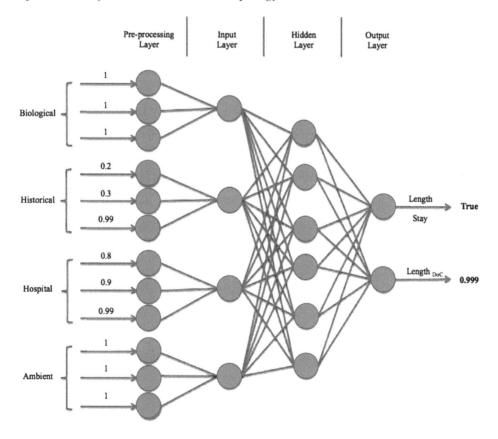

knowledge representation and reasoning techniques to set the structure of the information and the associate inference mechanisms. This representation is above everything else, very versatile and capable of covering every possible instance by considering incomplete, contradictory, and even unknown data. The main contribution of this work is to be understood in terms of the evaluation of the *DoC*, and the possibility to address the issue of incomplete information. Indeed, the new paradigm of knowledge representation and reasoning enables the use of the normalized values of the interval boundaries and their *DoC* values, as inputs to the ANN. The output translates the necessity of keeping a patient in a hospital order to improve their health and the degree of confidence that one has on such a happening. Future work may recommend that the same problem must be approached using other computational frameworks like Case Based Reasoning or Particle Swarm, just to name a few.

REFERENCES

Caldeira, A. T., Martins, M. R., Cabrita, M. J., Ambrósio, C., Arteiro, J., Neves, J., & Vicente, H. (2010). *Aroma Compounds Prevision using Artificial Neural Networks Influence of Newly Indigenous Saccharomyces SPP in White Wine Produced with Vitis Vinifera Cv Siria*.

Ferreira Maia Neves, J. C. (1984, January). A logic interpreter to handle time and negation in logic databases. *Proceedings of the 1984 annual conference of the ACM on The fifth generation challenge* (pp. 50-54). ACM. 10.1145/800171.809603

Fry, J. (1993). *General practice: the facts*. Radcliffe Medical Press.

Gelfond, M., & Lifschitz, V. (1988, August). *The stable model semantics for logic programming* (Vol. 88, pp. 1070–1080). ICLP/SLP.

Halpern, J. Y. (2003). *Reasoning about uncertainty* (Vol. 21). Cambridge: MIT press.

Kakas, A. C., Kowalski, R. A., & Toni, F. (1998). The role of abduction in logic programming. Handbook of logic in artificial intelligence and logic programming, 5, 235-324.

Kovalerchuk, B., & Resconi, G. (2010, July). Agent-based uncertainty logic network. *Proceedings of the 2010 IEEE International Conference on Fuzzy Systems (FUZZ)* (pp. 1-8). IEEE. 10.1109/FUZZY.2010.5584836

Liu, Y., & Sun, M. (2007, November). Fuzzy optimization BP neural network model for pavement performance assessment. *Proceedings of the IEEE International Conference on Grey Systems and Intelligent Services GSIS '07* (pp. 1031-1034). IEEE.

Lucas, P. (2004). *Quality checking of medical guidelines through logical abduction* (pp. 309–321). Springer London. doi:10.1007/978-0-85729-412-8_23

Machado, J., Abelha, A., Novais, P., Neves, J., & Neves, J. (2010). Quality of service in healthcare units. *International Journal of Computer Aided Engineering and Technology, 2*(4), 436–449. doi:10.1504/IJCAET.2010.035396

Neves, J., Machado, J., Analide, C., Abelha, A., & Brito, L. (2007). The halt condition in genetic programming. In *Progress in Artificial Intelligence* (pp. 160–169). Springer Berlin Heidelberg. doi:10.1007/978-3-540-77002-2_14

Pereira, L. M. (2009). Evolution prospection. In *New Advances in Intelligent Decision Technologies* (pp. 51–63). Springer Berlin Heidelberg. doi:10.1007/978-3-642-00909-9_6

Pritchard, P. M. (1981). *Manual of primary health care: its nature and organization.* Oxford University Press.

Vicente, H., Dias, S., Fernandes, A., Abelha, A., Machado, J., & Neves, J. (2012). Prediction of the quality of public water supply using artificial neural networks. *Journal of Water Supply: Research & Technology - Aqua, 61*(7), 446–459. doi:10.2166/aqua.2012.014

Vicente, H., Roseiro, J. C., Arteiro, J. M., Neves, J., & Caldeira, A. T. (2013). Prediction of bioactive compound activity against wood contaminant fungi using artificial neural networks. *Canadian Journal of Forest Research, 43*(11), 985–992. doi:10.1139/cjfr-2013-0142

World Health Organization, & Unicef. (1978). Primary health care: a joint report.

This research was previously published in Applying Business Intelligence to Clinical and Healthcare Organizations edited by José Machado and António Abelha; pages 153-168, copyright year 2016 by Medical Information Science Reference (an imprint of IGI Global).

Chapter 21

Radio Frequency Identification Technology in an Australian Regional Hospital:
An Innovation Translation Experience with ANT

Chandana Unnithan
Victoria University, Australia

Arthur Tatnall
Victoria University, Australia

ABSTRACT

Australian hospitals had begun exploring Radio Frequency Identification, a wireless automatic iden-tification and data capture technology for improving the quality of their services towards the end of 2000s. After many an unsuccessful pilots, a breakthrough for large hospitals came in 2010, with a key learning rendered by a large regional hospital that not only experimented with the technology, but also have made it all pervasive in their operations. In this chapter, we present the case study, through an innovation translation perspective, focusing on the socio-technical factors captured through elements of Actor-Network Theory.

INTRODUCTION

Healthcare has become a large part of expenditure in Australia, as in the case with many economies (Wamba, Anand & Carter, 2013). Using the Organisation for Economic Co-operation and Development's (OECD) methods, in 2011–12, Australia's health expenditure to GDP ratio was marginally above average compared with other OECD countries (AIHW, 2014). In 2010, the overall private and public spending on health was estimated at about 10% of the country's GDP or approximately about A\$ 65,000 million in annual spending (GS1-Australia, 2010). In 2011-12, A\$ 140.2 billion was spent on health, which is

DOI: 10.4018/978-1-7998-2451-0.ch021

Copyright © 2020, IGI Global. Copying or distributing in print or electronic forms without written permission of IGI Global is prohibited.

approximately 1.7 times higher in real terms (inflation adjusted) than in 2001-02 or expenditure has increased from A$ 4,276 per person in 2001-02 to A$ 6,230 in 2011-12 (AIHW, 2014).

Amongst the main stakeholders in Healthcare are large hospitals, which are trying to influence policies and governments to leverage the effective use of Information Communication Technologies (ICTs) to enable better quality of service (Payton et al, 2011). In the last decade, radio frequency identification (RFID) technology has captured the interest of hospitals worldwide (Ngai et al., 2009, Oztekin et al, 2010). Considered as a non-disruptive, open innovation, it is a technology that enables wireless automatic identification and data capture (Fosso Wamba et al., 2008, Foss Wamba, 2011).

RFID offers an improved means of reducing errors in patient care, such as adverse drug effects, allergies, patient–medication mismatches and medication dosage errors (Tu et al., 2009). Conversely, it promotes better management of critical healthcare assets (e.g., infusion pumps, wheelchairs) by enabling real-time identification, tracking and tracing (Bendavid et al., 2010). The capabilities of RFID technology have resulted in its potential to create value in health care (Dominguez-Péry et al., 2011). For example, (Najera et al., 2011) purports that the technology can enable healthcare stakeholders to monitor all steps related to the patient blood collection and transfusion process. This may include the identification of blood bags at the collection point, the tracking and tracing of products from the collection point to the hospital, and blood transfusion to a dedicated patient.

The value of RFID in the market rose from US$ 5.63 billion in 2010, to almost US$ 5.84 billion in 2011 (Das and Harrop, 2011). According to Pleshek (2011), there were approximately 150 million RFID tags in use within healthcare worldwide. It is no doubt, evident that the technology has high operational efficiencies and strategic potential in healthcare for improvement of quality services. A research conducted by Fosso Wamba et al (2013) found that the highest number of published research focuses on the technology issues of implementing RFID in hospitals (39.27%) . The research also found that organisational issues, focused on finance, was 37.24%, followed by data management, security and privacy issues that constituted 23.48%. These results are indicative of the fact that the focus is still remaining on the technical issues regarding RFID implementation, even in the year 2013.

Technical issues in implementing RFID had remained the main focus in many Australian hospitals (Unnithan and Tatnall, 2014). While adoption of this mobile technology has been investigated over a decade in hospitals (Coustasse et al., 2013), the focus is on using economic models (Yao, Chu and Li (2012) that try to explore the cost-benefits of the technology in relation to its rate of adoption. Conversely, RFID had only begun to be explored in Australian hospitals (Chowdhry & Khosla, 2007) since 2006, typically with vendor driven implementations that suited the cost-benefit analysis of hospitals (Chen, Wu, Su, & Yang, 2008; Unnithan and Tatnall, 2014).

In this chapter, we present the experience of a regional hospital in Australia, which focused on visualizing socio-technical factors that seem germane for the effective translation of RFID into hospital operations, through elements of Actor-Network Theory (ANT). This hospital has successfully jumpstarted the innovation translation of RFID in the regional public hospitals, while many pilots had been rendered unsuccessful.

HEALTHCARE CONTEXT IN AUSTRALIA

Prior to 2001, Australian health context was slow in adopting technologies in hospitals (Whetton, 2005; Duckett, 2007). As technologies had evolved over decades with patchy funding from government, hospitals had legacy systems that did not integrate or rather 'talk to each other'. It was in the decade 2001-2010 that technology refreshments had begun to occur in earnest, with the imminent national health records system (Muhammed, Teo & Wickramasinghe, 2012). Towards 2010, with the joint efforts of organisations such as Health Informatics Society of Australia (HISA, 2014), National E-health Transition Authority of Australia (NeHTA, 2014) and the Australasian College of Health Informatics (ACHI, 2014), hospitals in Australia had begun ardently testing and deploying technologies that would improve their quality of services to patients.

As Ho (2012) indicated, the demand for increased access to high-quality health care, an ageing population, shortage of clinicians in the regional areas, and increasing budgetary pressures have an impact on regional hospitals in particular. Two of the largest issues these hospitals face are enhancing worker productivity and reducing human error (Ho, 2012).

RFID IN AUSTRALIAN HOSPITALS

In Australia, health care is heavily affected by privacy regulations (Privacy Act of Australia 1988; Privacy.Gov 2013). While privacy and legal procedures do receive attention in many nations (for example, Fisher & Monahan point out that HIPAA significantly affects technology implementation, as well as health sector compliance in the USA), in Australia, the Privacy Act is more formidable (Privacy Act of Australia 1988, 2013). Often it is so doctrinaire that any data regarding an adult patient is not even provided to parents, unless they are named as carers, and if the patients are unable to handle themselves. This poses significant difficulties in emergencies, when an adult may be in perfectly good health, but not in a capacity to care about himself or herself at the time. Yet, the details of a condition may not even be immediately revealed to close relations (Duckett & Wilcox 2011).

In such restrictive conditions affecting the health sector, a piece of technology, such as RFID with its surveillance potential, was unacceptable in its original form to Australian hospitals. They had to be compliant with the existing privacy laws and standards. If not, perhaps similar to the USA (Fisher & Monahan 2008), organisations such as the nurse's union would have taken action and protested over the surveillance of people. Additional to this problem is the privacy of patients or individuals who may be moved using a wheelchair tagged by RFID.

The health care sector in Australia has received much attention from the government from the beginning of 2000s (Crompton 2002), when subsequent Productivity Commission (2005, 2006) reports recommended significant introductions of technologies in hospitals to improve processes. The National Health and Reforms Commission (2009) argued in favour of introducing technologies to improve efficiencies in the health sector. Novak and Judah (2011) suggest that the agenda for boosting productivity in the health sector is in progress. However, it may be noted that in the process of implementing technology agendas, state governments have to implement the policies and reforms enacted by the federal parliament (Gabbitas & Jeffs 2007; Goss 2008). In this continuum, many experiments occur. Often there are significant failures of implemented systems (Ducket & Willcox 2011). For example, the state of Victoria (Hopewell 2012) experimented with the HealthSmart system for refreshing technologies in hospitals; this was eventually cancelled being out of scope and overbudget. In the process, many new technologies were introduced, causing a lack of interoperability with existing systems and adding new ones (Dunlevy 2013).

RFID, as an innovation, was still being trialled towards the end of the 2000s, and was not yet fully accepted as a standard way of asset-tracking in hospitals. As Australian hospitals were on the pathway to e-health records at a national level, many large hospitals paused their proposed systems implementation projects, including RFID (Duckett & Wilcox 2011). An early report of RFID-enabled functions in Australia by Bacheldor (2006), reported that the Rockhampton Base Hospital in Queensland, Australia, used RFID to improve nurse safety in mental health ward buildings. Specifically, nurses in the hospital's mental health ward were using 'alarm cards, which combined a long-range wireless duress transmitter, a photo ID and proximity access control in one credit-card size device. The duress transmitter featured a battery-powered RFID tag. Any nurses in danger or in need of assistance pushed a button built into the back of the card, causing the transmitter to send a signal to an RFID reader, alerting co-workers. To make the process convenient, nurses received the cards when they signed in at the beginning of their shifts; the tag's unique ID numbers correlate in a database with the nurses' names and photos.

Chowdhury and Khosla (2007) provided an overview of the main components of an RFID-based patient management system, based on a model built for hospitals in Australian context. They argued that hospitals could track patients accurately and efficiently, improve the safety of clients by capturing basic data such as drug allergies, and prevent and reduce medical errors, as well as build a more collaborative environment with varied departments such as wards, medication and payments. Many pilot implementations, such as those at RMH and Barwon Health in Victoria (and others in Western Australia and Queensland) were introduced for not only asset-tracking but also patient tracking (infants, geriatrics & mentally disabled). However, most of these pilots did not result in full-scale implementation, or implementation was restricted to certain critical-care areas (Chowdhry & Khosla 2007).

Royal Adelaide Hospital in South Australia partnered with technology specialist Visionstream to deploy an integrated wireless network that combines tagging and tracking functionality to manage patient intake and care, as well as track availability of health care equipment throughout the hospital. The project is designed in conjunction with the South Australian government's new model of health care, which focuses on using technology to enable safe care solutions, reducing time spent on administration and increasing clinician-patient time (RFID 2012).

INNOVATION TRANSLATION AND ANT

In a systematics review of literature from 2002-2012, there was a gap that existed regarding socio-technical issues that impeded the successful translation of RFID into hospitals. Seminal work of academics as they reviewed RFID in the decade (Fisher & Monahan 2008; Roark & Miguel 2006; Hoskins 2006; Yao et al., 2012; Coustasse et al., 2013) pointed to mainly technical and economic issues relating to RFID, de-emphasising social and legal issues. Despite Australian hospitals piloting the technology towards the end of the decade, unsuccessful and abandoned examples persisted. Overall, research was still emerging regarding socio-technical issues in RFID adoption, even in 2013. RFID in Australia not only needed to be adopted widely, combatting all the interoperability and privacy issues, but also needed to be customised into this context, to be widely accepted. Rather, it was an innovation in the health sector that needed to 'translate' or become part of the context. Set in this premise, we explored the conceptual framework of 'innovation translation'.

Table 1. Questions for Moments of Translation

1.	**Problematisation:** What are the benefits defined by actors while introducing RFID? What are the roles of actors? What is the obligatory passage point?
2.	**Interessement:** How did the champions of RFID negotiate with other actors to establish and extend their network? How did they get others interested?
3.	**Enrolment:** Did key actors coerce, influence or impose on others to enrol them into the network of RFID acceptance?
4.	**Mobilisation:** Has the RFID solution/s gained wider acceptance? How was this achieved?

Callon (1986:196) outlined this novel approach to the study of power, the 'sociology of translation' using four moments of translation. We drew from this seminal work to build the conceptual framework, described as follows.

Moment 1: *Problematisation* is where key actors define the issues that RFID proposes to address in the hospital and their roles. The issue being addressed is 'translated' in terms of solutions offered by all actors, who then attempt to establish themselves as an 'obligatory passage point' (OPP) (Callon 1986), which must be negotiated as part of the solution. In other words, Callon (1986) refers to an OPP that has to occur for all the actors to satisfy the interests attributed to them by the focal actor. In this situation, we identified the actors, the issues they define and their defined roles. The idea of this *moment* is to foster relationships, to allocate or reallocate power between actors.

Moment 2: *Interessement* is whereby the actors defined in Moment one impose the identities and roles defined on other actors, thus building a network of relationships where all actors become involved. In this context, we studied how the champions or key actors negotiate with others in the network. *Interessement* is the set of actions by which an entity attempts to impose and stabilise the identities of actors in the same network for problematisation (Callon 1986). It involves a process of convincing other actors to accept the solution proposed. The actors are engaged in the process of confirming the OPP.

Moment 3: *Enrolment* occurs after the success of Moment 2, when a process of coercion, seduction and consent leads to the establishment of stable alliances. In this situation, we studied how the actors enrolled others into accepting the solution of RFID. More specifically, did they coerce, impose or influence others into enrolment? *Enrolment* involves consolidation of alliances through negotiations. It is the successful outcome of the first two moments.

Moment 4: *Mobilisation* occurs when the solution gains wider acceptance. In this situation, RFID gains wider acceptance as a solution for the proposed reason, within the hospital context. We investigated if this has occurred and how. *Mobilisation* of allies is a set of methods used to represent the group effectively or in other words 'who speaks for whom'? (Callon 1986) While some actors are used as initiators, others become spokespersons. This moment leads to stabilisation of the network. The questions we posed for eliciting the answers posed by these moments were as shown in Table 1.

The process of translation through the four moments may also be called a process of negotiation (Muhammad, Moghimi, Taylor, Redley, Nguyen, Stein, Kent, Botti & Wickramasinghe 2013). We considered a novel approach of visualising the data through a lens informed by ANT. Specifically, the presentation of interplay between all the factors (actors), while the solution of RFID as a technology was being considered and deployed, could be visualised better using elements of the ANT lens.

Table 2. ANT Depiction of Actors (Human and Non-Human) and Case Site

Actors/ Blackboxes	Name	Details (Non-Human Actors Have Been Given a Voice by a Human Actor)
Blackboxes	Regional hospital	The site where RFID entered into the context and has propagated successfully
	New Site	The new site of the regional hospital under construction
Non-Human Actors	DHS (Department of Health Services)	The external entity, which funded RFID implementation via a grant
	Symposium article	Voiced by CIO (Past)
	RFID tags/equipment, external entity (includes temperature tags)	Voiced by CIO (past and present)
	RFID results	Voiced by CIO (Current)
	RFID maps	Voiced by CIO (Current)
Considered Non-Human Actors	Nursing staff/orderlies	Voiced/represented by CIO in the focus group
	Pathology Food Services Engineering ICU OHS Infection Control	Voiced and represented by CIO (1) and CIO (2), Deputy Pharmacist
Human Actors	CIO (1) (The Champion)	The CIO is overall in-charge of all technology-based strategic decisions and drove the cause of RFID; the Godfather of RFID, who launched its career
	CIO (2) (reigning champion or current CIO—named as CIO)	This CIO was earlier the deputy head of ICT, second in command to the CIO; he is currently the CIO and also the champion of RFID who coaxed all the departments into trialling RFID and was successful
	Deputy Pharmacist	Deputy Head of Pharmacy Operation who drove RFID pioneering and propagation in the focus group
	Simpkin House Head	Voiced by the CIO in the focus group—followed up for confirmation by the Cameo
	Cameos (Researchers)	Researchers conducted direct interviews and focus group through a moderator, who then becomes the voice of cameos.

Actor-Network Theory (ANT), which was developed in 1980s by Bruno Latour (1986), and Law and Callon (1988), is an attempt to give voice to technical artefacts; they viewed that both social and technical determinism as flawed. ANT offers an advantage over other theories in that it does not have a dividing line between human and non-human entities nor an 'essence' attributed to either (Tatnall 2011). ANT has been applied to implementing and adopting different health care innovation studies (Berg 2001; Hall 2005; Bossen 2007; Cresswell, Worth & Sheikh 2010; Wickramasinghe, Bali, Tatnall, 2012; Muhmmed, Zwicker, Wickramasinghe, 2013).

The use of Actor–Network Theoretical conceptions has been used as a framework in narrating this case study. ANT uses the elements of blackboxes (or hospital/site in this instance), actors (human and non-human stakeholders), their relevant roles and the interplay between them, as the innovation (RFID) translates into the context of the hospital. In this case, RFID itself is considered the key actor (non-human) in this hospital. It debuts as an innovation, translates or 'integrates' itself into the context while re-negotiates the existing network of relationships within the hospital and establishes/sustains its presence, while evolving and emerging as a 'Star' that holds much promise in the future. In other words,

RFID technology entered the hospital (blackbox) as a key non-human actor and retained a position while enabling varied networks. In the continuum, it translated or integrated into this blackbox (hospital), transitioning into a more influential actor who has now become the 'Superstar', as it has been accepted as the 'key technology' for the new regional site.

CONTEXT AND PRECIS

The regional hospital in this research is situated in Victoria, in Australia, with more than 3,400 staff and 653 beds. It treats more than 37,000 in-patients annually; deals with more than 45,000 emergency cases and approximately 1,200 births annually. A 60-bed rehabilitation unit, eight-bed intensive care unit and five operating theatres complement the services, where almost 10,000 surgical procedures are performed annually. The organisation provides services in emergency, maternity, women's health, medical imaging, pathology, rehabilitation, community services, residential aged-care, psychiatric care, community dental, hospice, palliative care, cardiology, cancer services and renal dialysis.

In July 2010, the hospital began to roll out a Wi-Fi-based solution to manage the flow of patients through its surgical wards (Friedlos 2010). In 2011, it expanded the use of the system to include the temperature monitoring of pharmaceuticals and blood supplies, and a staff safety system for doctors and nurses. The system operates on a standard Wi-Fi network and utilises RFID tags and Real Time Location Systems (RTLS) software, as the hospital received funding to install Wi-Fi in its surgical theatre. Initially, the hospital wanted to obtain better real-time data regarding theatre and staff utilisation in its perioperative suite, which handles up to 10,000 surgical procedures annually. Upon arrival in the surgical theatre, orthopaedic patients are given a tag that provides information on the patients' location and movements, thereby enabling staff members to ensure that scheduled procedures start on time and that patients receive proper care.

The system collects data as it follows a patient's journey through theatre, from the admissions area to the waiting area to the theatre complex and the anaesthetic bay. This allows for business decisions to be merged into the complex flow of staff and resources to the perioperative suite. It was expected that the hospital would be able to process patients through the surgery more efficiently and use resources better. The system operates on the hospital's existing unified wireless network with access points throughout the hospital that act as RFID interrogators. This aspect resulted in a lower total cost of ownership for the hospital. The system utilises active tags, which are 802.11-compliant and operate at 2.4 GHz. Information is transmitted from the tags across the Wi-Fi network to MobileView software from AeroScout, which can be accessed by all employees on any computer monitor (Friedlos, 2010)

This regional hospital effectively gathered market information from the cases of failures in RFID implementation, while the technology was still evolving. In 2010, medical grade tags had evolved and technology costs had become lower. However, within the Australian health sector, interoperability issues and the strong resistance from hospital staff (particularly orderlies and nurses) was still impeding the innovation translation of this technology. It was at this time, the first author (and primary researcher) had met with the CIO of the hospital. A data collection ensued over a 2 year period with unstructured interviews including 2 CIOs, who succeeded each other (and worked together), and the department representatives in a focus group facilitated by a moderator.

FINDINGS AND DISCUSSION

Problematisation

We analysed the findings using the questions as follows:

What are the benefits perceived to be achieved by key actors while introducing RFID? What are the roles of the actors? What is the Obligatory Passage Point?

The case of RFID was introduced into this hospital via a pilot in 2010. However, a full-scale RFID implementation in the theatres/emergency area did not occur. The rationale is evident from the following excerpt:

HealthSmart in Victoria did not approve to send HL7 messages to iPM to enter data into the PAS in real time, and therefore, the project was abandoned, as efficiency was minimal. A nurse had to still physically enter details and be present throughout the patient journey, in addition to using the RFID system...The nurses accepted it at the beginning but—after six months they said, 'you've had a good trial, we don't need to do this any more, use the tags for something else', which is what we did, we just repurposed them and used them for something else, they weren't lost or anything...

Further probes into the situation revealed that RFID tags were repurposed for the ICU and related areas. Specifically, the initial problem was 'tracking the patient journey' in the orthopaedic surgeries. The problem owners were nurses. In the re-problematisation, the problem was owned by the ICU department, driven by nurses as the head of the department. Although it is a different department, nurse remained the problem owner. The solution owner did not change in this case; RFID was simply re-purposed. The problem was to track assets in the ICU using RFID (the OPP):

Asset management and some of them have actually gone up to the ICU for the bed tracking... ...high-value assets are tracked...Computers on wheels, ICU beds, emergency resuscitation equipment—it all came back from the fact that after Emergency Dept had their little rework last year, there was a $30,000 piece of equipment that no one could find anywhere—it had been submerged somewhere during the refit.

Clearly, a *re-problematisation* moment was visible. The benefits of RFID were realised not only by nurses who recommended that it be repurposed (almost six months after the trial), but ICU staff also accepted it. Two different departments—namely OHS and Infection Control—had to be involved in the trial, as it was a requirement. Thus, the tracking of equipment using RFID passed the OPP with a set of new actors. Then we discovered that RFID had taken another role in the hospital. Accidentally, a new form of tags—namely temperature tags that could monitor the temperature of equipment such as fridges—came into the hospital.

The supplier gave it to us...threw a box of temperature tags...said 'here have temperature tag to play with as well'...Well, once we got it and put it in the first fridge and found the fridge was faulty...results of this simple exercise was brilliant. We then went to Pharmacy and said 'would you like to be able to give a five-minute result on all your fridges?' and they said, 'yes, thank you'

The CIO and his team had taken the temperature tags concept to Pharmacy for a trial, outlining its benefits.

CIO: *... RFID tags to all pharmacy fridges were deployed. Data was logged in real time at five-minute intervals, which then set alarms to notify the Pharmacy when temperature varied outside a pre-set range. This data was then used to identify fault fridges. This project was successful.*

Pharmacist: *Wi-Fi gave us ability to set alarms, ability to have real-time monitoring...saved us at least a couple of hours a work week. Now, we get reports once a week and look at them, but if we get any alarms, basically we follow them up.*

There is a new problematisation moment visible here. Obviously, the two key actors here are the CIO and head of Pharmacy, who saw a clear benefit in the temperature tags. The Pharmacy decided to take up the trial, which was successful, and it decided to implement temperature tagging using RFID, which herein is the OPP. Problematisation was initiated by the CIO here and driven by Pharmacy (users), and the OPP was to use the RFID temperature tags to monitor temperatures.

Then we chanced upon the fact that 'staff tagging' had occurred to monitor staff duress in the high-care and mental health facility of the hospital. Upon exploring this further, we became aware that it was introduced by customising the regular RFID tracking tags that were used for patients and equipment, and were worn by staff. Thus, another problematisation moment was revealed. The key actors for problematisation were the OHS and ICT departments:

The OHS department had an audit...they needed a solution for managing staff duress. And there was also an incident. A theatre cleaner had a heart attach in the middle of the night and no one came running. So before he came back to work as part of his OH&S plan, they needed a process to be able to prevent further recurrence of being isolated.

It was evident that the problematisation occurred with the key actors planning to use RFID tags for staff in high-care facilities in order to reduce staff duress and isolation. The staff tagging using wearable RFID tags were fitted with a button that could trigger alarms elsewhere (the OPP). The problematisation moments continued to re-occur throughout the year.

Interessement

How did the champions of RFID negotiate with other actors to establish and extend their network? How did they get others interested?

It appeared that there was an interest among theatre nurses in a white paper from the US that discussed surgeons causing the delay in attending to patients from surgery by tracking the patient journey using RFID. The CIO indicated that in Australia, to track delays in attending to patients, the situation had to be handled differently. Specifically, if surgeons felt that their productivity was being tracked, that would raise privacy issues, and unions would also enter the fray. The following excerpt is relevant.

CIO: *... you can't tell surgeons they're the delay, so they ended up putting a big display board up, which tracked the patients through and after...so the surgeons could sit there and say, 'Hmm, there's a patient there waiting, and they're waiting for me—maybe I should be doing something, yes'. If someone is sat in the holding bay for a period of time...or say 10 patients are in the holding bay, alarms could be set up.*

The nurses who went into RFID tracking became interested by the white paper, which could monitor clinician productivity. Conversely, clinicians in Australia, who could not be tracked or monitored by law, were implicitly driven into interessement, as they could visualise the patients in the waiting bay. The CIO and the ICT department were consulted on this, and they felt that that they could improve efficiencies by facilitating RFID deployment. Thus, the ICT area became interested.

At another time, the conversation with the CIO revealed how the ICU became really interested in RFID tagging:

The biomedical people, we'd given them a little taste...tracked a few of their fusion pumps. When they go to do a service on the fusion pumps it can take them three and a half to four weeks to locate them all—they loved the fact that they can press a button and at least find four of them in a minute and a half. So they're quite happy to go down the 'yes let's tag everything' path because it saves them a lot of time. And we use the simplest interface—just have a webpage that shows you a picture of where they are ...

Thus, RFID was able to capture the attention and interest of related areas of emergency, namely ICU and wards. The champions of RFID were the CIO, his team and the pharmacist. The success of the Pharmacy area was shown to Pathology, which then became interested. In this case, it is the user (pharmacist, regarded in this investigation as clinical staff or equivalent to nurses).

CIO: *We mentioned the success of Pharmacy to Pathology. They decided to install tags for fridges, including sub-zero freezers.*

Subsequently, Food Services began using temperature tags for monitoring cabinet temperatures...it worked too.

Engineering...once they saw it in place and saw the results, they thought 'this is a good idea, we'll buy some of them ourselves'

Thus, it can be seen that multiple departments—Pharmacy, Pathology and Food Services—became interested in the concept, influenced initially by Pharmacy and enabled by the CIO/ICT department. The important fact is that each department saw the results from the earlier departments and subsequently decided to 'go for it'. The ICT department had been the champion, although it had worked indirectly. It was the actual users of the system who propagated and got others interested.

Subsequently, the OHS area was looking for options and negotiated the new tagging with the ICT department. The following quotations revealed that the actual users became interested through the negotiation of the ICT and OHS people. The key element in this conversation was that the CIO was influenced by the residential manager of nursing facilities to push the concept of duress alarms. This residential manager was also a nurse.

CIO: *The earlier residential manager of nursing facilities was pushing the concept of duress alarms at some stage…and here was an option, it works better.*

Subsequently, there was a question raised from the nursing staff about the use of RFID in staff tracking, when the CIO realised that they had the back end for RFID already, so they could make use of it. This resulted in three levels of tracking in high-care facility—namely Wi-Fi tracking, ward tracking as patients move in and out, and room tracking for accurate location. As they already had the RFID tags and Wi-Fi, they therefore had a roaming duress alarm that covered 2–3 areas with just one staff member.

CIO: *… the theatre cleaner had a heart attack and was on the job, and it was a couple of hours before anybody found him. He was quite happy, he was fine, but now he has a tag.*

More important was the fact that nurses recommended it and the staff user became interested because it assisted him to call for help when needed. He felt safe with an RFID tag.

Thus, the interessement was initiated by a nurse and always enabled by the CIO/ICT taking a supportive role; however, being proactive. While the nurses were able to get all other user groups convinced, the CIO/ICT department was also able to convince the pharmacist initially for a different type of tag to monitor temperatures. The pharmacist was also considered a key 'clinical' person in the hospital in charge of trauma fridges, emergency blood etc. Through this person, other related departments, such as Pathology, Food Services and Engineering, became interested. From another viewpoint, the interessement was really through the influence and propagation of nurses, who were also convinced about patient and clinician safety, using duress alarms. Here again, the nurse was the pivotal element in getting all others interested.

Enrolment

Did key actors coerce, influence or impose on others to enrol them into the network of acceptance?

The nurses influenced the decision of enrolment on the ICT department, theatres, nurses and clinicians. The theatre nurses were then responsible for word-of-mouth propagation to the ICU and wards, while the ICT department influenced the BioMed department. Regardless of the influence, it was an important finding that the key actors managed to influence and enrol everyone concerned into the network of acceptance. Specifically, the nurses and orderlies had transformed into the role of influencers for RFID. This transformation was empowering for the actual users of the system, who then continued to propagate it.

The key actors in the second part of the propagation of RFID were the ICT department and the pharmacist. These actors influenced other departments, namely Pathology, Food Services and Engineering, which enrolled into the network of acceptance. The enrolment was assisted by the fact that there was proof or evidence of success available to them, in addition to the word-of-mouth propagation.

CIO: *Pathology followed on from Pharmacy and then in Food Services, we just sort of gave them to them and they said, 'Yes we'll have that' because I had shown the some of the results coming out of Pharmacy.*

… Engineering…were the hardest but once they saw it in place and saw the results, they thought. 'this is a good idea, we'll buy some of them ourselves'…Engineering…have jumped on board…They use them

when people complain about air-conditioning, because you can put a tag there and within 24 hours they have a complete history of the temperature within that location.

If it is a the ED trauma fridge—it sends to the Pharmacy alert staff that this alert has been triggered, as well as sending to the ED shift manager, so not only the Pharmacy manager knows about it but the shift manager knows about it and can do something about it, probably before the pharmacy guy can ring the phone and say, 'what's wrong'?

It was evident that not only did the ICT people influence the decision, but the interlinked roles of Pharmacy and emergency nurses being linked together also affected the enrolment process. In an emergency, if blood is required in the operating theatres, the nurse calls for it by connecting to Pathology and Pharmacy (where blood is stored). Keeping the temperature of the fridges correct is a requirement for emergency blood bottles kept in the fridges.

When it came to Food Services and Engineering, it was more the convenience and efficiency gains that drove the enrolment. While Food Services wanted to gain efficiencies through less wastage of food, particularly when it was needed, Engineering was driven by an OHS audit. The OHS area was already in the milieu, having been involved with the first RFID-tracking enrolment. They were looking into maintaining 'location temperatures', and with the RFID tracking of temperature, it was possible to determine whether there was a problem with the equipment, or whether a fan was not working. Thus, four different areas were enrolled based on other departmental experiences.

It was also revealed that the key champions of RFID in the hospital sought a solution that was then recommended by nurses and given to them by the ICT department. The process of enrolment here was through continuous negotiations and influence. The enrolment process was successful, as the key actors were able to influence others into the network of acceptance. It is interesting to note that RFID itself, as a non-human actor, influenced the enrolment decisions.

CIO: *In high-care facilities—their existing duress system…basically a buzzer…makes a horrible noise… that upsets all the patients, so the patients come to see what the noise is and the incident increases. Whereas with the RFID version—they get Jamaica (software) on their phones and it tells them where to go to…basically it tells everybody that you need to know about it exactly where the staff member is when the button is pushed and it continues to track the button until that incident has ceased.*

In summary, the enrolment occurred smoothly, as it propagated through nurses in the first place. In this case, although the ICT/CIO was a strong champion of RFID, he never pushed the technology directly. Rather, he enlisted the nurses and pharmacist, who then propagated the cause of RFID throughout the entire hospital. One important aspect is clear; the nurse was the strongest influencer, or 'the voice', that everyone listened to. The ICT department had succeeded only when it made the nurses the mouthpiece for the cause.

Mobilisation

Has the solution gained wider acceptance? How was this achieved?

It was evident that RFID had already propagated into the hospital widely through the initial involvement of nurses, the OHS department and Infection Control, and supported by the ICT department. By involving a wider set of key actors, including strategists, technologists, medical staff (nurses, orderlies, clinicians), administrative and operations people (OHS, Infection Control), the solution was rapidly gaining a wider audience.

It was evident that the RFID solution was rapidly gaining wider acceptance. The take-up of temperature tags had proliferated into other areas of the hospital; two other departments were considering RFID as a solution for completely different purposes with temperature tagging. Indeed, mobilisation had occurred with temperature RFID tags as also reflected in the CIOs statements.

CIO: *... So it's expanding—so there's the theatre, there's another facility where there is just one staff member looking after low-care patients that are on their way home basically or going to go into surgery first thing in the morning, there's all of the food service people who work after hours, and it's just been expanded again—there's a ward that only has one staff member over night so that means a tag. We now also have the roaming duress alarm for staff involved in another facility, under maternity. A lot of young mothers come up here to deliver without telling their husbands in Melbourne for particular reasons that they're delivering up here, and the husband usually if he finds out...storms into the place. The reason is usually that there is an intervention order...so staff have to say 'go away'. For instances such as this, staff may be working out of hours...they use a roaming tag...*

Further, RFID had proved itself as a solution that fits in, integrates and is versatile. Minimal training was provided, but users (medical staff including nurses, orderlies, clinicians and administrative staff) did not need much training. The tracking used a web-based system and the tags were wearable and anonymous. Specifically, an RFID tag only had a number and was wearable around the neck. It only traced the person who was wearing it as the number on the day. When the day was over, the tags were returned, and the person could no longer be tracked. No individual names or persons could be stalked using the tags unless they chose to wear it for specific purposes within the hospital. For example, a person working in mental health facilities or a clinician in a highly sensitive area felt safer with a tag that could help him or her find assistance quickly. It was clear that mobilisation had occurred as the solution gained wider acceptance in the CIO's words.

CIO: *It's certainly in our specifications...We'll have the Wi-Fi system set up six months before if we can. And the equipment won't leave the loading bay until it is tagged and on the database...basically the tag will become ubiquitous across the entire hospital, and it's engineered at construction. And with the new electronic patient record, it fits in very—it's one arm of the new patient record—you need to have some form of patient tracking, so the only way to do that is with RFID.*

RFID as a solution assumed many forms, permeated into many departments and completed all moments of translation. The network of acceptance is now stabilised, as the hospital is planning to integrate RFID from the ground level into the architecture of the new building, and also with the e-health records' implementation. RFID has translated into the context of this hospital completely through all moments of translation. The acceptance of the solution across the hospital gained impetus from the onset, as the key users (nurses) recommended it to others. In addition, as the technology itself had advanced in 2010, there were other uses, such as tracking temperature movements, which helped the hospital's major departments, including Pharmacy, Pathology, Food Services and Engineering.

As this hospital had begun with the Wi-Fi infrastructure, it had the advantage of better accuracy in tracking and linking all departments. Conversely, they were also completing the e-health records implementation as recommended by the national government. At the onset, there was support from the government for implementing the technology within the emergency area, which is regarded as a crucial point for any technology take-up. Specifically, if the solution worked in emergency, most medical staff would accept the solution. In this case, that was indeed the experience.

Nurses, who are the key users of the system, instilled confidence in this technology to all other users within the hospital. Thus, it penetrated through to the ICU, wards and related areas. Conversely, the OHS and Infection Control, who were administratively involved with the implementation, also found different uses for RFID, as they were linked in from the beginning. While the nurses recommended and influenced its translation, the ICT department facilitated it.

Conversely, the new avatar of temperature tags that were incidentally left by the technology vendor implicitly found its way into other departments. OHS, which was seeking a solution to address staff duress subsequent to an audit, found a different use to RFID tags (i.e., to assist staff in duress situations by triggering alarms using a tag). A wearable tag is attached with a button that helped lodge the call for assistance without making a noise, which could upset the patients. This aspect of RFID made it beneficial to improve the quality of work processes within the hospital and made it popular among the staff.

Nurses did not find the process as a work intensification, as RFID was originally recommended by them and was well integrated into the hospital systems. Clinicians did not consider it a surveillance technology for monitoring their productivity, as the technology was used to track the patient journey rather than them. Patients in the waiting bay were tracked, and a screen indicated the number of people in the bay. If there was overcrowding in the waiting bay, clinicians could visualise it on the screen, which alerted them to their own duties without ordering them. This subtle persuasion helped to improve the quality of care.

Overall, the medical staff accepted the technology as a helpful solution for improving their workflows. Conversely, the enhancements over the past few years had improved the use of technology and its initial hiccups, making it conducive for hospitals as well. For example, the Wi-Fi infrastructure-based location helped remove additional tracking equipment, and it improved the accuracy of the location. The problematisation moment flowed into a 'closing the loop' each time, with the moment being completed through interessement, enrolment of actors and mobilisation.

By involving all key users of the technology, not only did RFID translate well into the hospital, but it is also gaining wider acceptance. Medical staff who were tagged with an RFID tag felt safer in high-care and certain areas where their safety was under threat. Clinicians did not feel monitored (which would have been against the privacy law in Australia), as they were not tagged. Rather, patients in the bay on a monitor indicated indirectly to them that their attention was needed. The hospital had thus found a way around the privacy implications in Australia. Further, by making the paramedical and other staff feel safer (rather than being monitored), they also worked around the potential union problems that could have emerged. The success of this hospital is the way in which RFID was introduced, negotiated through users and translated indirectly, thereby realising its versatility.

From the perspective of Innovation Translation and ANT, tokens exchanged between nurses, orderlies, clinicians, department heads and the ICT remained positive, resulting in the successful translation of RFID. The Emergency Department had the highest power in relation to implementation of RFID technology. Confirming the literature, the ED is the area where RFID technology has the largest effect. Having a strong network relationship with nurses, clinicians and orderlies across all departments, the positive exchange of tokens was done with ease. In this case, the ICT department played a supportive, facilitating role, and an evidence-based coaxing strategy to implement the technology. In addition to all nurses and clinicians being aware of the use of RFID (being initiated by them), the ICT department was also conversant with the health and hospitals sector for many years. The confidence of the varied department heads in the suggestions made for RFID implementation by the ICT regarding temperature tags were taken positively because there was evidence supporting it that was visible almost immediately. The positive exchange of tokens between medical staff (nurses, clinicians, orderlies) and IT staff resulted in correct punctualisation. The web of relationships is invisible but strong in enabling the translation of RFID.

EMERGING THEMES FROM THE MOMENTS OF TRANSLATION

Theme 1: The key to innovation translation in the health context is its introduction and involvement by influential caregivers.

In Innovation Translation theory (Callon 1986; Tatnall 2011,), problematisation is a key moment where a group of one or more key actors attempts to define the nature of the problem and the roles of other actors. This is done in such a way that the key actors are seen as indispensible to solving the problem. The problem is often refined by the terms of solutions offered by these key actors. To pass through the OPP, all actors need to accept a set of specific assumptions and ways of operation specified by the assorted engineers. If this occurs, a stable network of relationships will result (Callon 1986).

Although RFID was imposed by the CIO and his ICT department, the RFID solution was initiated via the orthopaedics department, which had successfully applied for a grant from the Department of Health Services to track the patient journey into operating theatres. The caregivers (nurses) had the solution in mind for enhancing the quality of care rendered to patients. For operational reasons relating to the PMS, they could not continue the adoption of technology at the time. However, the nurses influenced the decision to pass on the RFID tags to the ICU for asset-tracking, which did not require the use of PMS. It should be noted that the decision to deploy and repurpose was initiated and influenced by caregivers in this context. Further, the ICT and other administrative departments were facilitating the technology by demonstrating it and on the recommendation of nurses. This supportive attitude to caregivers also helped the permeation of the technology in the hospital.

As a result, this hospital site is progressing rapidly towards the adoption of RFID more completely, rather than as a sporadic deployment within some areas.

Theme 2: Innovation translation in hospitals occurs through persuasive champions who understand the context of care.

Innovation Translation theory purports 'interessement', which is a series of processes which attempt to impose identities and roles defined in the problematisation, on other actors. This process means interesting another participant by coming between the proposed technology and the actor. According to Law (1986), the 'enrollers' attempt to lock the other actors into roles proposed for them. Gradually existing networks are dissolved and replaced with networks created by the enrollers.

This hospital revealed the success of champions and the persuasive power. CIO (1), who was the champion of the technology in the hospital, did not introduce it himself or impose it on the hospital. Nonetheless, the CIO and the ICT department were not only aware, but also championed the technology by providing the results of the successful deployment to other departments sequentially. One success followed the other due to the subtle persuasive skills of the champions—namely the CIO and ICT staff in this hospital.

The ANT purports tokens, which are successful outcomes or functions of actors that are passed on to other actors within the network. When the token is increasingly transmitted, it becomes increasingly punctualised and reified. The results of successful implementation and improvement in the workflow were passed on as a token to other departments by the champions. These tokens resulted in increased punctualisation. The ANT also suggested that an incorrect passage of token could break down the social network. The nurses correctly passed on word-of-mouth recommendations as well as actual results through the ICT department to other actors in the network, which in turn stabilised the network.

Theme 3: The strength of innovation translation in hospitals is in number of caregivers enrolled in the network.

In the Actor–Network Theory (Latour 1986) purported that:

Power vested in a person or technology does not automatically confer the ability to change or cause change in a context. Potential adopters need to be persuaded to adopt a technology. The more the number of people willing to adopt in the situation, the better is the proposed adoption.

Conversely, as McMaster, Vidgen & Wastell (1997) pointed out, innovations do not wait passively to be invented or discovered, but are created from chains of weaker or stronger human and non-human associations. Each actor enrolled in the translation influences the innovation to shape it into the ultimate form, which is adopted in the blackbox. The ANT purported that a network of materially heterogeneous actors that is achieved by a great deal of work that both shapes those varied social and non-social elements and disciplines them so they work together is necessary for successful technology adoption.

The initial network was formed 'circumstantially' by a set of actors influential actors who were enrolled selectively in the context. From this network, a set of coaxing relationships ensued into other departments, via the ICT department. These coaxing relationships ultimately resulted in a harmonious heterogeneous networks and successful translation of the technology. The key to innovation translation is the creation of a powerful consortium of actors to carry it through and the ability of those involved to construct the necessary alliances amongst other actors (McMaster, et al., 1997).

From the view point of innovation translation, if interessement is successful, enrolment will follow through a process of coercion, seduction or consent (Grint & Woolgar 1997), leading to establishment of a stable network of alliances. However, enrolment involves more than one actor to impose their will on others, and others do need to yield (Singleton & Michael 1993).

The champion of RFID, namely the CIO was able to enrol 4–5 departments of care-givers beginning with nurses. It would be correct to suggest that enrolment occurred initially through the consent/persuasion of nurses; and other departments through 'seduction' where the participants yielded willingly. The strength increased in numbers as the number of participants rose. As reflected in this voice: 'basically RFID will become ubiquitous across the entire hospital, and it's engineered at construction'.

Innovation translation theory also purport the concept of mobilisation when the proposed solution gains wider acceptance and even larger network of absent entities is created through some actors acting as spokespeople for others, mobilisation is said to have occurred. The champions continue to propagate RFID to other areas such as 'high and low care'—where a new adaptation of the technology is being initiated for 'duress alarms'.

Theme 4: Technologies had to be customised before being adapted into the health context.

Innovation Translation theory suggests that innovations have to be customised before being translated into any context. RFID tags were accepted into the pilot only after validation by Infection Control and OHS departments of the hospital, as being medical grade—customised to the context for tracking. The 'incidental RFID tags' supplied in addition to the original customised RFID tags, resulted in a set of new functions for RFID. This had resulted in the technology being translated into the context faster.

Technology had to be customised to fit the perceptions of the caregivers (users) before being adopted into the context. Specifically, the caregivers had to be satisfied that the technology will enhance their workflows and empower them with the ability to provide better care, with efficiency. As endorsed by, only real results from implementation as a token passed on successfully in the network, could effectively help in successful adoption of the technology.

From the emerging themes it is clear that in health care, as against other regular businesses, technology adoption is not based on a business case acceptance. The context of health care makes it unique in that the current processes cannot be disrupted as it involves human life. Strategists and technologists may be able to build a business case and deploy it successfully after a pilot in other businesses. However, in hospitals, the acceptance of a technology would depend on caregivers. The involvement of caregivers or frontline medical staff, who may initiate and propagate the technology is a necessity in this complex and dynamic environment.

Any technology that is deployed in hospitals is best adopted when initiated by a caregiver. Familiarity of the technology within the context by caregivers is also a necessity, before it can be considered for deployment. The rationale is that in the context of saving human life or patient care, no mistakes can be made by technology. In other words, technology and human beings are considered equal in the context—no mistakes can be made by both, which may affect lives. In such complex environment, technology adoption can only occur if customised to suit the needs of caregivers and their perceptions of care, as technology can only help extend the quality of care.

In this first successful case of RFID translation in Australian hospitals, a large hospital in the regional area of the State of Victoria had implemented it. The users and all supportive administrative departments were involved in the design and implementation of this technology in the emergency areas. Beginning with tracking patient journey into theatres and then wards, the technology permeated to all across the hospital. Nurses recommended it, clinicians accepted it as it impacted their moral conscience indirectly, and all users accepted the recommendations of key users—the nurses. The technology was negotiated in a different format by key departments, with the ICT department supporting its promulgation. It had to be noted that unlike a large hospital in the State of New South Wales, the State of Victoria had additional hurdles in terms of ethics to cope with, where RFID technology was implemented. There are State imposed regulations such as an additional check on the privacy issues touched by this technology, which had the potential to permeate everywhere.

Although many technology vendors had attempted to push technologies in Australian hospitals, the success of this hospital indicates that key in translation of the technology smoothly was the social factors (users of the technology). This highly ignored or dismissed factors are pivotal in the translation of RFID in Australian hospitals. Social factors include users of the technology (mainly nurses, Patient Care Orderlies or Patient Care Assistants or simply Orderlies) as well as the Champions (namely IT department and other administrative areas) of the technology, who understand the context of care and legal issues associated with technology implementation that may be specific to Australian hospitals.

KEY LEARNING

The first factor that emerged was timing of introduction of RFID into the hospital. RFID did translate well into the hospital because the *timing* was indeed *appropriate* by the time of implementation in this environment. It was already 2010 when RFID had evolved as a technology. Hospital grade tags were already in the market and the technology standards had stabilised. Australia was rapidly transitioning into e-health records systems and many hospitals had refreshed their existing legacy systems with the help of national and State level government grants. The timing being a factor also involved infrastructure issues before Wi-Fi had become common as well as handheld devices that could be used for tracking. As the nation is gearing up for e-health record systems, having technology refreshments in all hospitals nationwide, enabled by Wi-Fi and handheld devices; RFID will emerge as a versatile technology.

The biggest influencing factor was the actor-network relationships between caregivers in hospitals. The findings reveal that the negotiation and network of relationships between the users are pivotal in promulgating the technology. The network of actors in hospitals are complex. Nurses and orderlies are the life of hospital operations. They are the key social actors (factors) who impacted the translation of any technology in the system. These factors need to be involved at the onset as any introduction of technologies impact their workflows. If the users were able to negotiate changes in the workflow successfully, that would enable translation of the technology into the milieu.

In this case, the negotiations between nurses and other medical staff were facilitated by the champions. The hospital champions also considered the privacy regulations of the Australian environment, and successfully worked around them such that the technology did not alter the workflows of medical staff. As a result, there was successful negotiation/interaction between all the social factors (actors) and also the non-human actor, namely RFID technology. Clearly, there are significant indictors that the socio-technical factors do impact the successful translation of RFID technology in the Australian context.

More significantly, the findings reveal that there is a complex, yet silent web of relationships between the key actors in hospitals, in relation to promoting RFID technology. In this case, the nurse–nurse, nurse–clinician and nurse–ICT relationships, which are not clearly visible at the onset, is indeed the most powerful social factor for RFID implementation. The findings indicate that a nurse-led approach would work for RFID implementation, as they are listened to by all actors. While the ICT department feels imposed upon by medical directors, if the nurse is the person raising the issue, they will accept take it on board and enable it. Doctors do not question nurses neither do the patient care orderlies. Nurse happens to be the *lynchpin* in Australian hospitals.

While most people say that technology needs to be clinician led, it needs to be translated into context by the key actors (or social factors), namely the nurses. A doctor may be listened to initially for reasons of obtaining a funding, but ICT department may not be really happy about the situation, as reflected in the comments. However, if the nurse is leading an issue and taking it up to the ICT department, it usually is taken on board and given sufficient consideration or immediate attention. Conversely, the nurses always seem to have 'one voice' no matter which department they are based in. None of the nurses seem to contradict any others. In terms of ANT, the nurse becomes the pivotal actor, who can stabilise the network and enable all other actors to pass through the OPP.

Amongst the factors that emerged is the dynamic nature of the technology itself that helped it emerge as the superstar. RFID was already an accepted technology in many industry sectors although it is relatively new to hospitals. From tracking assets to patients using location tracking ability, it evolved into 'monitoring temperatures' for fridges and spaces. In hospitals, refrigeration is indeed a key element that supports quality of services. Keeping blood and life support medicines in certain temperatures is critical to emergencies. This was enabled through temperature monitoring tags—an evolution of the technology towards 2010. The technology presented a solution as an alarm device, that is non-interventional in high-care facilities within hospitals. An alarm device, if pressed made a buzzing noise, which could adversely affect patients. An RFID tag worn with a button to be pressed, reported the staff in need request as a 'call for help' silently. The staff member in need was tracked without upsetting the rest of the patients in the hospitals. The technology thus integrated itself into the environment, being supportive, yet evolving in its uses.

The versatility of RFID technology, as visible in the case with regular and temperature tags, helped its propagation. In summary, RFID has evolved as a technology, it has become versatile in a way that it can be worn by people, embedded into equipment or tagged for tracking assets. These forms of tracking are now accepted by Australian hospitals and are slowly being trialled. While the technology itself has now progressed to the level of bio-degradable RFID tags used in Oncology (Yang & Halvorsen 2010), in the US, Australia has still a long way before the technology is permeated and accepted in healthcare completely. Nonetheless, the encounters of RFID technology with its users have instilled a level of confidence in its technical location tracking ability, enabling its successful translation into Australian hospitals.

LIMITATIONS

This chapter is focused on one regional hospital in Australia and captures a view of a decade. While it is still the single successful case in Australia, as the technology evolves and becomes part of the fabric in Australia, the findings and recommendations may eventually need to be revisited. A generalisation is not possible, although the case provides very good indication on what is relevant in the Australian hospitals in relation to RFID technology translation.

CONTRIBUTIONS

As pointed out when answering the research questions, the key contribution of this research thesis is for Australian hospitals which are considering or have been unsuccessful in RFID technology implementation thus far. RFID is still considered an innovation for Australian hospitals, and to an extent an intrusion to existing workflows, due to the existing privacy controlled environment. In such an environment, the users of the system—mainly nurses, orderlies need to accept and propagate the technology—so that it can successfully translate realising its potential to improve efficiency of workflows and effectively, improving quality of care.

The chapter would help hospital administrators and decision-makers to better understand the factors that make RFID implementation more difficult, in particular, convincing hospitals to use it to the fullest ability. The successful case revealed that the dynamic versatile nature of the technology where it can be integrated well with the support of users. The socio-technical factors, or interaction between the technology and the users became positive as the findings revealed.

Implementing innovative technologies is not a concept that is unfamiliar in any industry sector. As against other industry sectors such as retail or manufacturing supply chains, where RFID has been deployed over the last decade for tracking based on location, health sector is different. Initially, RFID as a technology was not accepted because of potential apprehensions regarding its interference with medical equipment. This was addressed easily as the technology evolved. Over the past decade, there was much research and implementation of this technology in hospitals all over the world. However in Australia, it is still a nascent technology for the hospitals.

The unique proposition in Australian hospitals is the current transition into e-health records and moving away from the legacy systems. This transition preordained that many legacy systems needed to co-exist until all health-related systems are linked and updated over time. In the milieu, RFID was thrown in as an innovation which was seen more as another piece of technology, although useful, but creating further upheaval within frenzied hospitals. In addition, Australian hospital sector and the environment is privacy regulated by law, and culturally, this has had a significant impact of introducing any new technology that is interventional. While the technology was meant to only locate equipment initially, the potential of location tracking with patients and staff made it susceptible to reluctant acceptance.

The views in academic literature were mainly from the USA, where the privacy regulation and the environment of hospitals is quite different. In the Australian context, RFID was still a new concept being accepted or rather translating slowly into the environment. The socio-technical aspects of translation have been rather ignored largely in terms of this technology. In the Australian context in particular, while there are RFID implementation models being constructed, studies that elicited factors that contributed to successful translation are still to emerge (at the time of this thesis submission). Therefore, the main contribution of this chapter is that it studied the process of translation (or negotiation) as RFID translates into the hospital and elicited success factors.

The theory framework of Innovation Translation was confirmed using the data analysis and moments of translation. There are 'problematisation' moments that occurred and went through *interessement, enrolment and mobilisation* sequentially. Here is an indication of successful translation of the technology. In addition, the conceptual framework presented with the ANT lens strengthens the ability of Innovation Translation theory to recommend future strategies for successful translation of technology.

Moreover, the contributions in this chapter reflects real-life experiences and successes where the key learning could be used for better translation of RFID in Australian hospitals. The successful translation as reported in subsequent publication that arose from the thesis is a good vaulting point for other hospitals that are considering RFID implementation. It is clear that making nurses the 'mouth piece' for the technology, and enabling it from ICT department (indirectly), is the best way to realise the benefits from this powerful technology. Industry expert validation is also supportive of this view, and in particular that nurses are the lynchpin in Australian hospitals.

The chapter also brought out the views from ICT department view (including implementation managers, CIO, consultant) and from clinician viewpoint (nurses, orderlies). These different perspectives that form the foundation of the web of network relationships that need to be stabilised for successfully translating the technology into Australian hospitals becomes apparent to hospital decision-makers. In turn, it helps them to better understand the process of successful translation and enable the process. For Australian hospitals, practitioners and technology vendors, the insights from this chapter is a start off point for incorporating better implementation processes within their own area. For academia, there is scope for study using ANT in the health sector, with a focus on Australian context.

REFERENCES

ACHI. (2014). *Australasian College of Health Informatics*. Retrieved from http://www.achi.org.au

AIHW. (2014). Australian Institute of Human Welfare, Australian Hospital Statistics report 2013-14, Australia. AIHW.

Bacheldor, B. (2006). RFID Fills Security Gap at Psychiatric Ward. *RFID Journal*. Retrieved October 24, 2007 from http://www.rfidjournal.com/article/articleview/2750/1/1

Bendavid, Y., Boeck, H., & Philippe, R. (2010). Redesigning the replenishment process of medical supplies in hospitals with RFID. *Business Process Management Journal, 16*(6), 991–1013.

Berg, M. (2001). Implementing information systems in health care organizations: Myths and challenges. *International Journal of Medical Informatics, 64*(2–3), 143–156. doi:10.1016/S1386-5056(01)00200-3 PMID:11734382

Bossen, C. (2007). Test the artefact – develop the organization: The implementation of an electronic medication plan. *International Journal of Medical Informatics, 76*(1), 13–21. doi:10.1016/j.ijmedinf.2006.01.001 PMID:16455299

Callon, M. (1986). Some elements of a sociology of translation: domestication of the scallops and the fishermen of St Brieuc Bay. In *J. Law, Power, action and belief: a new sociology of knowledge?* (pp. 196–223). London: Routledge.

Chen, C.C., Wu, J., Su, Y.S., & Yang, S.C. (2008). Key drivers for the continued use of RFID technology in the emergency room. *Management Research News, 31*(4), 273–288.

Chowdhury, B., & Khosla, R. (2007, July). RFID based Real Time Patient Management System. Computer and Information Science, 363–368.

Coustasse, A., Tomblin, S., & Slack, C. (2013). A review of Radio Frequency Identification Technologies and Impacts on the Hospital Supply Chain: 2002-2012. In *Proceedings of Academic and Business Research Institute (AABRI) International Conference*. MMM Track.

Cresswell, K. M., Worth, A., & Sheikh, A. (2010). Actor-network theory and its role in understanding the implementation of information technology developments in healthcare. *BMC Medical Informatics and Decision Making, 10*(1), 67. doi:10.1186/1472-6947-10-67 PMID:21040575

Crompton, M. (2002). *Privacy, Technology and the Healthcare Sector, Federal Privacy Commissioner Report*. Paper presented at the Australian Financial Review—4th Annual Health Congress, Sydney, Australia.

Dominguez-Pery, C., Ageron, B., & Neubert, G. (2013). A service science framework to enhance value creation in service innovation projects - An RFID case study. *International Journal of Production Economics, 141*(2), 440–451. doi:10.1016/j.ijpe.2011.12.026

Duckett, S. J. (2007). *The Australian Health Care System* (3rd ed.). Australia: Oxford University Press.

Duckett, S. J., & Willcox, S. (2011). *The Australian health care system* (4th ed.). Melbourne: Oxford University Press.

Dunlevy, S. (2013). *Outrage as eHealth record sign-up squads hit Australian hospital patients in bid to boost numbers*. News.com.au. Retrieved April 30 2013 from http://www.news.com.au/national-news/outrage-as-ehealth-record-sign-up-squads-hit-australian-hospital-patients-in-bid-to-boost-numbers/story-fncynjr2-1226619874616

Fisher, J. A., & Monahan, T. (2008). Tracking the social dimensions of RFID systems in hospitals. *International Journal of Medical Informatics, 77*(3), 176–183. doi:10.1016/j.ijmedinf.2007.04.010 PMID:17544841

Fosso Wamba, S. (2011). Positioning RFID technology into the innovation theorylandscape: A multidimensional perspective integrating case study approach. In *Proceedings of the 15th Pacific Asia Conference on Information systems (PACIS)*. Brisbane, Australia: PACIS.

Fosso Wamba, S., Anand, A., & Carter, L. (2013). A literature review of RFID-enabled healthcare applications and issues. *International Journal of Information Management, 33*(5), 875–891. doi:10.1016/j.ijinfomgt.2013.07.005

Fosso Wamba, S., Lefebvre, L. A., Bendavid, Y., & Lefebvre, E. (2008). Exploring the impact of RFID technology and the EPC network on mobile B2B eCommerce: A case study in the retail industry. *International Journal of Production Economics, 112*(2), 614–629. doi:10.1016/j.ijpe.2007.05.010

Friedlos, D. (2010, December). Australia's Bendigo Health Improves Efficiency Through RFID. *RFID Journal*.

GS1-Australia. (2010). *Healthcare Industry Report*. Author.

Gabbitas, O., & Jeffs, C. (2007). *Assessing productivity in the delivery of health systems in Australia: some experimental estimates*. Paper presented to the ABS-PC Productivity Perspectives 2007 Conference. Retrieved from http://www.pc.gov.au/research/conference-papers/health-service-productivity

Goss, J. (2008). *Projection of Australian health care expenditure by disease, 2003–2033, Cat. No. HWE 43*. Canberra: Australian Institute of Health and Welfare.

Grint, K., & Woolgar, S. (1997). *The machine at work- technology, work and organisation*. Cambridge: Polity Press.

Hall, E. (2005). The 'geneticisation' of heart disease: A network analysis of the production of new genetic knowledge. *Social Science & Medicine, 60*(12), 2673–2683. doi:10.1016/j.socscimed.2004.11.024 PMID:15820579

Health and Hospitals Reform Commission. (2009). *A healthier future for all Australians: Final Report.* Canberra: Commonwealth of Australia. doi:10.4018/978-1-60960-197-3.ch004

HISA. (2014). *Health Informatics Society of Australia.* Retrieved from http://www.hisa.org.au

Ho, G. (2012, April 27). *Can technology help overcome Australia's healthcare challenges?* Australian Broadcasting Corporation (ABC) - Technology and Games.

Hoskins, R. (2006). *InfoLogix Announces HealthTrax RFID Asset Tracking Software for Hospital Mobile Assets Management.* Retrieved 12 February 2006 from http://www.bbwexchange.com/pubs/2006/02/11/page1395-98309.asp

Latour, B. (1986). Article. In J. Law (Ed.), The power of association, Power, Action and Belief – a new Sociology of Knowledge, Sociological Review Monograph 32 (pp. 264–280). London: Routledge and Kegan Paul.

Law, J., & Callon, M. (1988). Engineering and Sociology in a Military Aircraft project: A network analysis of Technological Change. *Social Problems, 35*(3), 284–297. doi:10.2307/800623

McMaster, T., Vidgen, R. T., & Wastell, D. G. (1997). *Towards an understanding of technology in transition - Two conflicting theories.* Paper presented at Information Systems research in Scandinavia, IRIS20 Conference, Hanko, Norway.

Muhammad, I., Moghimi, F. H., Taylor, N. J., Redley, B., Nguyen, L., Stein, M., ... Wickramasinghe, N. (2013). Using ANT to uncover the full potential of an intelligent operational planning and support tool (IOPST) for acute healthcare contexts. *International Journal of Actor-Network Theory and Technological Innovation, 5*(2), 29–49. doi:10.4018/jantti.2013040103

Muhammed, I., Teoh, S., & Wickramasinghe, N. (2012). Why Using Actor Network Theory (ANT) Can Help to Understand the Personally Controlled Electronic Health Record (PCEHR) in Australia. *International Journal of Actor-Network Theory and Technological Innovation, 4*(2), 44–60. doi:10.4018/jantti.2012040105

Muhmmed, I., Zwicker, M., & Wickramasinghe, N. (2013). How Using ANT Can Assist to Understand Key Issues for Successful e-Health Solutions. *International Journal of Actor-Network Theory and Technological Innovation, 5*(3), 1–17.

Najera, P., Lopez, J., & Roman, R. (2011). Real-time location and inpatient care systems based on passive RFID. *Journal of Network and Computer Applications, 34*(3), 980–989. doi:10.1016/j.jnca.2010.04.011

NEHTA. (2014). *National E-Health Transition Authority of Australia.* Retrieved from http://www.nehta.gov.au

Ngai, E. W. T., Moon, K. K. L., Riggins, F. J., & Yi, C. Y. (2008). RFID research: An academic literature review (1995–2005) and future research directions. *International Journal of Production Economics, 112*(2), 510–520. doi:10.1016/j.ijpe.2007.05.004

Ngai, E. W. T., Poon, J. K. L., Suk, F. F. C., & Ng, C. C. (2009). Design of an RFID-based Healthcare Management System using an Information System Design Theory. *Information Systems Frontiers*, *11*(4), 405–417. doi:10.100710796-009-9154-3

Novak, J., & Judah, A. (2011). *Towards a health productivity reform agenda for Australia*. South Melbourne: Australian Centre for Health Research.

Oztekin, A., Foad, M. P., Delen, D., & Swim, L. K. (2010). An RFID network design methodology for asset tracking in healthcare. *Decision Support Systems*, *49*(1), 100–109. doi:10.1016/j.dss.2010.01.007

Payton, F. C., Pare, G., LeRouge, C., & Reddy, M. (2011). Health care IT: Process, people, patients and interdisciplinary considerations. *Journal of the Association for Information Systems*, *12*(2), i–xiii.

Privacy Act of Australia. (1988). Retrieved from http://www.privacy.gov.au/law/act

Privacy.Gov. (2013). *State and Territory Laws*. Office of the Australian Privacy Commissioner, Australia. Retrieved from http://www.privacy.gov.au/law/states

Productivity Commission. (2005). *Impacts of advances in medical technology in Australia*. Productivity Commission Research Report. Retrieved from http://www.pc.gov.au/study/medicaltechnology/finalreport/medicaltechnology.pdf

Productivity Commission (2006). *Potential benefits of the National Reform Agenda, Report to the Council of Australian Governments*. Canberra: Commonwealth of Australia.

Roark, D. C., & Miguel, K. (2006). Bar coding's replacement? *Nursing Management*, *37*(2), 29–31. doi:10.1097/00006247-200602000-00009 PMID:16452888

Singleton, V., & Michael, M. (1993). Actor-Networks and Ambivalence: General practitioners in the UK Cervical Screening Programme. *Social Studies of Science*, *23*(2), 227–264. doi:10.1177/030631293023002001

Tatnall, A. (2011). Innovation Translation, Innovation Diffusion, and the Technology Acceptance Model: Comparing three different approaches to Theorising Technological Innovation. In *Actor–Network Theory and Technology Innovation: Advancements and New Concepts*. IGI Global.

Tu, Y. J., Zhou, W., & Piramuthu, S. (2009). Identifying RFID-embedded objects in pervasive healthcare applications. *Decision Support Systems*, *46*(2), 586–593. doi:10.1016/j.dss.2008.10.001

Unnithan C, Tatnall A (2014). Actor-Network Theory (ANT) based visualisation of Socio-Technical Facets of RFID Technology Translation: An Australian Hospital Scenario. *International Journal of Actor-Network Theory and Technology Innovation, 2*(2).

Whetton, S. (2005). *Health Informatics*. Australia: Oxford University Press.

Wickramasinghe, N., Bali, R., & Tatnall, A. (2012). A Manifesto for e-health Success- The Key Role for ANT. *International Journal of Actor-Network Theory and Technological Innovation*, *4*(3), 24–35. doi:10.4018/jantti.2012070103

Yang, B., & Halvorsen, P. (2010). *Use of RFID to enhance the patient experience, increase safety and eliminate treatment errors, RFID in Oncology Clinics*. White Paper. Alliance Oncology.

Yao, W., Chu, C.-H., & Li, Z. (2012). The Adoption and Implementation of RFID technologies in Healthcare: A literature review. *Journal of Medical Systems*, *36*(6), 3507–3525. doi:10.100710916-011-9789-8 PMID:22009254

Yen Y, Lo N, Wu T (2012). *Two RFID based solutions for secure inpatient medication*. Academic Press.

Yu, Y. C. Y., Hou, T. W. T., & Chiang, T. C. T. (2012). Low cost RFID real lightweight binding proof protocol for medication errors and patient safety. *Journal of Medical Systems*, *36*(2), 823–828. doi:10.100710916-010-9546-4 PMID:20703651

KEY TERMS AND DEFINITIONS

Blood Cooler: Devices for keeping the blood cooled in hospitals.

BPM: Business Process Management (BPM) is the method of managing the redesign and redeployment of business processes within a given situation and organisation.

BPR: Business Process Redesign (BPR) is a process for assessing performance issues of a particular process and conducting radical redesign to the process, by redesigning the process itself and systems, policies or organisational structures.

Catheter: A thin tube used for medical purposes.

Defibrillator: Electric Shock Machine.

ED: Emergency Department.

Exciters: A device that uniquely extends the Real Time Location System of AeroScout, to provide robust and immediate Wi-Fi RFID tag detection capabilities. For example, the Exciter triggers AeroScout's RFID tags as they pass through a choke-point to transmit a message that is received by a standard Wi-Fi Access Point or AeroScout Location Receiver. This provides instant knowledge that a tagged asset or person passed through a gate, doorway or some other tightly defined area.

Implants: Something that is inserted into a human body during surgery.

Pacemaker: A device that regulates heartbeat.

PMS: Patient Management Systems.

This research was previously published in Maximizing Healthcare Delivery and Management through Technology Integration edited by Arthur Tatnall and Tiko Iyamu; pages 76-100, copyright year 2016 by Medical Information Science Reference (an imprint of IGI Global).

Chapter 22
Community Hospital Disaster Preparedness in the United States

Dan J. Vick
St. Vincent College, USA

Asa B. Wilson
Methodist University, USA

Michael Fisher
Regis University, USA

Carrie Roseamelia
SUNY Upstate Medical University, USA

ABSTRACT

Disasters are common events in the United States. They generally result in casualties and community hospitals play a critical role in caring for these victims. Therefore, it is critical that hospitals are prepared for disasters. There has been increased focus on hospital disaster preparedness in the United States because of events that have occurred in the 21st century. To determine the current state of disaster preparedness among community hospitals, a comprehensive review of the literature was conducted that focused on studies and other articles pertaining to disaster preparedness in U.S. community hospitals. The review showed mixed results as to whether hospitals are better prepared to handle disasters. Barriers to preparedness were identified. Opportunities for improvement may require additional study and involvement by federal and state governments, other agencies, and hospitals themselves to overcome barriers and assist hospitals in achieving a higher level of preparedness.

DOI: 10.4018/978-1-7998-2451-0.ch022

Copyright © 2020, IGI Global. Copying or distributing in print or electronic forms without written permission of IGI Global is prohibited.

INTRODUCTION

A disaster is defined as a "sudden, calamitous event that seriously disrupts the functioning of a community or society and causes human, material, and economic or environmental losses that exceed the community's or society's ability to cope using its own resources" (International Federation of Red Cross and Red Crescent Societies, n.d.). Natural disasters include weather-related phenomena, such as floods, hurricanes, and blizzards, and non-weather-related incidents, such as wildfires, tsunamis, and epidemics. Non-natural disasters include events such as mass transit mishaps, terrorist attacks, and chemical spills.

Disasters are common in the United States. Forty-three states have experienced earthquakes, all 50 states have encountered flooding, and approximately five hurricanes impact the southern and eastern coastlines every three years (McGlown & Robinson, 2011). Disasters are occurring more frequently; the average number per year increased around 60% from 2006 to 2015, compared with the average annual number in the two previous decades (U.S. Federal Emergency Management Agency, 2016). The number of people affected by disasters from 2006 to 2015 increased 44% over the number of people affected by disasters occurring in the previous decade (Centre for Research on the Epidemiology of Disasters, 2015). There have been a number of notable disasters in the 21st century, including the terrorist attacks of September 11, 2001; severe hurricanes, such as Katrina and Rita in 2005, Sandy in 2012, and Irma in 2017; and the tornado that devastated Joplin, Missouri in 2011.

Disasters inflict casualties, either from direct injuries or indirectly, such as from illnesses caused by contaminated water and food or toxic fume inhalation. Hospitals play a critical role in disaster response in affected communities. They represent an important component in a regional system for disaster preparedness and management. Disaster preparedness, as defined by the Department of Homeland Security (DHS) and the Federal Emergency Management Agency (FEMA), is "a continuous cycle of planning, organizing, training, equipping, exercising, evaluating, and taking corrective action in an effort to ensure effective coordination during incident response" which contributes to the ability to "prevent, respond to, and recover from natural disasters, acts of terrorism, and other disasters" (U.S. Department of Homeland Security, 2013, Plan and Prepare for Disasters).

It is important for hospital administrators and staff to improve their organizational ability to address disasters. This includes being able to handle large numbers of patients (surge) and to collaborate with outside agencies, community governments, and other healthcare facilities within the stricken area (Krizner, 2007).

Government resources are crucial for helping hospitals to achieve and maintain preparedness. Following the events of September 11th, the U.S. Department of Homeland Security (DHS) was established along with several other offices and agencies. A National Response System was developed to address terrorist attacks and natural disasters. The DHS issued a national strategy for homeland security in July 2002. This included creating the National Incident Management System (NIMS) and preparing health care providers to respond to incidents of catastrophic terrorism (Harrald, 2012).

The U.S. Department of Health and Human Services (HHS) established the Hospital Preparedness Program (HPP) in 2002 under the Health Resources and Services Administration (HRSA). The All-Hazards Preparedness Act of 2006 transferred the HPP from HRSA to the newly-created Assistant Secretary for Preparedness and Response (ASPR) (Cagliuso, 2014a). The HPP assists health systems and hospitals to prepare for public health emergencies and disasters (University of Pittsburgh Medical Center, 2009). It is the sole provider of federal funding for promoting regional healthcare system preparedness. Initially, the program awarded funds to hospitals for the purchase of preparedness-related equipment and supplies in order to improve their decontamination capability and surge capacity, increase vital supply quantities, and promote education and training (Kaji, Koenig, & Lewis, 2007; Meyers, 2006). Since 2012, the HPP has shifted to funding and facilitating the development of health care coalitions (HCCs) that encourage organizations to work with one another. The HPP's goals are to "improve patient outcomes, minimize the need for supplemental state and federal resources during emergencies, and enable rapid recovery" (U.S. Department of Health and Human Services, n.d.).

Given the added emphasis on disaster preparedness in recent years, have community hospitals in this country met with success in their attempts to improve preparedness for disasters? This article explores various studies and specific disaster incidents that have been described in the published literature to gain a better understanding of the current level of community hospital disaster preparedness in the U.S. The next section describes the methodology for this review. This is followed by a more detailed explanation of the essential role of hospitals in disaster management. Following sections address the objective question and identify barriers to preparedness. Hospital preparedness for natural and non-natural disasters is considered in subsequent paragraphs. Finally, disaster preparedness across various types of hospitals is evaluated. The Discussion offers an overall assessment of hospital disaster preparedness, areas of concern and potential focus for hospital administrators, and recommendations for further research.

REVIEW METHODOLOGY

The literature review was based on searches in proprietary library and public access Internet databases, such as PubMed, Medline, and Google Scholar. Various key words and phrases were used, such as: assessment, community hospitals, disaster planning, disaster preparedness, disasters, emergency preparedness, natural disasters, rural hospitals, and urban hospitals. The literature search included: books, journals, dissertations, reviews, magazine and newspaper articles, disaster preparedness survey databases, and reports from federal agencies and organizations such as the Centers for Disease Control and Prevention (CDC) and the American Hospital Association (AHA). Reference lists in journal articles and dissertations were also reviewed.

The focus was limited to disaster preparedness in the U.S. and in U.S. hospitals. An emphasis was placed on publications between January 2002 and March 2018 since articles published prior to 2002 do not reflect the increased attention given to disaster preparedness since September 11, 2001. Relevant articles were found in *JAMA, Prehospital and Disaster Medicine, American Journal of Infection Control, The Journal of Emergency Medicine*, and other journals.

For the purpose of this study, *community hospitals* are defined as "all nonfederal, short-term general and other special hospitals" including "academic medical centers or other teaching hospitals if they are nonfederal short-term hospitals" (American Hospital Association, January 2016).

COMMUNITY HOSPITAL DISASTER PREPAREDNESS

Significance and Essential Role of Hospitals

Hospitals are involved early on during a disaster. They are always open and are the place where victims of an event are most likely to seek treatment (Luband, 2006; Meyers, 2007). Hospitals take responsibility for healthcare disaster management and provide the majority of care for victims within their communities, even when they themselves are impacted by the disasters (Heine, 2011; World Health Organization, 2010). However, it is only in the last 30 years that hospitals have formalized a role for an Emergency/ Disaster Manager or Coordinator.

A basic principle of disaster management is preparing for unlikely events while acting to mitigate or prevent the possibility that they will actually occur (Reilly & Markenson, 2011). Given the low likelihood of such events, it is difficult to evaluate the strengths and weaknesses of hospital disaster preparedness. Hospitals are expected to respond to disasters and continue to provide non-disaster health services. They are viewed as a central care location for those with non-urgent medical and nonmedical needs, such as vaccinations, medication refills, food and water, and community shelter or refuge, during a disaster (Charney, Rebmann, Esguerra, Lai, & Dalawari, 2013). This was noted during the September 11th terrorist attacks and the Northeast Blackout of 2003 when people went to hospitals even though they were not in need of medical care. Disaster planning and response require hospitals to focus on population needs as opposed to the needs of individual patients - how hospitals usually deliver care (Reilly & Markenson, 2011).

Hospital disaster planning has assumed greater importance in this century because of domestic terrorist attacks and natural disasters. The emphasis has shifted to an all-hazards comprehensive disaster plan rather than planning for specific disasters or threats. There is a recognized need for hospitals to collaborate with community stakeholders in the planning process and to coordinate efforts with local and regional disaster management entities. Hospital disaster management can involve a variety of activities. Common focus areas include communication; surge capacity; preparation for chemical, biological, radiological, nuclear, and explosive (CBRNE) events; security measures; staff education and training; management of volunteers; and collaboration with public health agencies (Reilly & Markenson, 2011).

Mothershead (2004) stated that although most healthcare organizations have disaster plans, few actually have disaster preparedness programs. A sound program should include capability and capacity assessments, emergency operations planning, resource procurement and management, staff education and training, organizational exercises, and a focus on continuous quality improvement (CQI). Physician specialty societies and other professional organizations, including the American College of Emergency Physicians (2009) and the American College of Healthcare Executives (2014), have offered recommendations for hospital preparedness plans.

The Joint Commission (TJC) also recognized the importance of disaster preparedness and emphasized the need for facilities to assess risks, develop and test contingency plans, and demonstrate the ability to respond appropriately to a disaster. Since January 2001, TJC has required organizations to have a comprehensive emergency preparedness plan (Rubin, 2006). TJC urged hospitals to develop sustainable, community-integrated disaster response plans and conduct drills. They recommended that healthcare organizations perform at least two disaster plan tests per year (Steiert, 2007).

TJC developed new Emergency Management standards in 2010. These are designed to guide hospitals to a high level of preparedness and response capacity. The standards identified six focus areas for planning and developing response mechanisms: communication, resources and assets, staff responsibilities, safety and security, utilities, and patient clinical and support activities (Joint Commission Resources, Inc. & The Joint Commission, 2012; Response Systems, n.d.).

Are We Prepared?

The first decade of the 21st century was marked by high-profile natural and non- natural disasters. This led to a greater emphasis on disaster preparedness at all levels, from the Federal Government to the local community. Are hospitals more prepared as a result?

Following the September 11th attacks, hospitals on the West Coast indicated their preparedness as they mobilized relief efforts to provide cross-country assistance. At the same time, they increased their own security and conserved hospital supplies in case of similar attacks (Benko & Galloro, 2001). As the U.S. entered war in Iraq in 2003, concerns for a retaliatory attack in this country led senators to question whether hospitals were prepared. U.S. hospital and hospital association officials answered affirmatively, pointing to efforts such as more frequent checking of emergency supplies, holding regular emergency drills, and creating regional data repositories with information about supplies, bed availability, and staffing. They noted that preparedness was costing hundreds of millions of dollars and federal assistance funds were slow to arrive (Fong, 2003). However, testimony from emergency department (ED) physician and nurse leaders before a congressional subcommittee on emergency preparedness, just three years later, raised alarm over hospital ED overcrowding and lack of surge capacity (U.S. Congress, 2007).

Subsequent studies demonstrated mixed results. The CDC National Center for Health Statistics (NCHS) assessed hospitals for bioterrorism and mass casualty preparedness using a supplement to its 2003 and 2004 National Hospital Ambulatory Medical Care Survey (NHAMCS). The results from 739 responding facilities showed that 92% of hospitals had revised disaster preparedness plans following September 11th, but only 63% of the plans covered CBRNE events and natural disasters. Ten response plan components were evaluated and only 9% of hospitals addressed all 10 components (Niska & Burt, 2007). The 2008 NHAMCS included an expanded emergency preparedness supplement. Of the 294 responding hospitals, 99% had disaster plans that addressed chemical events, 98% addressed natural disasters, 93% had plans for biological incidents, 81% addressed nuclear or radiological events, and 80% had plans for explosive events. Only 68% of hospitals covered all six hazards. Although 51% held epidemic drills, just one-third of hospitals addressed medication distribution or mass vaccination (Niska & Shimizu, 2011).

A University of Pittsburgh Medical Center study for HHS assessed the impact of the HPP's first five years (2002-2007). Hospitals improved considerably in preparing for disasters with regard to senior leadership engagement, appointment of disaster coordinators, preparedness training and operations planning, and development of stockpiles of emergency supplies and medications. However, catastrophic emergency planning was still in the nascent stage and would require more federal assistance (University of Pittsburgh Medical Center, 2009). A later HHS report found that 85% of the nation's hospitals were participating in the HPP by 2009. More than 76% of those hospitals had met at least 90% of the program's all-hazard preparedness measures ("Study: U.S. Hospitals Better Prepared for Hazards," 2011).

Other organizations described similar findings. TJC evaluated collaboration between hospitals and community first responders in preparing for disasters and determined that more effective communication and planning were needed. TJC recommended the creation of healthcare organization coalitions, more realistic drills, and the development of national benchmarks for measuring improvement in disaster preparedness (Braun et al., 2006). A study of hospital chief nursing officers and chief human resources officers by Novation, a healthcare contracting company, showed 64% of hospitals were developing pandemic-specific disaster plans, but felt unprepared for a pandemic flu event. Only 29% believed that they could continue operating without external resources for at least four weeks ("Survey Shows Hospitals Could Operate", 2007).

The National Association of Public Hospitals and Health Systems (NAPH) surveyed its member hospitals and determined that 73% had cooperative aid agreements with local governments. The authors noted that public hospitals provide significantly more emergency services than non-public facilities and care for populations particularly at risk (e.g., chronically ill, pediatric patients) during an emergency. They do so despite limited preparedness planning resources and funding (Spieler, Singer, & Cummings, 2008). A study of 572 community hospital chief executive officers (CEOs) by the American Hospital Association (AHA) found that 85% of hospitals had taken part in large-scale community-wide drills within the previous year, 85% had formal agreements to share resources with other hospitals during a disaster, 87% were receiving federal or state aid for disaster preparedness, and 79% were able to add beds within 0 to 2 hours following a disaster (American Hospital Association, 2010, May 24).

Another study assessed disaster preparedness in Michigan hospital EDs from 2005 to 2012. Eighty-five percent of respondents believed they were better prepared to handle a natural disaster or terrorist attack in 2012 than they were in 2005. Yet, most expressed a desire for more equipment and training (Belsky, Klausner, Karson, & Dunne, 2013). Results of a survey of 127 hospitals by *Campus Safety* showed that facilities were "somewhat" to "very well prepared" for chemical disasters (85%) and biological events (84%). However, 35% of respondents were only "slightly prepared" or "not prepared at all" for a nuclear disaster. Only 59% felt that they had sufficient emergency plans ("Emergency Preparedness Survey Results", 2011).

Barriers to Preparedness

What are the perceived barriers to disaster preparedness in U.S. hospitals? A survey of more than 95 hospital and health system executives conducted by *Health Facilities Management* identified the following top five emergency preparedness challenges:

- Unfunded emergency preparedness mandates (39%);
- Time limitations (38%);
- Competing priorities for resources (36%);
- Government requirements and compliance issues (22%); and
- Training for staff (21%) (Vesely & Hoppszallern, 2014).

Other authors also identified funding issues as one of the most significant barriers (Barbera, Macintyre, & DeAtley, 2003). Preparedness efforts cost money, a challenge for facilities that generally operate on tight budgets and struggle to mitigate or prevent financial losses (Luband, 2006; Reilly & Markenson, 2011).

Cagliuso (2014a) noted that the HPP provided $3.7 billion for hospital emergency preparedness during its first nine years. This seems substantial, averaging approximately $100,000 per hospital per year. However, a hospital's pandemic event preparedness cost averages approximately $1 million. Additional recurring costs to maintain preparedness average $200,000 per hospital per year. In recent years, federal funding for disaster preparedness has declined. HPP funding in fiscal year 2014 was $255 million, one-half the funding level ten years earlier (Demko, 2014).

The Federal Government made disaster preparedness a Medicare and Medicaid Condition of Participation (CoP) in 2016 (U.S. Department of Health and Human Services, 2018). This requires facilities to have plans for continuing operations during power outages, conducting regular drills, and implementing systems to track and provide care for patients displaced during disasters. The calculated financial impact is approximately $8,000 per hospital. Critics believe this figure is unrealistically low and point out that disaster preparedness is an unfunded mandate, does not generate revenue, and has no traditional reimbursement. They suggest incentives, such as higher Medicare reimbursements, should be provided to hospitals demonstrating preparedness (Fink, 2016).

Various authors identified additional obstacles. Cagliuso (2014a) referred to chronic gaps in preparedness caused by inadequate surge capacity, confusing regulatory and accreditation requirements, and a lack of performance metrics. This same author conducted phenomenological interviews with hospital and other healthcare officials. Interviewees expressed a need for more coordination, collaboration, and communication among those involved in disaster preparedness, additional federal programs to support the preparedness mandates, and more hospital leadership buy-in, which may decline in the face of competing priorities (Cagliuso, 2014b).

Milsten (2000) evaluated disaster incidents over 22 years and identified hospital challenges, including communications, structural damage, power outages, and hospital evacuation. Rubin (2006) described the following pitfalls in hospital preparedness and response: communications, staff training, decontamination, staff protection from hazardous or infectious agents, security, and the design and implementation of exercises. ED personnel at hospitals with level 1 and level 2 trauma centers in Missouri revealed concerns regarding a lack of specialized equipment and training for certain events and insufficient dedicated time for instruction and drill participation (Rivera & Char, 2004).

Farmer and Carlton (2006) pointed to a lack of coordination between hospitals and government emergency management agencies, insufficient critical care resources, conflicts with competing priorities, and shortcomings in staff education. Other authors cited a need for additional disaster preparedness education and training for ED nurses (Miller, 2011; Baack & Alfred, 2013; Whetzel, Walker-Cillo, Chan, & Trivett, 2013). A full-scale regional exercise with a chemical attack scenario involving 16 hospitals revealed interagency communications deficiencies (Klima et al., 2012).

Hospital Preparedness for Natural Disasters

Several articles focused on hospital preparedness for natural disasters. Some described lessons learned following weather-related disasters while others dealt with preparedness for infectious disease outbreaks. Weather events may damage the hospital, impair its ability to operate, and generate an influx of patients who have been affected by the event.

Hurricanes

Berger (2006) assessed disaster preparedness at Charity Hospital in New Orleans following Hurricane Katrina. This storm and subsequent flooding forced the evacuation of 400 patients and 1,200 staff members over five days. The hospital's disaster preparedness director had previously secured federal preparedness funds and acquired portable generators, ventilators, an amateur radio system, and a stockpile of food. No patients died due to the flooding and patients and staff were safely evacuated.

Memorial Hermann Hospital (MHH) and other facilities in the Texas Medical Center in Houston were hit by Hurricane Allison in 2001 and Hurricane Rita in 2005. MHH's experience in 2001 prepared the facility to meet the challenges encountered with the 2005 storm. Hospital emergency preparedness personnel in both New Orleans and Houston believe that preparedness plans should address the following items: ·

- A simultaneous loss of water, sewage, power, and communication;
- Disaster drills;
- A unified community response with collaboration; and
- The need to determine the point during a disaster/catastrophe at which a hospital should be evacuated (Berger, 2006).

Rodriguez and Aguirre (2006) examined Hurricane Katrina's impact on New Orleans' hospitals and noted that this storm disrupted external supply systems, directly affected physical plants, and caused an influx of patients. Eight of 16 hospitals had to be closed, some permanently. The authors emphasized the need for healthcare organizations to develop resiliency, which will allow them to react appropriately to unanticipated crises and disruptions in service and rebound from these events. Resiliency requires establishing a more holistic and community-integrated approach to reducing vulnerability. It also involves learning from previous disasters, identifying possible threats within the area, and identifying internal vulnerabilities (Sullivan, 2014).

Staffing challenges may also adversely affect disaster response. In the aftermath of Hurricane Sandy in 2012, interviews were conducted with management officials in the Veterans Affairs New York Harbor Healthcare System. They identified barriers that hampered staff from reporting to work, including communication difficulties, personal property damage, and transportation issues (Morris, Ricci, Griffin, Heslin, & Dobalian, 2016).

Tornadoes

Tornadoes may directly affect hospitals. Sumter Regional Hospital in Georgia was heavily damaged by a tornado in 2007. An effective disaster plan and frequent drills enabled the staff to protect and move patients to safety within the hospital, prior to being hit by the tornado, and evacuate them all within a few hours following the storm. Resiliency allowed the hospital to resume operations in temporary facilities within a couple of months (Weinstock, 2007).

The 165-mph tornado that struck Joplin, Missouri in 2011 destroyed St. John's Regional Medical Center, killing five patients and a visitor. The staff resumed operations within days in a makeshift tent hospital (Overall, 2012). Given that the hospital's exterior and windows were unable to withstand the force of the storm, a stronger replacement hospital was built that features clay brick exteriors and precast concrete, high wind resistant windows, and "safe rooms" that are located well within the core of the facility ("New Joplin, Mo. Hospital Battles Tornadoes," 2013; Small, 2015).

Infectious Disease

Infectious disease outbreaks include old threats that continue to occur, such as influenza, as well as emerging infections, like Ebola hemorrhagic fever. Beigi, Davis, Hodges, and Akers (2009) surveyed preparedness planning for pandemic influenza among large maternity hospitals. The questionnaire assessed demographic characteristics, pandemic preparedness, and anticipated planning challenges. All of the responding hospitals had active pandemic planning committees. Seventy-eight percent had procedures for dealing with surge/overflow and backup communications. Only 44% had written plans concerning stockpiling resources and other supply chain issues. Challenges included staff and supply coordination, as well as coordination with government agencies.

Two studies involved surveys of hospital infection control professionals. The first (Rebmann, Carrico, & English, 2007) was a data analysis of a hospital emergency preparedness survey by Trust for America's Health (TFAH) and the Association for Professionals in Infection Control and Epidemiology (APIC). Responses were received from 1,745 hospitals. The goal was to understand U.S. hospitals' current preparedness to respond to either a bioterrorism attack or an outbreak of an emerging or re-emerging infectious disease. The authors developed two hypotheses. The first was that larger hospitals could care for a larger influx of patients than smaller facilities. The second was that most hospitals do not have the capacity (i.e., staff or equipment and supplies) to care for an influx of potentially infectious patients. Nearly 90% of responding facilities had an infection control professional. Sixty-eight percent had a surge capacity plan. This was not dependent upon hospital size or geographic location. However, smaller hospitals reported significantly less ability to accommodate patient influx than larger hospitals because of staffing, structure, and equipment issues.

The second study (Rebmann, Wilson, LaPointe, Russell, & Moroz, 2009) was conducted by APIC as a follow-up to the 2005 survey. Officials from 633 hospitals responded to a questionnaire that included components of hospital preparedness for infectious disease emergencies and personal preparedness measures. Hospital preparedness measures included the presence of infection control professionals on hospital disaster planning committees, hospital capacity to care for an influx of 50 to 100 infectious or potentially infectious patients, and plans for alternative/off-site care and cross-training of staff. The primary goal was to assess preparedness progress made by hospitals between 2005 and 2007. The hypotheses were the same as in the previous study. The findings suggested that U.S. hospitals had made little progress in infectious disease emergency planning since 2005 and that smaller hospitals are less prepared than are larger hospitals for this type of disaster.

The possibility of an influenza pandemic raises concern about hospital surge capacity to manage the demand for service and volume of patients. EDs would be greatly affected since they frequently care for underserved and uninsured patients and often serve as "safety nets" when primary care providers are overwhelmed (Rust et al., 2009). A pandemic might result in 25,000 to 50,000 cases of influenza for every 100,000 members of the population during a 3- to 4-month period, leading to 7,000 to 14,000 office visits and 1,000 to 2,000 hospital admissions (Great Britain Department of Health, 2009).

At the same time, 62% of U.S. EDs, including 79% of urban hospitals and 45% of rural hospitals, operate at capacity or over capacity (American Hospital Association and Lewin Group, 2002). This means longer wait times for patients to see healthcare providers and more hours of ambulance diversion, with the exception of most rural hospitals, which frequently cannot divert because they are the only hospitals in their communities. Healthcare providers and other department staff may become victims of the pandemic, which will also limit surge capacity. The fear of contracting influenza may deter healthcare workers from reporting to work, contributing further to personnel shortages (Irvin, Cindrich, Patterson, & Southall, 2008).

Hospital Preparedness for Non-Natural Disasters

Terrorist attacks, chemical spills, and other industrial accidents highlight the threat of deliberate and inadvertent biological, chemical, radiologic, and explosive disasters. Several authors consider terrorist-related disasters as "weapons of mass destruction" (WMD) incidents (Macintyre et al., 2000; Treat et al., 2001). These events raise many concerns. One concern is the large numbers of casualties that would be expected. Another is the risk to healthcare workers of infection or contamination from victims of these attacks. Finally, there is the concern that healthcare facilities themselves may be primary or secondary targets of the terrorists (Barbera, Macintyre, & DeAtley, 2003).

Various authors have suggested essential disaster plan components to address WMD. Macintyre et al. (2000) state that the plan should include prompt recognition of the type of event, protection for staff and the facility, decontamination and triage for patients, medical treatment, and coordination with external agencies. Perry and Lindell (2006) believe that the plan should address incident command, communications, patient surge, decontamination, mental health consequences of the event, and hospital security.

Bioterrorism

Bioterrorism events pose unique problems. One is the need to treat victims with antibiotics and vaccines, which requires availability and deployment of resources from the National Pharmaceutical Stockpile. Another is that the release of a biological agent causes delayed casualties over the course of days or weeks. Thus, such an attack might not be initially apparent (Johnson, 2001).

Helger and Smith (2002) surveyed all hospitals and long-term care (LTC) facilities in Nebraska. Only 49% of the 38 respondents felt that bioterrorism was something that could occur in their communities. Ninety-eight percent stated they were not prepared for such an incident. Hospitals acknowledged recognition of the potential threat more frequently than did the LTC facilities. This survey was conducted in March 2001, prior to the September 11th and subsequent anthrax attacks.

Lenaghan, Smith, and Gangahar (2006) surveyed 573 physicians, nurses, and other staff at a 689-bed urban Nebraska hospital in 2004. Seventy-five percent of respondents felt that a bioterrorist attack was likely or somewhat likely, but only 33% believed that their hospital's preparedness was excellent or good. Twenty-nine percent had received training for nuclear, biological, or chemical (NBC) attacks. Most felt that the hospital needed to provide more education, plans, and drills for these events.

Higgins, Wainright III, Lu, and Carrico (2004) evaluated bioterrorism preparedness in short-term and long-term hospitals in Kentucky through a mailed survey of CEOs. Ninety-nine percent of the 116 respondents were engaged in planning efforts. Hospitals reported being able to surge 27% of all licensed beds in the state. However, fewer hospitals had advanced planning and preparation capability. Regional differences were noted; areas that included large cities showed a greater level of preparedness.

TJC surveyed 68 hospitals in the Spring of 2001 to assess the effectiveness of their linkages with other agencies in collaborating and preparing for bioterrorism events. Following the September 11th attacks, TJC conducted another study of 97 hospitals in the Spring of 2002. Findings showed significant improvement in collaborative planning, particularly for surge capacity and pharmacy and laboratory issues. Hospital preparedness plans that included bioterrorism increased from 47% to nearly 91%. Nearly half (48%) of hospitals in 2002 had conducted a bioterrorism-related drill, compared with 19% of facilities in 2001 (Braun, Darcy, Divi, Robertson, & Fishbeck, 2004). Likewise, two government studies found that bioterrorism preparedness improved over time. The 2003 NHAMCS showed nearly 85% of approximately 500 general and short-stay hospitals had plans for responding to biological events (Niska & Burt, 2005), whereas 93% of 294 responding hospitals in the 2008 NHAMCS had bioterrorism plans (Niska & Shimizu, 2011).

The Agency for Healthcare Research and Quality (AHRQ) conducted a pilot survey of hospital preparedness for bioterrorism incidents. Responses from 111 hospitals showed that 97% had a designated bio-disaster coordinator and 91% had bioterrorism response plans. However, only 47% allocated funds for such preparedness. Larger hospitals were better prepared overall, and rural hospitals were less likely to participate in surveillance systems for emerging infectious agents. This led the authors to suggest that rural hospitals might be especially vulnerable to a bioterrorist attack (Thorne et al., 2006).

Chemical Exposures

Chemical production has greatly increased worldwide since the end of World War II, with 50,000 to 100,000 synthetic chemicals currently being used in most industrial countries. Thus, there is a greater likelihood of exposure to chemicals, many of which have toxic, corrosive, or explosive properties (Khorram-Manesh, 2015). Chemical disasters occur as a result of mishaps during production, storage, transportation, and disposal of such materials, as well as from manufacture and use by terrorists. They pose a unique threat because casualties of such events are contaminated and require special care, especially in the ED (Totenhofer & Kierce, 1999).

Madsen and Greenberg (2010) conducted an online survey of 89 medical directors of EDs in the 12 most populous cities in the U.S. to evaluate preparedness for mass casualty incidents involving the release of anticholinesterase compounds. They hypothesized that respondents would report inadequate preparation for this type of incident despite an increased focus on disaster planning in large cities. Fewer than 20% of the ED directors reported being very confident in the effectiveness of their preparation and training. Data from the 2003 and 2004 NHAMCS showed 85% of responding hospitals had emergency response plans for chemical events (Niska & Burt, 2007), whereas 99% of respondents to the 2008 NHAMCS had incorporated chemical incidents in their plans. However, less than 56% of the hospitals in this latter group included chemical accident or attack scenarios in their mass casualty drills (Niska & Shimizu, 2011).

Biological and Chemical Incidents

Several studies assessed hospital preparedness for both biological and chemical incidents. Treat et al. (2001) interviewed ED medical directors or nurse managers in 30 urban and rural hospitals in FEMA Region III to assess training needs of ED personnel for biological and chemical WMD preparedness. Nearly 75% of the respondents believed that their hospitals were not at all prepared to handle either a biological or a chemical attack. The 26% who felt somewhat prepared represented urban facilities. Only 27% of the hospitals included WMD preparedness in their disaster plans.

In 2001, the RAND Corporation surveyed public health departments, hospitals, and other local and state agencies. Eighty-five percent of hospitals had mutual aid agreements with other organizations for emergency response and disasters. However, only 10% of those agreements addressed WMD incidents. Thirty-two percent of hospital response plans addressed biological events and 54% covered chemical incidents. Counties with populations of at least one million were better prepared than were smaller counties (Davis & Blanchard, 2002).

Wetter, Daniell, and Treser (2001) conducted a cross-sectional survey of hospital ED directors in four northwestern states to examine the resources available for managing victims of biological or chemical weapons. Visits were made to a small sample of the 186 responding hospitals to verify certain responses. Although 80% of hospitals reported having a response plan to address hazardous materials events, less than 20% of hospitals had formal plans for biological or chemical weapons incidents, with urban hospitals being three times more likely than rural hospitals. Only 45% of hospitals possessed outdoor or indoor decontamination units. Bennett (2006) assessed preparedness for managing biological or chemical weapons incidents among all 102 acute care hospitals in Mississippi. Thirty-seven hospitals responded to a mailed survey. A majority of hospitals had preparedness plans (89%), provided specific preparedness education and training (89%), had dedicated facilities for decontamination (76%), and possessed pharmaceutical plans and supplies (57%). However, nearly 60% of the facilities could not increase surge capacity (in terms of supplies, equipment, staff, and beds) and nearly 92% lacked the appropriate laboratory resources to analyze and identify biological and chemical agents. Hospitals in urban areas were better prepared than rural hospitals. Bennett concluded that Mississippi hospitals were still not sufficiently prepared to take care of biological and chemical attack casualties.

Nuclear and Radiological Events

Nuclear events involve the detonation of a nuclear device with an accompanying explosion, whereas radiological events involve the release of radiation without a nuclear device detonation (U.S. Department of Health & Human Services, National Library of Medicine, 2016). Radiological events may include accidents at nuclear energy plants and terrorist attacks involving a radiological dispersal device (RDD), or "dirty bomb".

Hospital preparedness for radiological terrorism was assessed through a regional full-scale exercise involving 11 hospitals. The researchers found that hospitals were not prepared to handle and decontaminate mass casualties (Jasper et al., 2005). Becker and Middleton (2008) conducted 10 focus groups on radiological attack preparedness with 77 ED physicians and nurses at hospitals in three regions of the country. Participants uniformly felt that hospitals and their ED providers were not sufficiently prepared. They expressed concerns about lack of information, adequate surge capacity, contamination and harm to themselves or loved ones, and potential staffing and readiness issues. In the *Campus Safety* emergency preparedness survey, 35% of hospital officials indicated that their facilities were only slightly prepared (18%) or not prepared at all (17%) for responding to nuclear emergencies ("1 in 3 Hospitals Struggle With," 2011).

An online survey of 3,426 hospital workers at Johns Hopkins Hospital in Baltimore found that 39% were unwilling to assist if asked, but not mandated, during a RDD event. Only 50% were willing to respond if required. The willingness expressed by these survey participants was independent of their perception of threat, but appeared related to personal safety issues, perceived efficacy of response, and willingness of coworkers to respond. The authors recommended more education and training for employees to improve the likelihood that they will respond (Balicer et al., 2011). Approximately 75% of respondents in the 2003 and 2004 NHAMCS included nuclear-radiological events in their emergency plans (Niska & Burt, 2007). This number increased slightly to 81% of respondents in the 2008 NHAMCS, with less than 19% reporting the incorporation of these scenarios in their mass casualty drills (Niska & Shimizu, 2011).

Explosive-Incendiary Incidents

Preparedness for explosive-incendiary incidents is an area that presents challenges. Hospital burn centers have limited capacity and may become overwhelmed during a disaster. The 2003 and 2004 NHAMCS found that 78% of hospitals had response plans for explosive-incendiary incidents (Niska & Burt, 2007). This number increased only to 79% in the 2008 NHAMCS (Niska & Shimizu, 2011). Kearns, Holmes, & Cairns (2013) indicated the need for improved surge capacity, as well as improved capability and training for hospital staff to care for these patients.

Opportunities for improvement in overall disaster response were identified by Virginia Hospital Center in Arlington, Virginia following its response to the attack on the Pentagon. These included the need to develop specific role descriptions, identify specific staging areas for physicians and nurses, and designate additional treatment areas beyond the ED. Hospital officials also recognized the need to develop further plans, especially for hazardous material decontamination and bioterrorism response (Cyganik, 2003).

Disaster Preparedness Within and Across Various Types of Hospitals

Several researchers assessed disaster preparedness within a specific hospital category or across different types of hospitals. The most extensive study was conducted as part of the NHAMCS in 2003-2004 and evaluated disaster preparedness in 739 U.S. hospitals with emergency or outpatient departments. The goal was to determine features associated with emergency response planning and equipment and care unit availability (Niska & Burt, 2007). Hospitals were compared by location (urban or rural), bed capacity, and ownership category (nonprofit, state or local government, and proprietary). Urban hospitals addressed terrorist incidents (biological, chemical, radiological, and explosive) more frequently than did rural hospitals. A more expanded supplemental survey was added to the NHAMCS in 2008, but this focused primarily on aspects of the hospitals' response plans and not on a comparison of hospital types (Niska & Shimizu, 2011).

Beigi, Davis, Hodges, and Akers (2009) examined disaster preparedness in large maternity hospitals. Madsen and Greenberg (2010) evaluated urban hospitals in large population centers. Barfield and Krug (2017) discussed the disaster preparedness concerns in neonatal intensive care units. Rebmann et al. (2007, 2009) compared hospitals based upon the number of beds. Kaji and Lewis (2006) explored overall disaster preparedness in urban hospitals. They conducted a telephone survey of disaster coordinators at 45 hospitals in Los Angeles County, CA. Forty of these were community hospitals. The questionnaire assessed practice variation, plan characteristics, and surge capacity. Although all hospitals had detailed disaster plans and a high level of access to equipment and supplies, preparedness was limited by a lack of integration of interagency training and planning and an inability to achieve sufficient surge capacity.

Other studies have compared preparedness among urban and rural hospitals. Some of these found urban hospitals to be better prepared (Bennett, 2006; Treat et al., 2001; Wetter, Daniell, & Treser, 2001). Alshehri (2012) compared a rural hospital and an urban facility in the same region of New York for disaster response capabilities and perceptions of roles in the regional disaster response infrastructure. The urban hospital had more equipment and staff, a more detailed response plan, and better supply management. Both hospitals shared the view that their facilities served critical roles for their communities during a regional disaster. A similar study examined an urban versus a rural hospital in terms of their role within the community's disaster response system. Analysis showed that rural hospitals are felt to be more essential to the recovery of their communities than are hospitals in urban areas, since a rural hospital is often the sole hospital within a community, whereas an urban hospital likely will share disaster response efforts with other hospitals and community health care agencies (Li, 2012).

Rural community disaster preparedness has been the focus of increased attention during the past 15 years and concern has been expressed about the inherent challenges. Although large cities have a higher population at risk during a disaster, they have greater resources to deal with disasters. Rural communities have smaller populations at risk, but a higher proportion may be affected (Cross, 2001). Barriers to rural disaster preparedness include: resource limitations, low population density, communication challenges, and remote location and separation (Bryant, 2009). Barriers for the hospitals include: financial stress (smaller size, different patient mix), insufficient capital to invest in facilities and technology, lack of surge capacity, and shortages of health care workers (American Hospital Association, 2011; Gursky, 2004).

Rural communities are vulnerable to terrorist attacks because they possess desirable targets. These include: headwaters for urban water supplies, agricultural fields, and nuclear power and storage facilities. They often lack a strong public health infrastructure. These communities may not possess the expertise and tools to recognize bioterrorist infectious disease agents. Rural hospital providers may lack the training to respond to terrorist or other mass casualty events. EDs often are staffed with a solo physician and may be unable to handle a patient surge. This is troublesome given that attacks on nearby urban areas may result in a mass exodus of citizens to rural communities (Campbell, Frances, & Meit, 2004; Pennsylvania Rural Health Association, 2010; Schur, 2004; U.S. Department of Health and Human Services, 2002).

Manley et al. (2006) surveyed ED nurse managers in rural U.S. hospitals to evaluate attitudes and experiences of the ED staff regarding preparedness and response to natural and non-natural disasters. Ninety-five percent of the 941 respondents indicated limited surge capacity; even ten patients would overwhelm these hospitals in a disaster. Thirty-seven percent of the hospitals experienced a mass casualty incident within the previous two years that overwhelmed their EDs. Most respondents felt less confident in their ability to deal with larger casualty incidents or terrorist attacks. Another study of 307 nurses at a 222-bed rural hospital in Ohio found that a large percentage were not very familiar with components of disaster preparedness. Most had never experienced a significant disaster incident (Hodge, Miller, & Skaggs, 2017).

Edwards, Kang, and Silenas (2008) described a 3-hour tabletop exercise using a pandemic avian influenza scenario involving 17 rural Texas hospitals. Post-exercise observations found that participants felt underprepared for disasters and constrained by understaffing and facility issues. They expressed the need for more regional cooperation and inclusion in national preparedness initiatives.

Cliff, Morlock, and Curtis (2009) examined the association between risk perception and disaster preparedness in rural hospitals by analyzing survey data from the National Study of Rural Hospitals (2006-2007) from Johns Hopkins University. Seventy-eight percent of respondents from the 134 participating hospitals indicated a moderate level of overall preparedness. There were higher levels of preparedness in planning, communications, and training, with a lower level of preparedness in surge capacity. They reported greater perceived risk from natural disasters (79%) than non-natural disasters (23%). There was no significant association between risk perception and overall preparedness.

Jacobson et al. (2010) conducted a mailed survey to assess training needs and emergency readiness of nurses in rural North Texas and 941 nurses responded, 46% of whom worked in hospital settings. Less than 10% expressed confidence in their ability to diagnose or treat conditions caused by bioterrorist attacks. Only 30% indicated willingness to work with local and state authorities during such an incident. However, 69% expressed interest in attending or receiving additional related training.

Myers (2015) undertook a qualitative study involving hospital emergency management planners from seven rural hospitals across the U.S. to assess their planning, training, and capacity to respond to a disaster event. He found that rural hospitals still lack full capability to respond to internal or external emergencies. Obstacles included limited resources, lack of adequate administration support, and multiple responsibilities and higher priority tasks for the planners, leaving little time for planning activities.

DISCUSSION

Community hospitals have increased their disaster preparedness in recent years in response to the September 11th attacks and major natural disasters. However, the literature reviewed in this paper show hospital personnel reporting inconsistent levels of preparedness and a lack of confidence in their ability to manage disasters. Larger facilities seem better prepared than smaller organizations, and hospitals in urban communities report a higher level of preparedness than those in rural settings. The following paragraphs discuss some of the more frequently noted areas of concern, which merit increased attention by hospitals and other entities.

A number of facilities reported being unable to adequately increase surge capacity in the event of a disaster. Elements of surge capacity included beds, staff, equipment, and supplies. Further compounding surge issues, if external resources were unavailable for four weeks or longer, the vast majority of hospitals would be unable to continue operations. This is particularly troublesome since some disaster scenarios may overwhelm a hospital with large numbers of patients, but without access to outside assistance for several days or more, as was seen with Charity Hospital in New Orleans during Hurricane Katrina. Smaller hospitals were found to be less able to accommodate patient surge than larger facilities.

It is therefore important that hospital disaster plans address patient surge and all of its critical elements. This includes developing call back protocols for emergency staff augmentation, as well as identifying hospital units that can house more beds and non-clinical areas that can be set up as care units. Decisions need to be made as to what supplies and equipment can and should be stockpiled for use in a disaster, within the constraints of a given hospital's budget. Although a disaster may cut off access to external resources, it is highly recommended that hospitals develop memoranda of understanding and other collaborative agreements, such as patient transfer arrangements, with nearby health care institutions and other local agencies. These organizations may be able to provide additional resources to assist with a patient surge or help offload some of the surge when the originating hospital is simply too overburdened.

The literature review found that staff at many hospitals felt underprepared for dealing with non-natural disasters, particularly bioterrorism, chemical events, and nuclear disasters. Frequently, the staff felt less confident in dealing with these types of events than with natural disasters. This may be explained somewhat by the fact that natural disasters are more common and familiar events to which staff feel more comfortable in responding, whereas non-natural disasters are rare occurrences that may have an insidious onset and deliberate initiation. However, studies showed that many hospitals did not adequately address these types of events in their disaster plans, did not hold disaster drills or other training and education for their staffs involving these scenarios, or lacked the appropriate resources to identify things such as biological and chemical agents.

Hospital administrators should not overlook these less common disaster scenarios and should ensure that they are incorporated into their disaster plans. They must also endeavor to train staff to address these events, either through educational sessions, real-time drills, or a combination of both. Only then can the staff begin to develop a sense of preparedness and confidence to deal with these incidents. Finally, administrators need to acquire necessary resources to address these disasters, such as decontamination showers, and determine whether their hospitals will develop the expertise to identify biological and chemical agents or establish agreements with other facilities in their regions to perform these services.

Several studies demonstrated that urban hospitals are better prepared for disasters than are rural facilities. They generally have more comprehensive disaster plans, access to greater stores of equipment and supplies, larger numbers of personnel, and more facilities and agencies with which to collaborate.

Rural hospital staff, on the other hand, frequently reported being ill-equipped and under-trained to deal with various disaster scenarios.

Given the vital function that rural hospitals play in their communities, often serving as the only such facility for several miles around, it is imperative that their administrators make disaster preparedness a priority. Disaster planning is a critical function and should address alternative pathways for response and patient care, given that some equipment and supplies taken for granted in urban facilities may not be readily available to their rural counterparts. Staff need to be well-trained and drilled in order to develop the confidence to respond independently to disasters, with the understanding that external resources and support may take longer to arrive. Federal and state governments also must play a strong role in helping rural facilities to meet the challenge of disaster preparedness and response.

A number of barriers to preparedness were identified in studies cited in this review. Lack of sufficient funding was identified as the most frequent barrier. Although federal funding is provided through the HPP, this does not appear sufficient to fully address hospital preparedness needs. This raises a number of questions. Should Congress consider increasing funding levels for the HPP or should it promote development of other programs to support hospitals in their preparedness efforts? Should the responsibility for funding disaster preparedness be a shared federal-state venture, much like the Medicaid program, or should it be delegated solely to the individual states? Is there a role for public-private sector partnership? Finally, is it really the government's responsibility to prepare non-government hospitals for disasters or should the hospitals be held directly responsible for these endeavors? Although these authors assert that government involvement is essential, one may argue that government funding has been a failure and ought to be discontinued in favor of adopting strict regulatory standards to achieve preparedness among the nation's community hospitals. These are certainly issues that warrant further study and debate.

Recommendations for Additional Research

Hospitals have become more reliant on technology in the 21st century, especially with the development of electronic documentation systems and sophisticated communication devices. Loss of function of these technologies as a result of a natural disaster or deliberate event, such as a cyber-attack, certainly constitutes an internal disaster and could cause significant disruption of hospital operations. Yet, this literature review did not identify any comprehensive assessments of hospital preparedness for technology disasters. Such a study should be undertaken, and action plans developed to mitigate any risks that are identified.

Given the concerns expressed about disaster funding, there needs to be a review of all sources of monies available for this purpose to community hospitals. This should include identification of federal and state programs, as well as any non-governmental funds awarded as grants. An analysis should be undertaken to determine what are realistic levels of funding that need to be achieved so that hospitals can develop more satisfactory levels of preparedness.

Finally, hospitals need to act on the findings of this review and determine how to reshape their priorities so as to give greater emphasis to disaster preparedness. Staff education and training is a crucial element, and the use of regular and robust emergency drills will enable staff to maintain a level of expertise and confidence to deal with actual disasters when they arise. Collaborating with other community agencies is essential as well, especially for rural hospitals that may be sole health care providers within their communities. In order to make all of this happen, there needs to be senior executive buy-in to the importance of disaster preparedness. This increases the likelihood that hospitals will become better prepared, more resilient, and remain viable in the event of a disaster.

CONCLUSION

This review provides a current assessment of community hospital disaster preparedness in the United States. Consideration has been given to both natural and non-natural categories of disasters as well as disaster preparedness among various types of hospitals. Findings from the various studies and articles show an inconsistent level of preparedness among community hospitals, particularly with respect to non-natural disasters. Many hospitals express difficulty in developing surge capacity and rural hospitals are less prepared than their urban counterparts. Several barriers to preparedness have been identified, including a lack of sufficient preparedness funding. The findings suggest that there are more opportunities and a need to enhance disaster preparedness among the community hospitals in the United States.

Disaster preparedness requires more attention from federal and state governments, non-governmental agencies, policy makers, and advocacy bodies, as well as from hospital administrators. This, in turn, could lead to a re-evaluation of the funding process and allocation of funds for disaster preparedness, along with a greater emphasis by hospitals on staff education and training and other elements of preparedness. Collectively, these activities may lead to better disaster preparedness among our nation's community hospitals.

REFERENCES

Alshehri, A. (2012). *The hospital's role within a regional disaster response: A comparison study of an urban hospital versus a rural hospital* [Master's thesis].

American College of Emergency Physicians. (2009, April). *Best practices for hospital preparedness.* Retrieved from http://www.acep.org/WorkArea/DownloadAsset.aspx?id=45409

American College of Healthcare Executives. (2014, July/August). Healthcare executives' role in emergency preparedness. *Healthcare Executive, 29*(4), 90–91.

American Hospital Association. (2010, May 24). *The state of America's hospitals –Taking the pulse: Results of AHA survey of hospital leaders, March/April 2010.* Retrieved from www.aha.org/content/00-10/100524-thschartpk.pdf

American Hospital Association. (2011, April). *The opportunities and challenges for rural hospitals in an era of health reform.* Retrieved from http://www.aha.org/research/reports/tw/11apr-tw-rural.pdf

American Hospital Association. (2016, January). Fast facts on U.S. hospitals. Retrieved from http://www.aha.org/research/rc/stat-studies/fast-facts.shtml#community

American Hospital Association & Lewin Group. (2002, April). *Emergency department overload: A growing crisis: The results of the American Hospital Association survey of emergency department (ED) and hospital capacity.* Falls Church, VA: American Hospital Association.

Baack, S., & Alfred, D. (2013). Nurses' preparedness and perceived competence in managing disasters. *Journal of Nursing Scholarship, 45*(3), 281–287. PMID:23574544

Balicer, R. D., Catlett, C. L., Barnett, D. J., Thompson, C. B., Hsu, E. B., Morton, M. J., ... Links, J. M. (2011, October). Characterizing hospital workers' willingness to respond to a radiological event. *PLoS One, 6*(10), e25327. doi:10.1371/journal.pone.0025327 PMID:22046238

Barbera, J. A., Macintyre, A. G., & DeAtley, C. A. (2003). Ambulances to nowhere: America's critical shortfall in medical preparedness for catastrophic terrorism. In A. M. Howitt & R. L. Pangi (Eds.), *Countering terrorism: Dimensions of preparedness* (pp. 283–297). Cambridge, MA: The MIT Press.

Barfield, W. D., & Krug, S. E. (2017). Disaster preparedness in neonatal intensive care units. *Pediatrics, 139*(5), e20170507. doi:10.1542/peds.2017-0507 PMID:28557770

Becker, S. M., & Middleton, S. A. (2008, October). Improving hospital preparedness for radiological terrorism: Perspectives from emergency department physicians and nurses. *Disaster Medicine and Public Health Preparedness, 2*(3), 174–184. doi:10.1097/DMP.0b013e31817dcd9a PMID:18813129

Beigi, R. H., Davis, G., Hodges, J., & Akers, A. (2009). Preparedness planning for pandemic influenza among large US maternity hospitals. *Emerging Health Threats Journal, 2*(1), 2–5. doi:10.3402/ehtj. v2i0.7079 PMID:22460283

Belsky, J. B., Klausner, H. H., Karson, J., & Dunne, R. B. (2013, October). Disaster preparedness in Michigan 2005 to 2012: Are we more prepared? [Abstract]. *Annals of Emergency Medicine, 62*(4S), S15–S16. doi:10.1016/j.annemergmed.2013.07.324

Benko, L. B., & Galloro, V. (2001, September 17). West Coast facilities ready and waiting. *Modern Healthcare, 31*(38), 22. PMID:11586540

Bennett, R. L. (2006). Chemical or biological terrorist attacks: An analysis of the preparedness of hospitals for managing victims affected by chemical or biological weapons of mass destruction. *International Journal of Environmental Research and Public Health, 3*(1), 67–75. doi:10.3390/ijerph2006030008 PMID:16823078

Berger, E. (2006, January). Charity Hospital and disaster preparedness. *Annals of Emergency Medicine, 47*(1), 53–56. doi:10.1016/j.annemergmed.2005.12.004 PMID:16395776

Braun, B. I., Darcy, L., Divi, C., Robertson, J., & Fishbeck, J. (2004, October). Hospital bioterrorism preparedness linkages with the community: Improvements over time. *American Journal of Infection Control, 32*(6), 317–326. PMID:15454887

Braun, B. I., Wineman, N. V., Finn, N. L., Barbera, J. A., Schmaltz, S. P., & Loeb, J. M. (2006, June 6). Integrating hospitals into community emergency preparedness planning. *Annals of Internal Medicine, 144*(11), 799–811. doi:10.7326/0003-4819-144-11-200606060-00006 PMID:16754922

Bryant, D. (2009, April 8). Challenges of rural emergency management. *Homeland1.com*. Retrieved from http://www.homeland1.com/disaster-preparedness/articles/480917-Challenges-of-rural-emergency-management/

Cagliuso, N. V. (2014a). Stakeholders' experiences with US hospital emergency preparedness: Part 1. *Journal of Business Continuity & Emergency Planning, 8*(2), 156–168. PMID:25416377

Cagliuso, N. V. (2014b). Stakeholders' experiences with US hospital emergency preparedness: Part 2. *Journal of Business Continuity & Emergency Planning, 8*(3), 263–279. PMID:26591933

Campbell, P., Frances, J., & Meit, M. (2004, September 27-28). *Preparing for public health emergencies: Meeting the challenges in rural America.* Conference proceedings and recommendations from the First National Conference on Rural Public Health Emergency Preparedness, St. Paul, MN. Retrieved from https://www.upb.pitt.edu/uploadedFiles/about/sponsored_programs/Center_for_Rural_Health_Practice/conf_proceed_4.pdf

Campus Safety Magazine. (2011, March 23). 1 in 3 hospitals struggle with radiological disaster preparedness. Retrieved from http://www.campussafetymagazine.com/article/1-in-3-Hospitals-Not-Well-Prepared-for-Radiological-Disasters#

Centre for Research on the Epidemiology of Disasters. (2015). Country profile. Retrieved from http://emdat.be/country_profile/index.html

Charney, R. L., Rebmann, T., Esguerra, C. R., Lai, C. W., & Dalawari, P. (2013, October). Public perceptions of hospital responsibilities to those presenting without medical injury or illness during a disaster. *The Journal of Emergency Medicine, 45*(4), 578–584. doi:10.1016/j.jemermed.2013.05.010 PMID:23845529

Cliff, B. J., Morlock, L., & Curtis, A. B. (2009, December). Is there an association between risk perception and disaster preparedness in rural US hospitals? *Prehospital and Disaster Medicine, 24*(6), 512–517. doi:10.1017/S1049023X00007433 PMID:20301069

Cross, J. A. (2001). Megacities and small towns: Different perspectives on hazard vulnerability. *Environmental Hazards, 3*(2), 63–80. doi:10.3763/ehaz.2001.0307

Cyganik, K. A. (2003). Disaster preparedness in Virginia Hospital Center-Arlington after Sept 11, 2001. *Disaster Management & Response, 1*(3), 80–86. doi:10.1016/S1540-2487(03)00048-8 PMID:12888746

Davis, L. M., & Blanchard, J. C. (2002). *Are local health responders ready for biological and chemical terrorism?* Santa Monica, CA: RAND Corporation. doi:10.1037/e442162005-001

Demko, P. (2014, October 20). Ebola spotlights emergency-preparedness cuts. *Modern Healthcare, 44*(42), 12.

Edwards, J. C., Kang, J., & Silenas, R. (2008, Summer). Promoting regional disaster preparedness among rural hospitals. *The Journal of Rural Health, 24*(3), 321–325. doi:10.1111/j.1748-0361.2008.00176.x PMID:18643812

Emergency preparedness survey results: Hospitals. (2011, March 24). *Campus Safety.* Retrieved from http://www.campussafetymagazine.com/files/resources/ HospPrepCharts032411.pdf

Farmer, J. C., & Carlton, P. K. Jr. (2006). Providing critical care during a disaster: The interface between disaster response agencies and hospitals. *Critical Care Medicine, 34*(3 Suppl.), S56–S59. doi:10.1097/01.CCM.0000199989.44467.2E PMID:16477204

Fink, S. (2016, February 14). Can Hospitals Afford to Be Ready for Disaster? *New York Times*, p. 7(L). Retrieved from http://cmich.idm.oclc.org/login?url=http://go.galegroup.com.cmich.idm.oclc.org/ps/i.do?id=GALE%7CA443169114&v=2.1&u=lom_cmichu&it=r&p=SPN.SP00&sw=w&asid=bfba1646df68fde4e580c632a3103 306

Fong, T. (2003). Show them the money. *Modern Healthcare*, *33*(12), 8. Retrieved from http://cmich.idm.oclc.org/login?url=http://search.proquest.com.cmich.idm.oclc.org/docview/212002542?account id=10181 PMID:12687993

Great Britain Department of Health. (2009). *Pandemic flu: Managing demand and capacity in health care organisations: (Surge)*. London, UK: Department of Health.

Gursky, E. A. (2004, June). Hometown hospitals: The weakest link? Bioterrorism readiness in America's rural hospitals. *National Defense University*. Retrieved from http://ctnsp.dodlive.mil/files/2013/07/DTP-002.pdf

Harrald, J. R. (2012). Emergency management restructured: Intended and unintended outcomes of actions taken since 9/11. In C. B. Rubin (Ed.), *Emergency management: The American experience 1900-2010* (2nd ed.). Boca Raton, FL: CRC Press. doi:10.1201/b11887-7

Heine, G. R. (2011, June 3). Joplin proves need for disaster plans at local hospitals. *GazetteXtra*. Retrieved from http://www.gazettextra.com/news/2011/jun/03/joplin-proves-need-disaster-plans-local-hospitals/

Helger, V., & Smith, P. W. (2002). Bioterrorism preparedness: A survey of Nebraska health care institutions. *American Journal of Infection Control*, *30*(1), 46–48. doi:10.1067/mic.2002.122254 PMID:11852417

Higgins, W., Wainright, C. III, Lu, N., & Carrico, R. (2004). Assessing hospital preparedness using an instrument based on the mass casualty disaster plan checklist: Results of a statewide survey. *American Journal of Infection Control*, *32*(6), 327–332. doi:10.1016/j.ajic.2004.03.006 PMID:15454888

Hodge, A. J., Miller, E. L., & Skaggs, M. K. D. (2017). Nursing self-perceptions of emergency preparedness at a rural hospital. *Journal of Emergency Nursing: JEN*, *43*(1), 10–14. doi:10.1016/j.jen.2015.07.012 PMID:26454637

International Federation of Red Cross and Red Crescent Societies. (n.d.). What is a disaster? Retrieved from http://www.ifrc.org/en/what-we-do/disaster-management/about-disasters/what-is-a-disaster/

Irvin, C. B., Cindrich, L., Patterson, W., & Southall, A. (2008, July-August). Survey of hospital healthcare personnel response during a potential avian influenza pandemic: Will they come to work? *Prehospital and Disaster Medicine*, *23*(4), 328–335. doi:10.1017/S1049023X00005963 PMID:18935947

Jacobson, H. E., Mas, F. S., Hsu, C. E., Turley, J. P., Miller, J., & Kim, M. (2010, January/February). Self-assessed emergency readiness and training needs of nurses in rural Texas. *Public Health Nursing (Boston, Mass.)*, *27*(1), 41–48. doi:10.1111/j.1525-1446.2009.00825.x PMID:20055967

Jasper, E., Miller, M., Sweeney, B., Berg, D., Feuer, E., & Reganato, D. (2005, November). Preparedness of hospitals to respond to a radiological terrorism event as assessed by a full-scale exercise. *Journal of Public Health Management and Practice*, *11*(6 Suppl.), S11–S16. doi:10.1097/00124784-200511001-00003 PMID:16205528

Johnson, D. E. L. (2001, October). Hospitals and country are 'woefully unprepared' for bioterrorism attacks. *Health Care Strategic Management, 19*(10), 14–16. PMID:11683056

Joint Commission Resources, Inc.; Joint Commission. (2012). *Emergency management in health care: An all-hazards approach*. Oakbrook, IL: Joint Commission Resources.

Kaji, A. H., Koenig, K. L., & Lewis, R. J. (2007, November 14). Current hospital disaster preparedness. *Journal of the American Medical Association, 298*(18), 2188–2190. doi:10.1001/jama.298.18.2188 PMID:18000203

Kaji, A. H., & Lewis, R. J. (2006). Hospital disaster preparedness in Los Angeles County. *Academic Emergency Medicine, 13*(11), 1198–1203. doi:10.1197/j.aem.2006.05.007 PMID:16885400

Kearns, R., Holmes, I. V. J. IV, & Cairns, B. (2013, January). Burn disaster preparedness and the southern region of the United States. *Southern Medical Journal, 106*(1), 69–73. doi:10.1097/SMJ.0b013e31827c4d94 PMID:23263317

Khorram-Manesh, A. (2015). Preparedness for chemical threats: New challenges in management of trauma and disasters. *Bulletin of Emergency and Trauma, 3*(4), 115–117. PMID:27162914

Klima, D. A., Seiler, S. H., Peterson, J. B., Christmas, A. B., Green, J. M., Fleming, G., ... Sing, R. F. (2012, September). Full-scale regional exercises: Closing the gaps in disaster preparedness. *The Journal of Trauma and Acute Care Surgery, 73*(3), 592–598. doi:10.1097/TA.0b013e318265cbb2 PMID:22929489

Krizner, K. (2007, January). Hospital disaster preparedness plans become a necessity. *Managed Healthcare Executive, 17*(1), 33–34.

Lenaghan, P. A., Smith, P. W., & Gangahar, D. (2006, October). Emergency preparedness and bioterrorism: A survey of the Nebraska Medical Center staff and physicians. *Journal of Emergency Nursing: JEN, 32*(5), 394–397. doi:10.1016/j.jen.2006.06.001 PMID:16997027

Li, Y. (2012). *Hospital as a critical infrastructure in the community disaster response system* [Master's thesis].

Luband, C. (2006, Summer). Emergency preparedness for hospitals and the healthcare marketplace. *Administrative Law Review, 58*(3), 575–585.

Macintyre, A. G., Christopher, G. W., Eitzen, E. Jr, Gum, R., Weir, S., DeAtley, C., ... Barbera, J. A. (2000, January 12). Weapons of mass destruction events with contaminated casualties: Effective planning for health care facilities. *Journal of the American Medical Association, 283*(2), 242–249. doi:10.1001/jama.283.2.242 PMID:10634341

Madsen, J. M., & Greenberg, M. I. (2010, November/December). Preparedness for the evaluation and management of mass casualty incidents involving anticholinesterase compounds: A survey of emergency department directors in the 12 largest cities in the United States. *American Journal of Disaster Medicine, 5*(6), 333–351. PMID:21319552

Manley, W. G., Furbee, P. M., Coben, J. H., Smyth, S. K., Summers, D. E., Althouse, R. C., & Helmkamp, J. C. (2006, July-September). Realities of disaster preparedness in rural hospitals. *Disaster Management & Response, 4*(3), 80–87. doi:10.1016/j.dmr.2006.05.001 PMID:16904618

McGlown, K. J., & Robinson, P. D. (Eds.). (2011). *Anticipate, respond, recover: Healthcare leadership and catastrophic events.* Chicago, IL: Health Administration Press.

Meyers, S. (2006, February). Disaster preparedness: Hospitals confront the challenge. *Trustee, 59*(2), 12–19. PMID:16796230

Meyers, S. (2007, October). Disaster preparedness: When your community needs you most. *Trustee, 60*(9), 8–11. PMID:18030909

Miller, P. (2011). *An assessment of emergency department staff knowledge of emergency preparedness.* Retrieved from http://cmich.idm.oclc.org/login?url=http://search.proquest.com.cmich.idm.oclc.org/docview/861922980?accountid=10181

Milsten, A. (2000). Hospital responses to acute-onset disasters: A review. *Prehospital and Disaster Medicine, 15*(1), 32–45. doi:10.1017/S1049023X00024900 PMID:11066840

Morris, A. M., Ricci, K. A., Griffin, A. R., Heslin, K. C., & Dobalian, A. (2016). Personal and professional challenges confronted by hospital staff following hurricane Sandy: A qualitative assessment of management perspectives. *BMC Emergency Medicine, 16*(18), 1–7. doi:10.118612873-016-0082-5 PMID:27151172

Mothershead, J. L. (2004). Disaster planning for terrorism. In K. J. McGlown (Ed.), *Terrorism and disaster management: Preparing healthcare leaders for the new reality.* Chicago, IL: Health Administration Press.

Myers, H. (2015). *A qualitative study on the readiness of rural hospitals to respond to community disasters* [Doctoral dissertation].

New Joplin, Mo. hospital battles tornadoes with masonry walls: Mercy Hospital Joplin to replace medical center destroyed in May 2011. (2013, April 18). *PR Newswire.* Retrieved from http://cmich.idm.oclc.org/login?url=http://search.proquest.com.cmich.idm.oclc.org/docview/1328532478?accountid=10181

Niska, R.W., & Burt, C.W. (2005, September 27). Bioterrorism and mass casualty preparedness in hospitals: United States, 2003. In *Advance Data from Vital and Health Statistics* (No. 364). Hyattsville, MD: Centers for Disease Control and Prevention, National Center for Health Statistics.

Niska, R.W., & Burt, C.W. (2007, August 20). Emergency response planning in hospitals, United States, 2003-2004. In *Advance Data from Vital and Health Statistics* (No. 391). Hyattsville, MD: Centers for Disease Control and Prevention, National Center for Health Statistics.

Niska, R.W., & Shimizu, I.M. (2011, March 24). Hospital preparedness for emergency response: United States, 2008. In *National Health Statistics Reports* (No. 37). Hyattsville, MD: Centers for Disease Control and Prevention, National Center for Health Statistics.

Overall, M. (2012, May 20). Destroyed hospital helped lead Joplin recovery with optimism. *McClatchy-Tribune Business News.* Retrieved from http://cmich.idm.oclc.org/login?url=http://search.proquest.com.cmich.idm.oclc.org/docview/1014294824?accountid=10181

Pennsylvania Rural Health Association. (2010, August). *Pennsylvania rural health care.* Retrieved from http://www.paruralhealth.org/PARuralHealth_StatusCheck5.pdf

Perry, R., & Lindell, M. (2006, April-June). Hospital planning for weapons of mass destruction incidents. *Journal of Postgraduate Medicine, 52*(2), 116–120. PMID:16679675

Rebmann, T., Carrico, R., & English, J. F. (2007). Hospital infectious disease emergency preparedness: A survey of infection control professionals. *American Journal of Infection Control, 35*(1), 25–32. doi:10.1016/j.ajic.2006.07.002 PMID:17276788

Rebmann, T., Wilson, R., LaPointe, S., Russell, B., & Moroz, D. (2009). Hospital infectious disease emergency preparedness: A 2007 survey of infection control professionals. *American Journal of Infection Control, 37*(1), 1–8. doi:10.1016/j.ajic.2008.02.007 PMID:19081162

Reilly, M. J., & Markenson, D. S. (2011). *Health care emergency management: Principles and practice.* Sudbury, MA: Jones & Bartlett Learning.

Rivera, A. F., & Char, D. M. (2004, October). Emergency department disaster preparedness: Identifying the barriers. *Annals of Emergency Medicine, 44*(4 Suppl.), S94.

Rodriguez, H., & Aguirre, B. E. (2006, Fall). Hurricane Katrina and the healthcare infrastructure: A focus on disaster preparedness, response, and resiliency. *Frontiers of Health Services Management, 23*(1), 13–24. doi:10.1097/01974520-200607000-00003 PMID:17036849

Rubin, J. N. (2006). Recurring pitfalls in hospital preparedness and response. In J. H. McIsaac (Ed.), *Hospital preparation for bioterror: A medical and biomedical systems approach.* Burlington, MA: Academic Press. doi:10.1016/B978-012088440-7/50003-3

Rust, G., Melbourne, M., Truman, B. I., Daniels, E., Fry-Johnson, Y., & Curtin, T. (2009). Role of the primary care safety net in pandemic influenza. *American Journal of Public Health, 99*(Suppl. 2), S316–S323. doi:10.2105/AJPH.2009.161125 PMID:19797743

Schur, C. L. (2004, April). Understanding the role of the rural hospital emergency department in responding to bioterrorist attacks and other emergencies. *Walsh Center for Rural Health Analysis.* Retrieved from www.norc.org/PDFs/Walsh%20Center/Links%20Out/WalshCtr2004_LitRev_final.pdf

Small, L. (2015, March 12). After natural disasters, hospitals rebuild with "resilient design." *FierceHealthcare.* Retrieved from http://www.fiercehealthcare.com/story/after-natural-disasters-hospitals-rebuild-resilient-design/2015-03-12

Spieler, S.S., Singer, M.P., & Cummings, L. (2008, May). Emergency preparedness in public hospitals: Complete findings of the 2006-2007 emergency preparedness study. Washington, DC: National Association of Public Hospitals and Health Systems.

Steiert, M. J. W. (2007, August). Disaster preparedness. *AORN Journal, 86*(2), 175–176. doi:10.1016/j.aorn.2007.07.013 PMID:17683715

Study: U.S. hospitals better prepared for hazards. (2011, May 10). *Campus Safety.* Retrieved from http://www.campussafetymagazine.com/article/u-s-hospitals-meeting-more-hazard-preparedness-measures

Sullivan, K. (2014, July 8). Hospital resiliency most important after natural disaster, emergencies. *FierceHealthcare.* Retrieved from http://www.fiercehealthcare.com/story/hospital-resiliency-most-important-after- natural-disaster-emergencies/2014-07-08

Survey shows hospitals could operate one week with current disaster plans. (2007, July). *Healthcare Purchasing News, 31(*7), 10.

Response Systems. (n.d.). JCAHO compliance. Retrieved from http://www.disasterpreparation.net/resources.html

Thorne, C. D., Levitin, H., Oliver, M., Losch-Skidmore, S., Neiley, B. A., Socher, M. M., & Gucer, P. W. (2006, November-December). A pilot assessment of hospital preparedness for bioterrorism events. *Prehospital and Disaster Medicine, 21*(6), 414–422. doi:10.1017/S1049023X0000412X PMID:17334188

Totenhofer, R. I., & Kierce, M. (1999). It's a disaster: Emergency departments' preparation for a chemical incident or disaster. *Accident and Emergency Nursing, 7*(3), 141–147. doi:10.1016/S0965-2302(99)80073-3 PMID:10693383

Treat, K. N., Williams, J. M., Furbee, P. M., Manley, W. G., Russell, F. K., & Stamper, C. D. Jr. (2001, November). Hospital preparedness for weapons of mass destruction incidents: An initial assessment. *Annals of Emergency Medicine, 38*(5), 562–565. doi:10.1067/mem.2001.118009 PMID:11679869

University of Pittsburgh Medical Center. (2009, March). Hospitals rising to the challenge: The first five years of the U.S. Hospital Preparedness Program and priorities going forward. Baltimore, MD: UPMC Center for Biosecurity.

U.S. Congress, House of Representatives, Committee on Homeland Security. (2006). Emergency care crisis: A nation unprepared for public disasters: Hearing before the Subcommittee on Emergency Preparedness, Science, and Technology of the Committee on Homeland Security, House of Representatives, One Hundred *Ninth Congress, second session, July 26, 2006.* Washington, DC: U.S. Government Printing Office.

U.S. Department of Health and Human Services. (2018, January 15). Emergency preparedness rule. Retrieved from https://www.cms.gov/Medicare/Provider-Enrollment-and-Certification/SurveyCertEmergPrep/Emergency-Prep-Rule.html

U.S. Department of Health and Human Services, Health Resources and Services Administration, Office of Rural Health Policy. (2002, April). *Rural communities and emergency preparedness.* Retrieved from www.out-of-hospital.com/EMS1/documents/RuralPreparedness.pdf

U.S. Department of Health and Human Services, National Library of Medicine. (2016, January 12). Is it a radiological or nuclear incident? Retrieved from https://www.remm.nlm.gov/nukevsrad.htm

U.S. Department of Health and Human Services, Public Health Emergency. (n.d.). *Hospital preparedness program: An introduction.* Retrieved from http://www.phe.gov/Preparedness/planning/hpp/Documents/hpp-intro-508.pdf

U.S. Department of Homeland Security. (2013, December 27). Plan and prepare for disasters. Retrieved from http://www.dhs.gov/topic/plan-and-prepare-disasters

U.S. Federal Emergency Management Agency. (2016). Disaster declarations by year. Retrieved from https://www.fema.gov/disasters/grid/year? field_disaster_type_term_tid_1=All&=GO

Vesely, R., & Hoppszallern, S. (2014). Planning for disaster: Hospitals learn valuable lessons in responding to natural and man-made catastrophes. *Health Facilities Management, 27*(7), 16–23. PMID:25141441

Weinstock, M. (2007, May). Tornado's wrath, heroic response. *Hospitals & Health Networks, 81*(5), 24. PMID:17569445

Wetter, D. C., Daniell, W. E., & Treser, C. D. (2001, May). Hospital preparedness for victims of chemical or biological terrorism. *American Journal of Public Health, 91*(5), 710–716. doi:10.2105/AJPH.91.5.710 PMID:11344876

Whetzel, E., Walker-Cillo, G., Chan, G. K., & Trivett, J. (2013, January). Emergency nurse perceptions of individual and facility emergency preparedness. *Journal of Emergency Nursing: JEN, 39*(1), 46–52. doi:10.1016/j.jen.2011.08.005 PMID:21963139

World Health Organization. (2010, October 13). Protecting hospitals and health centres before disasters saves lives. Retrieved from http://who.int/mediacentre/news/notes/2010/disaster_reduction_20101013/en/

This research was previously published in the International Journal of Disaster Response and Emergency Management (IJDREM), 1(2); edited by Dean Kyne and William Donner; pages 1-22, copyright year 2018 by IGI Publishing (an imprint of IGI Global).

Chapter 23
E–Commerce and IT Projects:
Evaluation and Management Issues in Australian and Taiwanese Hospitals

Wenqi Jacintha Hee
Curtin University, Australia

Geoffrey Jalleh
Curtin University, Australia

Hung-Chih Lai
National Chi Nan University, Taiwan

Chad Lin
Curtin University, Australia

ABSTRACT

Hospitals and healthcare organizations are facing an increasingly competitive business environment which demands the efficient use and appropriate evaluation of their tangible and intangible resources and competencies in order to continuously improve their organizational performance. The management of e-commerce/IT outsourcing is a crucial management issue for hospitals and healthcare organizations in recent years since only a small proportion of these organizations have reaped the expected benefits from their outsourcing projects. Therefore, the main objective of this article is to better understand the investment evaluation and benefits realization practices and processes of Australian and Taiwanese hospitals that have outsourced their e-commerce/IT systems. This article provides the opportunity to examine outsourcing practices of a highly developed economy (Australia) and a newly industrialized economy (Taiwan). Some e-commerce/IT outsourcing issues and challenges confronted by hospitals in Australia and Taiwan will be identified, discussed and presented. The findings of this study will assist hospitals and other healthcare organizations to formulate appropriate strategies to better handle the potential issues and challenges in undertaking e-commerce/IT outsourcing projects.

DOI: 10.4018/978-1-7998-2451-0.ch023

Copyright © 2020, IGI Global. Copying or distributing in print or electronic forms without written permission of IGI Global is prohibited.

INTRODUCTION

It is becoming increasingly important for organizations to take advantage of electronic commerce (e-commerce). Retail e-commerce sales worldwide have been estimated to rise by 23.2% to $2.29 trillion in 2017 and are likely to account for 10% of total global retail sales (eMarketer, 2017). Sales are likely to hit $4.48 trillion which will account for 16% of total global retail sales in 2021 (eMarketer, 2017). E-commerce includes trade between business-to-consumers (B2C), consumer-to-consumer (C2C) as well as business-to-business (B2B) trade and utilizes technologies such as the Web, the Internet, intranets, extranets, and electronic data interchange (EDI) to support commercial activities (Cao, Lu, Gupta, & Yang, 2015; Osmonbekov, Zhang, & Dang, 2016; Tan & Ludwig, 2016). E-commerce provides hospitals with increased opportunities for enhancing organizational activities such as exchanging information, coordinating logistics and communications via international hospital supply chains (Elbeltagi, Hamad, Moizer, & Abou-Shouk, 2016; Kurnia, Choudrie, Mahbubur, & Alzougool, 2015). Commonly adopted e-commerce technologies include the Internet, EDI, Electronic Funds Transfer (EFT) and barcodes (Kurnia, Choudrie, Mahbubur, & Alzougool, 2015; Zeng, Wen, & Yen, 2003). E-commerce uses the open Internet and existing information technology to expand customer value by giving organizations easier access to their internal business systems (Lee, Lim, & Tan, 1999; Yeh, Lee, & Pai, 2015). It also provides the opportunity for organizations to attain a greater degree of Internet connectivity at a fraction of the cost of an in-store trade, and it is an effective mean to share and exchange data and information (Hoque & Boateng, 2017; Lee et al., 1999; Tsao, Lin, & Lin, 2004). In addition, it assists organizations such as hospitals and healthcare organizations to purchase medical supplies in real time as well as to utilize it as a cheaper alternative to enter into new markets (Kurnia, Choudrie, Mahbubur, & Alzougool, 2015; Raisinghani et al., 2005).

Outsourcing of e-commerce/IT systems has often been used by hospitals and healthcare organizations to control their costs and remain competitive. According to Gartner, global the IT outsourcing service market grew by 4.6% to reach approximately US$285.5 billion in 2016 (Huntley & Blackmore, 2017). The percentage of the total IT budget spent on IT outsourcing increased from 10.6% in 2016 to 11.9% in 2017 (Computer Economics, 2017). However, only 28% of healthcare organizations engage in IT outsourcing activities, which is well below the average for all industries at 53% (Computer Economics, 2017). Nevertheless, IT outsourcing has increasingly become a popular business strategy for all types of organizations (Moon, Choe, Chung, Jung, & Swar, 2016). In particular, it has more impact on hospital productivity in the short run, with the optimal level of IT outsourcing being between 50% and 80% of overall IT spending (Lee, 2017). However, difficulties in quantifying the intangible benefits of e-commerce/IT outsourcing projects are the major concern for hospitals (Cutler & Sterne, 2000; Standing & Lin, 2007; Stockdale, Lin & Stoney, 2005; Torres, 2017). Although the adoption of e-commerce/IT projects can be seen as a strategic move to gain a competitive advantage and boost organizational performance, the difficulty in measuring the less precisely defined technology of e-commerce is problematic for organizations since the physical boundaries between trading partners are usually difficult to separate (Barua, Konana, & Whinston, 2004; Liu, Huang, & Lin, 2012; Melville, Kraemer, & Gurbaxani, 2004; Zhuang, 2005). Organizations need to adopt appropriate evaluation methodologies and approaches to evaluate the new type of organizational capabilities in order to improve productivity of the e-commerce/IT outsourcing investments (Lin, Pervan, Lin, & Tsao, 2008).

The success of benefits realization has been made to link change management, business strategies with the targeted e-commerce/IT investments (Breese, Jenner, Serra, & Thorp, 2015). It is also firmly connected with organizational performance and the main focus has been on value creation (Chih, & Zwikael, 2015). The benefits realization methodologies or processes have not been widely utilized by most organizations and among those that have adopted such practices, their usage might be limited (Lin & Pervan, 2000). There has been a lack of research on benefits realization practices (Breese, Jenner, Serra, & Thorp, 2015; Hellang, Flak, & Päivärinta, 2013). More research is required on the issue of benefits realization of e-commerce/IT projects to address the 'Information Paradox' where there has been a long-running debate in the relevant literature among IT practitioners and researchers (Brynjolfsson & Hitt, 2003; Hellang et al., 2013; Lin, Pervan, & McDermid, 2002). Researchers and practitioners (e.g., Brynjolfsson & Hitt, 2003; Byrd, Lewis, & Bryan, 2006) have argued that the uncertainty over the realization of e-commerce/IT benefits is possibly attribute to difficulty in adopting a proper IT investment evaluation methodology, poor outsourcing management practices, and poor IT investment evaluation processes. Particularly, the practices of e-commerce/IT outsourcing and evaluation in Australian and Taiwanese hospitals and healthcare organizations remain poorly understood and relatively under-researched. Therefore, the main objective of this study is to better understand the investment evaluation and benefits realization practices and processes of those Australian and Taiwanese hospitals that have outsourced their e-commerce/IT systems. One key contribution of this study is that some e-commerce/IT outsourcing issues and challenges confronted by hospitals in Australia and Taiwan will be identified and discussed. The findings will assist hospitals and other healthcare organizations to formulate appropriate strategies to better handle potential issues and challenges in undertaking e-commerce/IT outsourcing projects.

LITERATURE REVIEW

The socio-technical systems theory aims to examine the fit between the social and technical subsystems when innovations are introduced within an organization (e.g. electronic commerce and IT outsourcing) (Clegg, 2000; Trist, Murray, & Pollack, 1963). Therefore, the theory was drawn in this research study to understand and address the difficulties and opportunities arising from the interactions between social (e.g., human behavior) and technical (e.g., e-commerce) (Shani & Sena, 1994). The socio-technical systems theory has great relevance to help us understand social and technical issues that have been identified in the adoption of e-commerce/IT outsourcing projects within hospitals and healthcare organizations (Doherty, 2014; Heeks, 2002). The theory provides the foundation for an examination of the social and technical views (e.g. e-commerce/IT investment evaluation, benefits realization and outsourcing, top management support, user involvement, perceived time pressure, user information requirements determination, and cultural similarity, and strategic fit) which may have some impact on the adoption of e-commerce/IT outsourcing projects in hospitals and healthcare organizations.

Evaluation and Benefits Realization of E-Commerce/IT Projects

Evaluation of e-commerce/IT projects is important for hospitals and healthcare organizations since it is used to define whether each project is successful (Claxton, Paulden, Gravelle, Brouwer, & Culyer, 2011; Lin et al., 2014; Peute, Aarts, Bakker, & Jaspers, 2010; Serra & Kunc, 2015). The evaluation of e-commerce/IT projects measures how well these projects deliver the expected value as well as meet business objectives and strategies (Chao, Lin, Lin, Shen, & Wang, 2012; Karthik & Kumar, 2013; Lin, 2002; Mitra, Sambamurthy, & Westerman, 2011). Although substantial research has been conducted in evaluation and benefits realization in e-commerce/IT domain (Lin & Huang, 2007), limited work has been done in the area of healthcare (Brender, 1997). Traditionally, e-commerce/IT evaluation studies in the healthcare setting focuses mainly on improving efficiency in administrative or clinical processes (Brender, 1997; Coiera, 2003). Evaluation of e-commerce/IT is generally conducted in systems development life cycle stages (Brender, 1997; Norton, Coulson-Thomas, Coulson-Thomas, & Ashurst, 2013). However, recent e-commerce/IT evaluation and benefits realization studies in healthcare have started to examine technical and social aspects which involve various stakeholders such as system users, IT professionals, patients, clinicians, medical suppliers, and medical professionals (Walston, Bennett, & Al-Harbi, 2014; Yusof, Papazafeiropoulou, Paul, & Stergioulas, 2008). They are important in identifying benefits of e-commerce/IT and how benefits criterial have been produced (Casey, Wainwright, & Waring, 2015). The effective adoption of e-commerce/IT evaluation and benefits realization practices can help organizations to provide benefits to existing and new suppliers and customers (Ababneh, Shrafat & Zeglat, 2017; McGaughey, 2002). The integration of proper IT investment evaluation methodologies into the organizational governance process can assist hospitals and healthcare organizations to improve the effectiveness of health information systems, deliver quality healthcare for patients in a required schedule and budget, achieve greater clinical efficiency, improve business strategic fit and organizational outcomes, and reduce operating costs (Friedman & Wyatt, 1997; Kuhn, Giuse, & Talmon, 2003). However, the use of IT investment evaluation methodologies by hospitals alone is not sufficient (Lin et al., 2014; Liu and Lin, 2008). In order to make the value and strategic relevance of each project clearer, benefits realization methodologies must be adopted by hospitals in conjunction with the proper governance of other key organizational factors in order to realize expected benefits (Lin et al., 2014; Serra & Kunc, 2015).

The realization of benefits from e-commerce/IT and outsourcing projects is an increasing concern for hospitals and healthcare organizations that rely on projects for enhancing organizational performance (Keeys & Huemann, 2017; Lin, Lin, Huang, & Jalleh, 2011). Many organizations have simply failed to meet project objectives and realize expect benefits from their e-commerce/IT projects (Badewi, 2016; Coombs, 2015; Lin, Huang, & Cheng, 2007). Project managers within these organizations often do not have a good understanding of how to obtain benefits and values from their e-commerce/IT projects (Marnewick, 2017). The formulation and use of appropriate evaluation and benefits realization methods or frameworks can help organizations in successfully managing and obtaining expected project benefits and goals (Chih & Zwikael, 2015; Ozkan, Baykal, & Sincan, 2012; Sadoughi & Aminpour, 2011). However, evaluation and benefits realization have not been conducted effectively by hospitals and healthcare organizations (Yusof et al., 2008) as well as organizations in other industries (Terlizzi, & Albertin, 2017). Only a small portion of e-commerce/IT investments have been considered to be successful (Doherty, 2014).

A review of the literature confirms that many organizations did not conduct any post-implementation reviews of their e-commerce/IT investments because the costs to identify, manage and review these benefits can be large and uncertain (Marnewick, 2017; McKay & Marshall, 2004). Moreover, research has shown contradictory findings on the effect of the e-commerce/IT spending on organizational productivity (Thatcher & Pingry, 2004). More than ever before, many business executives are skeptical about the contribution of their e-commerce/IT investments on the overall business and financial performance (Chaysin,

Daengdej, & Tangjitprom, 2016). Indeed, the actual dollar returns of e-commerce/IT investment have been the subject of heated debate by many researchers (Sugumaran & Arogyaswamy, 2004). Some of the barriers to the adoption of evaluation and benefits realization of e-commerce/IT and outsourcing projects identified included use of informal evaluation and benefits realization methodologies, bureaucracy, lack of use of evaluation criteria, staff resistance to change, difficulties in quantifying intangible benefits, poor IT adoption practices, and lags in learning and adjustments (Stratopoulos & Dehning, 2000; Terlizzi, & Albertin, 2017; Turner & Ledwith, 2016). Literature has shown that effective evaluation and benefits realization of e-commerce/IT investments is directly linked to organizational performance (Brynjolfsson & Hitt, 2003; Melville et al., 2004; Serra & Kunc, 2015; Terlizzi, & Albertin, 2017). Indeed, e-commerce/IT projects must focus on the delivery of business benefits in order to develop competitive advantages (Lee & Runge, 2001; Lin, Huang, Cheng & Lin, 2007; Marnewick, 2016).

Although benefits realization practices have been linked to e-commerce/IT project success (Hafeez, Hussain, Javed & Saeed, 2016), their adoption and the benefits delivery are notoriously difficult to manage and measure particularly when they are linked electronically to the supply chain (Giaglis, Paul, & Doukidis, 1999; McKay & Marshall, 2004). The difficulty in measuring the less precisely defined technology of e-commerce in particular are problematic for organizations since the physical boundaries between trading partners are usually difficult to separate (Torkzadeh & Dhillon, 2002). Hence, failure to take into account technical and social aspects of the organizational/business strategies and objectives which involve main stakeholders in the process of measuring the benefits from e-commerce/IT projects can have damaging effects on business performance (Doherty, 2014).

The adoption of an evaluation methodology for e-commerce/IT projects is insufficient for ensuring the delivery of expected benefits for organizations (Remenyi & Whittaker, 1996; Ward & Griffiths, 1996). Careful management of benefits realization for each project ensures the delivery of the expected benefits and thus creates strategic value to organizations (Love, Irani, Standing, Lin, & Burn, 2005; Serra & Kunc, 2015; Ward & Griffiths, 1996). Benefits and costs need to be continuously justified, prioritized, tracked, reviewed and monitored throughout the life of the e-commerce/IT projects as the benefits and costs are not as clearly defined as they are with other type of investments (Doherty, 2014; Tallon, Kraemer, & Gurbaxani, 2000).

Outsourcing of E-Commerce/IT

Rising healthcare costs, increasing competition, and tighter legal legislations can all have a huge influence on the decision of hospitals to outsource some of their e-commerce/IT systems (Ferdosi et al., 2013; Kahouei, Farrokhi, Abadi, & Karimi, 2016). Due to these constraints, hospitals and healthcare organizations often are unable to invest sufficient resources to main their e-commerce/IT infrastructure (Kahouei, Farrokhi, Abadi, & Karimi, 2016). The main benefits of e-commerce/IT outsourcing in the healthcare industry include quicker development cycle time, access to a larger pool of skills, cost saving, improved patient satisfaction, increased organizational flexibility, focus of core competencies, improved services and efficiency, economies of scale, and reduction in staff turnover (Danvers & Nikolov, 2010; Hsiao, Pai, & Chiu, 2009; Johnson, Murphy, McNeese, Reddy, & Purao, 2013; Kahouei, Farrokhi, Abadi, & Karimi, 2016; Menachemi, Burke, & Diana, 2007; Patil & Wongsurawat, 2015; Sujata, Reddy, & Jayalakshmi, 2013). However, despite the expected benefits and savings from the e-commerce/IT outsourcing for hospitals and healthcare organizations, costs and risks arising from this also need to be taken into account. These include increased government regulations, hidden costs, costs increase for patients, user resistance, the risk of losing sensitive patient data, poor strategic similarity between outsourcing hospitals and external outsourcing vendors, inability to manage outsourcing contracts, reduced quality control, loss of core business focus, and inexperienced employees by external vendors (Hsiao et al., 2009; Karimi, Agharahimi, & Yaghoubi, 2012; Lawrence & Firth, 2013; Ondo & Smith, 2006).

Many organizations believe e-commerce/IT outsourcing can bring numerous benefits such as cost savings, reduced training costs, improved quality of patient care, increased patient satisfaction, improved patients' privacy, more cash flow, access to required technical expertise and knowledge, better relocation of resources, reduction of risks, reduced medical errors, and enhanced competitive advantage (Aggelidis & Chatzoglou, 2012; Alaghehband, Rivard, Wu, & Goyette, 2011; Gorla & Somers, 2014; Moon, Choe, Chung, Jung, & Swar, 2016; Mudambi & Tallman, 2010; Samantra, Datta, & Mahapatra, 2014; Sujata et al., 2013; Yu, 2010). However, the scope, variety, and complexity of e-commerce/IT outsourcing are generally the main challenges in IT investment evaluation and benefits realization practices (Doherty, Ashurst, & Peppard, 2012; Tallon et al., 2000). This is often due to the fact that most hospitals and healthcare organizations do not regularly measure and review their e-commerce/IT outsourcing since formal evaluation methodologies are difficult to understand and operationalize (Low & Chen, 2012). Therefore, many organizations rely on informal methodologies such as cost/benefit analysis and return on investment (ROI) calculations to evaluate their e-commerce/IT and outsourcing projects (McIvor, 2000). Organizations that adopt formal evaluation methodologies for their e-commerce/IT investments tend to achieve better business (Tallon et al., 2000). Outsourcing organizations are advised to choose evaluation methodologies which are: easy to adopt and understand by both outsourcing organizations and external vendors; aligned with mutual strategic fits, business objectives, and expectations; measurable by objective criteria; controllable by external vendors; able to produce the desirable results and conducts by both outsourcing organizations and external vendors (Misra, 2004).

Top Management Support and User Involvement

As e-commerce/IT outsourcing projects become increasingly complicated both organizationally and technically, more emphasis has been placed on human relationship and management issues (Gantman & Fedorowicz, 2016; Wiener, Remus, Heumann, & Mähring, 2015). One of the leading human management issues is top management support for e-commerce/IT outsourcing. Top management support has been defined as the degree to which senior management understand the significant nature of the e-commerce/IT operations and the relative importance to which it is involved in e-commerce/IT projects (Kurnia, Choudrie, Mahbubur, & Alzougool, 2015; Ragu-Nathana, Apigian, Ragu-Nathana, & Tu, 2004). It may affect an organization's e-commerce/IT capacities as well as the adoption of IT/business strategies (Yeh, Lee, & Pai, 2015). It is often being considered as one of the most critical contributing factors for e-commerce/IT success (e.g., Norton et al., 2013; Young & Jordan, 2008). Several studies indicate that top management support is critical and will very likely contribute to the e-commerce/IT success (e.g., Ragu-Nathana et al., 2004). Other research studies indicate that successful launching of new or outsourced e-commerce/IT projects is difficult without top management support and such support is required to overcome interdepartmental communication challenges within an organization (Lee & Kim, 2007). Top management support is also vital in evaluating and assessing e-commerce/IT benefits (Chugh, Sharma, & Cabrera, 2017). Another benefit of top management support is in relation to employee resistance to the adoption of new or outsourced e-commerce/IT projects.

The other main issue contributing to failures of e-commerce/IT outsourcing projects is the lack of user involvement. It is difficult to outsource e-commerce/IT outsourcing projects without understanding the values and beliefs of users (Kahouei, Farrokhi, Abadi, & Karimi, 2016). Executives in hospitals and healthcare organizations need to make every effort to understand how the outsourcing decisions would affect the users given that previous research has shown a clear association between users' commitment and satisfaction and organizational performance (Kahouei, Farrokhi, Abadi, & Karimi, 2016). By failing to involve relevant users throughout system development stages, they might feel disappointed, threatened, and disenchanted. This usually results in resistance and disputes between the executives and the users (Abelein & Paech, 2014; Bano & Zowghi, 2015; Durugbo, 2012). Lack of user involvement can also result in suspicion and distrust between executives and users, leading to job dissatisfaction and less than ideal e-commerce/IT systems (Lin & Lin, 2011). In particular, job insecurity among users may generate negative feelings which can result in low morale, job turnover, loss of commitment, and increased absenteeism (Kahouei, Farrokhi, Abadi, & Karimi, 2016). On the other hand, there are a number of benefits that can result from users being involved in the decision-making process such as increased system quality, enhanced system efficiency, and greater user acceptance and knowledge about the system (Abelein & Paech, 2014; Durugbo, 2012; de Waal & Batenburg, 2014).

Perceived Time Pressure

The process of e-commerce/IT outsourcing involves a more complicated adjustment to the workplace environment which has the potential to create a sense of stress and confusion for the entire IT project team (Kahouei, Farrokhi, Abadi, & Karimi, 2016; Saorín-Iborra, Redondo-Cano, Revuelto-Taboada, & Vogler, 2015). Several studies have been conducted on the negative outcomes of coping with perceived time pressure in e-commerce/IT since meeting the deadline for completion is one of the most used measures for e-commerce/IT project success (Thomas, Fugate, & Koukova, 2011; Syrek, Apostel, & Antoni, 2013). Perceived time pressure happens when the time given to accomplish a job is unachievable (Schick, Gordon, & Haka, 1990; Thomas et al., 2011). This can lead to negative effects for the entire e-commerce/IT project team including errors, passivity, stress, avoidance and incorrect decision-making process and performance (Kocher & Sutter, 2006; Rissler, 1994). However, it can also be an important driving force for work progress (Zika-Viktorsson, Sundstrom, & Engwall, 2006).

Several coping mechanisms have been suggested to deal with the perceived time pressure. For instance, Schultze & Vandenbosch (1998) who studied LotusNotes users in an organization suggested the utilization of filtering mechanisms. The use of appropriate decision tools such as schema that synthesized previous decisions can help to reduce decision overload (Paul & Nazareth, 2010). Hence, an increase in the perceived time pressure may have a positive impact on e-commerce/IT outsourcing by hospitals. However, failure to cope with perceived time pressure may have a negative impact on the establishing of better communication relationship/trust with external outsourcing vendors.

Cultural Similarity and Strategic Fit

Research has been conducted on the impact of culture similarity on organizational performance (Hahn & Bunyaratavej, 2010; Ralston, Holt, Terpstra, & Kai-Cheng, 2008; Peute et al., 2010). The cultural divergence between two different entities can be understood in terms of elements such as individualism/collectivism, masculinity/femininity, power distance, and uncertainty avoidance (Hofstede, 1997).

Cultural differences between two organizations can be substantial as employees from different cultures understand and judge the nature of the world differently (Han & Lee, 2012; Licht, 2004). In the context of e-commerce/IT outsourcing, this can increase the risks, uncertainty, and transaction costs because it is likely that external outsourcing vendors might not fully understand outsourcing hospitals' organizational culture or its requirements (Han & Lee, 2012).

The fit between different organizational functions is important for the successful implementation of any e-commerce/IT system (Rahim, Kurnia, Samson, & Singh, 2014). The lack of strategic fit between various organizational functions may have a negative impact on the benefits realization for e-commerce/IT outsourcing initiatives (Aversano, Grasso, & Tortorella, 2013; Lin, 2002). Strategic alignment acknowledges that both business and IT functions should be managed and operated in their respective focuses in order to complement each other. Functional integration centers on the association among business/IT strategies, IT execution, and business operations which assist in delivering the expected benefits to the organizations when they are working well together. Yayla & Hu (2012) have concluded that organizations with higher levels of fit of their control and strategies components perform better than those with lower levels of fit. Proper alignments between outsourcing hospitals and external vendors can help in integrating various IT resources effectively to support their business strategies and to achieve the expected benefits and better business outcomes from their outsourcing projects (Chan, Huff, Barclay, & Copeland, 1997; Huang, Lin, Liu, & Tung, 2013; Kuo, Lin, Hsu, & Huang, 2006; Li, 2012).

Information Requirements Determination

Organizations which collect feedback about users' information requirements are likely to better comprehend their task needs (Babar, Wong, & Abedin, 2014; Dutot, Bergeron, & Raymond, 2014; Shuraida & Barki, 2013). The information requirements determination (IRD) process is an important element within the system development life cycle. IRD has been put forward as a means for improving the success rate of e-commerce/IT projects (Hsu, Lin, Zheng, & Hung, 2012; Liu et al., 2011; Wu & Shen, 2006). The IRD process has been defined by Browne & Ramesh (2002, p. 625) as "…a set of activities used by a systems analyst when assessing the functionality required in a proposed system…" With rapid changes of technology and customer driven requirements, however, IRD process has become an increasingly difficult exercise for organizations (Gorschek, Svahnberg, Borg, Loconsole, & Sandahl, 2007). This IRD uncertainty can lead to conflicts between different stakeholders as users prefer changes to reflect their environmental instabilities whereas IT professionals prefer to lock-in their information requirements so they are able to complete their e-commerce/IT projects on time and within budget (Liu et al., 2011). Hence, the success of e-commerce/IT projects depends heavily on how well the IRD process has been carried out.

Many research studies have pointed out that the IRD process is problematic, and in many cases, project failures have nothing to do with technical issues (Lin & Lin, 2011; Urquhart, 2001). Some of the reasons behind many of these problems include lack of user involvement, incomplete information requirement specifications, lack of flexible information systems, poor communication, and lack of common knowledge. Incomplete information requirements specifications can result in identifying the wrong information needs and this may ultimately lead to e-commerce/IT project failures (Hsu et al., 2012; Khalil & Elkordy, 2005). Humans' limited ability to process information and solve problems is yet another reason for failure during the IRD stage (Land, 1987).

RESEARCH METHODS

Despite the importance of e-commerce/IT investment evaluation and benefits realization processes within organizations, the literature lacks empirical evidence about how organizations are adopting these processes. Therefore, the main objective of this study is to better understand the investment evaluation and benefits realization practices and processes of those Australian and Taiwanese hospitals that decide to outsource their e-commerce/IT systems. This study provides the opportunity to examine outsourcing practices of a highly developed economy (Australia) and a newly industrialized economy (Taiwan). Hospitals in Australia and Taiwan were chosen for this study because e-commerce/IT outsourcing in hospitals has been extremely popular in both countries. Despite this, e-commerce/IT investment evaluation and benefits realization processes remain poorly understood in these hospitals. To the best of our knowledge, no comparative studies have been published in the literature focusing on e-commerce/IT investment evaluation and outsourcing in both Taiwanese and Australian hospitals. Hence, a better understanding of the e-commerce/IT investment evaluation and outsourcing processes is warranted. Case studies were conducted with e-commerce/IT stakeholders from 20 Australian and Taiwanese hospitals. All of the hospitals interviewed have adopted e-commerce systems for at least five years and had outsourced at least part of the systems and functions. To remain competitive, Australian and Taiwanese hospitals need to make good use of their IT resources such as e-commerce systems and health information systems.

To follow the non-random sampling strategy suggested by Eisenhardt (1989), 20 cases were intentionally selected to focus on theoretically useful cases. The data collection process continued until the benefit of an additional interview was seen as too small (Eisenhardt, 1989). The interviews allowed the authors to probe how hospitals measure their e-commerce/IT investments and to what extent their expected e-commerce/IT benefits were achieved. The topics covered in the interviews included: various e-commerce/IT implementation and outsourcing management issues, the processes of e-commerce/IT investment evaluation and benefits realization, and the impacts of evaluation processes on e-commerce/ IT benefits and user satisfaction.

Multiple data sources were collected and these included hospital documents, meeting minutes, and annual reports. Interview notes and transcripts were analyzed and coded using the qualitative content analysis outlined by Miles and Huberman (1994). The analysis of the findings was conducted in a cyclical manner and the external experts had checked and examined the findings first by tracing the logical flow of the research objectives, questions, variables, results and then by identifying gaps in the chain of evidence (Yin, 2002). Questions and responses for a specific research cluster or theme, for example, level of user satisfaction, were sorted and grouped as a category. Various opinions and responses within the same hospital were assessed in terms of the relative power of the views in accordance with the numbers of responses in specific categories in order to enhance the validity, reliability and overall quality of this research (Yin, 2002).

RESEARCH FINDINGS

Drawing on the socio-technical systems theory, this research attempts to examine the following management and organizational issues: user involvement, top management support, e-commerce/IT investment evaluation and benefits realization, strategic fit, e-commerce/IT outsourcing, cultural similarity, user information requirements determination, and perceived time pressure. The findings indicated that a large percentage of Australian and Taiwanese hospitals (70% and 80%, respectively) had used a formal or semi-formal e-commerce/IT investment evaluation methodology or process to evaluate their outsourced e-commerce/IT investments. However, around 60% of Australian hospitals had used a formal or semi-formal e-commerce/IT benefits realization methodology or process on their electronic commerce investments and only 40% of Taiwanese hospitals had done so. Of those who had adopted the methodologies or processes, several indicated that they were in most cases neither effective in adopting successful e-commerce/IT systems nor widely used within their hospitals.

For both Australian and Taiwanese hospitals, efficiency improvement and cost reduction were the two major reasons to outsource their e-commerce/IT systems. Other major reasons included decreased power of the union, greater business focus, and increased justification of costs against business outcomes. On the other hand, outsourcing was often employed to overcome lack of resources and to reduce their labor force for Taiwanese hospitals. A number of the key issues in managing the e-commerce/IT outsourcing projects are identified and presented in the following sub-sections.

Lack of User Involvement and Management Support

The results revealed that there were a general lack of strong top management support and commitment for most of the new and outsourced e-commerce/IT projects in most hospitals. Those e-commerce/IT projects which had gained strong support from top management tended to provide more training and assistance to users. More training provided by top management had resulted in greater user skill in dealing with e-commerce/IT systems. This in turn had led to more user participation and familiarity with the e-commerce/IT systems and projects. Users who were deeply involved with the projects tended to perceive fewer system barriers and more benefits than those with less involvement. In addition, strong top management support was positively related to the adoption of e-commerce/IT investment evaluation and benefits realization processes/methodologies. For example, one hospital IT manager stated: "…… the methodology has allowed us to produce the evidence and key performance measures to show our top management that these projects will have long-term strategic benefits to the hospital……" Indeed, the use of these methodologies had permitted hospital management to determine if a particular project had resulted in significant benefits for the hospital.

Generally, the outsourcing and implementation of new e-commerce/IT systems were forced upon employees or users by top management. Most employees and users felt that they were not involved with the initial decision-making process for outsourcing and this had resulted in user resistance. Furthermore, many users indicated that most of the expected benefits arising from the outsourcing of new e-commerce/IT systems were designed for top management. There was a positive relationship between hospitals that involved their users during the initial decision-making process for outsourcing and those that implemented IT investment evaluation and benefits realization methodologies.

Inability to Cope with Perceived Time Pressure

High level of perceived time pressure from participants in Taiwanese hospitals had resulted in high level of stress and turnover in the workplace. Generally, the participants attempted to work faster and this had appeared to have a negative impact on their relationships with external outsourcing vendors. For example, one IT manager in a Taiwanese hospital stated that: "…we simply do not have enough manpower and time to complete the many projects we have at the moment… this is a real problem for us and our external outsourcing contractors." A lot of participants indicated that no proper procedures and training were put in place by top management to help them to cope with perceived time pressure. The ambiguity in task distribution by hospitals did not assist in reducing the level of perceived time pressure for those involved in e-commerce/IT outsourcing and this in turn had a negative impact on establishing better relationship, trust, and communication with external outsourcing vendors. This seemed to be more prevalent among Taiwanese hospitals.

Cultural Divergence between Outsourcing Hospitals and Vendors

Participating hospitals generally outsourced their e-commerce/IT systems to external outsourcing vendors in order to save costs, deliver better service, and improve efficiency. However, several hospitals were not able to deliver the expected benefits due to cultural divergence between themselves and the external outsourcing vendors. Australia is an individualistic society whereas Taiwan has a collectivistic culture under the individualism-collectivism index proposed by Hofstede (1997). Taiwanese culture is characterized by high collectivism and this was particularly the issue for the Taiwanese hospitals where their e-commerce/IT outsourcing market was mostly dominated by Western vendors. Organizations from different cultures understand, and assess the worldview differently (Han & Lee, 2012). Problems came across by the Taiwanese hospitals and their external outsourcing vendors included different values and methods of managing projects and objectives. Although for Taiwanese hospitals to enter into e-commerce/IT outsourcing contracts with Western vendors were likely to gain global synergies, however this resulted in a high level of uncertainty and cultural clash for them because the external outsourcing vendors did not fully comprehend their organizational values and cultures. This was especially the case for the Taiwanese public hospitals which required efficient services in line with government legislation and regulations. For example, an IT manager from a Taiwanese public hospital said: "As a public hospital, the reason for outsourcing was often more to do with providing better services in line with government directives rather than simply cost saving and generating revenue… but our outsourcing contractor appears to be only interested in making money out of us from the outsourced… system… we also seem to have different cultures in managing things and achieving the stated goals…" Furthermore, selecting appropriate external outsourcing vendors was an integral component of e-commerce/IT investment evaluation and benefits realization processes. The decision to select a particular outsourcing vendor often came down to whether the bilateral relationship would work out and whether the cultural distance between the two parties was small. Those hospitals which did not undertake proper e-commerce/IT investment evaluation and benefits realization processes at the initial stage of their outsourcing projects to determine the cultural distance between both parties appeared to have more cultural related problems later on. On the other hand, this was not a significant problem for Australian hospitals where the Australian e-commerce/IT outsourcing market was dominated by domestic or Western vendors which had overall smaller cultural distances.

Lack of Mutual Strategic Fit

Mutual fit between hospitals and external outsourcing vendors can help to integrate their e-commerce/IT resources more effectively to support business/IT strategies as well as to realize the expected benefits from their outsourcing contracts (Li, 2012; Lin & Lin, 2011). Despite this, most hospitals indicated that it was not an easy task because external outsourcing vendors were assessed and selected based not only on hospitals' business and service requirements but also on areas of similarity in terms of strategic fit between both parties during the initial pre-project justification phase. One hospital IT manager stated: "...a lot of time and resources had been spent... to make sure that our (outsourcing hospital and contractor's) strategies and control mechanism are properly aligned..." Indeed, appropriate amount of resources and time required for e-commerce/IT investment evaluation methodologies or processes had to be expended at the initial pre-project justification phase. The lack of mutually agreed strategic fit, goals, and visions between the outsourcing hospitals and their external vendors could result in problems later down the track for both parties. This could also affect the system quality and user satisfaction. For Taiwanese hospitals, the most often mentioned reason was the lack of time and expertise in carrying out an e-commerce/IT investment evaluation and benefits realization process at the pre-project justification phase to ensure that a contractor with similar strategic alignment was selected, whereas for Australian hospitals the lack of appropriate funding was often the number one reason for not achieving such strategic fit.

Inaccurate Information Requirements Determination Process

Most of the errors from the e-commerce/IT projects can be traced back to the IRD phase (Hsu et al., 2012; Lin & Lin, 2011). This is important since the main objective of users involved in the e-commerce/IT projects is to share their expertise and experience to determine actual requirements of new systems (He & King, 2008). Despite this, it seemed that only a few participating hospitals had paid sufficient attention to the user IRD process. For instance, one hospital IT procurement manager revealed that: "...It was difficult to obtain complete requirements from users... they were changing all the time... We couldn't do much about it." In many cases, this had resulted in the mismatch between user requirements and business outcomes from the e-commerce/IT outsourcing projects because most of hospital expertise and experience integration process (e.g., corporate memory not retained) was not conducted successfully. One main reason for this was that the outsourcing hospitals often did not budget sufficient organizational resources to manage the IRD process for their e-commerce/IT outsourcing projects. Other reasons for the IRD failure included: (1) lack of experienced IT professionals in getting accurate and complete user information requirements; (2) lack of communication between top management and users; (3) conflicting agendas and requirements between outsourcing hospitals and external outsourcing vendors; (4) unstable and changing user requirements; and (5) failure to allocate sufficient resources to set up governance mechanism to manage the IRD process. There were differences for the Australian and Taiwanese hospitals in involving users and stakeholders during the e-commerce/IT outsourcing stage. Australian hospitals executives tended to budget more resources and time in eliciting user requirements than their Taiwanese counterparts. For Australian hospitals, outsourcing was often conducted to justify increased spending against business outcomes. For Taiwanese hospitals, outsource was often carried out without user consultation and used to overcome lack of resources as well as to reduce their labor force.

DISCUSSIONS

This study found that having a greater business focus was one of the main motivations for Australian hospitals to outsource their e-commerce/IT systems, whereas for Taiwanese hospitals e-commerce/IT outsourcing was implemented to address lack of resources and reduce their labor force. In addition, the findings demonstrated that most Australian and Taiwanese hospitals had implemented an e-commerce/

IT investment evaluation process or methodology to assess their projects. However, only 60% of Australian and 40% of Taiwanese hospitals had implemented an e-commerce/IT benefits realization process or methodology. Furthermore, the findings revealed that there may be roadblocks in implementing an e-commerce/IT investment evaluation and benefits realization methodologies for participating hospitals.

Some key management and evaluation issues identified in this research included: lack of user involvement and management support; inaccurate information requirements determination process; inability to cope with perceived time pressure; lack of mutual strategic fit; cultural divergence between outsourcing hospitals and vendors. The findings revealed that the hospital management had forced their employees and users to use the new systems without first involving them in the initial pre-project justification phase. Moreover, there was a general lack of strong top management support for most of the new outsourced e-commerce/IT projects in most participating hospitals. There appeared to be more training provided to the users for those e-commerce/IT projects which had obtained strong top management support and commitment. Obtaining accurate user information requirements is crucial for having a successful e-commerce/IT project and most of the errors during the development stages can be traced back to the IRD stage. The findings suggested that only a few participating hospitals had invested sufficient resources and time in the IRD process. Australian hospitals appeared to invest more resources and time in getting accurate and complete user information requirements than their Taiwanese counterparts. For Australian hospitals, outsourcing was often conducted to justify increased spending against business outcomes. For Taiwanese hospitals, outsourcing was often carried out without user consultation and used to overcome lack of resources as well as to reduce their labor force.

The findings of this study also demonstrated that there was a level of high perceived time pressures among participants within Taiwanese hospitals, and in many instances they responded by attempting to work faster and this had a negative effect on the relationships and trust with their external outsourcing vendors. To reduce the perceived time pressure among users, hospitals and healthcare organizations can give timely assistance in critical situations, minimize task ambiguity, and provide adequate training. Strategic objectives, expectations, and visions of the outsourcing projects should be communicated and discussed by both parties during the contract negotiation process and these should also be included in the service level agreements. Additionally, outsourcing hospitals should make every effort in strengthening the communication process with their external vendors and put in place a control mechanism to continuously assess and track the expectations and goals in outsourcing their e-commerce/IT systems. This is important given that performance of the contracts may deteriorate quickly if the expectations and goals are not met.

Another aspect which may impact on comparisons of the identified key management and evaluation issues between countries is the cultural divergence. A deeper understanding of these differences allows hospital executives to cross-borders e-commerce/IT outsourcing projects because similar evaluation practices can be perceived differently by different cultures. Cultural divergence was particularly apparent for Taiwanese hospitals where the Taiwanese e-commerce/IT outsourcing market was mostly dominated by Western vendors. Some of the problems they and external outsourcing vendors encountered were having different visions, goals, and processes of accomplishing and managing projects. Although for Taiwanese hospitals to enter into e-commerce/IT outsourcing contracts with Western vendors were likely to gain global synergies, this had resulted in a high level of uncertainty and cultural clash for them because the external outsourcing vendors did not fully comprehend their organizational values and cultures. This was especially the case for the Taiwanese public hospitals which required efficient services in line with government legislation and regulations. On the other hand, this was not a significant problem for the

Australian hospitals where the Australian e-commerce/IT outsourcing market was dominated by domestic or Western vendors which had overall smaller cultural distances. Overall, it was generally difficult for hospitals to achieve strategic fit with their external outsourcing vendors and this had often resulted in unfulfilled requirements and goals for both parties.

Potentially, the results of this study can assist hospitals and healthcare organizations in getting a better understanding of their e-commerce/IT investment evaluation and benefits realization practices. It is critical for senior management to look at these key issues in order to deliver the expected e-commerce/IT benefits from their outsourcing projects. In addition, other behavioral, attitudinal, and organizational issues should be examined by hospital management. For instance, there must be open discussion among users and other stakeholders on the benefits of the new e-commerce/IT systems since their subsequent behaviors and attitudes can help hospital management to formulate appropriate intervention strategies and policies to maximize their use within the hospitals. After all, a benefit to one group of users can be considered detrimental to another group. Only through such openness can users and other stakeholders understand the implications of e-commerce/IT projects and the impact upon their work. Furthermore, project champions should be identified to reduce the uncertainty in using new e-commerce/IT systems.

This research study's contribution is not only to examine and identify key e-commerce/IT management and evaluation issues, but also to highlight the barriers by which hospitals and healthcare organizations can overcome in order to deliver the expected benefits. There are similarities between the Australian and Taiwanese hospitals. For instance, a large proportion of Australian and Taiwanese hospitals had adopted an e-commerce/IT investment evaluation methodology and the outsourcing of e-commerce/IT system enabled these hospitals to communicate with key stakeholders such as patients, external outsourcing vendors or users at a lower cost. Hence, hospital management need to understand the factors influencing users' perceptions about the utilization of outsourced systems in order to clearly identify their benefits and then support improvements of their e-commerce/IT investment evaluation and benefits realization processes. Hospitals should spend appropriate resources, time, and effort to establish effective long-term e-commerce/IT marketing strategies in order to improve stakeholder loyalty and improve efficiency.

Similar to those programs and strategies adopted in health promotion and marketing, through the use of social networking sites (e.g., Snapchat, Pinterest, Tumblr, Facebook, LinkedIn, Google+, Twitter), intensive public awareness campaigns, the awareness and positive images of services offered by the hospitals and healthcare organizations can be improved for stakeholders (Donovan, Boulter, Borland, Jalleh, & Carter, 2003; Economo et al., 2010; Heydon, Kennington, Jalleh, & Lin, 2012; Jalleh et al., 2010; Jalleh, Donovan, Lin, & Slevin, 2008; Johnson et al., 2013). These strategies may assist stakeholders in developing a sense of identity for being a valuable employee, resulting in increased loyalty towards the hospitals. The intervention content (e.g., personalized messages and online word-of-mouth recommendations) is accessible by the targeted users as they can be accessed anywhere and at any time (Carter, Donovan, & Jalleh, 2011; Donovan, Jalleh, Clarkson, & Giles-Corti, 1999; Donovan, Jalleh, & Henley, 1996; Jalleh et al., 2001; Stringam & Gerdes Jr., 2010).

CONCLUSION, LIMITATIONS, AND FUTURE RESEARCH DIRECTIONS

Australian and Taiwanese hospitals have invested a lot of time and resources in adopting new e-commerce/IT systems in recent years. However, e-commerce/IT systems are generally not yet mature within the hospital industry. As e-commerce/IT systems are replacing manual human tasks in supporting innovative tasks it becomes a challenge for hospitals and other healthcare organizations to manage these key management and evaluation issues. Despite this, e-commerce/IT systems and applications are producing a more level playing field for all industry players. In the foreseeable future, it is expected that e-commerce/IT systems will result in more efficient operations of hospitals and healthcare organizations. For example, they can be used to manage relationships with external entities such as e-intermediaries and other members of product and service value chain.

Some limitations in this study need to be acknowledged. While there has much research on e-commerce/IT evaluation, there has been limited research on the relationships between the e-commerce/IT evaluation, benefits realization and e-commerce/IT outsourcing, particular in the healthcare sector. As a result, comparisons are difficult to make. Future research can focus on identifying common patterns in e-commerce/IT benefits realization methodology usage and commitment across different organizations and studies. Moreover, our study took place at a particular point in time and the findings are based on 20 hospitals in Australia and Taiwan only. Further research can be conducted to capture opinions of participants at various stages of e-commerce/IT outsourcing project development process across different industries and countries. Furthermore, more research is required to identify and examine other critical factors that may affect the management and evaluation of e-commerce/IT outsourcing projects. Finally, this study can be replicated in a few years time to examine how e-commerce/IT outsourcing evaluation and benefits realization practices in hospitals are being managed and evaluated.

REFERENCES

Ababneh, H., Shrafat, F., & Zeglat, D. (2017). Approaching information system evaluation methodology and techniques: A comprehensive review. *International Journal of Business Information Systems*, *24*(1), 1–30. doi:10.1504/IJBIS.2017.080943

Abelein, U., & Paech, B. (2013). Understanding the Influence of User Participation & Involvement on System Success–a Systematic Mapping Study. *Empirical Software Engineering*.

Abelein, U., & Paech, B. (2014). State of Practice of User-Developer Communication in Large-Scale IT Projects. In *Requirements Engineering: Foundation for Software Quality* (pp. 95–111). USA: Springer International Publishing. doi:10.1007/978-3-319-05843-6_8

Aggelidis, V. P., & Chatzoglou, P. D. (2012). Hospital information systems: Measuring end user computing satisfaction (EUCS). *Journal of Biomedical Informatics*, *45*(3), 566–579. doi:10.1016/j.jbi.2012.02.009 PMID:22426283

Alaghehband, F. K., Rivard, S., Wu, S., & Goyette, S. (2011). An Assessment of the Use of Transaction Cost Theory in Information Technology Outsourcing. *The Journal of Strategic Information Systems*, *20*(2), 125–138. doi:10.1016/j.jsis.2011.04.003

Aversano, L., Grasso, C., & Tortorella, M. (2013). A Literature Review of Business/IT Alignment Strategies. *Lecture Notes in Business Information Processing*, *141*, 471–488. doi:10.1007/978-3-642-40654-6_28

Babar, A., Wong, B., & Abedin, B. (2014). Investigating the role of business analysts competencies into strategic business requirements gathering. In *Proceedings of the 18th Pacific Asia Conference on Information Systems (PACIS 2014)*, Chengdu, China.

Badewi, A. (2016). The impact of project management (PM) and benefits management (BM) practices on project success: Towards developing a project benefits governance framework. *International Journal of Project Management, 34*(4), 761–778. doi:10.1016/j.ijproman.2015.05.005

Bano, M., & Zowghi, D. (2015). A systematic review on the relationship between user involvement and system success. *Information and Software Technology, 58*, 148–169. doi:10.1016/j.infsof.2014.06.011

Barua, A., Konana, P., & Whinston, A. B. (2004). An Empirical Investigation of Net-Enabled Business Value. *Management Information Systems Quarterly, 28*(4), 585–620.

Breese, R., Jenner, S., Serra, C. E. M., & Thorp, J. (2015). Benefits management: Lost or found in translation. *International Journal of Project Management, 33*(7), 1438–1451. doi:10.1016/j.ijproman.2015.06.004

Brender, J. (1997). Methodology for Assessment of Medical IT-Based Systems, vol. 42, IOS Press, Amsterdsam, 1997.

Browne, G. J., & Ramesh, V. (2002). Improving Information Requirements Determination: A Cognitive Perspective. *Information & Management, 39*(8), 625–645. doi:10.1016/S0378-7206(02)00014-9

Brynjolfsson, E., & Hitt, L. M. (2003). Computing Productivity: Firm-Level Evidence. *The Review of Economics and Statistics, 85*(4), 793–808. doi:10.1162/003465303772815736

Byrd, T. A., Lewis, B. R., & Bryan, R. W. (2006). The Leveraging Influence of Strategic Alignment on IT Investment: An Empirical Examination. *Information & Management, 43*(3), 308–321. doi:10.1016/j.im.2005.07.002

Cao, Y., Lu, Y., Gupta, S., & Yang, S. (2015). The effects of differences between e–commerce and m–commerce on the consumers' usage transfer from online to mobile channel. *International Journal of Mobile Communications, 13*(1), 51–70. doi:10.1504/IJMC.2015.065890

Carter, O., Donovan, R. J., & Jalleh, G. (2011). Using Viral e-mails to Distribute Tobacco Control Advertisements to Young Adults: An Experimental Investigation. *Journal of Health Communication, 16*(7), 698–707. doi:10.1080/10810730.2011.551998 PMID:21432712

Casey, R., Wainwright, D., & Waring, T. (2015). Benefits Realisation of Information Technology in the National Health Service: A Paradigmatic Review. In *Proceedings of the European Conference on Information Management and Evaluation* (pp. 37-44). Reading: Academic Conferences International Limited.

Chan, Y. E., Huff, S. L., Barclay, D. W., & Copeland, D. G. (1997). Business strategy orientation. *Information Systems Research, 8*(2), 125–150. doi:10.1287/isre.8.2.125

Chao, C. J., Lin, C., Lin, K., Shen, C. L., & Wang, C. H. (2012). Using the Analytic Hierarchy Process Methodology to Assess the Drivers Affecting the Implementation of Interactive Digital Television as a Commerce Platform. *International Journal of Wireless Networks and Broadband Technologies, 2*(3), 42–51. doi:10.4018/ijwnbt.2012070104

Chaysin, P., Daengdej, J., & Tangjitprom, N. (2016). Survey on Available Methods to Evaluate IT Investment. *Electronic Journal Information Systems Evaluation, 19*(1), 71–82.

Chih, Y. Y., & Zwikael, O. (2015). Project benefit management: A conceptual framework of target benefit formulation. *International Journal of Project Management, 33*(2), 352–362. doi:10.1016/j.ijproman.2014.06.002

Chugh, R., Sharma, S. C., & Cabrera, A. (2017). Lessons Learned from Enterprise Resource Planning (ERP) Implementations in an Australian Company. *International Journal of Enterprise Information Systems, 13*(3), 23–35. doi:10.4018/IJEIS.2017070102

Claxton, K., Paulden, M., Gravelle, H., Brouwer, W., & Culyer, A. J. (2011). Discounting & Decision Making in the Economic Evaluation of Health-Care Technologies. *Health Economics, 20*(1), 2–15. doi:10.1002/hec.1612 PMID:21154521

Clegg, C. W. (2000). Sociotechnical principles for system design. *Applied Ergonomics, 31*(5), 463–477. doi:10.1016/S0003-6870(00)00009-0 PMID:11059460

Coiera, E. (2003). *Guide to Health Informatics* (2nd ed.). Boca Raton, Florida, USA: CRC Press. doi:10.1201/b13618

Computer Economics. (2017) *IT Outsourcing Statistics: 2017/2018*, Computer Economics Inc., Irvine, CA, USA.

Coombs, C. R. (2015). When planned IS/IT project benefits are not realized: A study of inhibitors and facilitators to benefits realization. *International Journal of Project Management, 33*(2), 363–379. doi:10.1016/j.ijproman.2014.06.012

Cutler, M., & Sterne, J. (2000). *E-Metrics: Business Metrics for the New Economy*, NetGenesis, Source: [On-Line]: http://www.netgen.com/emetrics/

Danvers, K., & Nikolov, P. (2010). Does Outsourcing Affect Hospital Profitability? *Journal of Health Care Finance, 37*(1), 13–29. PMID:20973370

de Waal, B. M., & Batenburg, R. (2014). The process & structure of user participation: A BPM system implementation case study. *Business Process Management Journal, 20*(1), 107–128. doi:10.1108/BPMJ-05-2012-0045

Doherty, N. F. (2014). The Role of Socio-technical Principles in Leveraging Meaningful Benefits from IT Investments. *Applied Ergonomics, 45*(2), 181–187. doi:10.1016/j.apergo.2012.11.012 PMID:23305923

Doherty, N. F., Ashurst, C., & Peppard, J. (2012). Factors Affecting the Successful Realisation of Benefits from Systems Development Projects: Findings from Three Case Studies. *Journal of Information Technology, 27*(1), 1–16. doi:10.1057/jit.2011.8

Donovan, R. J., Boulter, J., Borland, B., Jalleh, G., & Carter, O. (2003). Continuous Tracking of the Australian National Tobacco Campaign: Advertising Effects on Recall, Recognition, Cognitions, & Behaviour. *Tobacco Control, 12*(Suppl. 2), ii30–ii39. doi:10.1136/tc.12.suppl_2.ii30 PMID:12878771

Donovan, R. J., Jalleh, G., Clarkson, J., & Giles-Corti, B. (1999). Evidence for effectiveness of sponsorship as a health promotion tool. *Australian Journal of Primary Health, 5*(3), 82–92.

Donovan, R. J., Jalleh, G., & Henley, N. (1996). Effective Road Safety Advertising: Symposium on mass media campaigns in road safety. In *Proceedings of the Public Health Association National Conference*, Perth, Australia.

Durugbo, C. (2012). Modelling User Participation in Organisations as Networks. *Expert Systems with Applications*, *39*(10), 9230–9245. doi:10.1016/j.eswa.2012.02.082

Dutot, V., Bergeron, F., & Raymond, L. (2014). Information management for the internationalization of SMEs: An exploratory study based on a strategic alignment perspective. *International Journal of Information Management*, *34*(5), 672–681. doi:10.1016/j.ijinfomgt.2014.06.006

Economo, K., Stewart, S., Sullivan, D., Jalleh, G., Carter, O., & Lin, C. (2010). The Importance of Public Education Campaigns in Raising Awareness & Support for Smoke-free Car Legislation in Western Australia. *Australian and New Zealand Journal of Public Health*, *34*(1), 92–93. doi:10.1111/j.1753-6405.2010.00483.x PMID:20920115

Eisenhardt, K. M. (1989). Building Theories From Case Study Research. *Academy of Management Review*, *14*(4), 532–550.

Elbeltagi, I., Hamad, H., Moizer, J., & Abou-Shouk, M. A. (2016). Levels of Business to Business E-Commerce Adoption and Competitive Advantage in Small and Medium-Sized Enterprises: A Comparison Study Between Egypt and the United States. *Journal of Global Information Technology Management*, *19*(1), 6–25. doi:10.1080/1097198X.2016.1134169

eMarketer. (2017). *Worldwide Retail and Ecommerce Sales: eMarketer's Estimates for 2016–2021.*

Ferdosi, M., Farahabadi, E., Mofid, M., Rejalian, F., Haghighat, M., & Naghdi, P. (2013). Evaluation of Outsourcing in Nursing Services: A Case Study of Kashani Hospital, Isfahan in 2011. *Materia Socio-Medica*, *25*(1), 37–39. doi:10.5455/msm.2013.25.37-39 PMID:23678338

Friedman, C. P., & Wyatt, J. C. (1997). *Evaluation Methods in Medical Informatics*. New York, USA: Springer-Verlag. doi:10.1007/978-1-4757-2685-5

Gantman, S., & Fedorowicz, J. (2016). Communication and control in outsourced IS development projects: Mapping to COBIT domains. *International Journal of Accounting Information Systems*, *21*, 63–83. doi:10.1016/j.accinf.2016.05.001

Giaglis, G. M., Paul, R. J., & Doukidis, G. I. (1999). Dynamic Modelling to Assess the Business Value of Electronic Commerce. *International Journal of Electronic Commerce*, *3*(3), 35–51. doi:10.1080/10864415.1999.11518340

Gorla, N., & Somers, T. M. (2014). The Impact of IT Outsourcing on Information Systems Success. *Information & Management*, *51*(3), 320–335. doi:10.1016/j.im.2013.12.002

Gorschek, T., Svahnberg, M., Borg, A., Loconsole, A., & Sandahl, K. (2007). A controlled empirical evaluation of a requirements abstraction model. *Information and Software Technology*, *49*(7), 790–805. doi:10.1016/j.infsof.2006.09.003

Hafeez, S., Hussain, S., Javed, Y., & Saeed, B. B. (2016). Influence of Benefits Realization Management on Business Strategies and Project Success in Pakistan's Construction Projects. *International Review of Management and Marketing, 6*(3).

Hahn, E. D., & Bunyaratavej, K. (2010). Services cultural alignment in offshoring: The impact of cultural dimensions on offshoring location choices. *Journal of Operations Management, 28*(3), 186–193. doi:10.1016/j.jom.2009.10.005

Han, J., & Lee, S. T. (2012). Impact of Vendor Selection on Firms' IT Outsourcing: The Korea Experience. *Journal of Global Information Management, 20*(2), 25–43. doi:10.4018/jgim.2012040102

He, J., & King, W. R. (2008). The role of user participation in information systems development: Implications from a meta-analysis. *Journal of Management Information Systems, 25*(1), 301–331. doi:10.2753/MIS0742-1222250111

Heeks, R. (1999). *Reinventing government in the information age: international practice in IT-enabled public sector reform*. London, New York: Routledge. doi:10.4324/9780203204962

Hellang, Ø., Flak, L. S., & Päivärinta, T. (2013). Diverging Approaches to Benefits Realization from Public ICT Investments: A Study of Benefits Realization Methods in Norway. *Transforming Government: People, Process & Policy, 7*(1), 93–108.

Heydon, N., Kennington, K. S., Jalleh, G., & Lin, C. (2012). Western Australian Smokers' Strongly Support Regulations on the Use of Chemicals and Additives in Cigarettes. *Tobacco Control, 21*(3), 381–382. doi:10.1136/tobaccocontrol-2011-050302 PMID:22170334

Hofstede, G. H. (1997). *Cultures & organizations: Software of the mind*. New York, NY: McGraw-Hill.

Hoque, M. R., & Boateng, R. (2017). Adoption of B2B e-Commerce in Developing Countries: Evidence from Ready Made Garment (RMG) Industry in Bangladesh, *Pacific Asia. Journal of the Association for Information Systems, 9*(1), 55–74.

Hsiao, C., Pai, J., & Chiu, H. (2009). The Study on the Outsourcing of Taiwan's Hospitals: A Questionnaire Survey Research. *BMC Health Services Research, 9*(1), 78. doi:10.1186/1472-6963-9-78 PMID:19435526

Hsu, J. S., Lin, T., Zheng, G., & Hung, Y. (2012). Users as knowledge co-producers in the information system development project. *International Journal of Project Management, 30*(1), 27–36. doi:10.1016/j.ijproman.2011.05.008

Huang, Y., Lin, C., Liu, Y., & Tung, M. (2013). The Effects of IT Resource Alignment and Organizational Dynamism on Alliance Performance in Hemodialysis Centers, *International Technology. Management Review, 3*(2), 105–115.

Huntley, H., & Blackmore, D. (2017, June 12). Market Share Analysis: IT Outsourcing Services, Worldwide, 2016 (*Gartner Report # G00322204*). Gartner Inc.

Jalleh, G., Donovan, R. J., Clarkson, J., March, K., Foster, M., & Giles-Corti, B. (2001). Increasing mouthguard usage among junior rugby and basketball players. *Australian and New Zealand Journal of Public Health, 25*(3), 250–252. doi:10.1111/j.1467-842X.2001.tb00571.x PMID:11494994

Jalleh, G., Donovan, R. J., Lin, C., & Slevin, T. (2008). Changing Perceptions of Solaria & Cancer Risk: The Role of the Media. *The Medical Journal of Australia, 188*(12), 735–735. PMID:18558905

Jalleh, G., Donovan, R. J., Lin, C., Slevin, T., Clayforth, C., Pratt, S., & Ledger, M. (2010). Beliefs about Bowel Cancer among the Target Group for the National Bowel Cancer Screening Program in Australia. *Australian and New Zealand Journal of Public Health, 34*(2), 187–192. doi:10.1111/j.1753-6405.2010.00505.x PMID:23331364

Johnson, N., Murphy, A., McNeese, N., Reddy, M., & Purao, S. (2013). A Survey of Rural Hospitals' Perspectives on Health Information Technology Outsourcing. In *Proceedings of the AMIA Annual Symposium* (pp. 732-741).

Johnson, R., Jalleh, G., Pratt, I. S., Donovan, R. J., Lin, C., Saunders, C., & Slevin, T. (2013). Online advertising by three commercial breast imaging services: Message takeout and effectiveness. *The Breast, 22*(5), 780–786. doi:10.1016/j.breast.2013.01.013 PMID:23422256

Kahouei, M., Farrokhi, M., Abadi, Z. N., & Karimi, A. (2016). Concerns and hopes about outsourcing decisions regarding health information management services at two teaching hospitals in Semnan, Iran. *The HIM Journal, 45*(1), 36–44. doi:10.1177/1833358316639455 PMID:28691564

Karimi, S., Agharahimi, Z., & Yaghoubi, M. (2012). Impacts of Outsourcing in Educational Hospitals in Iran: A Study on Isfahan University of Medical Sciences-2010. *Journal of Education and Health Promotion, 1*(1), 25. doi:10.4103/2277-9531.99959 PMID:23555128

Karthik, V., & Kumar, S. (2013). Investigating 'Degree of Adoption' Effects on e–procurement Benefits. *International Journal of Procurement Management, 6*(2), 211–234. doi:10.1504/IJPM.2013.052470

Keeys, L. A., & Huemann, M. (2017). Project benefits co-creation: Shaping sustainable development benefits. *International Journal of Project Management, 35*(6), 1196–1212. doi:10.1016/j.ijproman.2017.02.008

Khalil, O. E. M., & Elkordy, M. M. (2005). EIS Information: Use & Quality Determination. *Information Resources Management Journal, 18*(2), 68–93. doi:10.4018/irmj.2005040104

Kocher, M. G., & Sutter, M. (2006). Time is Money: Time Pressure, Incentives, & the Quality of Decision Making. *Journal of Economic Behavior & Organization, 61*(3), 375–392. doi:10.1016/j.jebo.2004.11.013

Kuhn, K. A., Giuse, D. A., & Talmon, J. L. (2003). The Heidelberg Conference: Setting an Agenda for the IMIA Working Group on Health Information Systems. *International Journal of Medical Informatics, 69*(2–3), 77–82. doi:10.1016/S1386-5056(02)00097-7 PMID:12810112

Kuo, W., Lin, C., Hsu, G., & Huang, Y. (2006). An Empirical Study of Resource Contribution in SMEs Alliance. *Journal of Global Business Management, 2*(2), 103–111.

Kurnia, S., Choudrie, J., Mahbubur, R. M., & Alzougool, B. (2015). E-commerce technology adoption: A Malaysian grocery SME retail sector study. *Journal of Business Research, 68*(9), 1906–1918. doi:10.1016/j.jbusres.2014.12.010

Land, F. (1987). Adapting to Changing User Requirements. In R. D. Galliers (Ed.), *Information Analysis: Selected Readings*. Sydney: Addison - Wesley.

Lawrence, C., & Firth, D. (2013). Improving Healthcare Administration: Real Time Locations Systems or Outsourcing? *Information Systems Education Journal, 11*(5), 49.

Lee, J. (2017). Strategic risk analysis for information technology outsourcing in hospitals. *Information & Management*. doi:10.1016/j.im.2017.02.010

Lee, J., & Runge, J. (2001). Adoption of Information Technology in Small Business: Testing Drivers of Adoption for Entrepreneurs. *Journal of Computer Information Systems, 42*(1), 44–57.

Lee, K. S., Lim, G. H., & Tan, S. J. (1999). Dealing with Resource Disadvantage: Generic Strategies for SMEs. *Small Business Economics, 12*(4), 299–311. doi:10.1023/A:1008085310245

Lee, S., & Kim, K.-J. (2007). Factors affecting the implementation success of Internet-based information systems. *Computers in Human Behavior, 23*(4), 1853–1880. doi:10.1016/j.chb.2005.12.001

Li, J. J. (2012). The alignment between organizational control mechanisms & outsourcing strategies: A commentary essay. *Journal of Business Research, 65*(9), 1384–1386. doi:10.1016/j.jbusres.2011.09.020

Licht, A. N. (2004). Legal plug-Ins: Cultural distance, cross-listing, & corporate governance reform. *Berkeley Journal of International Law, 22*, 195–239.

Lin, C. (2002) *An Investigation of the Process of IS/IT Investment Evaluation & Benefits Realisation in Large Australian Organisations* [PhD Thesis]. Curtin University of Technology, Western Australia. Retrieved from http://adt.curtin.edu.au/theses/available/adt-WCU20030826.094151/

Lin, C., & Huang, Y. (2007). An Integrated Framework for Managing eCRM Evaluation Process. *International Journal of Electronic Business, 5*(4), 340–359. doi:10.1504/IJEB.2007.014782

Lin, C., Huang, Y., & Cheng, M. (2007). The Adoption of IS/IT Investment Evaluation and Benefits Realization Methodologies in Service Organizations: IT Maturity Paths and Framework. *Contemporary Management Research, 3*(2), 173–194. doi:10.7903/cmr.88

Lin, C., Huang, Y., Cheng, M., & Lin, W. (2007). Effects of Information Technology Maturity on the Adoption of Investment Evaluation Methodologies: A Survey of Large Australian Organizations. *International Journal of Management, 24*(4), 697–711.

Lin, C., Lin, H. K., Huang, Y., Jalleh, G., Liu, Y. C., Huang, Yueh-Hsia, Su, S., & Chao, C. (2014) Towards a B2B E-Commerce Evaluation Management Model to Assess Organizational Drivers in Hospitals, *International Technology Management Review, 4*(3), 115-132.

Lin, C., & Lin, K. (2011). A Study of Information Requirement Determination Process of an Executive Information System. In Enterprise Information Systems: Concepts, Methodologies, Tools & Applications (pp. 1030-1038). Hershey, PA: IGI Global.

Lin, C., Lin, K., Huang, Y., & Jalleh, G. (2011). The Fit Between Organizational B2B E-commerce Policy, IT Maturity and Evaluation Practices on B2B E-commerce Performance in Australian Healthcare Organizations. *African Journal of Business Management, 5*(5), 1983–2005.

Lin, C., & Pervan, G. (2000) Realising the Benefits of IS/IT Investments in Australian Organisations. In *Proceedings of the Eleventh Australasian Conference on Information Systems (ACIS 2000)*, Brisbane, Australia, December 6-8.

Lin, C., Pervan, G., Lin, K., & Tsao, H. (2008). An Investigation into Business-to-Business Electronic Commerce Organizations. *Journal of Research and Practice in Information Technology*, *40*(1), 3–18.

Lin, C., Pervan, G., & McDermid, D. (2002). Research on IS/IT Investment Evaluation & Benefits Realization in Australia. In W. Van Grembergen (Ed.), *Information Systems Evaluation Management* (pp. 244–254). Hershey, PA: IGI Global. doi:10.4018/978-1-931777-18-6.ch015

Liu, Y., Huang, Y., & Lin, C. (2012). Organizational Factors' Effects on The Success of E-Learning System & Organizational Benefits - An Empirical Study in Taiwan. *International Review of Research in Open and Distance Learning*, *13*(4), 130–151. doi:10.19173/irrodl.v13i4.1203

Liu, Y., & Lin, C. (2008). How are public sector organizations assessing their it investments & benefits - an understanding of issues for benchmarking. *International Journal of Advanced Information Technologies*, *2*(2), 86–100.

Love, P. E. D., Irani, Z., Standing, C., Lin, C., & Burn, J. (2005). The Enigma of Evaluation: Benefits, Costs & Risks of IT in Small-Medium Sized Enterprises. *Information & Management*, *42*(7), 947–964. doi:10.1016/j.im.2004.10.004

Low, C., & Chen, Y. H. (2012). Criteria for the Evaluation of a Cloud-based Hospital Information System Outsourcing Provider. *Journal of Medical Systems*, *36*(6), 3543–3553. doi:10.100710916-012-9829-z PMID:22366976

Marnewick, C. (2016). Benefits of information system projects: The tale of two countries. *International Journal of Project Management*, *34*(4), 748–760. doi:10.1016/j.ijproman.2015.03.016

Marnewick, C. (2017). The reality of adherence to best practices for information system initiatives. *International Journal of Managing Projects in Business*, *10*(1), 167–184. doi:10.1108/IJMPB-05-2016-0045

McGaughey, R. E. (2002). Benchmarking Business-to-business Electronic Commerce, *Benchmarking*. *International Journal (Toronto, Ont.)*, *9*(5), 471–484.

McIvor, R. (2000). A practical framework for understanding the outsourcing process. *Supply Chain Management*, *5*(1), 22–36. doi:10.1108/13598540010312945

McKay, J., & Marshall, P. (2004). Strategic Management of eBusiness. Australia, Queensland: John Wiley & Sons.

Melville, N., Kraemer, K., & Gurbaxani, V. (2004). Review: Information Technology & Organizational Performance: An integrative Model of IT Business Value. *Management Information Systems Quarterly*, *28*(2), 283–322.

Menachemi, N., Burke, D., & Diana, M. (2007). Characteristics of Hospitals that Outsource Information. System Functions. *Journal of Healthcare Information Management*, *19*(1), 63–69. PMID:15682678

Miles, M. B., & Huberman, A. M. (1994). *Qualitative Data Analysis: An Expanded Sourcebook*. California: Sage Publications.

Misra, R. B. (2004). Global IT Outsourcing: Metrics for Success of All Parties. *Journal of Information Technology Cases & Applications*, 6(3), 21–34. doi:10.1080/15228053.2004.10856047

Mitra, S., Sambamurthy, V., & Westerman, G. (2011). Measuring IT Performance & Communicating Value. *MIS Quarterly Executive*, 10(1), 47–59.

Moon, J., Choe, Y. C., Chung, M., Jung, G. H., & Swar, B. (2016). IT outsourcing success in the public sector: Lessons from e-government practices in Korea. *Information Development*, 32(2), 142–160. doi:10.1177/0266666914528930

Mudambi, S. M., & Tallman, S. (2010). Make, buy or ally? Theoretical perspectives on knowledge process outsourcing through alliances. *Journal of Management Studies*, 47(8), 1434–1456. doi:10.1111/j.1467-6486.2010.00944.x

Norton, A. L., Coulson-Thomas, Y. M., Coulson-Thomas, C. J., & Ashurst, C. (2013). Ensuring Benefits Realisation from ERP II: The CSF Phasing Model. *Journal of Enterprise Information Management*, 26(3), 218–234. doi:10.1108/17410391311325207

Ondo, K., & Smith, M. (2006). Outside IT the Case for Full IT Outsourcing: Study Findings Indicate Many Hospitals Are Turning to Full IT Outsourcing to Achieve IT Excellence. What's the Best Approach for Your Organization? *Healthcare Financial Management*, (February).

Osmonbekov, T., Zhang, Y. G., & Dang, Y. M. (2016). Investigating essential factors of reseller perceived inequity and reseller performance in e-business. *Journal of Electronic Commerce Research*, 17(3), 205.

Ozkan, S., Baykal, N., & Sincan, M. (2012). *Process-Based Evaluation of Hospital Information Systems: Application of an Information System Success Model (PRISE) in the Healthcare Domain. In Health Information Systems: Concepts, Methodologies, Tools, and Applications* (pp. 339–355). Hershey, PA: IGI Global.

Patil, S., & Wongsurawat, W. (2015). Information technology (IT) outsourcing by business process outsourcing/information technology enabled services (BPO/ITES) firms in India: A strategic gamble. *Journal of Enterprise Information Management*, 28(1), 60–76. doi:10.1108/JEIM-09-2013-0068

Paul, S., & Nazareth, D. L. (2010). Input information complexity, perceived time pressure, & information processing in GSS-based work groups: An experimental investigation using a decision schema to alleviate information overload conditions. *Decision Support Systems*, 49(1), 31–40. doi:10.1016/j.dss.2009.12.007

Peute, L. W., Aarts, J., Bakker, P. J., & Jaspers, M. W. (2010). Anatomy of a failure: A sociotechnical evaluation of a laboratory physician order entry system implementation. *International Journal of Medical Informatics*, 79(4), e58–e70. doi:10.1016/j.ijmedinf.2009.06.008 PMID:19640778

Ragu-Nathana, B. S., Apigian, C. H., Ragu-Nathana, T. S., & Tu, Q. (2004). A path analytic study of the effect of top management support for information systems performance. *Omega*, 32(6), 459–471. doi:10.1016/j.omega.2004.03.001

Rahim, M. M., Kurnia, S., Samson, D., & Singh, P. (2014). Developing an IT Maturity Model for Sustainable Supply Chain Management Implementation. In *Proceedings of the 18th Pacific Asia Conference on Information Systems (PACIS 2014)*, Chengdu, China.

Raisinghani, M. S., Melemez, T., Zhou, L., Paslowski, C., Kikvidze, I., Taha, S., & Simons, K. (2005). E-Business Models in B2B: Process Based Categorization & Analysis of B2B Models. *International Journal of E-Business Research*, *1*(1), 16–36. doi:10.4018/jebr.2005010102

Ralston, D. A., Holt, D. H., Terpstra, R. H., & Kai-Cheng, Y. (2008). The impact of national culture & economic ideology on managerial work values: A study of the United States, Russia, Japan, & China. *Journal of International Business Studies*, *39*(1), 8–26. doi:10.1057/palgrave.jibs.8400330

Remenyi, D., & Whittaker, L. (1996). The Evaluation of Business Process Re-engineering Projects. In L. Willcocks (Ed.), *Investing in information systems: evaluation & management* (Ch. 7, pp. 143–167). UK: Chapman & Hall.

Rissler, A. (1994). Extended periods of challenging demands in high tech work. Consequences for efficiency, quality of life & health. In G. E. Bradley & H. W. Hendrick (Eds.), *Human factors in organizational design & management* (pp. 727–732). Amsterdam: Elsevier.

Sadoughi, F., & Aminpour, F. (2011). A Review on the Evaluation Methods of Health Information Systems. *Indian Journal of Medical Education*, *10*(5), 1077–1086.

Samantra, C., Datta, S., & Mahapatra, S. S. (2014). Risk Assessment in IT Outsourcing using Fuzzy Decision-making Approach: An Indian Perspective. *Expert Systems with Applications*, *41*(8), 4010–4022. doi:10.1016/j.eswa.2013.12.024

Saorín-Iborra, M. C., Redondo-Cano, A., Revuelto-Taboada, L., & Vogler, É. (2015). Negotiating behavior in service outsourcing. An exploratory case study analysis. *Service Business*. doi:10.100711628-014-0259-5

Schick, A. G., Gordon, L. A., & Haka, S. (1990). Information overload: A temporal approach. *Accounting, Organizations and Society*, *15*(3), 199–220. doi:10.1016/0361-3682(90)90005-F

Schultze, U., & Vandenbosch, B. (1998). Information overload in a groupware environment: Now you see it, now you don't. *Journal of Organizational Computing and Electronic Commerce*, *8*(2), 127–148. doi:10.120715327744joce0802_3

Serra, C. E. M., & Kunc, M. (2015). Benefits realisation management and its influence on project success and on the execution of business strategies. *International Journal of Project Management*, *33*(1), 53–66. doi:10.1016/j.ijproman.2014.03.011

Shani, A. B., & Sena, J. A. (1994). Information technology & the integration of change: Sociotechnical system approach. *The Journal of Applied Behavioral Science*, *30*(2), 247–261. doi:10.1177/0021886394302007

Shuraida, S., & Barki, H. (2013). The Influence of Analyst Communication in IS Projects. *Journal of the Association for Information Systems*, *14*(9), 482–520.

Standing, C., & Lin, C. (2007). Organizational Evaluation of the Benefits, Constraints & Satisfaction with Business-To-Business Electronic Commerce. *International Journal of Electronic Commerce*, *11*(3), 107–153. doi:10.2753/JEC1086-4415110304

Stockdale, R., Lin, C., & Stoney, S. (2005). The Effectiveness of SME Websites in a Business To Business Context. In *Proceedings of the IADIS International Conference E-Commerce 2005*, Porto, Portugal, December 15 - 17 (pp. 259-266).

Stratopoulos, T., & Dehning, B. (2000). Does Successful Investments in Information Technology Solve the Productivity Paradox? *Information & Management*, *38*(2), 103–117. doi:10.1016/S0378-7206(00)00058-6

Stringham, B. B., & Gerdes, J. Jr. (2010). An Analysis of Word-of-Mouse Ratings & Guest Comments of Online Hotel Distribution Sites. *Journal of Hospitality Marketing & Management*, *19*(7), 773–796. doi:10.1080/19368623.2010.508009

Sugumaran, V., & Arogyaswamy, B. (2004). Measuring IT Performance: "Contingency" Variables & Value Modes. *Journal of Computer Information Systems*, *44*(2), 79–86.

Sujata, T. L., Reddy, B. K., & Jayalakshmi, C. (2013). Hospitals Outsourcing Complete Departments: A Study. *International Journal of Research in Commerce & Management*, *4*(9), 1–4.

Syrek, C. J., Apostel, E., & Antoni, C. H. (2013). Stress in Highly Demanding IT Jobs: Transformational Leadership Moderates the Impact of Time Pressure on Exhaustion & Work–life Balance. *Journal of Occupational Health Psychology*, *18*(3), 252–261. doi:10.1037/a0033085 PMID:23834443

Tallon, P. P., Kraemer, K. L., & Gurbaxani, V. (2000). Executives' Perceptions of the Business Value of Information Technology: A Process-Oriented Approach. *Journal of Management Information Systems*, *16*(4), 145–173. doi:10.1080/07421222.2000.11518269

Tan, J., & Ludwig, S. (2016). Regional Adoption of Business-to-Business Electronic Commerce in China: Role of E-Readiness. *International Journal of Electronic Commerce*, *20*(3), 408–439. doi:10.1080/10864415.2016.1122438

Terlizzi, M. A., Albertin, A. L., & de Moraes, H. R. O. C. (2017). IT benefits management in financial institutions: Practices and barriers. *International Journal of Project Management*, *35*(5), 763–782. doi:10.1016/j.ijproman.2017.03.006

Thatcher, M. D., & Pingry, D. E. (2004). Understanding the Business Value of Information Technology Investments: Theoretical Evidence from Alternative Market & Cost Structure. *Journal of Management Information Systems*, *21*(2), 61–85. doi:10.1080/07421222.2004.11045804

Thomas, R. W., Fugate, B. S., & Koukova, N. T. (2011). Coping with Time Pressure & Knowledge Sharing in Buyer-Supplier Relationships. *The Journal of Supply Chain Management*, *47*(3), 22–42. doi:10.1111/j.1745-493X.2011.03229.x

THRF. (2011). *Hospital Finance: The Financial Supervision for the Health Institutions in Taiwan*. Taipei, Taiwan: Taiwan Healthcare Reform Foundation.

Torkzadeh, G., & Dhillon, G. (2002). Measuring Factors that Influence the Success of Internet Commerce. *Information Systems Research*, *13*(2), 187–204. doi:10.1287/isre.13.2.187.87

Torres, A. R. (2007). The hot potato game: Roles and responsibilities for realizing IT project benefits. *The Journal of Modern Project Management, 5*(2).

Trist, E. H., Murray, B. J., & Pollack, A. (1963). *Organizational Choice*. London: Tavistock.

Tsao, H., Lin, K., & Lin, C. (2004). An Investigation of Critical Success Factors in the Adoption of B2BEC by Taiwanese Companies. *The Journal of American Academy of Business, Cambridge, 5*(1/2), 198–202.

Turner, R., & Ledwith, A. (2016). Project Management in Small to Medium-Sized Enterprises: Fitting the Practices to the Needs of the Firm to Deliver Benefit. *Journal of Small Business Management*. doi:10.1111/jsbm.12265

Urquhart, C. (2001). Analysts & Clients in Organizational Context: A Conversational Perspective. *The Journal of Strategic Information Systems, 10*(3), 243–262. doi:10.1016/S0963-8687(01)00046-4

Walston, S. L., Bennett, C. J., & Al-Harbi, A. (2014). Understanding the Factors Affecting Employees' Perceived Benefits of Healthcare Information Technology. *International Journal of Healthcare Management, 7*(1), 35–44. doi:10.1179/2047971913Y.0000000051

Ward, J., & Griffiths, P. (1996). *Strategic Planning For Information Systems*. Chichester, UK: John Wiley & Sons Ltd.

Wiener, M., Remus, U., Heumann, J., & Mähring, M. (2015). The effective promotion of informal control in information systems offshoring projects. *European Journal of Information Systems, 24*(6), 569–587. doi:10.1057/ejis.2014.16

Wu, I., & Shen, Y. (2006). A Model for Exploring the Impact of Purchasing Strategies on User Requirements determination of e-SRM. *Information & Management, 43*(4), 411–422. doi:10.1016/j.im.2004.11.004

Yayla, A. A., & Hu, Q. (2012). The impact of IT-business strategic alignment on firm performance in a developing country setting: Exploring moderating roles of environmental uncertainty & strategic orientation. *European Journal of Information Systems, 21*(4), 373–387. doi:10.1057/ejis.2011.52

Yeh, C. H., Lee, G. G., & Pai, J. C. (2015). Using a technology-organization-environment framework to investigate the factors influencing e-business information technology capabilities. *Information Development, 31*(5), 435–450. doi:10.1177/0266666913516027

Yin, R. K. (2002). *Case Study Research, Design & Methods* (3rd ed.). Newbury Park: Sage Publications.

Young, R., & Jordan, E. (2008). Top management support: Mantra or necessity. *International Journal of Project Management, 26*(7), 713–725. doi:10.1016/j.ijproman.2008.06.001

Yu, P. (2010). A multi-method approach to evaluate health information systems. In *Proceedings of the World Congress on Medical Informatics* (pp. 1231-1235). Amsterdam: IOS Press.

Yusof, M. M., Papazafeiropoulou, A., Paul, R. J., & Stergioulas, L. K. (2008). Investigating Evaluation Frameworks for Health Information Systems. *International Journal of Medical Informatics, 77*(6), 377–385. doi:10.1016/j.ijmedinf.2007.08.004 PMID:17904898

Zeng, Y. E., Wen, H. J., & Yen, D. C. (2003). Customer Relationship Management (CRM) in Business-to-business (B2B) E-commerce. *Information Management & Computer Security*, *11*(1), 39–44. doi:10.1108/09685220310463722

Zhuang, Y. (2005). Does Electronic Business Create Value For Firms? An Organizational Innovation Perspective. *Journal of Electronic Commerce Research*, *6*(2), 146–159.

Zika-Viktorsson, A., Sundstrom, P., & Engwall, M. (2006). Project overload: An exploratory study of work & management in multi-project settings. *International Journal of Project Management*, *24*(5), 385–394. doi:10.1016/j.ijproman.2006.02.010

This research was previously published in the International Journal of Public Health Management and Ethics (IJPHME), 2(1); edited by Qiang (Shawn) Cheng; pages 69-90, copyright year 2017 by IGI Publishing (an imprint of IGI Global).

Chapter 24

Operations Project and Management in Trauma Centers:
The Case of Brazilian Units

Thais Spiegel
Rio de Janeiro State University, Brazil

Daniel Bouzon Nagem Assad
Rio de Janeiro State University, Brazil

ABSTRACT

Topic of discussions over the last decades, the literature related to the care of patients suffering from poly-trauma, under the assistance point of view, is sufficiently consolidated concerning to the adoption of best practices, what, usually are conducted and disseminated by accrediting organizations. However, expanding the search frontier beyond the assistance dimension, it's noticed the divergences between the recent researches or theoretical shortcomings regarding to the design and management of these operations. In face of this finding, noticed from a literature review in the most important bases of operations management and health, it's adopted a conceptual model which covers relevant elements of the project of an operation, such as: strategy, capacity, human resources, incentive systems, organizational structure and decision making; in order to systematize the current stage of the field, highlighting the differences between recent studies and proposing a set of practices and premises, which are necessary for the operationalization of the proposed model.

INTRODUCTION

Topic of discussions over the last decades, the literature related to the care of patients suffering from poly-trauma, under the assistance point of view, is sufficiently consolidated concerning to the adoption of best practices, what, usually are conducted and disseminated by accrediting organizations (for

DOI: 10.4018/978-1-7998-2451-0.ch024

Copyright © 2020, IGI Global. Copying or distributing in print or electronic forms without written permission of IGI Global is prohibited.

example, ACS). However, expanding the search frontier beyond the assistance dimension, it's noticed the divergences between the recent researches or theoretical shortcomings regarding to the design and management of these operations.

In face of this finding, noticed from a literature revision in the most important bases of operations management and health, it's adopted a conceptual model which covers relevant elements of the project of an operation, such as: strategy, capacity, human resources, incentive systems, organizational structure and decision making; in order to systematize the current stage of the field, highlighting the differences between recent studies and proposing a set of practices and premises, which are necessary for the operationalization of the proposed model.

BACKGROUND

The origin of the word" trauma" comes from the Greek trauma (plural: traumathos, traumas) whose significant is "wound". In medicine, the word accepts different meanings, all of them linked to unforeseen and undesirable events, which, in a more or less violent way, affect individuals involved therein, causing them any kind of lesion or damage (SBAIT, 2015). It has an agent (energy), a vector (i.e. fire gun, motor vehicle, etc.) and a host (patient). As a disease, it must be approached by prevention strategies, an early diagnosis, an appropriated treatment and rehabilitation, targeting the reduction of the related morbidity and mortality (ACS, 2014a).

Figure 1. Incidence of deaths due to traffic accidents
Source: DataSUS (2014).

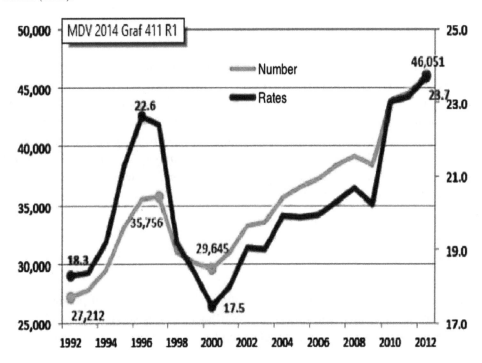

In Brazil, from the 80s on, it constitutes one of the most important points of the epidemiological transition (Azevedo, 2010: 25). Despite being a disease that traditionally focuses on the younger population, the rate of death by trauma and the estimated recovery time increases with age. This generates a significant increase in the use of resources for these older patients (Beilman et al., 2004), and which must be managed in the allocation of resources in a trauma unit. Neto & Malik (2011) reinforce the issue of the demand and argue that each patient behaves in a certain way, hindering the rigid standardization of the work process and a rationalization of service delivery.

Enhancing the criticality of this type of operation, the first hour after the accident is said as critical to perform the rescue, patient referral and design of treatment that will be applied and that's why it's considered "The Gold Hour". The initial treatment done in an appropriate way and in timely can significantly improve the prognosis of severe trauma.

According to Brohi, Parr & Coats (2009), understand the incidence of the trauma and specially the major trauma in the region, is critical for the design and development of the systems. Generally, according to the same author, there is no strong population data that support the design of this kind of system. In the Brazilian case, researches performed by the DataSUS show in Figure 1 in an aggregated way, the relationship between the number and the death rate due to traffic accidents, which may be the start point for the development of this system.

THE RESEARCH

This text present results of a research project about the Organizational Solutions of treatment to the polytrauma patients in public hospitals in Brazil. Embrace their projects, their ways of management, resource allocation and the key processes and protocols adopted. The Figure 2 show the research method adopted.

Contextualization: The Trauma Hospital Type 3 in Brazil

According to the Ordinance 1.366 (2013), the trauma Hospitals or Centers play the role of specialized reference for the care of the patients who are victims of trauma and must have as a target the improvement

Figure 2. Research method
Source: Authors.

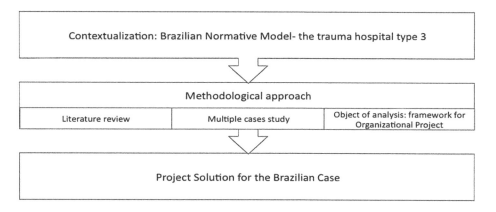

of these patients' care besides universalization and standardization of a service model in all its stages in order to reduce mortality and sequels of trauma patients. Therefore, the same ordinance defines the minimum requirements in terms of human resources, facilities and equipment, left to the discretion of each County, State and Council of the involved professional classes (CRM and CONFEN) the establishment of the necessary standards and contingents.

Regarding the division by specialties for the treatment of trauma patients, the same Ordinance stablishes three types of Trauma Center, whose physical distribution; complexity and variety of the offered treatments are defined from the size of the population that should be treated.

In case the referred specialty is not available 24 hours a day in the hospital, it must be activated by it. Yet, in this Ordinance, it's not specified, for example, the waiting reference time for the arrival of the specialist at the hospital; neither the Number of beds by type or size of the Trauma Centers.

Methodological Approach

The research methods are the basis for the creation of knowledge, being the tools that lend themselves to understand the reality (Pinsonneault & Kraemer, 1993). To investigate how the Health Units design and manage their trauma centers, it was adopted an exploratory methodology (Jonsen & Jehn, 2011), aiming to obtain descriptive information of these organizations' practices; and that there is little recent literature devoted to discussion of the design and management of trauma centers.

On the other hand, there is a vast literature approaching the welfare aspects of this type of unit. What it at stake is exactly the development of a theoretical and conceptual perspective, empirically effective (MASON, 2006) to guide the designers and the decision makers when they have to face the demands of this kind of Health Unit's reality.

To get an insight of how the different characteristics of the models of management of trauma centers interact and interrelate with their organizational project's development and about the approach and parameters effectively used by the Health Units, it was adopted as a methodological approach the Multiple Cases Study (Yin, 2005; Eisenhardt, 1989), in the context of a comprehensive systematic review of the literature (Van Aken et al., 2007) on the basis: Science Direct, PubMed e ISI Web of Science.

Object of Analysis: Organizational Solution

Bensabat et al. (1987) highlight the relevance of the definition of the analysis unit that is most appropriated for the study. Different analysis units imply in distinct ways to gather data and which results and conclusions might be withdrawn from the research (Patton, 2002), namely, the definition of what is waited to be said at the end of the study.

The Organizational Structure defines the units that an organization will have and the relationship among them. It has several degrees of aggregation: from the organization as a whole up to the position filled by the individuals/employees (Baligh, 2005); and define the lines of authority and responsibility of an organization (Burton et al., 2008). This means power to allocate resources, to increase or reduce the staff, to define the directions and/or strategies of the organization (Burlton, 2010). These formal structures are complemented by a myriad of arrangements, which help the everyday conduct of organizations, such as commissions, committees, communities of practice, organizational processes (Markus & Jacobson, 2010).

During the research, it's adopted the model Star of Galbraith et al. (2003).

Figure 3. Star mode
Source: Galbraith et al. (2003).

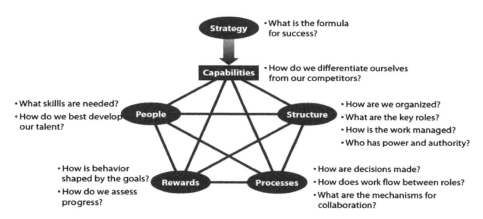

Research Protocol

To YIN (2005), the protocol is much more than just an information-gathering tool; it has not only the tool, but also the procedures and the general rules that must be followed. The author highlights that is essential to have a protocol in the case of a conduction of multiple cases' studies.

The content of this tool must include a general vision of the cases' study design (Mason, 2006), the field procedures, the issues of the research that the work aims to answer and a guide for the preparation of the case study report (Yin, 2005).

The research protocol considers a set of issues to be worked with the stakeholders of companies and guide the collection of documents and evidence.

Research Sample

In terms of the chosen cases, the focus of research is in the public units that currently take care the multiple trauma patients in a state in Brazil. To make the overall sample of the entire project research the following starting criteria were used: guided by the Ordinance 1.366 (2013), therefore, inserted in the no SUS/Brazil; number of beds offered to the patient victim of polytrauma; number of operating rooms dedicated to the care of the patient victim of polytrauma; number of professionals, by specialty allocated to the care of patients of polytrauma (ideal team); Promotion or monitoring of the patient in the rehabilitation phase.

Two State General Hospitals, reference in trauma, with 'open doors' units, were studied. Additionally, although it is a 'closed door' unit, the practices of the Federal Institute of Trauma Reference, were also analyzed. The three units are inserted in that State. Table 1 provides a summary of the cases.

Table 1. Summary of the visited units with reference in trauma

	State Hospital 1	State Hospital 2	Federal Institute
Education and research (residence)	Yes	No	Yes. Also offers Masters programs and has partnerships with some universities
Beds of ICU	8 dedicated	35 (shared)	48 (shared)
Operating Rooms	7 (being1 exclusively dedicated to trauma emergency)	3 for trauma and 4 in the Surgery Center	21
Time spent in the Trauma Center	4 hours	1:30 hours	Not applicable
Problems with the blood supply	Yes	No	There is, but it's not very serious, since they have their own blood bank and the collect is done at the very Institute.
Health professionals contracting model	"CLT", outsourced	"CLT", outsourced	Gazetted of the Ministry of Health
Remuneration (R$)	R$ 8.500,00 per 24 hours/week	*Information not available*	R$ 3.500,00 per 20 hours/week
Care (patient per month)	1.000	335	834
In-hospital rehabilitation	Yes	Yes	Yes
Ideal team to serve the greater trauma	3 surgeons 3 anesthetists 4 nurses 4 nursing technicians	2 surgeons 1 anesthetists 1 nurse 1 nursing technician	*Information not available*
Access to the Hospital	Own means and regulated by the centrals State regulation	Own means and regulated by the centrals State regulation	Regulated by the centrals State or Federal regulation

Source: Authors.

SOLUTIONS AND RECOMMENDATIONS

Facing the object of analysis of this research, in this section, there will be presented under the optical of its five dimensions: the points not yet established in the literature, the points for which the literature is already established and the points for which the present document launches proposals in order to have a continuous improvement.

Strategy: Training

A system of trauma care consists of an organized approach to facilitate and coordinate an answer from the multidisciplinary system to take care of those who have been serious injured (HRSA, 2006). The Trauma Center, serving as installation of definitive specialized care, is key component and differs from the other hospital units of the system insofar as it ensures the availability of all necessary specialties for the evaluation and handle of the patient with multiple lesions. These centers must be integrated with the other components of the system to allow the best use of the resources according to the patients' necessity. The coordinated care system involves all the facilities' levels, so the rapid and efficient integration of hospital resources may occur according to the needs of the patient (Boffard, 2003).

Figure 4. Typical inputs and outputs of a trauma center
Source: Demetriades & Asensio (2000:4).

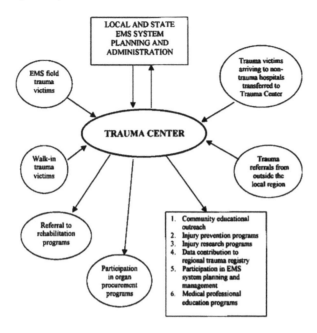

In order to enable the operation of this coordinated system as proposed above, the resource management strategy must reflect the relationship between the resources demand and its supply. Depending on the availability of these resources (abundant or scarce), different strategies of allocation might be adopted, such as, cancel one or more elective surgeries to meet a peak of demand (accident with multiple victims) or creating tools to solve the systemic deficiencies of significant resources (Christian et al., 2009).

Deriving from the possibility of the imbalance between supply and demand inherent to the nature of the transaction, it's possible that the professionals from this kind of organization face a scenery of limited resources, and for these cases, the doctors will be required to decide the best way of deal with a potential of saving lives. It makes a difference the complexity involved in this decision and its orientation according to an ethical sight, there are common ways to share scarce resources, considering as main factors, the patient's condition and the result potential of the medical care medico (Christian et al., 2009).

In conditions of operation for which the care demand doesn't exceed the offer, the objectives of a trauma care system are (HRSA, 2006):

- Reduce the incidence and severity of the traumas;
- Assure equitable and accessible care for all persons with trauma;
- Avoid unnecessary deaths and disability resulting from trauma
- Contain costs and improve efficiency;
- Implement the improvement of quality and performance of the trauma care at the whole system;
- Assure that the designated facilities have the appropriate resources to meet the injured' needs

Figure 5. Organizational solution for the trauma unit
Source: From Hyer et al. (2009)'s Description.

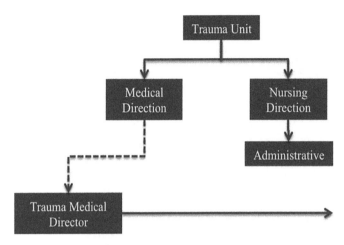

Structure

Under the organizational perspective, the literature supports that a focused Trauma Unit is an administrative one inside a bigger organization, where the resources are allocated, and seen as a planning and controlling point and accountable for performance and improvement (Hyer et al., 2009).

Organizationally, the Trauma Unit tends to be a dominant part, multi-functional, since it encompasses a range of activities such as, for instance, the pain management, small surgeries, some laboratory tests, several therapies, case management, patient safety, among others. The care with the critical trauma patients also includes the burn unit and the unit of neurosciences (ACS, 2014a; Hyer et al., 2009).

In some configurations, as Figure 5, the Director of Trauma provides the care to the patients, while the Trauma Unit itself is managed by an administrative director ("subordinated" to the Nursing Direction) and a medical director (trauma surgeon) (Hyer et al., 2009).

In other configurations, the trauma's medical Director and the coordination of the trauma's program provide the care to the Trauma Center's patients, as Figure 6.

In another configuration, as Figure 7, in units with resources dedicated to trauma, there is:

In the reference manuals, it's highlighted that the trauma service must be dedicated and previously idealized according to the organizational structure of the hospital, taking into consideration some aspects, such as:

- A Medical Director, hired to run and supervise the operation of the trauma service;
- A manager of the trauma program (usually, nursing coordination), specifically designed for trauma service;
- At least one surgeon qualified in trauma (ATLS, etc.) and be a part of the primary trauma care, in all moments;
- At least one surgeon qualified in trauma ready to provide backup in all moments of the trauma service;
- At least one surgeon qualified in pediatric trauma for the trauma service;

Figure 6. Organizational solution for the trauma unit
Source: From ACS (2014a)'s description.

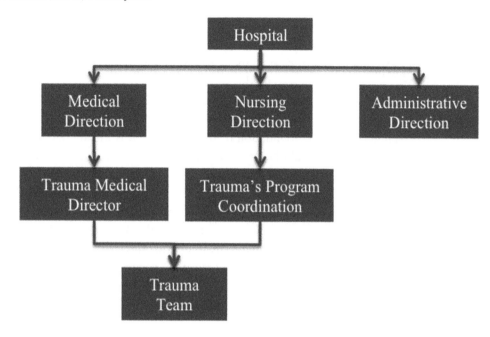

The trauma program should involve several disciplines and transcend normal departmental hierarchies (Alo & Griffith, 2000). As the best care extends itself since the place of a wound through the establishment of sharp care until the rehabilitation center, the trauma program must count with the appropriate specialties in all phases of treatment. Representatives of all disciplines provide the appropriate competencies as members of a team that work together to implement a treatment based on a priority plan of care (ACS, 2014b).

Figure 7. Organizational solution for trauma program
Source: Peterson (2013).

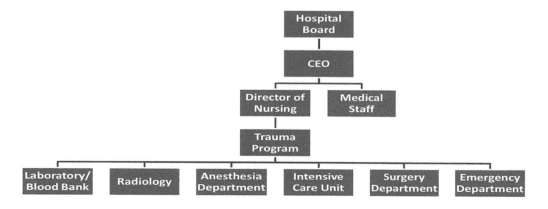

Processes

In the Trauma Centers, there must be places with easily access for the rescue vehicles that will be used in the initial care of the polytrauma patient, and these places are called trauma rooms, in other words, places where the initial emergency procedures may be performed, and even offering the possibility of performing small surgery procedures, once essential.

Aiming to define the patient's initial prognostic (viable or not) in the shortest time possible (it's recommended that the patients should not remain in the room for longer than 60 minutes), the trauma room requires great technical skill and scientific foundation from the team that works there (Freire, 2001).

The activation of the room trauma should be done based on the patient's condition. By easing the activation criteria, the great demand can lead to patients with severe lesions not having the necessary care, as well as too strict criteria can lead to avoidable deaths. The literature highlights several protocols for the emergency care. The most established ones are found in the package of the course/certification *Advanced Trauma Life Support* – ATLS, which has been offered by the *American College of Surgeons* – ACS – in 1978. The use of the ATLS's recommendation assure that the level of care offered does not deteriorate at no time during the evaluation, resuscitation and initial care, besides preparing appropriately for the inter or intra hospital transfer of the patient.

The macro process proposed by ATLS – used as reference in the trauma room – consist of 9 stages, which are:

1. Preparation,
2. Screening,
3. Primary Survey (ABCDE),
4. Resuscitation,
5. Auxiliary measures to the primary survey and resuscitation,
6. Secondary examination (from head to toe),
7. Auxiliary measures to the secondary examination,
8. Reevaluation and continuous monitoring,
9. Definitive Care.

The accountability of the Emergency Department with the patient ends, when he/she is sent to the definitive care and there are three main ways for that: Release; Routing for performing a surgical procedure; Transfer to another care center.

Despite the convergence of literature regarding the sequence of activities throughout the care process, it's not conclusive regarding the flow of decision making where the model to be adopted will vary according to the necessity of the patient. As an example, Sarcevic (2011) illustrates in the following Figure 8, the alternatives of interdisciplinary decision models, considering that many Trauma Centers also incorporated the doctors who are shared with the emergency department and the surgery center.

System of People

Patients of trauma may need care from specialists, besides the one provided by the general surgeons, emergency doctors, orthopedists and neurosurgeons. The efficacy of a Trauma Center is reinforced by the commitment of these additional people. These specialists must be promptly available and qualified in

Figure 8. Leadership decision models of the trauma team
Source: Sarcevic (2011).

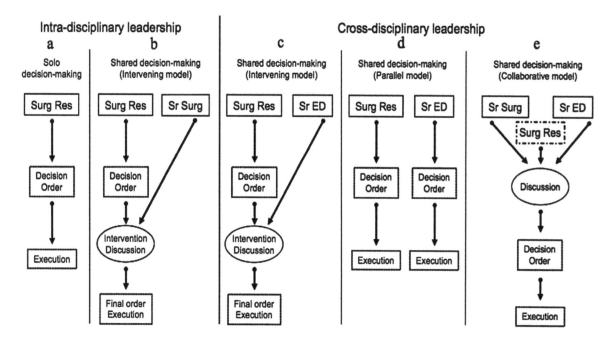

their specialization areas. The ready availability is defined as being available within 30 minutes counting from the notification (ACS, 2014a). For Stürmer & Neugebauer (2002) this response time should be from 15 to 20 minutes. So, the trauma service access other clinic services by the demand and needs to deal with ways to manage the resources. The perspective of the coordinated system involving all dimensions of this type of organization, as proposed by Boffard (2013), is translated, in the people's system dimension, in the role of the health unit coordinator. This role has as attributions (Peterson, 2013):

- Activate the trauma team after the notification from the pre hospital;
- Confirm the arrival of all team members;
- Determine if additional medical staff will be necessary;
- Keep direct contact with emergency service;
- Gather and copy all documentation for the transport team, for instance, letters, laboratories, X-rays;
- Prepare forms of patients transfer and get the signature from the emergency service provider, in case the patient needs to be transferred;
- Security request to ensure the heliport;

By meeting the welfare nature of the assignments, Murphy et al. (2011) highlight that the increasing complexity associated to the care to the polytrauma patient that assume operations in complex and dynamic environments, characterized by multifaceted decisions, information overload and great time restrictions with severe consequences for errors, require, not only the domain of knowledge and procedural's skills, but also the ability of communicating effectively with the patients and other care providers from where derives the necessity of develop and improve the strong skills of the interdisciplinary team.

As part of the continuous improvement, an efficient technique in the perspective of communication, quality perception and improvement of the teams' competences (knowledge, skills and attitudes) is the learning through training and simulation that directly impacts the performance, providing: timely responses, high quality decisions' taking and reduction of the patient's safety risk. As an example, one may cite the "TraumaMan", which has been used in the ATLS courses in order to enable practical training of various surgical procedures in an anatomical dummy.

Reward System

Trauma systems are complex organizational structures, with the evolution of the methods and care standards. It's necessary to have an ongoing evaluation mechanism, based on: self-monitoring and external evaluation (Boffard, 2003). Boffard (2003) suggests that the trauma system would be monitored and evaluated through a continuous measurement of the results of the care providing process. Alo & Griffith (2000) argue that programs of trauma development improvement should provide a structured approach for the continuous improvement of the trauma care. The main target is to reduce an inappropriate variation and unwanted results in the care.

The following components are important for the efforts in the trauma development improvement:

1. Identification of the trauma patients' characteristics (epidemiological study):
   a. During the visits to these Brazilian State Trauma Centers, it was noticed a great variability of the demand by geographical and seasonal issues. While in some centers, the most recurrent problem was the ones that have been stabbed, and particularly, on Sundays, those who were shot, in others there were traffic accident victims coming from the nearby expressways. New changes in the macro environment may affect the operation of a trauma center such as, for instance, the construction of new expressways, installation of new companies, great events among others.
2. Problem Identification:
   a. **Concurrent Review:** Revision of the patient assistance while it's been provided.
   b. **Retrospective Review:** Revision the care provided to the patient after their release.
   c. Revision of the problems related to the care in multiple patients over time.
   d. Indicators for improving the trauma performance.
   e. **Evaluation:** Multidisciplinary evaluation of the individual care to the patient in a detailed way during the whole process of the trauma care.
   f. **System of Analysis of the Root Cause:** Detailed evaluation of the problem, including all the related stages and processes, which could potentially affect the issue.
   g. **Conclusions:** Consensual assessment as to whether there is an opportunity for improvement. A causal factor should be determined, to help the planning of the appropriate corrective actions, whenever possible.
   h. **Corrective Actions:** An action is necessary only if there is an improving opportunity. It must correspond to a determined root cause. It may include, education, counseling, change in protocol, resource enhancement, refers to another area for further evaluation and disciplinary action.

i.   **Return and Loop Closure**: Assure that the corrective action was concluded and it was compatible with the desired effect. If the desired effect didn't occur, it may be necessary additional actions until the improvement is reached.

Alo & Griffith (2000) argue that programs of trauma development improvements should provide a structured and multidisciplinary approach for the continuous improvement to the trauma care, aiming to reduce the inadequate variation and undesirable results in the care. Therefore, it's necessary the development of a indicators chart that allows:

- Surveillance procedures and processes;
- Analysis of the protocols' adequacy;
- Analysis of material and technologies;
- Analysis of personal development;
- Suggestion of new practices based on scientific evidences;
- Analysis and release of statistic data related to the assistance quality and the patients' safety;
- Suggestion of training to the division of continuous education;

FUTURE RESEARCH DIRECTIONS

Throughout this document, it was clear several point where the literature, about the dimensions proposed in the Galbraith's model et al. (2003) was inconclusive or unexplored. Even not being the scope of this text, it's worth to highlight that the literature lacks quantitative models that relate the amount of the necessary resources to the care of polytrauma victim patients to a determined level of service. This kind of studies could be worth in the perspective of the trauma's network, where, by knowing for which number of patients such trauma center was firstly designed, the 'trauma coordinator' could trigger contingency plans or ask for help to units geographically close to it.

CONCLUSION

In this document, it's been developed a theoretical and conceptual perspective, which, from the dimensions proposed by the Galbraith's model et al. (2003), it was evident the consolidated and open points in the literature, reinforced by empiric researches, guided by a protocol extracted from the literature revision and the present regulatory mark, allowed the understanding of the practices and challenges of the three studied organizations.

From this understanding, it contributed to the body of knowledge on the subject by synthesizing the cross-organizational variables to the departments, which should be considered in the context of design and management of a line of trauma care.

REFERENCES

ACS. (2014a). *Resource for Optimal Care of the Injured Patient*. Committee on Trauma American College of Surgeons.

ACS. (2014b). *ATLS - Suporte Avançado de Vida no Trauma*. ACS Committee on Trauma.

Alo, K. E., & Griffith, P. M. (2000). Trauma Program Manager. In D. Demetriades & J. A. Asensio (Eds.), *Trauma Management* (pp. 655–662).

Azevedo, A. L. D. C. S. (2010), *Gerencimento do cuidado de enfermagem em unidade de urgência traumática* [Doctoral dissertation]. Universidade de São Paulo.

Baligh, H. H. (2005). *Organization Structures: Theory and Design, Analysis and Prescription* (1st ed.). Springer.

Beilman, G. J., Taylor, J. H., Job, L., Moen, J., & Gullickson, A. (2004). Population-based prediction of trauma volumes at a Level 1 trauma centre. *Injury*, *35*(12), 1239–1247. doi:10.1016/j.injury.2004.03.018 PMID:15561113

Benbasat, I., & Weber, R. (1996). 'Research commentary: Rethink 'diversity' in information system research'. *Information Systems Research*, *7*(4), 389–399. doi:10.1287/isre.7.4.389

Boffard. (2003). *Manual of Definitive Surgical Trauma Care*. CRC Press.

Brohi, K., Parr, T., & Coats, T. (2009). *Regional trauma systems. Interim guidance for commissioners* (pp. 1–60). London: Royal College of Surgeons of England.

Burlton, R. (2010). Delivering Business Strategy Through Process Management. In: J. Vom Brocke & M. Rosemann (Orgs.). Handbook on Business Process Management 2: Strategic Alignment, Governance, People and Culture (1st ed., pp. 5-38). Springer. doi:10.1007/978-3-642-01982-1_1

Christian, M., Farmer, J., & Young, B. (2009). *Disaster triage and allocation of scarce resources. Fundamentals of Disaster Management* (3rd ed., pp. 1–18). Mount Prospect, IL: Society of Critical Care Medicine.

Demetriades, D., & Asensio, J. A. (2000). *Trauma Management*. Georgetown, Texas: Landes Biosciences.

Eisenhardt, K. M. (1989). Building theories from case study research. Academy of Management Review, 14(4), 532–550.

Freire, E. (2001). Trauma: a doença dos séculos. São Paulo: Atheneu.

Galbraith, J., Downey, D., & Kates, A. (2003). *Designing Dynamic Organizations: a hand-on guide for leaders at all levels*. New York: Amacon.

HRSA. (2006). *Model Trauma System Planning and Evaluation*. U.S. Department of Health and Human Services Program Support Center.

Hyer, N. L., Wemmerlöv, U., & Morris, J. A. Jr. (2009). Performance analysis of a focused hospital unit: The case of an integrated trauma Center. *Journal of Operations Management, 27*(3), 203–219. doi:10.1016/j.jom.2008.08.003

Jonsen, K., & Jehn, K. A. (2011). Using triangulation to validate themes in qualitative studies. *The Learning Organization, 4*(2), 123–150.

Markus, M. L., & Jacobson, D. D. (2010). Business Process Governance. In J. Vom Brocke & M. Rosemann (Orgs.). Handbook on Business Process Management 2: Strategic Alignment, Governance, People and Culture (1st ed., pp. 201-222). Springer. doi:10.1007/978-3-642-01982-1_10

Mason, N. (2006). Is operations research really research? *Orion, 22*(2), 155–180.

Murphy, M. M., Edwards, C. M., Seggie, J. Z., & Curtis, K. (2011). Emergency Department Trauma Redesign in a Level 1 Trauma Centre. *Australasian Emergency Nursing Journal, 14*(1), 50–58. doi:10.1016/j. aenj.2010.10.003

Neto, G. V., & Malik, A. M. (2011). Gestão em Saúde.

Ordinance No 1.366. (2013, July 8). *Estabelece a organização dos Centros de Trauma, estabelecimentos de saúde integrantes da Linha de Cuidado ao Trauma da Rede de Atenção às Urgências e Emergências (RUE) no âmbito do Sistema Único de Saúde (SUS)*. Retrieved from http://www.brasilsus.com.br/legislacoes/legislacoes-recentes/legislacoes/gm/119738-1366.html

Patton, M. Q. (2002). *Qualitative Research & Evalutation Methods, 3 Edition*. Sage Publications.

Peterson, T. (2013). *Trauma Hospital Resource Manual*. Minnesota Statewide Trauma System.

Pinsonneault, A., & Kraemer, K. L. (1993). Survey research methodology in a management information systems: An assessment. *Journal of Management Information Systems, 10*(2), 75–105. doi:10.1080/07 421222.1993.11518001

Sarcevic, A., Marsic, I., Waterhouse, L. J., Stockwell, D. C., & Burd, R. S. (2011). Leadership structures in emergency care settings: A study of two trauma centers. *international journal of medical informatics, 80*(4), 227-238.

SBAIT. (2015). *Trauma*. Retrieved from http://www.sbait.org.br/trauma.php

Stürmer. Klaus Michael, & Neugebauer, Edmund. (2002). S3 – Guideline on Treatment of Patients with Severe and Multiple Injuries. Berlin. German Trauma Society (DGU) (lead) Office in Langenbeck-Virchow House Luisenstr.

Van Aken, J. E., Berends, H., & Bij, H. V. D. (2007). Problem Solving in Organizations: A Methodological Handbook for Business Students (1st ed.). Cambridge University Press. doi:10.1017/CBO9780511618413

Yin, R. K. (2005). *Case Study Research: Design and Methods*. New York: Sage Publications.

KEY TERMS AND DEFINITIONS

Operations Management: Set of goals, policies and restrictions that describe how the organizations aims to direct and develop all the resources invested in the production to better accomplish the mission.

Organizational Structure: Administrative tools that guided to a determined objective, groups activities, resources, hierarchical levels and decision-making processes of an organization.

People: Decision-makers, who, by facing a set of information, match their will and previous experience to conduct an action.

Process: Activities sequenced logical and temporally.

Rewards: Award that is granted or obtained from satisfactory result in the execution of a task.

Strategy: Most appropriate action or path to be executed to achieve a goal.

Trauma Center: Health Unit dedicated to the care line of the trauma patients.

Trauma: External nature event to an individual, in a more or less violent manner and that could produce any lesion or damage.

This research was previously published in the Handbook of Research on Healthcare Administration and Management edited by Nilmini Wickramasinghe; pages 104-119, copyright year 2017 by Medical Information Science Reference (an imprint of IGI Global).

Section 4
Quality and Performance

Chapter 25
Quality Evaluation of Health Care Establishment Utilizing Fuzzy AHP

Mohammad Azam
Career Institute of Medical Sciences & Hospital, India

Mohamed Rafik Noor Mohamed Qureshi
King Khalid University, Saudi Arabia

Faisal Talib
Aligarh Muslim University, India

ABSTRACT

Quality evaluation of healthcare establishment (HCE) is a difficult process as it involves multiple components of quality criteria with various factors and sub-factors therein. Further, the quality criteria are not universally standardized. The subjective evaluation in itself is not reliable as a tool so that available HCEs may be investigated for selecting the best among them. Thus, to avoid vagueness and imprecision due to process of human cognition the need to evolve a useful method for evaluation of quality of HCE was essentially required. To achieve such an objective three well established HCEs from northern cities of India have been studied. An Integrated Quality Model designed for HCE (Azam et al., 2012a, 2012b) and specifically tested previously with the AHP study by the authors (Azam et al., 2015) with its components, parameters and factors sub-factors has been utilized to evaluate the quality aspects of HCEs forming subjects of the current study. Further, the standard formula of Fuzzy AHP methodology with the application of fuzzy set theory was applied to the multiple components of the quality criteria with various factors and sub-factors therein pertaining to various HCEs forming the subject of the study. Quality of the HCEs thus could be evaluated empirically avoiding vagueness due to human cognition factors. Utilizing this methodology respective rankings of HCEs could also be assigned among them with practical utility to maintain the required quality of their services. Quality evaluation of Health Care Establishment utilizing Fuzzy AHP along with fuzzy set theory is a unique method which will benefit the client patients to select the best HCE among the available alternatives of HCEs. It also helps the managers to improve the business by allocating scarce resources wherever critically required to improve various quality components criteria factors and sub-factors of their HCEs.

DOI: 10.4018/978-1-7998-2451-0.ch025

Copyright © 2020, IGI Global. Copying or distributing in print or electronic forms without written permission of IGI Global is prohibited.

INTRODUCTION

The multi criteria decision model (MCDM) such as Analytic Hierarchy Process (AHP) is a hierarchy or a set of structure at integrated levels and is empirically constructed for complex problems with criteria and sub-criteria of multiple nature therein to achieve the intended objectives of the organization (Talib et al., 2011a; Talib and Rahman, 2015a; Hassanien et al., 2015). It thus, seeks consistency of judgment with a user-friendly approach. Along with operations research techniques it may also deal with intricate problems to find appropriate solutions (Azam et al., 2015). Multiple criteria thus, can be dealt with relative ease (Dura'n and Aguilo, 2008; Hassanien et al., 2014). AHP however, is found to be deficient to deal with the ambiguity creeping in due to conceptual aspects as a result of subjective judgment attributable to the human beings (Talib et al., 2011a). This deficiency resulting vagueness may be rectified through the Fuzzy AHP method. The quality aspects of any Health Care Establishment (HCE) is important both from the point of view of clients as also from the point of view of managers. The judgments in AHP are likely to be faced with human cognitive problems due to subjectivity creeping therein. This problem however, is avoided in Fuzzy AHP method which is combined with Fuzzy set theory as an extension of AHP model.

In recent past studies, a number of approaches have been proposed to assess the performance of service organizations. They can be broadly classified into three fundamental clusters: stated importance methods (SIMs), derived importance methods (DIMs) and the MCDM based approaches (Lupo, 2016). As regards to the above techniques, MCDM methodologies such as AHP, Technique for Order of Preference by Similarity to Ideal Solution (TOPSIS), Interpretive Structural Modeling (ISM) and others are recognized as favorite development approaches which have ability to evaluate and/or select service alternatives (Lupo, 2016; Saaty, 2008; Li et al., 2014; Chang, 2014; Talib and Rahman, 2017; Kumar and Talib, 2017; Faisal and Talib, 2016a, 2016b; Khanam et al., 2016). Several recent applications of MCDM based approaches especially Fuzzy AHP in the HCEs are described and implemented by researchers. Few of them are as follows. Lupo (2016) applied a fuzzy framework to evaluate service quality in the public healthcare sector based on SERVQUAL disconfirmation paradigm and incorporated the AHP method to draw out reliable estimates of service quality expectations. Aloui and Touzi (2015) developed a new flexible querying approach using fuzzy ontological knowledge based platform. This approach presents fuzzy clustering algorithm (FCA) based methodology for building ontologies from scratch then integrating them intelligently through the fusion of conceptual clustering, fuzzy logic and FCA. Kouah and Saidouni (2015) developed a large dynamic system named as fuzzy labeled transaction refinement tree which provides a formal specification framework for designing multi agent systems among other collection and internal agent's behavior. Salama and Hassanien (2014) proposed a modified fuzzification of Euclidian space calculated for the Fuzzy C-means and support vector machine techniques based on the ranking of features extracted from evaluating the features. Ghallab et al. (2014) studies the analysis, classification, mining and predictions based on fuzzy as an intelligent system called the strictness petroleum prediction system (SPPS). Ho (2012) developed a construct factor evaluation model of health management center selected by customers with fuzzy AHP. He made the weight assessment on evaluation indexes of health management center. Five major perspectives for customer's selection of health management center were used. They are: health management department, personal management department, health examination service department, market department and environment department. Hillerman et al. (2017) presents a model for the analysis of suspicious claims data from healthcare providers with the use of different clustering algorithm and the application of the AHP multicriteria method for prioritizing the identified suspects entitles for subsequent auditing. Handayani et al. (2015) studied the strategic hospital services quality in Indonesia by analyzing the dimensions that are required by the hospital to increase the quality of hospital services to meet the stakeholders needs and expectations. Woldegebriel et al. (2015) proposes a fuzzy logic integrated with AHP to consider the uncertainties to prioritize service quality improvement in the healthcare by considering the SERVQUAL dimensions. Ahmadi et al. (2014) identified, categorized and analyzed meso-level dimensions for the adoption of Electronic Medical Records (EMR) in the healthcare establishments and developed a MCDM framework and adoption of EMR in HCE. Similarly, in the area of healthcare quality evaluation, several research works described by Akdag et al. (2014), Buyukozkan and Cifci, (2012), Cebeci (2009); Lin et al. (2008) are of interest too.

In light of the above studies, a novel evaluation model is herein developed and presented to overcome the know weaknesses with the aim of evaluating the quality in HCEs. In this study, it has been attempted to present Fuzzy AHP method analyzing an integrated quality model for HCE with its components, factors and sub-factors developed earlier by the authors (Azam et al., 2012b). Thus, Fuzzy AHP method has been utilized as a quality evaluation method to select the best HCE among the HCEs under study. Fuzzy AHP therefore provides a mechanism to select potentially the best HCE among alternative available choices of HCEs, with the ability to avoid vagueness. Fuzzy AHP mechanism enables the clients to confidently select and enjoy the services of a potentially best HCE. It also provides opportunities for the managers to improve any deficiency of service of HCE by allocating scarce resources appropriately to improve it (Ryan et al., 2014). At the same time it further also validates the specifically designed integrated quality model for the HCE by the authors (Azam et al., 2012a, 2012b).

After the introduction of the subject paper, in the subsequent section of the paper research objective of the study is presented. Thereafter, an extant literature review on Fuzzy AHP has been brought out. After literature review section, a detailed methodology adopted for this study is explained followed by results and discussion sections. The paper ends by highlighting some recommendations, limitations, future scope and prospects in conclusion section.

RESEARCH OBJECTIVE

To enable clients to select potentially the best HCE among group of HCEs a simple and reliable selection methodology avoiding vagueness of human subjective judgment is required to be evolved to evaluate the quality aspects of the available alternative HCEs. The following objective therefore, has been considered for this research work along with literature review:

To develop an empirical model as an evaluation method using Fuzzy Analytic Hierarchal Process (Fuzzy AHP) combined with Fuzzy Set Theory, by utilizing Integrated Quality Model factors for HCEs which have already been validated with the application of an AHP model (Azam et al., 2015).

REVIEW OF LITERATURE

AHP (Saaty, 2000) as a process has been utilized successfully to seek solutions for unstructured decisions of complex nature (Partovi, 1994; Talib et al., 2011a). AHP is a process with number of steps. The first step is to construct hierarchies of components, sub component of the multiple criteria. The second step is to achieve comparative judgment and in the last step the priority synthesis and consistency checking is undertaken. In AHP one faces vagueness due to cognitive and language perception of the observer and bias on account of his/her emotional feelings which may be empirically affecting their judgment itself. Thus, the overall results may be affected. It has been emphasized that the fixed value judgments are difficult to arrive at in comparison to interval judgments which may be presented reliably, (Chan and Kumar, 2007). It is also difficult to evaluate the service quality concept being intangible phenomenon with a number of criteria. However, in such situations, the 'Fuzzy AHP' approach may adequately deal with the human preferences and the uncertainty associated with them. By combining the Saaty's AHP with the 'Fuzzy Set Theory' evolved by Zadeh (1965) the process of AHP is extended and is called as Fuzzy AHP methodology. Fuzzy set theory deals the classes whose boundaries are vague and notwell defined, (Azar, 2010a, 2010b; Azar and Vaidyanathan, 2015; Ayag, 2005). In a fuzzy set an element has a degree of membership (Negoita, 1985; Zimmermann,1985; Zhu and Azar, 2015) where the vagueness and uncertainty is mathematically represented. The problem of vagueness and uncertainty in real life situations are thus resolved through use of Fuzzy AHP method with effective decisions (Chan and Kumar, 2007) along with utilization of Fuzzy set theory (Azar, 2012) and 'Triangular Fuzzy Numbers" for criterion preferences. Thus, imprecision in decision making is avoided by use of Fuzzy AHP as has been brought out in relevant studies and literature thereof (Kahraman et al., 2004; Ayag, 2005; Fu et al., 2006; Chan and Kumar, 2007; Kang and Lee, 2007; Dura'n and Aguilo, 2008; Huang et al., 2008; Celik et al., 2009; Cebeci, 2009; Chamodrakas et al., 2010, Golpira, 2015).

Constructing hierarchies; comparative judgment and priority synthesis with consistency checking similar to AHP methodology are three broad steps of the Fuzzy AHP model too considering the decision problems. These steps in detail have been explained and presented in the study of AHP to select best HCE among available alternatives by Azam et al. (2015). Use of 'Triangular Fuzzy Numbers (TFN)', 'Fuzzy Set Theory', 'Priority synthesizing' and 'Consistency checking' in Fuzzy AHP with standard formulae, processes and techniques are described in detail within Appendix A attached.

METHODOLOGY

The most important objective of the present research is to identify best HCE among alternative HCEs with Fuzzy AHP method. The Fuzzy AHP method is utilized to avoid vagueness of human judgment by constructing an empirical model. This has been achieved by extending the model of AHP further through the use of Triangular Fuzzy Numbers with Fuzzy Set Theory. For achieving the stated objective of this research study following methodology was adopted:

1. An in-depth literature review has been undertaken as above explaining the Fuzzy AHP approach through the use of Triangular Fuzzy Numbers with Fuzzy Set Theory (Appendix A). The same has been utilized for empirical evaluation of multiple criteria with regard to decision making, avoiding thus, the vagueness and uncertainty of human preferences.
2. Quality Model for HCE (Azam et al., 2012a, 2012b) was selected for the study through Fuzzy AHP method. This quality model for HCE with the components, parameters, factors, sub-factors and criteria therein as evaluated earlier by the authors within their study of AHP to select best HCE (Azam et al., 2015) was fully adopted for the present study. The same has been attached as Appendix B depicting the designed quality model along with the codes for its components, parameters, fac-

tors, sub-factors and criteria therein with groupings in accordance with their relative importance (see Tables 3, 4, and 5).

3. Three HCEs formed the subject of current study. The profile of HCEs and relevant details are attached as Appendix C. The HCEs which formed the subject of this study have been designated as HCE-A, HCE-B and HCE-C. This has been done to maintain the confidentiality aspects of the results of the study which may affect their business reputation.

4. Seniorexperts in Medicine, Surgery and Community Medicine with Hospital Management qualifications were chosen to evaluate various aspects of quality parameters, factors, sub-factors and criteria therein as per Appendix B.

5. To the quality parameters, factors, sub-factors and criteria of various HCEs as observed and evaluated by the experts the standard Fuzzy AHP formula with use of Triangular fuzzy numbers have been applied for bringing out the preferences of one criterion over another along with utilization of Fuzzy Set theory in AHP. This process with the application of 'Standard Fuzzy AHP method' as brought out within the above-mentioned Appendix A was used with the objective to eliminate vagueness on account of human cognition factors.

6. The results finally obtained have been utilized for comparative evaluation of various quality components, parameters, factors, sub-factors and criteria of HCEs according to the Quality Model for HCE (Azam et al., 2012a&b) with application of Fuzzy AHP along with Fuzzy set theory. Thus avoiding vagueness on account of human cognition factors, the best HCE quality-wise could be empirically selected among the HCEs forming the subject of current study.

RESULTS

The quality components of HCEs which were evaluated using Fuzzy AHP along with Fuzzy set theory therein have been undertaken after disintegrating them at various hierarchal levels as shown within Figure12 (Appendix C). Thereafter, at each level, pair wise matrices for comparison have been formed. Thus, at level II seven quality components have been pair-wise compared as per matrices. Further, the sub-components of above mentioned seven quality components have also been pair-wise compared at level III matrix. The results of which are depicted in Table 6, 7 and 8 (Appendix D). The composite relative weights and global weight of each quality components of potential HCEs along with their overall ratings were thus obtained using standard Fuzzy AHP method as shown in Tables 9 and 10 (Appendix D).

Based on their overall ratings, the HCE-A, HCE-B and HCE-C could be easily compared and assessed for selecting the best HCE among them. The respective ranks of HCE-A, HCE-B and HCE-C could thus be indicated clearly as is discernible with in Table 10 (Appendix D). The likely vagueness therefore, which creeps in AHP model could be avoided by use of Fuzzy AHP. According to ratings and rankings of HCEs as shown in Figure 1 below, it could be observed that the *HCE-A(0.3848)> HCE-C(0.3677)>HCE-B(0.2475)*.

In the present case study, HCE-A may be selected when compared to HCE- C and HCE- B. Thus, it is easy for the clients to choose the best HCE among the alternative HCEs by comparing them according to their ratings and rankings. Managers too could improve their respective HCEs by detecting the deficient aspects and allocating the resources appropriately.

Figure 1. Overall ratings and ranking of HCEs- A, B and C

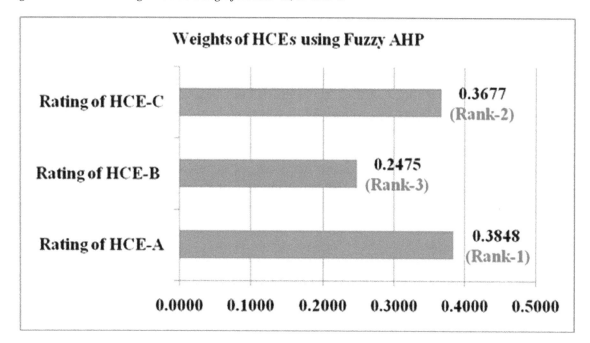

DISCUSSION

The clients and managers of the HCEs often face the difficult situation to choose the best HCE quality wise from among various HCEs. It is due to the fact that the functional structure of any HCE is a complex matrix of a number of quality components, sub-components criteria and sub - criteria factors therein. The functional structure of a HCE involves not only the core subjects of medical sciences but also the managerial aspects of it with inherent quality factors required to be maintained keeping pace with contemporary knowledge of the applicable subjects. Thus, considering the quality dimensions of the HCE a reliable mechanism is required to be developed to comparatively assess the HCE especially from functional quality point of view (Talib and Rahman, 2015b; Talib et al., 2011b). The procedure will require a quality model for HCE covering the functional areas of HCE well integrated. Keeping in view this aspect therefore, an integrated quality model for a HCE as described by the authors (Azam et al., 2012b) was selected after an in-depth review of literature on the subject. The other aspect is to apply a reliable methodology to obtain the relative ratings of the HCEs so that clients may easily choose the highest ranking HCE among the alternative HCEs obviating vagueness thereof likely to be there due to human cognition problems of judgment. To achieve this objective therefore, an appropriate methodology of Fuzzy AHP model has been chosen. The chosen Fuzzy AHP methodology was further applied to the duly coded quality components, sub-components criteria and sub - criteria factors of the selected integrated quality model for the study. In case of Fuzzy AHP the fuzzy numbers are utilized to achieve pair wise comparisons of the quality criteria and the sub-criteria at various hierarchal levels. Through this method weights for the comparative rankings of HCE are obtained and the best HCE may then be selected easily. The earlier study of authors (Azam et al., 2015) utilizing AHP model has thus been extended to this study of Fuzzy AHP model in combination with Fuzzy set theory where triangular fuzzy numbers are applied.

The degree of membership (Negoita, 1985; Zimmermann, 1985) of an element within Fuzzy set theory being a theory of classes with boundaries which are not well defined (Ayag, 2005) helps in clearing vagueness due to process of human cognition. There are intrinsic numerical methods within Fuzzy set theory to obviate vagueness, uncertainty and imprecision of problems. Chan and Kumar (2007), emphasized the importance of Fuzzy AHP to achieve results with effective decision making process. To achieve several theoretical results, Fuzzy set theory in AHP has been utilized (Kahraman et al., 2004; Ayag, 2005; Fu et al., 2006; Chan and Kumar, 2007; Kang and Lee, 2007; Dura'n and Aguilo, 2008; Huang et al., 2008; Celik et al., 2009; Cebeci, 2009; Chamodrakas et al., 2010).

The quality evaluation of HCEs applying the Fuzzy AHP methodology has distinct advantages. The multiple quality criteria of HCEs are quantified after coding of factors/sub-factors therein, followed by application of standard formula of Fuzzy AHP and integration of Fuzzy set theory with mathematical precision. The results of the study are thus obtained with clear rankings of HCEs, indicating that quality wise HCE A > C > B. Therefore, a choice regarding best HCE i.e. HCE- A may be accordingly recommended by the management.

The results of various factors/ sub-factors may also be compared and shortcoming thus found, may be improved with prioritization of allocation of resources to the deficient areas of the organization. Thus, improvement of service quality of concerned HCE may then be achieved.

The main focus of this research work thus has been to formulate Fuzzy AHP based methodology as an extension of AHP model along with use of Fuzzy set theory and Triangular Fuzzy numbers. The objective was to find overall priority and rank of the respective HCEs understudy to select the best HCE among them. This has been achieved successfully in three broad steps i.e. constructing hierarchies; comparative judgment and priority synthesis with consistency checking.

This study of HCEs with application of Fuzzy AHP method coupled with Fuzzy set theory therefore, is unique with utilization of novel quality model developed and tested with AHP model earlier by the authors (Azam et al., 2012 b and Azam et al., 2015). The present Fuzzy AHP study thus has been essentially undertaken to obviate the cognition error of observers to improve reliability of results.

Managerial Impact

The Fuzzy AHP has clear advantage for clients as well as for management elaborated as under:

Implications for Clients

The Fuzzy AHP model is a robust mechanism to enable clients to evaluate the available HCEs and to choose the best among them. It helps to achieve this objective by clearing vagueness due to human cognition factors and judgmental imprecision. Thus, the clients will be able to avail best of the quality services of HCE chosen by them.

Implications for Manager

Development of the Fuzzy AHP model to select potential HCE is also useful for the management point of view apart from serving the interests of the clients. Using fuzzy AHP methodology, the manager is able to obviate the vagueness of human imprecision due to cognition problems of judgment by the decision makers evaluating the HCEs. The manager at the same time is able to pin point the deficient quality criteria affecting the satisfaction of the patients. Accordingly, such identified specific quality criteria may be maintained suitably by allocating adequate resources to the affected HCE and its deficient functional areas. Thus, services of the concerned HCE may be improved qualitatively to achieve patient satisfaction appropriately, thereby enhancing its reputation as well as the business prospects.

CONCLUSION, RECOMMENDATIONS, LIMITATIONS, FUTURE APPLICATION, SCOPE AND PROSPECTS

The focus of the present study is to ensure that the evaluation of HCEs is undertaken without any vagueness on account of imprecision due to human cognition process of the evaluating experts which is likely common problem of any evaluation methodology. The vagueness aspect in the study has been taken care of by avoiding it through adoption of Fuzzy AHP process with the Fuzzy set theory where the evaluation parameters, criteria and sub criteria factors of a HCE are mathematically converted to numerical values. Thus comparisons, allocation of overall priority and rankings of various HCEs are achieved avoiding the vagueness and the best HCE may be chosen in a most reliable manner. This is an improvement by extension of AHP model through application of Fuzzy AHP and Fuzzy set theory to avoid vagueness. Potential HCE if selected through the Fuzzy AHP method obviating vagueness allows the clients to enjoy quality services and at the same time, it also enables the management to improve shortcomings enhancing reputation of the HCE. Thus, management is able to improve business opportunity and help to grow in the global market in the long run.

Recommendations

The standard Fuzzy AHP method along with the designed integrated quality model for the HCE (Azam et al., 2012 b) is recommended for evaluation of HCEs to help the clients to select potentially the best HCE to enjoy its quality services. It is also recommended for use by the managers to help them to determine shortcomings of service quality at various hierarchal levels and functional areas of the HCE. It will thereby help the managers to allocate resources appropriately to improve the quality of affected services. Thus, managers may optimize costs improving profitability to enhance the reputation as well as the business of the HCE.

Limitations

The HCEs practically utilizable by the clients especially on account of accessibility factors may be studied in short period of time to select the best HCE through Fuzzy AHP method. However, to find the best HCE among a large number of HCEs a long-term study as a project work only may be undertaken.

Future Application, Scope and Prospects

Evaluation of quality of a HCE is a difficult task as there is always a chance of vagueness with regard to the results of evaluation of its various parameters, criteria and sub criteria factors. The integrated quality model for HCE and its parameters, criteria and sub criteria factors utilized within AHP model study (Azam et al., 2012b and Azam et al., 2015) may also be utilized for evaluation of HCEs through application of Fuzzy AHP and Fuzzy set theory. Thus, vagueness on account of human judgmental errors due to cognition process may be avoided. Further, it will allow the clients to reliably select the best HCE from among various available HCEs. The Fuzzy AHP method simultaneously will also enable the manager to improve services of the concerned HCE with optimization of costs by allocation of scarce resources to the deficient functional areas of the concerned HCE. Thus, the satisfaction of clients, stakeholders and society at large may be achieved.

REFERENCES

Ahmadi, H., Nilashi, M., Darvishi, M., Ibrahim, O., Zakaria, R., Zolghadri, A.H. and Alizadeh, M. (2014). Fuzzy Multi-Criteria Approaches for Evaluating the Critical Factors of Electronic Medical Record Adoption. *Review of Contemporary Business Research, 3*(2), 01-24.

Akdag, H., Kalayci, T., Karagöz, S., Zülfikar, H., & Giz, D. (2014). The evaluation of hospital service quality by fuzzy MCDM. *Application of Software Computations., 23*, 239–248. doi:10.1016/j. asoc.2014.06.033

Aloui, A., & Touzi, A. G. (2015). A Fuzzy Ontology-Based Platform for Flexible Querying. *International Journal of Service Science, Management, Engineering, and Technology, 6*(3), 12–26. doi:10.4018/ IJSSMET.2015070102

Ayag, Z. (2005). A fuzzy AHP-based simulation approach to concept evaluation in a NPD environment. *IIE Transactions, 37*(9), 827–842. doi:10.1080/07408170590969852

Azam, M., Qureshi, M. N., & Talib, F. (2015). AHP Model for Identifying Best Health Care Establishment. *International Journal of Productivity Management and Assessment Technologies, 3*(2), 34–66. doi:10.4018/IJPMAT.2015070104

Azam, M., Rahman, Z., & Talib, F. (2012a). Core Quality and Associated Supportive Quality Parameters/ Dimensions: A Conceptual Quality Framework in Health Care Establishment. *International Journal of Business Excellence, 5*(3), 238–277. doi:10.1504/IJBEX.2012.046641

Azam, M., Rahman, Z., Talib, F., & Singh, K. J. (2012b). A critical study of quality parameters in health care establishment: Developing an integrated quality model. *International Journal of Health Care Quality Assurance, 25*(5), 387–402. doi:10.1108/09526861211235892 PMID:22946239

Azar, A. T. (2010a). *Fuzzy Systems*. Vienna, Austria: IN-TECH.

Azar, A. T. (2010b) Adaptive Neuro-Fuzzy Systems. In: A.T Azar (ed.), Fuzzy Systems. IN-TECH, Vienna, Austria, Azar AT (2012). Overview of Type-2 Fuzzy logic systems. International Journal of Fuzzy System Applications, 2(4), 1-28. doi:10.5772/7220

Azar, A. T., & Vaidyanathan, S. (2015). *Computational Intelligence applications in Modeling and Control. Studies in Computational Intelligence, 575*. Germany: Springer-Verlag.

Büyüközkan, G., & Cifc, G. (2012). A combined fuzzy AHP and fuzzy TOPSIS based strategic analysis of electronic service quality in healthcare industry. *Expert System Application, 39*(3), 2341–2354. doi:10.1016/j.eswa.2011.08.061

Cebeci, U. (2009). Fuzzy AHP-based decision support system for selecting ERP systems in textile industry by using balanced scorecard. *Expert Systems with Applications*, *36*(5), 8900–8909. doi:10.1016/j.eswa.2008.11.046

Celik, M., Er, I. D., & Ozok, A. F. (2009). Application of fuzzy extended AHP methodology on shipping registry selection: The case of Turkish maritime industry. *Expert Systems with Applications*, *36*(1), 190–198. doi:10.1016/j.eswa.2007.09.004

Chamodrakas, I., Batis, D., & Martakos, D. (2010). Supplier selection in electronic market places using satisficing and fuzzy AHP. *Expert Systems with Applications*, *37*(1), 490–498. doi:10.1016/j.eswa.2009.05.043

Chan, F. T. S., & Kumar, N. (2007). Global supplier development considering risk factors using fuzzy extended AHP-based approach. *Omega*, *35*(4), 417–431. doi:10.1016/j.omega.2005.08.004

Chang, T. H. (2014). Fuzzy VIKOR method: A case study of the hospital service evaluation in Taiwan. *Information Science*, *271*, 196–212. doi:10.1016/j.ins.2014.02.118

Cheng, C. H., & Mon, D. L. (1994). Evaluating weapon system by analytical hierarchy process based on fuzzy scale. *Fuzzy Sets and Systems*, *63*(1), 1–10. doi:10.1016/0165-0114(94)90140-6

Duran, O., & Aguilo, J. (2008). Computer-aided machine-tool selection based on a fuzzy-AHP approach. *Expert Systems with Applications*, *34*(3), 1787–1794. doi:10.1016/j.eswa.2007.01.046

Faisal, M. N., & Talib, F. (2016a). Implementing traceability in Indian food supply chains: An interpretive structural modeling approach. *Journal of Foodservice Business Research*, *19*(2), 171–196. doi:10.1080/15378020.2016.1159894

Faisal, M. N., & Talib, F. (2016b). E-government to m-government: A study in a developing economy. *International Journal of Mobile Communications*, *14*(6), 568–592. doi:10.1504/IJMC.2016.079301

Fu, H. P., Ho, Y. C., Chen, R. C. Y., Chang, T. H., & Chien, P. H. (2006). Factors affecting the adoption of electronic marketplaces: A fuzzy AHP analysis. *International Journal of Operations & Production Management*, *26*(12), 1301–1324. doi:10.1108/01443570610710560

Ghallab, S. A., Badr, N. L., Salem, A. B., & Tolba, M. F. (2014). Strictness Petroleum Prediction System Based on Fuzzy Model. *International Journal of Service Science, Management, Engineering, and Technology*, *5*(4), 44–65. doi:10.4018/ijssmet.2014100104

Golpîra, H. (2015). Extended Earned Value Management Based on Fuzzy Multi-Criteria Decision Making. *International Journal of Service Science, Management, Engineering, and Technology*, *6*(4), 16–32. doi:10.4018/IJSSMET.2015100102

Handayani, P. W., Hidayanto, A. N., Sandhyaduhita, P. I., Kasiyah, & Ayuningtyas, D. (2015). Strategic hospital services quality analysis in Indonesia. *Expert Systems with Applications*, *42*(6), 3067–3078. doi:10.1016/j.eswa.2014.11.065

Hassanien AE, Azar AT, Snasel V, Kacprzyk J, Abawajy JH (2015) Big Data in Complex Systems: Challenges and Opportunities, Studies in Big Data, 9, Springer-Verlag GmbH Berlin/Heidelberg.

Hassanien, A. E., Tolba, M., & Azar, A. T. (2014) Advanced Machine Learning Technologies and Applications. In *Proceedings of the Second International Conference AMLTA 2014*, Cairo, Egypt. Springer-Verlag GmbH Berlin/Heidelberg.

Hillerman, T., Souza, J. C. F., Reis, A. C. B., & Carvalho, R. N. (2017). Applying clustering and AHP methods for evaluating suspect healthcare claims. *Journal of Computational Science*, *19*, 97–111. doi:10.1016/j.jocs.2017.02.007

Ho, C. C. (2012). Construct factor evaluation model of Health Management Center selected by customers with Fuzzy Analytic Hierarchy Process. *Expert Systems with Applications*, *39*(1), 954–959. doi:10.1016/j.eswa.2011.07.094

Huang, C. C., Chu, P. Y., & Chiang, Y. H. (2008). A fuzzy AHP application in government sponsored R&D project selection. *Omega*, *36*(6), 1038–1052. doi:10.1016/j.omega.2006.05.003

Kahraman, C., Cebeci, U., & Ruan, D. (2004). Multi-attribute comparison of catering service companies using fuzzy AHP: The case of Turkey. *International Journal of Production Economics*, *87*(2), 171–184. doi:10.1016/S0925-5273(03)00099-9

Kang, H. Y., & Lee, A. H. I. (2007). Priority mix planning for semiconductor fabrication by fuzzy AHP ranking. *Expert Systems with Applications*, *32*(2), 560–570. doi:10.1016/j.eswa.2006.01.035

Khanam, S., Siddiqui, J., & Talib, F. (2016). A DEMATEL approach for prioritizing the TQM enablers and IT resources in the Indian ICT industry. *International Journal of Applied Management Sciences and Engineering*, *3*(1), 11–29. doi:10.4018/IJAMSE.2016010102

Kouah, S., & Saïdouni, D. E. (2015, July). (2105). Application of Fuzzy Labeled Transition System to Contract Net Protocol. *International Journal of Service Science, Management, Engineering, and Technology*, *6*(3), 27–46. doi:10.4018/IJSSMET.2015070103

Kumar, S., & Talib, F. (2017). Modelling the psychological and design attributes of innovative product using interpretive structural modeling. *International Journal of Intelligent Engineering Informatics*, *5*(2), 139–166. doi:10.1504/IJIEI.2017.084169

Li, Y., Hu, Y., Zhang, X., Deng, Y., & Mahadevan, S. (2014). An evidential DEMATEL method to identify critical success factors in emergency management. *Applied Soft Computational Journal*, *22*, 504–510. doi:10.1016/j.asoc.2014.03.042

Lin, C.-T., Wu, C.-R., & Chen, H. C. (2008). The Study of Construct Key Success Factors for the Taiwanese Hospitals of Location Selection by Using the Fuzzy AHP and Sensitivity Analysis. *International Journal of Information and Management Sciences*, *19*(1), 175–200.

Lupo, T. (2016). A fuzzy framework to evaluate service quality in the healthcare industry: An empirical case of public hospital service evaluation in Sicily. *Applied Soft Computing*, *40*, 468–478. doi:10.1016/j.asoc.2015.12.010

Partovi, F. Y. (1994). Determining What to Benchmark: An Analytic Hierarchy Process Approach. *International Journal of Operations & Production Management*, *14*(6), 25–39. doi:10.1108/01443579410062068

Ryan, L., Tormey, D., & Share, P. (2014). Cultural Barriers to the Transition from Product to Product Service in the Medical Device Industry. *International Journal of Service Science, Management, Engineering, and Technology, 5*(2), 36–50. doi:10.4018/ijssmet.2014040103

Saaty, T. L. (1980). *The analytic hierarchy process: Planning, priority setting.* New York: Mc Graw-Hill.

Saaty, T. L. (2000). *Fundamentals of Decision Making and Priority Theory* (2nd ed.). Pittsburgh, PA: RWS Publications.

Saaty, T. L. (2008). Decision making with the analytic hierarchy process. *International Journal of Service Science, 1*(1), 83–98. doi:10.1504/IJSSCI.2008.017590

Salama, M. A., & Hassanien, A. E. (2014). Fuzzification of Euclidean Space Approach in Machine Learning Techniques. *International Journal of Service Science, Management, Engineering, and Technology, 5*(4), 29–43. doi:10.4018/ijssmet.2014100103

Talib, F., Azam, M., & Rahman, Z. (2015). Service Quality in Healthcare Establishments: A Literature Review. *International Journal of Behavioural and Healthcare Research, 5*(1&2), 1–24. doi:10.1504/IJBHR.2015.071465

Talib, F., & Rahman, Z. (2013). Current health of Indian healthcare and hospitality industries: A demographic study. *International Journal of Business Research and Development, 2*(1), 1–17. doi:10.24102/ijbrd.v2i1.242

Talib, F., & Rahman, Z. (2015a). Identification and prioritization of barriers to total quality management implementation in service industry: An analytic hierarchy process approach. *The TQM Journal, 27*(5), 591–615. doi:10.1108/TQM-11-2013-0122

Talib, F., & Rahman, Z. (2015b). An interpretive structural modeling for sustainable healthcare quality dimensions in hospital services. *International Journal of Qualitative Research in Services, 2*(1), 28–46. doi:10.1504/IJQRS.2015.069780

Talib, F., & Rahman, Z. (2017). Modeling the barriers of Indian telecom services using ISM and MIC-MAC approach. *Journal of Asia Business Studies, 11*(2), 188–209. doi:10.1108/JABS-11-2015-0196

Talib, F., Rahman, Z., & Azam, M. (2011b). Best practices of total quality management implementation in healthcare setting. *Health Marketing Quarterly, 28*(3), 232–252. doi:10.1080/07359683.2011.5956 43 PMID:21815741

Talib, F., Rahman, Z., & Qureshi, M. N. (2011a). Prioritising the practices of total quality management: An analytic hierarchy process (AHP) analysis for the service industries. *Total Quality Management and Business Excellence, 22*(12), 1331–1351. doi:10.1080/14783363.2011.625192

Woldegebriel, S., Kitaw, D., & Rafele, C. (2015). Application of Fuzzy Logic for Prioritizing Service Quality Improvement in Healthcare. *International Journal of Scientific & Engineering Research, 6*(5), 530–537.

Zadeh, L. A. (1965). Fuzzy set. *Information and Control, 8*(3), 338–353. doi:10.1016/S0019-9958(65)90241-X

Zhu, Q., & Azar, A. T. (2015). *Complex system modelling and control through intelligent soft computations. Studies in Fuzziness and Soft Computing, 319*. Germany: Springer-Verlag.

Zimmermann, H. J. (1985). *Fuzzy set theory and its applications*. Boston, MA: Kluwer. doi:10.1007/978-94-015-7153-1

This research was previously published in the International Journal of Service Science, Management, Engineering, and Technology (IJSSMET), 8(4); edited by Ahmad Taher Azar and Ghazy Assassa; pages 83-120, copyright year 2017 by IGI Publishing (an imprint of IGI Global).

APPENDIX A

Fuzzy AHP Approach: Use of Triangular Fuzzy Numbers (TFN) and Fuzzy Set Theory

Zadeh (1965) introduced the operations with triangular fuzzy numbers (TFN). TFN among various types of the fuzzy numbers are the widely used numbers. Triangular fuzzy number may be defined as a triplet (a1, a2, a3); the membership function of the fuzzy number $\tilde{A}$ is defined in Figure 2. TFN can be represented with three points $A = (a_1, a_2, a_3)$.

Figure 2.α -cut operations and membership function of triangular fuzzy number (TFN)

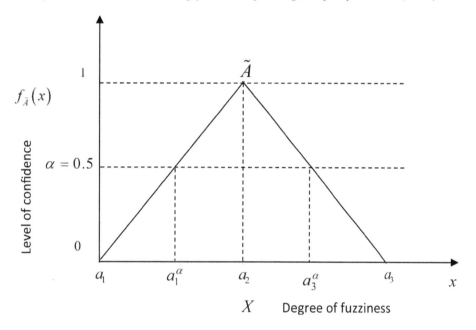

Let X be the universe of discourse, $X = \{x_1, x_2, ..., x_n\}$. A fuzzy set $\tilde{A}$ of X is a set of order pairs

$$\left\{\left(x_1, f_A^"(x_1)\right), \left(x_2, f_A^"(x_2)\right), ..., \left(x_n, f_A^"(x_n)\right)\right\} \text{ where } f_A^" : X \rightarrow [0,1],$$

is the membership function of $\overset{\text{Ů}}{A}$, and $f_{\tilde{A}}(x_i)$ stands for the membership degree of x_i in $\tilde{A}$.

The $\propto$-cut $\tilde{A}_\propto$ and strong α-cut $\tilde{A}_{\propto+}$ of the fuzzy set $\overset{\text{Ů}}{A}$ in the universe of discourse, X is defined by

$$\tilde{A}_\propto = \left\{x_i \setminus f_{\tilde{A}}(x_i) \geq \propto, x_i \in X\right\}, \; Where \propto \in [0,1] \tag{1}$$

$$\tilde{A}_{\alpha+} = \left\{ x_i \setminus f_{\tilde{A}}\left(x_i\right) > \alpha, x_i \in X \right\}, \quad Where\, \alpha \in \left[0,1\right] \tag{2}$$

A fuzzy set $\overset{\cup}{\tilde{A}}$ of the universe of discourse X is convex if and only if every $\tilde{A}_\alpha$ is convex, that is $\tilde{A}_\alpha$ is close interval of $\Re$. It can be written as

$$\tilde{A}_\alpha = \left[P_1^{(\alpha)}, P_2^{(\alpha)}\right], where \quad \alpha \in \left[0,1\right] \tag{3}$$

$$f_{\tilde{A}}\left(x\right) = \begin{cases} 0, & x < a_1, \\ {(x - a_1)} \big/ {(a_2 - a_1)}, & a_1 \le x \le a_2, \\ {(a_3 - x)} \big/ {(a_3 - a_2)}, & a_2 \le x \le a_3, \\ 0, & x > a_3, \end{cases} \tag{4}$$

Further:

Let $\tilde{A}_\alpha$ and $\tilde{B}$ be two triangular fuzzy numbers parameterized by the triplet (a_1, a_2, a_3) and (b_1, b_2, b_3) respectively, and then the operational laws (Zimmermann, 1985) of these two triangular fuzzy numbers are as follows:

$$\overline{A\left(+\right)\tilde{B}} = \left(a_1, a_2, a_3\right)\left(+\right)\left(b_1, b_2, b_3\right) = \left(a_1 + b_1, a_2 + b_2, a_3 + b_3\right) \tag{5}$$

$$\overline{A\left(-\right)\tilde{B}} = \left(a_1, a_2, a_3\right)\left(-\right)\left(b_1, b_2, b_3\right) = \left(a_1 - b_3, a_2 - b_2, a_3 - b_1\right) \tag{6}$$

$$\tilde{A}\left(\times\right)\tilde{B} = \left(a_1, a_2, a_3\right)\left(\times\right)\left(b_1, b_2, b_3\right) = \left(a_1 b_1, a_2 b_2, a_3 b_3\right) \tag{7}$$

$$\tilde{A}\left(\div\right)\tilde{B} = \left(a_1, a_2, a_3\right)\left(\div\right)\left(b_1, b_2, b_3\right) = \left(\frac{a_1}{b_1}, \frac{a_2}{b_2}, \frac{a_3}{b_3}\right) \tag{8}$$

$$k\tilde{A} = \left(ka_1, ka_2, ka_3\right) \tag{9}$$

$$(\tilde{A})^{-1} = \left(\frac{1}{a_3}, \frac{1}{a_2}, \frac{1}{a_1}\right) \tag{10}$$

To get crisp interval by α-cut operation, interval A_α shall be obtained as $\forall \alpha \in [(0,1)]$. From

$$\frac{a_1^{(\alpha)} - a_1}{a_2 - a_1} = \alpha, \qquad \frac{a_3 - a_3^{(\alpha)}}{a_3 - a_2} = \alpha,$$
$$a_1^{(\alpha)} = \left(a_2 - a_1\right) \alpha + a_1$$
$$a_3^{(\alpha)} = \left(a_3 - a_2\right) \alpha + a_3$$

(11)

may be obtained.

$$A_\alpha = \left[a_1^{(\alpha)}, a_3^{(\alpha)}\right] = \left[\left(a_2 - a_1\right) \alpha + a_1, -\left(a_3 - a_2\right) \alpha + a_3\right]$$

(12)

Considering the numerical example as shown in the Figure 3.

Figure 3. α = 0.5 cut of triangular fuzzy number (TFN) A = (-5,-1,1)

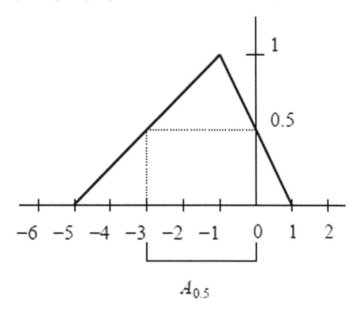

α -cut interval from the above TFN will be:

$$A_\alpha = \left[a_1^{(\alpha)}, a_3^{(\alpha)}\right]$$
$$A_\alpha = \left[4 \alpha - 5, 2 \alpha + 1\right]$$

(13)

If α=0.5, substituting 0.5 for α,

$$A_{0.5} = [a_1^{(0.5)}, a_3^{(0.5)}]$$

(14)

$$A_{0.5} = [-3,0] \tag{15}$$

The main operations for positive fuzzy numbers are described below (Cheng and Mon, 1994):

$$\forall a_1, a_3, b_1, b_3 \in R^+, \tilde{A}_\alpha = \left[a_1^{(\alpha)}, a_3^{(\alpha)} \right], \tilde{B}_\alpha = \left[b_1^{(\alpha)}, b_3^{(\alpha)} \right] \in \left[0,1 \right],$$

$$\tilde{A}_\alpha \oplus \tilde{B}_\alpha = \left[a_1^{(\alpha)}, a_3^{(\alpha)} \right] \oplus \left[b_1^{(\alpha)}, b_3^{(\alpha)} \right] = \left[a_1^{(\alpha)} + b_1^{(\alpha)}, a_3^{(\alpha)} + b_3^{(\alpha)} \right], \tag{16}$$

$$\tilde{A}_\alpha - \tilde{B}_\alpha = \left[a_1^{(\alpha)}, a_3^{(\alpha)} \right] - \left[b_1^{(\alpha)}, b_3^{(\alpha)} \right] = \left[a_1^{(\alpha)} - b_1^{(\alpha)}, a_3^{(\alpha)} - b_3^{(\alpha)} \right], \tag{17}$$

$$\tilde{A}_\alpha \otimes \tilde{B}_\alpha = \left[a_1^{(\alpha)}, a_3^{(\alpha)} \right] \otimes \left[b_1^{(\alpha)}, b_3^{(\alpha)} \right] = \left[a_1^{(\alpha)} b_1^{(\alpha)}, a_3^{(\alpha)} b_3^{(\alpha)} \right], \tag{18}$$

$$\tilde{A}_\alpha / \tilde{B}_\alpha = \left[a_1^{(\alpha)}, a_3^{(\alpha)} \right] / \left[b_1^{(\alpha)}, b_3^{(\alpha)} \right] = \left[a_1^{(\alpha)} / b_1^{(\alpha)}, a_3^{(\alpha)} / b_3^{(\alpha)} \right], \tag{19}$$

Priority Synthesizing and Consistency Checking in Fuzzy AHP

Pair wise comparison provides relative importance of the criteria. Therefore, using the Saaty scale as in Table 1, (Saaty, 1980), along with consistency checks various comparisons may be made which is described as under:

1. A pair wise comparison matrix is constructed using a scale of relative importance. The judgments are entered using the fundamental scale of the AHP proposed by Saaty (1980). Using pair wise comparison intensity of relative importance between two criteria can be established using Table 1 and the same is also depicted in Figure 4.

Table 1. Saaty's scale

Intensity of Relative Importance	Fuzzy Number	Definition	Membership Function
1	1	Equally preferred	(1,1,2)
3	3	Moderately preferred	(2,3,4)
5	5	Essentially preferred	(4,5,6)
7	7	Very strongly preferred	(6,7,8)
9	9	Extremely preferred	(8,9,10)

(Source: Saaty, 1980)

Figure 4. Fuzzy membership function for linguistic values for attributes or alternatives

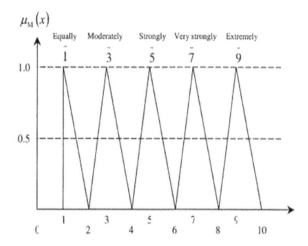

Assuming M criteria, the pair wise comparison of criterion i with criterion j gives a square matrix $A1_{M \times M}$ where *aij* denotes the relative importance of criterion i with respect to criterion j.

In the matrix $a_{ij} = 1$, when $i = j$ and $a_{ji} = 1/a_{ij}$

2. Find the relative normalized weight (*Wi*) of each criterion by calculating the geometric mean of ith row and normalizing the geometric mean of rows in the comparison matrix.

$$GM_i = \left(\prod_{j=1}^{M} a_{ij} \right)^{1/M} \tag{20}$$

and

$$W_i = \frac{GM_i}{\sum_{j=1}^{M} GM_j} \tag{21}$$

3. Calculate matrix A3 and A4 such that A3 = A1*A2 and A4 = A3/A2, where

$$A2 = [W_1, W_2, W_3, \ldots, W_t, W_N]^T \tag{22}$$

4. Find out the maximum Eigen value λ_{max} which is the average of matrix A4.
5. Calculate the consistency index

$$CI = (\lambda_{max} - M)/(M - 1) \tag{23}$$

The smaller the value of C.I., the smaller is the deviation from the consistency.

Table 2. Average random index (RI)

n	1	2	3	4	5	6	7	8	9	10
RI	0	0	0.52	0.89	1.11	1.25	1.35	1.40	1.45	1.49

(Source: Saaty, 1980)

6. Obtain the random index (R.I.) using Table 2, according to the number of criteria used in decision making. Average R.I. based on matrix size is shown in Table 2.
7. Calculate the consistency ratio

$$CR = CI/RI \qquad (24)$$

Usually, a C.R. of 0.1 or less is considered as acceptable as an informed judgment is reflected through the attributed knowledge of the analyst about the specific problem under consideration. The evaluation within the matrix is acceptable or indicates a good level of consistency in the comparative judgments represented in that matrix if the value of CR is either equal to, or less than the CR value of 0.1. However, if the CR is more than the acceptable value, it is presumed that inconsistency of judgments within that matrix has taken place and the evaluation process is required to be reviewed, reconsidered and improved. Matrix with less than 10% consistency have to be dropped formulating fresh comparisons matrix with the use of knowledge of the expert decision maker. In determining the priorities of a set of criteria, an acceptable consistency property therefore, helps in ensuring the reliability of the decision-maker.

Table 3. Summary of codes for components and parameters of the designed integrated quality model for HCE

Components of Integrated Quality Model for HCE with details	Code	Parameters							
Burden of Disease management in Society (BD) **BD-1** State of awareness, preparedness, adequacy and effectiveness of awareness Programme regarding Disease burden Management of HCE	**BD-1**	State of Awareness of organization regarding priority of treatment and management according to burden of disease in population	State of preparedness of organization plan to manage burden of disease of population	State of adequacy of Resources and efforts utilized for management of the disease burden	State of effectiveness of awareness programme for populations concerned regarding prevention of disease burden				
BD-2 Management of General and Deficiency Diseases	**BD-2**	State of Management of Unsafe water sanitation / hygiene and risk of infection and parasite disease like diarrhea, dysentery, viral hepatitis.	State of Management of Underweight/ Malnutrition	State of Management of Iron and zinc deficiencies especially in mothers	State of Management of Vit. A deficiency	State of management Obesity/high cholesterol, Diabetes			
BD-3 Management of Preventable Disease	**BD-3**	State of Management of Alcohol effects	State of Management of Blood Pressure	State of Management of Tobacco effects	State of Management of Indoor smoke effect due to its solid fuel and its effects, chronic Bronchitis	State of Management of Respiratory infection, TB	State of Management of Trauma/ accidents /Road accidents	State of Management of Unsafe sex – STD/HIV	
Knowledge Management in HCE(KM) **KM-1** State of Identification of knowledge	**KM-1**	Identification of competencies	Assessment of knowledge professional/ technical/ Managerial	Education/ training programme regarding Professional / Technical/ Managerial	Overall State				
KM-2 State of Collection, of Knowledge	**KM-2**	Relevant Data Base	Employee Suggestion Programme	Overall State					
KM-3 State of Selection of Knowledge	**KM-3**	Validation of Knowledge	Overall State						
KM-4 State of Storage of Knowledge	**KM-4**	Use of expert system	Documentation	Reports	Computer Data	Storage of Data Relevant to Organizational Requirement	Overall State		
KM-5 State of Sharing of Knowledge	**KM-5**	Person to person communication	Inter Departmental communication	Electronic sharing (a) Individual Email	(b)Organizational Email/Web site	Word of mouth overall	Formal written reports	Organizational magazine/ journal	Formal Training and Motivation Programme & Overall state
KM-6 State of Application of Knowledge	**KM-6**	Application for performance of tasks (professional/ technical/ management)	Use of specialized System for application- Integrated Performance and Support system	Overall State					

continued on following page

Table 3. Continued

Components of Integrated Quality Model for HCE with details	Code	Parameters							
KM-7 State of Creation of Knowledge	**KM-7**	Discovery of new Knowledge by insight: a) Professional/ Technical Field	Managerial Field	Automation/ data mining tools/ query tools	Overall State				
KM-8 State of Selling of Knowledge	**KM-8**	New Product	New Services	Overall State					
KM-9a State of External Initiative for KM	**KM-9a**	Health Education	Meetings	Seminars	Overall State				
KM-9b State of Internal Initiative for KM	**KM-9b**	Appointment and Functioning of Knowledge Officer	Knowledge Management Structure within organization	Overall State					
KM-10 State of Competence initiative for KM	**KM-10**	Localized Environment for Knowledge Transfer and Learning through Simulation & Pilot scale Activities	Other methods: (a)Tutorials / lectures/ demonstration	Formal training of interns/PG training/Nurse Diploma paramedical training.	Practical training programme Doctors Nurses, Paramedics and Managers.	Overall State			
Core Qualities & Associated Supportive Qualities (CQ&AQ) **AQ: CR-1** State of conceptual requirements of associated supportive quality parameters	**AQ: CR-1**	Continuous education policy for staff	Respectful treatment to client	Information to potential clients on treatment	Information on treatment and other activity to environment	Anticipation of changing demand	Integration of activities	Realization of aim related to cost of treatment	
CQ: CR- 1 State of Conceptual requirement of Core quality Parameters	**CQ:CR- 1**	Structured patient oriented treatment on the basis of thorough diagnosis	Client satisfaction of treatment						
AQ: OSR-1 State of operational stakeholders requirement: Associated supportive Quality parameters (AQ:OSR)	**AQ:OSR-1**	Treatment tuned to client requirement	Client can express his needs and wishes	Clinic is free for all clients	Clinic is only for those who can pay	Excellence of information flow in health care process			
AQ: OSR-2	**AQ:OSR-2**	Optimal budget allocated for each treatment	Respectful treatment of clients	Image of health care and treatment of clients	Image of health care establishment / clinic	Clients image of hospital	Satisfaction of clients (patients)		
AQ: OSR-3	**AQ:OSR-3**	Clients(system external customers patient) well informed about treatment	Clients (system external customers patient) well informed about specific treatment	Visually attractive and comfortable physical facilities (waiting rooms, chairs etc.)					

continued on following page

Table 3. Continued

Components of Integrated Quality Model for HCE with details	Code	Parameters						
AQ: OSR-4	**AQ:OSR-4**	Convenient office location	Professional appearance and appropriate dress of staff, doctors, nurses paramedics and others etc	Physician reputation	Consistency of fees and other charges			
CQ: OSR-1 State of operational stakeholders requirement: Core quality parameters (professional technical qualities) (CQ:OSR)	**CQ:OSR-1**	Correct diagnosis	Treatment tuned to diagnosis	Objective of treatment is specialized to clients requirement	Objective of treatment clear to all	Result of treatment continuously improved	Treatment tuned/timed to following treatment	
CQ: OSR-2	**CQ:OSR-2**	Match between clinical and outpatient help	Clients (system internal customers) level of satisfaction	Clients (system internal customers) well informed about available treatment	Clients (system internal customers) well informed about specific treatment	Correct performance of services first time		
CQ: OSR-3	**CQ:OSR-3**	Maintaining accurate and neat records of patient case history	Prescription of efficient reliable and affordable medicine	Physician compliance with universal precaution	Modern medical equipment	GP's referral contacts		
CQ: OSR-4	**CQ:OSR-4**	Positive medical outcome of treatment	Feeling good emotionally and psychologically	Emphasis on patient education	Knowledgeable and skilled support staff			
CQ: OSR-5	**CQ:OSR-5**	Qualified doctors(GPs), specialists	Familiarity of doctors, specialists with latest advancement in medical science knowledge	Clear display of doctors' qualification	Implementation of mandatory regulatory provisions(e.g.) Pre Natal Diagnostic Test Act (PNDT Act), hospital waste management and other related laws/ regulations			
Priority Areas Management for critical care(PAM): State of quality attributes in operation room (OR) / operation theatre (OT)	**PAM:OT-1**	Service in OR/OT	Surgery in time	Outcome improvement	Appropriate scheduling IT Based scheduling and communication programme (Hardware, software, networking and security system) for OR/OT Management with Trained OR/OT Management Team			
PAM: OT-2 State of Human resources available for surgery	**PAM OT-2**	Motivated Nurses, Doctors and support staff	New recruitment policy	Fair Salaries	Promotion and reward system	Team Development		
PAM: OT-3 Efficient OR/OT	**PAM:OT-3**	Dynamic Maintenance programme for equipment in Total Productive Maintenance frame work.	Dynamic inspection and maintenance of OR/OT with proper record.	Purchasing all state of the art equipment	Improving Bio Medical Engineering Department with standardization	Measures for prevention of hospital borne infection		

continued on following page

Table 3. Continued

Components of Integrated Quality Model for HCE with details	Code	Parameters							
PAM: Cas.D(A&E)-1 Priority Areas Management for critical care: State of Quality attributes in Causality Department (Accident and Emergency)	**PAM: Cas.D (A&E)-1**	Use of accident and emergency by the population	Treatment on time	Decreased adverse patient outcome	On time consultation- Motivated Nurses	On time consultation- Motivated Doctors	On time consultation- Motivated Support Staff	On time consultation- Recruitment, Team building and training activities for all Nurses, Doctor, Support Staff	Effective patient disposal with Problems of related units solved
PAM: Cas.D(A&E)-2 State of Quality Attributes in Casualty Department (Accident and Emergency):Adequacy of infrastructure	**PAM: Cas.D (A&E)-1**	Efficient pre-hospital services	Adequate material resources- Optimum layout	Adequate material resources- Adequate consultation rooms	Adequate material resources- State of art equipment	Adequate material resources- Adequate supply of drugs	Adequate material resources- IT based communication infrastructure		
PAM: Cas.D(A&E)-3 Referral & Evacuation of patient (Ambulance Services and In-transit Treatment Facilities during evacuation/ transfer of patient)	**PAM: Cas.D (A&E)-1**	State of equipment	Free/fully subsidized by Organization/ Govt.	Partially subsidized by the Organization/ Govt.	Prepaid insurance	Reimbursement after insurance	Full out of pocket expense by patient family.	State of total cases referred and/ total deaths in last one year in transit	
PAM: ICU-1 Priority Areas management for critical care: state of quality attributes in intensive care units (ICUs)	**PAM: ICU-1**	Satisfaction level of ICU stake holders	State of Services in ICU	Reduced Adverse patient outcome (i.e. state of reduction level of Morbidity/ Mortality)					
PAM: ICU-2 (Improved patient comfort)	**PAM: ICU-2**	Motivated Doctors Nurses (Recruitment Training Team building activities)	Adequate ICU drug/equipment (Purchasing state of art equipment Adequate supply of drug.)	Maintenance Management in total productive maintenance frame work	Efficient functioning of related units (On line lab reports, Organizing logistics for intra-hospital transfer of patients).				
PAM: ICU-3 (Presence of treatment protocol)	**PAM: ICU-3**	Designing IT Based admission/ discharge protocol.	Objectively organized daily round	Antibiotic protocol established	Standardized review/ audit				
PAM: ICU-4 (Proper communication)	**PAM: ICU-4**	Communication Design IT based,	Frequent communication with patients and their surrogate/family members.)						
Clinical Governance (CG) CG (i)-1 State of clinical governance quality in HCE organizational dimensions- Input	**CG (i)-1**	Financial resources (Additional commitments)	Infrastructure (New buildings, equipments)	Human resources (creation of new posts, clinical governance leadership, new recruitment to fill vacancies)	Policy (recognition of quality as statutory duty of organization)	Latest information on evidence based medicine			

continued on following page

Table 3. Continued

Components of Integrated Quality Model for HCE with details	Code	Parameters							
CG (s)-2 State of clinical governance quality in HCE organizational dimensions- Structure	CG (s)-2	Clinical governance committee	Performance	Management for total quality of care	Protocols and guidelines for clinical care	Education, training and career planning development	Clinical audit	System to integrate all quality activities in healthcare.	Clinical risk management strategies
		Reporting system for errors and adverse incidents	System to receive patient feed back.	Promoting evidence based medicine	Leadership development programme				
CG (p)-3 State of clinical governance quality in HCE organizational dimensions- Process	CG (p)-3	Implementation, monitoring and evaluation of risk	Job descriptions to include quality as an individual responsibility	IT training and access for use of latest electronics information.	Multidisciplinary management of clinical care	Recognition of human resource for quality.	Regular multi disciplinary clinical audit.	Sharing information, communication and coordination.	Systematic clinical supervision to deal with underperformance.
		Training to help health staff cope with their changing role in organization.	Promoting increased coordination among different professional groups.	Training to share information with patients (obtain patients consent and understand the willingness of patients to participate in treatment).	Management of patient's information and safeguarding its confidentiality.	Systematic evaluation of clinical errors and adverse incidents	Regular collection of data on clinical care.		
CG (o)-4 State of clinical governance quality in HCE organizational dimensions- Outcome	CG (o)-4	Continuous quality improvement.	Reduced waiting lists.	Patient satisfaction	Reduced numbers of adverse incidents.	Better patient -clinician relationship	Informed coordination between professionals and managers	Increased treatment based on evidence based medicine	
Treatment chain management quality in HCE (TCM) **TCM: IC-1** Treatment chain management quality in HCE: Internal customer Inputs between Outpatient departments to Investigation Departments & Vice-versa: (Treatment Chain Management inputs through Doctor's core competence for various departments to which the patient is referred during management process)	TCM: IC-1	Outpatient to Investigation Departments: To Laboratory	Outpatient to Investigation Departments: To Radiology	Investigation to outpatient departments: From Laboratory	Investigation to Outpatient departments: From Radiology				

continued on following page

Table 3. Continued

Components of Integrated Quality Model for HCE with details	Code	Parameters						
TCM: IC-2 Treatment chain management quality in HCE/ referral among internal customers; professional Doctors: Inpatient Departments to Investigation Departments& vice versa	**TCM: IC-2**	Inpatient to Investigation departments:To Laboratory	Inpatient to Investigation departments: To Radiology	Investigation to Inpatient departments: From Laboratory	Investigation to Inpatient departments: From Radiology			
TCM: IC-3 Treatment chain management quality in HCE/ referral among internal customers: professional Doctors (Other Inter-Departmental treatment chain management including with other hospitals & specialty centers)	**TCM: IC-3**	Inpatient to operation theater	Operation theatre to inpatient department.	Out patient/ Inpatient to Intensive Care Units (ICUs)	Inpatient convalescence to Rehabilitation Unit/ physiotherapy	Institutional to home/ domiciliary care/ convalescence	Referral (General to Specialty Department to Super Specialty to other Specialized Centers).	
TCM: EVC-1 Treatment chain management quality in HCE: Referral/ Evacuation chain management	**TCM: EVC-1**	Need based essential referral to save life and limbs of patient in emergency and for diagnostic / opinion purpose	Facilities of evacuation through well equipped Ambulances.	Ambulance staff/attendant training in resuscitation.	In-transit treatment facilities.	Cost of transfer by Ambulance		
TCM: Doc&R-1 Treatment chain management quality in HCE: Documentation and Maintenance of Records	**TCM: Doc&R-1**	Maintenance system: Conventional (Paper work)	Maintenance system: Use of Computers	Maintenance quality	Retrieval system promptness quality	Quality of Audit of patient record: Carried out at the time of discharge	Quality of Audit of patient record: After discharge at fixed time	Advices and rectification for future cases.
Patient Satisfaction assessment (PS) through Patient expectation / Patient Perception and Overall Patient perception of services Patient Expectation (PE) of services PE (tan)-1 Patient Expectation of services: Tangibility	**PE (tan)-1**	Up-to-date and well maintained medical facilities and equipments	Well maintained support service (canteen, dietary, Laundry & Linen, telecommunication	Well maintained waste disposal system	Clean and comfortable environment with good directional sign.	Doctor/staff professional and neat in appearance.	Informative Brochure/ booklet about services.	Privacy during treatment	Treatment facilities available (General/ Multi-specialty/ super-specialty).
PE (rel)-2 Patient Expectation of services: Reliability	**PE (rel)-2**	Service should be provided at appointed time	Services should be carried out right the first time	Doctor/staff should be professional and competent	Error free and fast retrieval of documents			
PE (fin)-3 Patient Expectation of services: Fair Financing	**PE (fin)-3**	Consistency of charges (distributions of risk of cost of health system according to ability to pay)	Paid out of pocket while utilizing service(Not applicable in the Government Hospital except non entitled cases)	Sliding scale as per ability to pay/income level	Insurance (Pre-payment, Reimbursement)			

continued on following page

Table 3. Continued

Components of Integrated Quality Model for HCE with details	Code	Parameters							
PE (resp)-4 Patient Expectation of services: Responsiveness	PE (resp)-4	Patient should be given prompt services.	Responsive doctors/staff	Attitude of doctors/staff should instill confidence in patients	Waiting time of not more than one hour.	Desired waiting time less than half an hour			
PE (asrc)-5 Patient Expectation of services: Assurance	PE (asrc)-5	Friendly and courteous staff / doctors	Doctors possess a wide spectrum of knowledge	Patient treated with dignity and respect	Thoroughness of explanation of medical condition to patient				
PE (emp)-6 Patient Expectation of services: Empathy	PE (emp)-6	Obtain feed back from patients.	Complaint resolution promptly.	24 Hours service availability	Doctor/staff should have patient's best interest at heart.	Doctor/ staff should understand the specific needs of patients.			
PE (acs & aff) – 7 Patient Expectation of services: Access& Affordability	PE (acs & aff)-7	Location accessibility	Adequacy of parking facilities.	Affordability of charges for service rendered.					
PE (per. fct)-8 Patient Expectation of services: Performance Factors	PE (per. fct)-8.	Outcome (achievement of better health)	Responsiveness to people's expectation	Fair financing	Over all rating of service provision	Health awareness and education programmes	Outreach health programmes to homes		
Patient Perception (PP) of services PP (tan)-1 Patient Perception of services: Tangibility	PP (tan)-1	Up-to-date and well maintained medical facilities and equipments	Well Maintained support service (canteen, dietary, Laundry & linen, Telecom-munication)	Well maintained waste disposal system	Clean and comfortable environment with good directional Sign.	Doctor/staff professionals and personnel neat in Appearance	Informative Brochure/ booklet about services	Privacy during treatment.	Treatment facilities availabe (General/ Multi-specialty/ Super-specialty).
PP (rel)-2 Patient Perception of services: Reliability	PP (rel)-2	Service should be provided at appointed time.	Services should be carried out right the first time.	Doctor/staff should be professional and competent.	Error free and fast retrieval of documents.				
PP (fin)-3 Patient Perception of services: Fair financing	PP (fin)-3	Consistency of charges (distributions of risk of cost of health system according to ability to pay)	Paid out of pocket while utilizing service(Not applicable in the Government Hospital except non entitled cases)	Sliding scale as per ability to pay/income level	Insurance (Pre-payment, Reimbursement)				
PP (resp)-4 Patient Perception of services: Responsiveness	PP (resp)-4	Patient should be given prompt services.	Responsive doctors/staff	Attitude of doctors/staff should instill confidence in patients	Waiting time of not more than one hour.	Desired waiting time less than half an hour			
PP (asrc)-5 Patient Perception of services: Assurance	PP (asrc)-5	Friendly and courteous staff / doctors	Doctors possess a wide spectrum of knowledge	Patient treated with dignity and respect	Thoroughness of explanation of medical condition to patient				
PP (emp)-6 Patient Perception of services: Empathy	PP (emp)-6	Obtain feed back from patients.	Complaint resolution promptly.	24 Hours service availability'	Doctor/staff should have patient's best interest at heart.	Doctor/ staff should understand the specific needs of patients.			

continued on following page

Table 3. Continued

Components of Integrated Quality Model for HCE with details	Code	Parameters						
PP (acs & aff)-7 Patient Perception of services: Accessibility& affordability	**PP (acs& aff)-7**	Location accessibility	Adequacy of parking facilities.	Affordability of charges for service rendered.				
PP (per. fct)-8 Patient Perception of services: Performance factors	**PP (per. fct)-8**	Outcome (achievement of better health)	Responsiveness to people's expectation	Fair financing.	Over all rating of service provision	Health awareness and education programmes	Outreach health programmes to homes	
PPO Overall Patient Perception of services	**PPO**	Very Good	Good	Fair	Poor	Very Poor		

(Source: Azam et al., 2015)

Table 4. Summary of codes for components, parameters and their relative importance (RI) in respect of the designed integrated quality model for HCE

Components of designed integrated quality model for HCE						
Burden of Disease	**Knowledge Management**	**Core Qualities & Associated Supportive Qualities**	**Priority Areas Management of Operation Room (OR/ OT), Intensive Care Unit (ICU), Casualty Department (Accident & Emergency) (CD: A&E)**	**Clinical Governance**	**Treatment Chain Management, Referrals Evacuation (Ambulance services & in-transit care), Maintenance of Records**	**Patient satisfaction (PS) {Patient Expectation & Patient Perception (PE&PP) (by Gap: PE& PP) & Overall(O) Patient Perception of Hospital Services (PPO)}**
Code BD	**Code KM**	**Code CQ&AQ**	**Code PAM**	**Code CG**	**Code TCM**	**Code PS**
RI-7	**RI-6**	**RI-4**	**RI-1**	**RI-5**	**RI-2**	**RI- 3**
BD-1: State of awareness, preparedness, adequacy and effectiveness of awareness programme regarding disease burden management of HCE	**KM-1** State of Identification of knowledge	**AQ: CR-1** State of conceptual requirements of associated supportive quality parameters	**PAM: OT-1 to PAM: OT-3** Priority area quality attributes: State of quality attributes in operation room (OR) / operation theatre (OT)	**CG (i)-1** State of clinical governance quality in HCE organizational dimensions- Input	**TCM: IC-1 to TCM: IC-3** Treatment chain management quality in HCE Internal customer Inputs: (Treatment Chain Management inputs through Doctor's core competence for various departments to which the patient is referred during management process)	**PE -1to8** Patient expectation of services {PE (tan)-1 PE (rel)-2 PE (fin)-3PE (resp)-1 PE (asrc)-5 PE (emp)-6 PE (acs & aff) -7 PE (per fct)-8}
BD-2 Management of General and Deficiency Diseases	**KM-2 to 4** State of Collection, Selection & Storage Of Knowledge	**CQ: CR- 1** State of Conceptual requirement of Core quality parameters	**PAM: Cas. D (A&E)-1 to PAM: Cas.D(A&E)-3 7** Priority area quality attributes: State of quality attributes in causality department (accident and emergency)	**CG (s)-2** State of clinical governance quality in HCE organizational dimensions- Structure	**TCM: EVC-1** Treatment chain management quality in HCE referral/evacuation chain management	**PP -1to8** Patient Perception of services {PP (tan)-1 PP (rel)-2 PP (fin)-3 PP (resp)-1 PP (asrc)-5 PP (emp)-6 PP (acs & aff) - 7 PP (per fct)-8}

continued on following page

Table 4. Continued

Components of designed integrated quality model for HCE						
Burden of Disease	**Knowledge Management**	**Core Qualities & Associated Supportive Qualities**	**Priority Areas Management of Operation Room (OR/OT), Intensive Care Unit (ICU), Casualty Department (Accident & Emergency) (CD: A&E)**	**Clinical Governance**	**Treatment Chain Management, Referrals Evacuation (Ambulance services & in-transit care), Maintenance of Records**	**Patient satisfaction (PS) {Patient Expectation & Patient Perception (PE&PP) (by Gap: PE& PP) & Overall(O) Patient Perception of Hospital Services (PPO)}**
BD3 Management of Preventable Disease	**KM-5&KM5a** State of Sharing of Knowledge including sharing of Knowledge by word of mouth	**AQ: OSR-1 to AQ: OSR-4** State of operational stakeholders requirement: Associated Supportive quality parameters (Managerial logistics qualities)	**PAM: ICU-1 to PAM: ICU-4** Priority area quality attributes ICUs: state of quality attributes in intensive care units (ICUs)	**CG (p)-3** State of clinical governance quality in HCE organizational dimensions-Process	**TCM: Doc&R-1** Treatment chain management quality in HCE including referral/evacuation chain management: Documentation and records)	**PPO** Overall Patient Perception of services (Very Good, Good, Fair, Poor & Very Poor)
	KM-6 &7 State of Application & Creation Of Knowledge	**CQ: OSR-1 to CQ: OSR-5** State of operational stakeholders requirement: Core quality parameters (professional technical qualities)		**CG (o)-4** State of clinical governance quality in HCE organizational dimensions-Outcome		
	KM-8 State of Selling of Knowledge					
	KM-9a, 9b & KM-10 State of Initiative (External, Internal & Competence initiative) for KM					

Note: The above groupings in order of relative importance (RI) of components from RI-1 to R-7 in decreasing order with highest being RI-1 have been indicated considering the potential to save life and limb, importance of the management process and its impact on outcome of disease management affecting patient care and satisfaction. These have been further summarized as shown in Appendix C so that the same could be conveniently utilized to develop an AHP model. (Source: Azam et al., 2015)

Table 5. Summary of codes for components and parameters of the designed integrated quality model of HCE along with groupings in order of relative importance(RI)

Burden of Disease RI-7	Knowledge Management RI-6	Core Qualities & Associated Supportive Qualities RI-4	Priority Areas Management of Operation Room (OR/OT), Intensive Care Unit (ICU), Casualty Department (Accident & Emergency) (CD:A&E) RI-1	Clinical Governance RI-5	Treatment Chain Management, Referrals Evacuation (Ambulance services &in-transit care), Maintenance of Records RI-2	Patient satisfaction (PS) {Patient Expectation & Patient Perception (PE&PP) (by Gap: PE& PP) & overall (O) Patient Perception of Hospital Services (PPO)} RI-3
BD-1	KM-1	AQ: CR-1	PAM: OT-1to 3	CG (i)-1	TCM:IC-1to 3	PE -1to8
BD-2	KM-2 to 4	CQ: CR- 1	PAM: Cas. D (A&E)-1to 3	CG (s)-2	TCM: EVC-1	PP -1to8
BD3	KM-5&5a	AQ:OSR-1to4	PAM: ICU-1to4	CG (p)-3	TCM: Doc&R-1	PPO
	KM-6 &7	CQ: OSR-1to5		CG (o)-4		
	KM-8					
	KM-9a,9b &10					

Note: RI - Relative Importance of components with highest being RI-1(refer Appendix B, Table 3 for details of components) The above groupings in order of relative importance (RI) of components from RI-1 to RI-7 in decreasing order with highest being RI-1 have been indicated considering the potential to save life and limb, importance of the management process and its impact on outcome of disease management affecting patient care and satisfaction. These have been further summarized as shown in Appendix C so that the same could be conveniently utilized to develop an AHP model (Source:Azam et al., 2015)

APPENDIX C

(Adopted from Azam et al., 2015)

CASE STUDY: PROFILE OF HCEs A, B &C

Step1. Evaluation framework: The Fuzzy AHP is utilized to find the best healthcare establishment among the alternative choices of available HCEs with basic objectives to avoid vagueness of human judgment due to problems of cognition.

For this study, three alternative HCEs of north India as in earlier study by the authors (Azam et al., 2015) regarding the use of AHP model to select the best HCE were chosen for evaluating and selecting the best HCE among them through Fuzzy AHP method also. Criteria components of the integrated quality model for the HCE, designed and developed by Azam et al., (2012a&b) were similarly utilized for the evaluation purposes. The attached Appendix B as above reproduced from the earlier study by the author (Azam et al., 2015) regarding AHP model to select best HCE provide details of various parameters, factors and sub-factors pertaining to the components of the above suggested integrated quality model for HCE. These have been utilized with specific codes as essential criteria and sub-criteria along with their groupings in order of relative importance to develop the requisite hierarchy for the proposed Fuzzy AHP model.

For maintaining the confidentiality of the HCEs and to protect their market reputation due to their comparative assessment within the study their profiles have been described labeling them as HCE -A, HCE- B, and HCE- C the details of which are reproduced from the earlier study by the authors (Azam et al., 2015) as under:

HCE – A: It is a government hospital of North India located in the city of Roorkee. The hospital established in July 1947 with an initial bed capacity of 100 grew in stages over a period of time to 440 beds by the year 1989. It has 22 major departments providing multispecialty hospital services with adequate logistics support. There are approximately 40 specialists including general duty doctors with adequate number of nursing staff and other paramedical staff working round the clock to provide comprehensive health care to dedicated government employees of central government, their dependent parents as well as children and other relatives as per government rules. It has on an average, a patient turn over of 600 to 800 per month, with seasonal variations. It is a training hospital for doctors and paramedical staff. It has affiliated dental and health units. The hospital operates with assigned zonal role including for disaster management under strict government rules and regulations. Facilities for dedicated engineering services with adequate staff to maintain equipments avoiding any break down has been provided with constant monitoring by the engineering staff. Strict auditing is carried out regarding the financial grants received from the government to maintain the hospital. Higher authorities both administrative as well as medical and health professionals carry out periodically their scheduled inspection of the hospital to assess its functional status. The existing facilities for transfer of patients to higher referral hospitals in chain with readily available transport including air transport on call at short notice is also especially assessed to check the preparedness for any eventuality.

HCE – B: It is a large corporate hospital of metropolis of Delhi like the HCE- A with a total bed capacity of 210 established in January 1984. There are 30 departments of the hospital providing multispecialty services. The logistics support to sustain them is adequate. At any time a total number of 30 specialists and doctors are working round the clock employed by the hospital. A patient turn over of 1719 per month has been achieved by the hospital, however it has no integral dental or health unit. Empanelled facilities for dental care have been arranged on as required basis.

HCE – C: This HCE is a private commercial hospital situated in the metropolis of Delhi. Established in January 1997, it was started with a total bed capacity of 170. The 40 departments of the hospital provide multispecialty services. Adequate logistics support has been created to sustain and support these departments with a total of 75 specialists and doctors employed by the hospital, however a number of specialists have been employed on call on as required basis according to type of cases required to be dealt. A patient turn over of approximately 2000 per month has been achieved however, dental or health units are not there. Dental cover is provided through referrals to other nearby dental care establishments.

Step2. Decision making group: Doctors of several hospitals with specialist qualification and experience of their own subjects including hospital working knowledge formed the decision making group (Talib and Rahman, 2013). Thus, five experts of medicine, surgery, obstetrics & gynecology and health expert in social and preventive medicine with sufficient experience of working as medical officer in charge of hospital and at directorial level provided the data. Quality of the service in healthcare sector was recognized as an important aspect by all these experts with experience as doctors of accomplished hospitals (Talib et al., 2015). To avoid any ambiguity the author himself administered the standard questionnaire prepared specifically for the study of fuzzy AHP and interviewed the respondents and the department staff obtaining first hand information regarding the functioning and the facilities of the HCE. Consensus of opinion existed among the expert group. For the numerical evaluation Expert Choice software -2010 finally may be utilized. The standard questionnaire for the study covered the overall goal of meeting criteria components of integrated quality model to find out the best HCE. Similarly sub-criteria of component criteria were individually dealt with as is coded and depicted in Appendices A, B and C. The Fuzzy AHP method including above focused areas are described in detail hereinafter.

Coding the Factors of Components of Integrated Quality Model for Use Within AHP model

The components and factors of integrated quality model for HCE (Azam et al., 2012 b) therein, to act as criteria and sub-criteria within fuzzy AHP model, have been developed after coding them as within the earlier study by the authors (Azam et al., 2015) regarding the use of AHP model to select the best HCE. These have been depicted in detail within Appendices A, B, and C in tabulated formats.

Grouping of Components of Integrated Quality Model for Use in Fuzzy AHP According to their Relative Importance

The components of the integrated quality model for HCE (Azam et al., 2012b) and the parameters, factors therein are required to be grouped to act as criteria and sub criteria as the case may be for their use in Fuzzy AHP methodology as extension of AHP to fine tune it. According to the relative importance of the components these have been grouped as under as have been shown duly coded within Appendices A to C which are reproduced from the earlier study by the authors (Azam et al., 2015) as under.

1. Priority Areas Management (PAM) of Operation Room (OR/OT), Intensive Care Unit (ICU), Casualty Department-Accident & Emergency (Cas. D (A&E) are grouped as indicated in Figure 5.

Figure 5. Coding, grouping and hierarchy of PAM

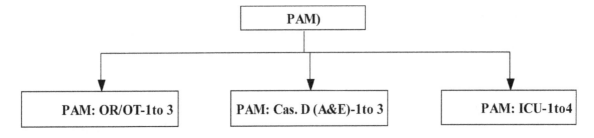

2. Treatment Chain Management, Referrals, Evacuation (Ambulance services &in-transit care), Maintenance of Records (TCM) are further broadly evaluated and grouped as TCM-Internal Customer (TCM-IC), TCM- Evacuation including referral (TCM: EVC) and TCM–Documentation and Records (TCM: Doc &R) shown in Figure 6.

Figure 6. Coding, grouping and hierarchy of TCM

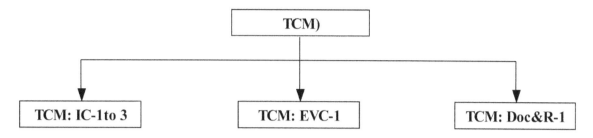

3. Patient satisfaction (PS) through evaluation of Patient Expectation & Patient Perception (PE & PP) by Gap study of PE& PP and overall Patient Perception of Hospital Services (PPO) are grouped as depicted in Figure 7.

Figure 7. Coding, grouping and hierarchy of PS

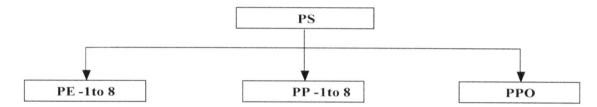

4. Core Qualities & Associated Supportive Qualities (CQ & AQ) comprising Associated quality–Conceptual requirement (AQ-CR), Core quality–Conceptual requirement (CQ-CR), Associated quality–Operational stakeholder requirement (AQ-OSR), Core quality– Operational stakeholder requirement (CQ- OSR) are grouped as shown in Figure 8.

Figure 8. Coding, grouping and hierarchy of CQ & AQ

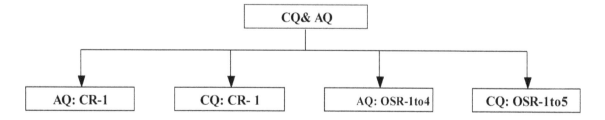

5. Clinical Governance (CG) including CG-input (CG(i)), CG-structure (CG(s)), CG-process (CG (p)), CG- output (CG(o)) are grouped as presented in Figure 9.

Figure 9. Coding, grouping and hierarchy of CG

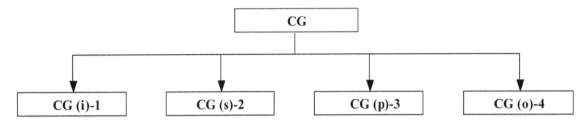

6. Knowledge Management (KM) including State of Identification of knowledge (KM-1), State of Collection, Selection & Storage of Knowledge(KM-2 to 4), State of Sharing of Knowledge including sharing of Knowledge by word of mouth (KM-5&KM5a), State of Application & Creation of Knowledge (KM-6 &7), State of Selling of Knowledge (KM-8), State of Initiative (External, Internal & Competence initiative) for KM (KM-9a, 9b & KM-10) are grouped as indicated in Figure 10.

Figure 10. Coding, grouping and hierarchy of KM

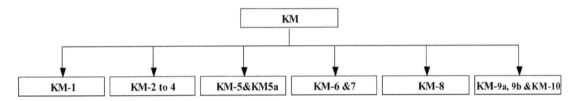

7. Burden of Disease (BD) including State of awareness, preparedness, adequacy, and effectiveness of awareness programme regarding disease burden management of HCE (BD-1), Management of General and Deficiency Diseases (BD-2) and Management of Preventable Diseases (BD-3) have been grouped as shown in Figure 11.

Figure 11. Coding, grouping and hierarchy of BD

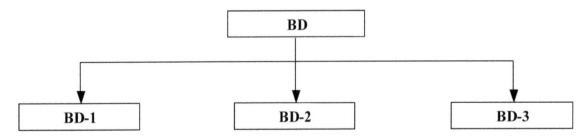

Within Appendices A, B and C as above are depicted the components, parameters, criteria and sub criteria of the designed integrated quality model for HCE utilized for the study.

Developing a Fuzzy AHP with Use of Integrated Quality Model its Components, Parameters, Criteria and Sub Criteria for the HCE

The level of quality of the components and parameters of the integrated quality model applied to the HCEs being studied as yardstick of quality services rendered to the patients in view of their relative importance may be assessed by utilizing AHP model. The results of AHP model will assist patients and stakeholders to select the best among the available HCEs. The managers of the HCEs will also be able to further improve the quality of services by allocating adequate resources to the deficient areas. The AHP study may be further fine tuned through Fuzzy AHP methodology. The model of AHP applied by the authors (Azam et al., 2015) for selecting best HCE earlier has been further utilized through case study method for analysis using Fuzzy AHP along with Fuzzy set theory to avoid vagueness creeping in due to human cognition problems.

The Proposed Potential HCE Selection Model Using Fuzzy AHP

The model using Fuzzy AHP at various hierarchal levels is depicted as under in Figure 12. The hierarchy for the fuzzy AHP method without difference is maintained on similar level as those for the AHP method (Azam et al., 2015).

Figure 12. The Fuzzy AHP proposed model for selection of potential HCE

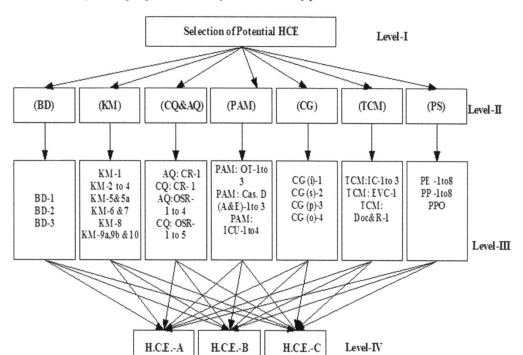

The selection of potential HCE at level I based on the main issue of selection parameters at level II are as under:

(1) Burden of Disease (BD)
(2) Knowledge Management (KM)
(3) Core Qualities & Associated Supportive Qualities (CQ&AQ)
(4) Priority Areas Management of Operation Room (OR/OT), Intensive Care Unit (ICU), Casualty Department (Accident & Emergency) (CD:A&E) (PAM)
(5) Clinical Governance (CG)
(6) Treatment Chain, Management, Referrals Evacuation (Ambulance services &in-transit care), Maintenance of Records, (TCM)
(7) Patient satisfaction (PS) {Patient Expectation & Patient of this research work. Perception (PE&PP) (by Gap: PE& PP) & overall (O) Patient Perception of Hospital Services (PPO)} (PS).

At level III sub components of each of above quality parameters of level II have been shown along with alternative potential HCEs under consideration have been depicted at level IV.

APPENDIX D

Application of Fuzzy AHP Methodology with the Integrated Quality Model for HCE

The procedure adopted for application of Fuzzy AHP methodology involved disintegration of various quality components of the quality model earlier developed by the author (Azam et al., 2012b). The same has been shown within appendices A-C duly coded.

These quality components therein have been disintegrated at various levels and at each level pair wise matrix for comparison have been formed. At level II seven quality components have been pair wise compared as per matrices which are as depicted in Table 6, 7, and 8.

Table 6. Pair-wise comparison of Quality components of Potential HCE

Potential HCE	BD	KM	CQ & AQ	PA	CG	TCM	PS
BD	1	1	1	1	1	1	3^1
KM	1^1	1	1^1	1^1	1	1	3^1
CQ & AQ	1^1	1	1	1^1	1	1	1^1
PA	1^1	1	1	1	3	1	1^1
CG	1^1	1^1	1^1	3^1	1	1	1^1
TCM	1^1	1^1	1^1	1^1	1^1	1	1^1
PS	3	3	1	1	1	1	1

λ_{max}=7.7882, CI= 0.1313, CR=0.0995

Table 7. α-cuts fuzzy comparison matrix for the determinants (α= 0.5)

Quality Components	BD	KM	CQ&AQ	PAM	CG	TCM	PS
BD	[1,1]	[1,2]	[1/2,1]	[1,2]	[1,2]	[1,2]	[1/4,1/2]
KM	[1/2,1]	[1,1]	[1/2,1]	[1/2,1]	[1,2]	[1,2]	[1/4,1/2]
CQ&AQ	[1,1]	[1,2]	[1,1]	[1/2,1]	[1,2]	[1,2]	[1/2,1]
PA	[1/2,1]	[1,2]	[1,2]	[1,1]	[2,4]	[1,2]	[1/2,1]
CG	[1/2,1]	[1/2,1]	[1/2,1]	[1/4,1/2]	[1,1]	[1,1]	[1/2,1]
TCM	[1/2,1]	[1/2,1]	[1/2,1]	[1/2,1]	[1/4,1/2]	[1,1]	[1/2,1]
PS	[2,4]	[2,4]	[1,2]	[1,2]	[1,2]	[1,2]	[1,1]

Table 8. Pair wise comparison matrix for the relative importance of the determinants (CR = 0.0995)

Quality Components	BD	KM	CQ&AQ	PAM	CG	TCM	PS	e-Vector
BD	1.000	1.500	0.750	1.500	1.500	1.500	0.375	0.136
KM	0.750	1.000	0.750	0.750	1.500	1.500	0.375	0.109
CQ&AQ	1.500	1.500	1.000	0.750	1.500	1.500	0.750	0.145
PA	0.750	1.500	1.500	1.000	3.000	1.500	0.750	0.169
CG	0.750	0.750	0.750	0.375	1.000	3.000	0.750	0.120
TCM	0.750	0.750	0.750	0.750	0.375	1.000	0.750	0.095
PS	3.000	3.000	1.500	1.500	1.500	1.500	1.000	0.226

λ_{max}=7.7882, CI= 0.1313, CR=0.0995

Further, the sub-components of above mentioned seven quality components have been pair wise compared at level III matrix. The composite relative weights and global weight of each quality components of potential HCEs were finally subjected to calculation for the purpose of finding their overall rating based on which HCE-A, HCE-B and HCE-C could be assessed for selecting the best HCE among them (Table 9 and 10).

Table 9. Composite relative weights of Quality components of potential HCE using Fuzzy AHP

Sr. No.	Quality Components Factors	Code	Relative Weights	Sub factor Code	Relative Weights
1	Burden of Disease	(BD)	0.1365	BD-1	0.1160
				BD-2	0.5293
				BD-3	0.3547
2	Knowledge Management	(KM)	0.1089	KM-1	0.1680
				KM-2 to 4	0.1511
				KM-5 & 5a	0.1359
				KM-6 & 7	0.1358
				KM-8	0.1397
				KM-9a, 9b& 10	0.2695
3	Core Qualities & Associated Supportive Qualities	(CQ&AQ)	0.1451	AQ: CR-1	0.1241
				CQ;CR-1	0.2669
				AQ:OSR-1 to4	0.5509
				CQ:OSR-1 to 5	0.0581
4	Priority Areas Management of Operation Room (OR/ OT), Intensive Care Unit (ICU), Casualty Department (Accident & Emergency) (CD:A&E)	(PAM)	0.1687	PAM:OT-1 to 3	0.1160
				PAM: Cas. D (A&E)-1to3	0.5293
				PAM:ICU-1 to 4	0.3547
5	Clinical Governance	(CG)	0.1203	CG (i)-1	0.1241
				CG (i)-2	0.2669
				CG (i)-3	0.5509
				CG (i)-4	0.0581
6	Treatment Chain Management, Referrals Evacuation (Ambulance services &in-transit care), Maintenance of Records	(TCM)	0.0949	TCM:IC-1to 3	0.1160
				TCM: EVC-1	0.5293
				TCM: Doc&R-1	0.3547
7	Patient satisfaction (PS) {Patient Expectation & Patient Perception (PE&PP) (by Gap: PE& PP)& overall(O) Patient Perception of Hospital Services (PPO)}	(PS)	0.2256	PE -1 to 8	0.1160
				PP -1 to 8	0.5293
				PPO	0.3547

Table 10. Overall all rating of potential HCE –A, HCE –B and HCE –C being considered for selection

Sr. No.	Code	Relative Weights	Sub factor Code	Relative Weights	Global Weights	HCE –A	HCE -B	HCE -C	HCE -A	HCE -B	HCE -C
1	(BD)	0.1365	BD-1	0.1160	0.0158	0.1409	0.2158	0.6433	0.0022	0.0034	0.0102
			BD-2	0.5293	0.0722	0.6433	0.1409	0.2158	0.0465	0.0102	0.0156
			BD-3	0.3547	0.0484	0.7044	0.1305	0.1651	0.0341	0.0063	0.0080
2	(KM)	0.1089	KM-1	0.1680	0.0183	0.0914	0.5063	0.4023	0.0017	0.0093	0.0074
			KM-2 to 4	0.1511	0.0165	0.1080	0.1533	0.7387	0.0018	0.0025	0.0122
			KM-5 & 5a	0.1359	0.0148	0.1409	0.2158	0.6433	0.0021	0.0032	0.0095
			KM-6 & 7	0.1358	0.0148	0.1160	0.3547	0.5293	0.0017	0.0052	0.0078
			KM-8	0.1397	0.0152	0.1160	0.3547	0.5293	0.0018	0.0054	0.0081
			KM-9a, 9b& 10	0.2695	0.0294	0.1080	0.1533	0.7387	0.0032	0.0045	0.0217
3	(CQ&AQ)	0.1451	AQ: CR-1	0.1241	0.0180	0.0908	0.2493	0.6599	0.0016	0.0045	0.0119
			CQ;CR-1	0.2669	0.0387	0.6433	0.1409	0.2158	0.0249	0.0055	0.0084
			AQ:OSR-1 to4	0.5509	0.0799	0.1160	0.3547	0.5293	0.0093	0.0283	0.0423
			CQ:OSR-1 to 5	0.0581	0.0084	0.1409	0.2158	0.6433	0.0012	0.0018	0.0054
4	(PAM)	0.1687	PAM:OT-1 to 3	0.1160	0.0196	0.1409	0.2158	0.6433	0.0028	0.0042	0.0126
			PAM: Case. D (A&E)-1to3	0.5293	0.0893	0.6599	0.0908	0.2493	0.0589	0.0081	0.0223
			PAM:ICU-1 to 4	0.3547	0.0598	0.1160	0.5293	0.3547	0.0069	0.0317	0.0212
5	(CG)	0.1203	CG (i)-1	0.1241	0.0149	0.0769	0.3832	0.5399	0.0011	0.0057	0.0081
			CG (i)-2	0.2669	0.0321	0.1409	0.2158	0.6433	0.0045	0.0069	0.0207
			CG (i)-3	0.5509	0.0663	0.6599	0.2493	0.0908	0.0437	0.0165	0.0060
			CG (i)-4	0.0581	0.0070	0.1160	0.5293	0.3547	0.0008	0.0037	0.0025
6	(TCM)	0.0949	TCM:IC-1to 3	0.1160	0.0110	0.4134	0.5204	0.0662	0.0046	0.0057	0.0007
			TCM: EVC-1	0.5293	0.0503	0.1160	0.5293	0.3547	0.0058	0.0266	0.0178
			TCM: Doc&R-1	0.3547	0.0337	0.6433	0.1409	0.2158	0.0217	0.0047	0.0073
7	(PS)	0.2256	PE -1 to 8	0.1160	0.0262	0.5293	0.3547	0.1160	0.0138	0.0093	0.0030
			PP -1 to 8	0.5293	0.1194	0.6433	0.1409	0.2158	0.0768	0.0168	0.0258
			PPO	0.3547	0.0800	0.1409	0.2158	0.6433	0.0113	0.0173	0.0515
Overall priority									0.3848	0.2475	0.3677
Rank									1	3	2

Chapter 26
TQM Practices in Public Sector:
Case of Finnish Healthcare Organizations

Mian M. Ajmal
Abu Dhabi University, UAE

Ville Tuomi
University of Vaasa, Finland

Petri T. Helo
University of Vaasa, Finland

Maqsood Ahmad Sandhu
UAE University, UAE

ABSTRACT

This study aims to discuss the evolution, principles, and stages of total quality management (TQM) in public health care organizations. It also makes a comparison that how case organizations think about quality and TQM along with its applicability within public sector. The study can be categorized as qualitative research. The data is collected from semi structural interviews of the informants and the concerning documents, which consist of strategy, policy papers and audit reports of the case organizations. Altogether there are two case organizations. Furthermore, data is analyzed with the help of content analysis. Most vital issues in TQM practices are its comprehensiveness, and its application in such a way which is appropriate for the organization, with a logical way of operation and the participation of management and personnel. Training, guidance, teamwork, involvement and learning are imperative for achieving a continuous improvement culture and are vital elements when adopting TQM. Managers should learn from the experience of TQM implementers by studying expected challenges and pitfalls. They should also pay more attention to the crucial role of all stakeholders in the TQM implementation. The study could be quite valuable from a strategic perspective in providing guidelines to build up a proper plan for TQM practices more promptly. The paper also manages to shed light on TQM practices of public service organizations by comparing their current approaches to quality.

DOI: 10.4018/978-1-7998-2451-0.ch026

Copyright © 2020, IGI Global. Copying or distributing in print or electronic forms without written permission of IGI Global is prohibited.

INTRODUCTION

In the past TQM used to be implemented in the manufacturing sector, but now it has also been widely applied in service organizations and the public sector (Fryer et al., 2007) e.g. health care. All kinds of organizations in the private as well as the public sector are looking to be customer-oriented organizations to carry on their operations in a globally competitive environment. Therefore to compete as customer-oriented organizations it is necessary to offer quality products and services to their customers. Subsequently, TQM is such a philosophy that provides the tools and the direction to improve the quality of their products and services.

However, TQM implementation in manufacturing firms is not considered a novel and multifaceted strategy, but TQM implementation and practice particularly in public service organizations like health-care is really quite a recent and composite undertaking. The introduction of the TQM term in health care is well established, but there is still lack of such a supporting framework that can make it easier for newcomers to follow the boulevard.

Therefore, the objective of this research is to study which kinds of TQM practices there are in public sector services, whether they are applying a fully-fledged TQM approach or only some parts of the TQM are being employed? More specifically, this research proceeds to examine the implementation of TQM in the public service organizations in the attempts to:

- Present an overview of TQM initiatives in service organizations
- Identify the level of understanding and knowledge about TQM in health care

To accomplish the objective mentioned above and to achieve sub goals of the study, the paper will analyze the distinctiveness of the TQM practices in each target organization. First, it will carry on by providing an up to date literature review of the associated terms individually with more emphasis on quality, TQM and its applicability in service organizations. Second, it will elaborate on the methodological approach which has been employed during this study and a description of all target organizations. Third, it will illustrate the results along with discussion and managerial implications. Finally, it draws some conclusions based on the present results and discussions in light of previous literature. It also includes an appendix that portraits an overview of TQM practices and approaches of all case organizations.

LITERATURE REVIEW

Service Quality

Quality is concerned with fulfilling the needs, wants and expectations of the valued customers. One of the key and stable definitions may be that, 'quality is suitability for purpose'. Quality is also defined as 'satisfying customer's requirements' or 'fitness for purpose' (Ghobadian et al., 1994). However, it is complex to define service quality rather than the quality of goods. Service quality can be defines as an attitude of the consumer relating to the results from comparisons between expectations of service with his perceptions of actual performance (Grönroos, 2007). The quality of services executed can only be appraised during or after consumption (Audhesh et al., 2004). The more composite and personal the service, the more detective effort customers will perform (Berry et al., 2006). The primary source of value creation for a service quality is performance by the service provider. It is often the small things that influence a customer's overall perception of service quality, be it the tangibility associated with the service or the behavior or technical performance by the service provider (Kumar et al., 2010).

Service Quality Dimensions

The most commonly stated set of service quality was offered by Zeithaml et al. (1990), who using factor analysis, condensed the dimensions of service quality into five categories:

1. Tangibles (facilities, equipment and appearance of staff);
2. Reliability (ability to perform the promised service dependably and accurately);
3. Responsiveness (willingness to help customers and provide prompt service);
4. Assurance (knowledge and courtesy of staff and their ability to convey trust and confidence);
5. Empathy (caring, individualized attention the organization provides to its customers).

Total Quality Management

According to British Standard BS 7850, TQM is defined as management philosophy and company practices that endeavor to strap up the human and material resources of an organization in the most efficient way to accomplish the organizational objectives. In general, the overall scope of quality, total quality and TQM can be classified as follows (Kanji, 1991):

- **Quality:** Is to satisfy customer's requirement persistently;
- **Total Quality:** Is to achieve quality at low cost;
- **Total Quality Management**: Is to obtain total quality by involving everyone's daily commitment.

According to Vouzas and Psychogios (2007) there are two substantial aspects of TQM that can be identified; the 'hard' side and the 'soft' side. The hard (or technical) side refers to management tools and practices, while the soft (or philosophical) is associated with management concepts and principles. The hard aspects of TQM consist of clear and well documented methods while the soft aspects compose its whole theory, combining its background and philosophical elements. It is argued that TQM has to evolve. Four stages can be identified in the evolution of TQM:

- Inspection-based System;
- System of Quality Control;
- Quality Assurance;
- Total Quality Management.

Quality Management initiated with a simple Inspection-based system, where a product was compared with a product standard by a team of inspectors. First revolutionary charge – System of Quality Control came along with World War II. At that time quality was achieved through control systems, product testing and documentation control. In the Quality Assurance stage, there was a change from product quality to systems quality. Typical of this stage were quality manuals, quality planning and advanced document control. Quality assurance is prevention-based. The fourth stage of development was TQM. A clear and unambiguous vision, few interdepartmental barriers, staff training, excellent customer relations, emphasis on continuous improvement, and quality of the company as a whole are typical in a TQM environment.

Over time the definitions of quality management have been widened to incorporate the wellbeing of society, the environment and future generations. A large part of the development of quality concept and quality management has taken place without much consideration of what quality management really is or should be. It has been claimed, that quality management should focus on customers and their satisfaction and not concentrate on stakeholders and interest parties who are affected by the products and processes (Klefsjö et al., 2008), but on the other hand TQM is in many researches said to be implemented with the help of quality awards, which are considered as excellence models (Bou-Lusar et al., 2008; Vernero et al., 2007).

TQM can be described as the development of an organizational culture, which is defined by, and supports, the constants attainment of customer satisfaction through an integrated system of techniques and tools. TQM is a way of managing to improve the effectiveness, efficiency, flexibility, and competitiveness of a business as a whole. There are eight most common principles in the TQM: leadership and management, strategic planning, focus on customer, focus on employees, focus on suppliers, focus on material resources, process management and performance results (Rad, 2005).

Total Quality Management in Healthcare

In exceedingly competitive healthcare environments, hospitals similar to all other public or private organizations and institutions, are confronted with the stipulation of measuring both their financial (costs, revenues, profitability) and non-financial performance (quality of their services), in order to improve their functions and increase their competitiveness (Chaniotakis and Lymperopoulos, 2009). Performance measurement is not an easy task in health services, where a wide range of stakeholders are involved. Lim and Tang (2000) argue that customer based determinants and perceptions of service quality play an important role in hospitals. Hence, Wisniewski and Wisniewski (2005) revealed that service quality from the patients' perspective should be consistently monitored and assessed. Silvestro (2005) proposes the development of a tool for measuring the gap between patients' priorities and their perceptions and the match between the patient and management perspective.

Ovretveit (2001) has found seven components in integrated quality development in hospitals, which is an application of total quality management in a hospital. The components are based on longitudinal empirical research in European hospitals. The components are as follows:

1. Four coordinated organization-wide programs to develop professionals' competencies, managers' competencies, organization and processes, and a new role for patients;
2. Three-dimensional definition of quality (patient, professional and management quality);
3. Patient pathway and process development;
4. Quality data gathering;
5. Team quality projects;
6. Patient focused system development; and
7. Creating 'soulful spirals' and preventing 'soulless spirals'.

These seven components aim to combine effective established professional quality assurance methods with newer quality improvement methods, simultaneously by improving patient, professional and management quality, and describing and developing the system of care experienced by the patient in a soulful way.

Conceptualization of Critical Dimensions of TQM in Hospitals

An instrument that identifies the operating elements of TQM in hospitals from the viewpoint of the health-care service providers has been developed and validated in the study by Duggirala et al., (2008). It has also identified critical factors of provider-perceived TQM in hospitals:

1. Top management commitment and leadership;
2. Human resource management in the hospital:
    a. Selection;
    b. Training;
    c. Employee involvement;
3. Process management:
    a. Ease of access to the hospital, and ease of admission processes and procedures;
    b. Administrative services;
    c. Processes: administrative and clinical;
    d. Exit;
    e. Clinical outcomes of medical care;
4. Hospital facilities and infrastructure;
5. Patient focus;
6. Employee focus;
7. Measurement of hospital performance;
8. Hospital information system;
9. Errors, safety and risk management;
10. Service culture;
11. Continuous improvement;
12. Benchmarking;
13. Union influence;
14. Governance and social responsibility.

According to Bassand et al., (2007) TQM in healthcare is a relative concept that requires comparison either with the performances of others or with the standards. The measurement of quality needs to be relevant for both service providers and patients, and also the process of care should be measured. There should be regional and/or national programs to measure performance indicators systematically and provide feedback to individual hospitals.

METHODOLOGY

This study is qualitative because of its subject, quality management that is a vague subject, with many dimensions (Garvin, 1988) and a hospital is also complex organization with multiple goals (Kast & Rosenzweig, 1970). A qualitative approach allows a researcher to deal with complexity, context and fuzzy phenomena. For example, holistic case studies are applicable in these kinds of situations (Gummesson 2006, 167). Qualitative methods are also very suitable for studies concerning organizational change, because they allow the detailed analysis of the change and by using the qualitative methods we can assess how (what processes are involved) and why (in terms of circumstances and stakeholders) the change has occurred (Cassell & Symon, 1994- 5). However this research process consists of the following steps applied from the study of Lukka (2003):

1. Find a practically relevant problem which also has potential for theoretical contribution;
2. Examine the potential long-term research co-operation with the target organization(s);
3. Obtain deep understanding of the topic area both practically and theoretically;
4. Innovate a solution idea and develop a problem solving construction, which also has potential for theoretical contribution;
5. Implement a solution and test how it works;
6. Ponder the scope of applicability of the solution;
7. Identify and analyze the theoretical construction.

The study material consists of semi structural interviews of the informants, audit reports, strategies and other documents available. The material is analyzed with the help of content analysis. Some previous studies, which have used the same approach, are for example Kunkel & Westerling (2006). Interview made from the following informants:

- Central Hospital of the Vaasa Hospital District (CHV); general manager, manager doctor, quality manager, manager of the heart unit, politician;
- Central Hospital of the Keski-Pohjanmaa Hospital District (CHK); general manager, manager doctor, quality manager, manager of the heart unit and worker (group interview), politician.

The content analysis can be defined as any methodological measurement applied to text (or other symbolic materials) for social science purposes (Duriau et al., 2007). Content analyzes are most successful when they focus on facts that are constituted in language, in the uses of particular texts which the content analysts are analyzing. Such linguistically constituted facts can be divided into four classes: attributions, social relationships, public behaviors and institutional realities. Attributions are concepts, attitudes, beliefs, intentions, emotions, mental states and cognitive processes which ultimately manifest themselves in the verbal attributes of behavior. They are not observable as such. Institutional realities, like the government, are constructions that rely heavily on language. See the exact description of the content analysis of the study in appendix.

Target Organizations

Altogether there are two target organizations. These are regional hospitals and in both hospitals managers of the units are chosen for examples of sub-units of hospitals because of their supposed quality management experiences. Below is a short overview of each exploring their strengths, weaknesses, possibilities and threats regarding TQM practices.

Table 1. Strengths, weaknesses, possibilities and threats concerning TQM

Strengths	
Strengths • Enough know-how • A tradition of systematic working • Easy to learn new theories and models • Well educated personnel • Ethical background • Language of the SHQS is suitable for the health care industry • Much experience of development work • Commitment towards TQM (nursing staff) • Sufficient human resources • Planning of strategies, security policy and risk management (*) • Customer focus(*) • Meeting practices (*) • Human resources management practices, like well-being of the personnel, recruitment • Benchmarking (*)	**Weaknesses** • Insufficient know-how concerning quality work • Every patient and diagnosis is considered as unique cases • Multidimensionality of health care, lack of standardized products, rapidly increasing amount of knowledge • A big organization • Everything must be communicated in Swedish and in Finnish communication • Lack of commitment of physicians and other personnel • Quality systems in primary health care • Modeling and measurement of processes in hospital and unit levels (*) • Goals and measures of operation and levels (*) • Part of planning practices (*)
Possibilities • Changes in the operation environment force to improve the organization • Changes in the structure of municipalities and services can help hospitals to improve their operations • All the social- and health care units use the same kind of (quality) system and thus it is possible to create a unitary system • To find the process owner for the social and health care services across the organization boundaries • Top management of the central hospital is committed to quality work • Functionality of communication among the special fields	**Threats** • Border lines between professions • The aim has been to offer almost everything to essentially everybody for free. This leads to a continuous gap between the needs and possibilities of the whole public administration and falls heavily on health care. • Operation environment is changing and resources are needed to follow-up the changes. Maintenance of a quality system requires work on an almost daily basis. • Lack of resources • Cooperation between hospital districts and outpatient care: there is no motivation to improve quality in every place. • More and more specialized health care leads to a situation in which the patient's viewpoint disappears and totality becomes vague

(*) = audit report (SHQuality 2010)

Central Hospital of the Vaasa Hospital District, (CHV)

The Central Hospital of the Vaasa has an administrative role in the Vaasa Hospital District, which consists of three hospitals. The District is owned by 23 municipalities and it is a bilingual organization (both Swedish and Finnish speaking personnel, customers, and owners). The number of the personnel in the year 2010 was 1997, which consisted of nursing staff (1060), physicians (183), research staff (240), and maintenance staff (109). Services are offered for 166,000 inhabitants in the area of the municipalities (SHQuality, 2010). This Hospital District is one of the 20 Finnish hospital districts. See Tables 1 and 2 for strengths and weaknesses charts concerning TQM.

According to the quality policy and strategy, good quality in CHV is defined as service processes which are from the customer's or patient's point of view, high level, available, efficient and economic, and during which the well-being of the personnel and expectations of the stakeholders are taken into consideration (Vaasa Hospital District, 2007). In the strategy there is a decision to establish a quality system for the hospital (Vaasa Hospital District, 2003). In the heart unit of the CHV (8.10.2004) there is a quality manual which is made according to ISO 9001:2000 quality management standard. However, the hospital is still using the SHQS quality system (SHQuality, 2010).

Table 2. Strengths, weaknesses, possibilities and threats concerning TQM

Strengths	Weaknesses
• Electronic appointment in the laboratory • Citizen's acceptance • Networking with educational institutions • Long traditions of SHQS since the year 1996 • Qualified and committed internal audit group • Positive attitude of the personnel towards development (**) • Small organization (flexibility) • Big volumes and clear procedures of operations • Commitment of the personnel (*) • Customer focus (*) • Cost awareness (*) • Regional cooperation (*) • Commitment to values (*) • good job satisfaction survey (*)	• Funding system and attitudes concerning it • Appointment problems • Lack of commitment • Quality management is not applied on daily basis • No full-time development and quality manager • Small size of the organization • It is difficult to change (bureaucracy, trade-unions, etc.) • Complicated organization • Lack of physicians • No consideration about the totality of the social- and health care services • Lack of quality policy (*) • Information systems and knowledge management (*) • risk management (*) • process measurement (*)
Possibilities • Integrated clinical pathways can become more flexible and efficient while the organization is growing • Quality management may encompass the whole social and health care services	**Threats** • Belief in extremely big organizations • Recruitment of competent personnel fails • Municipalities don't understand SHQS • Cure is improved on an economic basis instead of the need of patients • Quality management is applied only partially and the totality is forgotten

(*) = audit report (SHQuality, 2010), (**) = both audit report (SHQuality, 2010) and interviews

Central Hospital of the Keski-Pohjanmaa Hospital District (CHK)

The Keski-Pohjanmaa Central Hosital has an administrative role in the Keski-Pohjanmaa Hospital District. The District is owned by 13 municipalities and it is a bilingual organization (both Swedish and Finnish speaking personnel, customers, and owners) (Keski-Pohjanmaa hospital District 19.11.2010). The number of the personnel in the year 2010 was 1143 and in the year 2011 it was 1164 (Keski-Pohjanmaa hospital District 2010).

In the strategic plan of the hospital, high service quality was mentioned as one of the key values of the hospital. The service quality is based on hearing the needs of the customer and patient, high-quality services, effectiveness, and taking care of knowledge, readiness of operation and facilities of operation (Keski-Pohjanmaa Hospital District, 19.11.2010).

FINDINGS

The development of a quality system is the most adopted initiative in all the case organizations. The least adopted TQM initiative is the application of statistical process control. This can be explained by the respondents' lack of knowledge about the exact control methods used by the Quality Improvement departments or, because some hospitals lack the financial resources and expertise to implement these statistical process control methods.

According to the interviews the most important issues in TQM practices is comprehensiveness, a systematic way of operation, the participation of management and personnel, high quality cure processes, reporting and reacting, the implementation of high-level goals (ethics and values), focus on development as well as measurement and goal levels. TQM is seen as quite applicable or very applicable to (a) hospitals and libraries but there are several issues, which foster the implementation of TQM. Language used in the implementation should be familiar and suitable to the target organizations, and unfamiliar language should not be used by force. SHQS is an example of translating the language of TQM into a language familiar to the healthcare industry. This requires it to be accommodated to healthcare.

In all the case organizations, they claimed that there is no TQM but simultaneously ISO quality standard is implemented there. TQM is usually seen as a method for practicing quality. However, TQM is not applied in every single part of the organization. In every organization they applied TQM in a way that is typical to the industry: in hospitals they used SHQS. In the heart unit of the Vaasa Central Hospital, they also applied ISO quality management standard. Furthermore, the heart units were evaluated by medical experts.

It is visible that everybody is talking about quality assurance instead of quality management or TQM. The most important issue in TQM is the totality, participation, continuous improvement and organizational learning process. In the interviews most problems were seen in the measurement processes of the TQM in such organizations.

DISCUSSION AND IMPLICATIONS

TQM is considered to be a generic management model that is applicable to every organization, but on the other hand it is also suggested that the operation environment of an organization should be taken into consideration while implementing quality management. It is crucial to persuade quality as early as possible, preferably at the initial stage of organizational operations. Organizational structure modification supports the success of TQM which must always be considered. Leadership and top management support are keys to TQM implementation and practice. Upper management must always conduct continuous improvement activities with the consensus of all employees. They should also make use of selective application of TQM tools and techniques by appraising their suitability with the organization. There must also be sufficient financial resources available for TQM initiatives (Tuomi, et al., 2013). Healthcare organizations must integrate quality indicators into their operational strategy with the aim of increasing customer satisfaction and safeguard competitive advantage (Ahmed, 2014).

Training, tutoring, teamwork and staff involvement are important for achieving a continuous improvement culture and are vital elements when adopting TQM. This claim is supported by Fung's (1998) study which showed that the learning team approach assists in accomplishing an educational organization and attains TQM. It is noted from the findings that most of the staff members from case organizations are not familiar with the approach of TQM, so providing appropriate training for employees and support from top management are considered vital success factors by most researchers (Ennis & Harrington, 1999). This result is consistent with the results of Rad (2005) concerning the key success factors for TQM implementation.

Successful TQM implementation requires top management commitment, employee involvement and empowerment, customer focus and continuous improvement, training for TQM throughout the organization and increased communication (Tuomi, et al., 2013). Furthermore, there is a need for patience and tolerance as it is a time-consuming process and it is not easy to change an organization. An increased focus on the area of organizational change related to TQM is also needed. To conclude, the successful

TQM implementation requires a thorough understanding of critical success factors, barriers to achieving these factors, and managerial tools and techniques to overcome these barriers along with continuous organizational learning. The barriers of the implementation of the TQM are resistance to change and people's attitudes, problems in finding funding and time for training, while maintaining current services in the library. It is also difficult to make a change in organizational structures, yet TQM requires institutions to restructure themselves (Moghaddam & Mogalleghi 2006) and be ready to learn each and every thing that occurs over the passage of time.

Finally, the results of research argue that TQM initiative implementation may seem to be an easy task, but this is a very illusory deliberation. The dilemma is not only how to implement the agenda, but how to make it work effectively and efficiently. Managers as well as quality policy makers should pay more attention to the vital role of all stakeholders in the TQM implementation and success stages. A non-implementer of the TQM philosophy should learn about the expected challenges and pitfalls from the experiences of TQM implementers.

REFERENCES

Ahmed, S. (2014). Simulation Method to Improve Hospital Service Quality. *International Journal of Information Systems in the Service Sector*, 6(3), 96–117. doi:10.4018/ijisss.2014070106

Audhesh, K. P., Spears, N., Hasty, R., & Gopala, G. (2004). Search quality in the financial services industry: A contingency perspective. *Journal of Services Marketing*, 18(5), 324–338. doi:10.1108/08876040410548267

Bassand, J.-P., Priori, S., & Tendera, M. (2007). Evidence-based vs. 'impressionist' medicine: How best to implement guidelines. *European Heart Journal*, 26(12), 1155–1158. doi:10.1093/eurheartj/ehi262 PMID:15870117

Berry, L. L., Wall, A. E., & Carbone, P. L. (2006). Service clues and customer assessment of the service experience: Lessons from marketing. *The Academy of Management Perspectives*, 20(2), 43–57. doi:10.5465/AMP.2006.20591004

Bou-Lusar, J. C., Escrig-Tena, A. B., Roca-Puig, V., & Beltrán-Martin, I. (2008). An empirical assessment of the EFQM Excellence Model: Evaluation as a TQM framework relative to the MBNQA Model. *Journal of Operations Management*, 27(1), 1–22. doi:10.1016/j.jom.2008.04.001

Cassell, C., & Symon, G. (1994). Qualitative research in work context. In Qualitative Methods in Organizational Research. A Practical Guide, Cassell, C. & Symon, G (ed.), 1–13. London: SAGE Publications. New Delhi: Thousand Oaks.

Chaniotakis, I. E., & Lymperopoulos, C. (2009). Service quality effect on satisfaction and word of mouth in the health care industry. *Managing Service Quality*, 19(2), 229–242. doi:10.1108/09604520910943206

Duggirala, M., Rajendran, C. & Anantharaman, R.N. (2008). Provider-perceived dimensions of total quality management in healthcare, *Benchmarking: an international journal*, 15(6), 693-722.

Duriau, V. I., Reger, R. K., & Pfarrer, M. D. (2007). A content analysis of the literature in organization studies: Research themes, data sources, and methodological refinements. *Organizational Research Methods*, 10(1), 5–34. doi:10.1177/1094428106289252

Ennis, K., & Harington, D. (1999). Factors to consider in the implementation of quality within Irish healthcare. *Managing Service Quality, 9*(5), 320–326. doi:10.1108/09604529910282508

Fryer, M., Antony, J., & Douglas, A. (2007). Critical success factors of continuous improvement in the public sector. A literature review and some key findings. *The TQM Magazine, 19*(5), 497–517. doi:10.1108/09544780710817900

Fung, M. (1998). A learning team approach for service organizations to achieve TQM and beat the competition. *Managing Service Quality, 8*(5), 367–374. doi:10.1108/09604529810235826

Garvin, D. A. (1988). *Managing Quality. New York*. Free Press.

Ghobadian, A., Speller, S., & Jones, M. (1994). Service quality: Concepts and models. *International Journal of Quality & Reliability Management, 11*(9), 43–66. doi:10.1108/02656719410074297

Grol, R., Baker, B., & Moss, F. (2002). Quality improvement research: Understanding the science of change in health care. *Quality & Safety in Health Care, 11*(2), 110–111. doi:10.1136/qhc.11.2.110 PMID:12448794

Gronroos, C. (2007). *Service management and marketing: customer management in service competition. Chisester*. Wiley.

Gummesson, E. (2006). Qualitative research in management: Addressing complexity, context and persona. *Management Decision, 44*(2), 167–176. doi:10.1108/00251740610650175

Heart unit of the Vaasa central hospital (8.10.2004). *Quality manual.* (in Finnish)

Juntunen, A., Ovaska, T., Saarti, J., & Salmi, L. (2005). Managing library processes: Collecting data and providing tailored services to end-users. *Library Management, 26*(8/9), 487–493. doi:10.1108/01435120510631774

Kanji, G. K. (1991). Education, training, research and consultancy – the way towards for total quality management. *Total Quality Management & Business Excellence, 2*(3), 207–212. doi:10.1080/09544129100000025

Kast & Rosenzweig. (1970). *Organization and Management. A Systems Approach. McGraw-Hill Series in Management*. New York: McGraw-Hill.

Keski-Pohjanmaa hospital District (2007). *Financial statement.* (in Finnish).

Keski-Pohjanmaa Hospital District (19.11.2007). *Budget and economic plan.* (in Finnish and Swedish).

Kunkel, S. T., & Westerling, R. (2006). Different types and aspects of quality systems and their implications. A thematic comparison of seven quality systems at a university hospital. *Health Policy (Amsterdam), 76*(2), 125–133. doi:10.1016/j.healthpol.2005.05.004 PMID:15982780

Lim, P. C., & Tang, N. K. H. (2000). A study of patients' expectations and satisfaction in Singapore hospitals. *International Journal of Health Care Quality Assurance, 1*(7), 290–299. PMID:11484647

Lukka, K. (2003). The constructive research approach. In Case Study Research in Logistics, L Ojala and O-P Hilmola (eds.), pp. 83–101. Turku: Publications of the Turku School of Economics and Business Administration. Series B 1/2003.

Moghaddam, G. G., & Mogalleghi, M. (2008). Total quality management in library and information sectors. *The Electronic Library*, *26*(6), 912–922. doi:10.1108/02640470810921664

Rad, A. (2005). A survey of total quality management in Iran: Barriers to successful implementation in health care organizations. *Leadership in Health Services*, *18*(3), 12–34. doi:10.1108/13660750510611189

SHQuality. (2006). *Audit report of the Keski-Pohjanmaa Hospital District*. Kokkola. (in Finnish)

SHQuality (2007). Audit report of the Vaasa Hospital District. 17 September. Vaasa (in Finnish).

Silvestro, R. (2005). Applying gap analysis in the health service to inform the service improvement agenda. *International Journal of Quality & Reliability Management*, *12*(3), 215–233. doi:10.1108/02656710510582462

Strategy of the Vaasa Hospital District 2003–2010. (2003). Vaasa: Vaasa Hospital District. (in Finnish)

Tuomi, V., Ajmal, M.M. & Helo, P.T. (2013). 'Implementing TQM initiatives in public service organizations: case of academic libraries', *International journal of productivity and quality management*, 11(4), 393–411.

Vaasa Hospital District. (2007). *Quality Policy and Quality Strategies of the Vaasa Hospital District*. Vaasa: Vaasa Hospital District. (in Finnish)

Vernero, S., Nabitz, U., Bragonzi, G., Rebelli, A., & Molinari, R. (2007). A two-level EFQM self-assessment in an Italian hospital. *International Journal of Health Care Quality Assurance*, *20*(3), 215–223. doi:10.1108/09526860710743354 PMID:17585618

Vouzas, F., & Psychogios, A. G. (2007). Assessing managers' awareness of TQM. *The TQM Magazine*, *19*(1), 62–75. doi:10.1108/09544780710720844

Wisniewski, M., & Wisniewski, H. (2005). Measuring service quality in a hospital colposcopy clinic. *International Journal of Health Care Quality Assurance*, *18*(3), 217–228. doi:10.1108/09526860510594776 PMID:15974517

Zeithaml, V. A., Parasuraman, A., & Berry, L. L. (1990). *Delivering quality service: balancing customer perceptions and expectations. New Your*. The Free Press.

This research was previously published in the International Journal of Information Systems in the Service Sector (IJISSS), 8(1); edited by John Wang; pages 34-44, copyright year 2016 by IGI Publishing (an imprint of IGI Global).

APPENDIX

Comparison of the Cases

Table 3. Definition of the quality and approach to TQM

	CHK	CHV
Definition of quality	Best possible cures in a cost-effective and appropriate way including the availability of the service. Small amount of defects, combination of different kinds of viewpoints, i.e. experience of the patient, technical quality of the cure, management and personnel; all good operations; systematic operations, enough documentation and well-defined regulations	Good available cure based on patients/customers' needs, effective and economic service processes, and operations in which the well-being of the personnel and expectations of the stakeholders are taken into consideration.
Approach to TQM VS strategy *Why quality is needed? *Most important issues in total quality	QM supports the establishment of a strategy by giving information. There has to be 4-6 key goals in a smaller unit and well thought out meanings to these goals in their operations. The goals in the units have to be concrete and connected to time, resources and economy. QM is needed because of the following reasons: • To get an overall view of operation: economy + personnel + process/customers viewpoint. • Operations can't be improved without evaluation and documentation. The most important issues in QM are the following: - patient centeredness, communication with personnel, being in the right place at the right time from the operations point of view - to find measures and to develop evaluation - follow-up - Clear management system based on information and documentation generated by quality management	Quality system and strategy are closely interconnected. The quality system calls for clear strategic goals and vision. Quality work is based on values, which in turn are included in strategy. QM is needed for the following reasons: • - to control totality • - to implement values • - On the other hand it is a management fad, but it is also needed a) to guarantee cure for customers and to show what kind of working place it is. • - low quality work must be avoided • - required regulations The most important issues in QM are the following: • - comprehensiveness • - applying QM in a way which is suitable for the organization • - systematic way of operation • - participation of management and personnel • - high quality cure processes • - reporting, reacting

Table 4. Applicability to the public sector

	CHK	CHV
How easy it is to apply in the public sector?	quite easy	quite easy or very easy
Reasons why it could be applicable	- the existence of an organization depends on quality	TQM –thinking is very applicable to public administration, if it is reconciled with health care
Issues which make it difficult to apply QM:	If innovativeness is decreasing because of the "quality". If the situation of a patient with multiple problems is not taken into consideration.	Organizational structure as a mixture of service and production organization, difficulties in standardization and more dramatic understanding of deficiencies.

Table 5. Total quality management in practice

	CHK	CHV
State of art	Quality work is both every day work as well as a separate project.	Quality work is both every day work (like in the heart unit) and distinct development work.
Practical implications in quality work	• Education and projects in which clinical pathways and service chains are identified and described together with stakeholders	Process improvement and documentation concerning risks.
Quality tools	SHQS and quality tools, which include flow charts and cause-and-effect diagrams	SHQS (includes self-evaluations and audits), ISO quality management standards, and group work methods

Table 6. The roles of the personnel and management in the TQM

	CHK	CHV
The role of personnel	Participation in development projects, work as a member of an expert team, consider feedback in an appropriate way and not emotionally	Commitment, good work and know how concerning continuous improvement
The role of management	To provide resources, emphasize the importance of quality and work as a role model. To provide information on statistics, and reward appropriately	To motivate personnel, commitment, work as a role model and provide resources

Table 7. Evaluation and measurement in the organization

	CHK	CHV
Measurement and evaluation in general	SHQS, and medical evaluations	SHQS (includes self-evaluations and audits), evaluations of authorities, follow-up of statistics, benchmarking etc.
Measurement of customer satisfaction	Common surveys; clinic specific evaluations, like questionnaires, calling to patients and feedback boxes; utilization of ICT will come in the future	• Twice annually with surveys. • Feedback is discussed in the different units of the hospital
Process measurement	delay (time), patient satisfaction, technical quality, economy/costs, personnel, lead time, efficiency, effectiveness, medical evaluation etc.,	- There should be measurement instruments with many viewpoints.
Problems in the utilization of the evaluations and measurements	• Technology is underdeveloped • Interpretation of the feedback is difficult • Finns are not in the habit of complaining (too polite)	• All the measures should not be chosen at the hospital level • The effectiveness of the units can't be measured and is the right thing being done

Table 8. Process improvement

	CHK	CHV
Importance of the processes for good quality. How to improve processes?	Processes are important It is important to increase service oriented development instead of diagnosis centeredness. A clinical pathway is a wider concept than a process; there must be compatibility between processes and clinical pathways.	Processes are important • • Processes should be improved by identifying, describing and measuring them. • • The goals of the hospital are vague: to make patients healthy.

Chapter 27

Hospital Service Quality from Patients Perspective:
A Case of Indonesia

Puspa Indahati Sandhyaduhita
Universitas Indonesia, Indonesia

Haya Rizqi Fajrina
Universitas Indonesia, Indonesia

Ave Adriana Pinem
Universitas Indonesia, Indonesia

Achmad Nizar Hidayanto
Universitas Indonesia, Indonesia

Putu Wuri Handayani
Universitas Indonesia, Indonesia

Kasiyah M. Junus
Universitas Indonesia, Indonesia

ABSTRACT

This study aims to identify and analyse strategic service quality as perception-minus-expectation from patient perspective using SERVQUAL-based Handayani et al.'s framework. The result from 297 respondents shows that the criteria gaps are given as follows in descending order from the biggest gap: (1) responsiveness, (2) assurance, (3) professionalism, (4) reliability, (5) empathy and (6) tangible. Apparently, the gap for each criterion transpires to be significantly different which straightforwardly indicates the quality of the service delivered by hospitals for each criterion is still below respondents' expectations. Recommendation towards hospitals is proposed from technological point of view in forms of IT support in order to significantly improve the process as the dimension of the responsiveness criterion. Nonetheless, suggestion towards the Ministry of Health as the policy maker is also addressed that urges the establishment of policy and its implementation concerning IT support for accelerating hospitals automation.

DOI: 10.4018/978-1-7998-2451-0.ch027

Copyright © 2020, IGI Global. Copying or distributing in print or electronic forms without written permission of IGI Global is prohibited.

INTRODUCTION

As a developing country with a projected population of 255 million in 2015 according to the Statistics Central Bureau[1], the Indonesian healthcare industry must also grow to serve its population. In order to provide healthcare services, the Indonesian Ministry of Health (Kemenkes) employs a Health Referral System which is authorized by the Health Minister Regulation No. 001 Year 2012 regarding Individual Healthcare Referral System (Hukor, 2014). In the Referral System, patients' health service is provided by three tiers; tier one is provided by primary healthcare facilities, e.g., Puskesmas, clinics or Pratama hospitals, that provide basic healthcare services; tier two is provided by hospitals both generals and specialized hospitals, that provide specialist healthcare services; and tier three is provided by hospitals that provide sub specialist healthcare services. Thus, it is evident that hospitals hold a vital role in providing healthcare services to the people.

According to Data Rumah Sakit Online[2], there are 2,333 hospitals with a total of 283,515 inpatient beds available. Although the overall ratio beds to population is still around the WHO standard (1:1000), there many areas in which the ratio is below standard[3][4][5]. This inpatient bed shortage will surely affect the healthcare service quality since hospitals have to reject the patients due to bed shortage. Moreover, many Indonesian hospitals in tier two also state that they endure health personnel shortages including general and specialist doctors, nurses and administrative staff[6][7][8][9][10]. Furthermore, besides those two there are some other factors that could hinder healthcare service quality, e.g., complex/time-consuming administration process in hospital, medicine or medical equipment unavailability, etc.[11].

On the 1st January 2014, the Indonesian Government launched the National Health Coverage (JKN)[12], authorized by Law No. 40 Year 2004 (SJSN, 2004), through BPJS which is established by Law No. 24 Year 2011 (BPJS, 2011), as a concrete effort to guarantee that the healthcare of all Indonesian citizens are covered. Consequently, this program will increase the number of patients in the hospitals. As hospitals in general are not well-prepared to anticipate the increase, hospitals capacity (facility and healthcare personnel) is unable to meet the demand for healthcare services[13]. Therefore, this event will further exacerbate the earlier situation in which services quality is already hindered by the lack of bed, health personnel, etc.

A poor health service quality is certainly undesirable, especially since the subject is a human being. As human beings and the prime consumers of health services, patients undoubtedly have their own expectations and perceptions of the health services they experience. Understanding patients' perception is deemed necessary because patient satisfaction is essential for quality assurance in medical services and hospitals (Laslet, 1994 in Sohail, 2003). Moreover, O'Connor et. al., (as cited in Shabila et. al., 2014) noted that "patients' perspective is increasingly viewed as a meaningful and important indicator of health service quality that should be taken into account as part of a comprehensive assessment of quality health care". Thus, understanding patients' expectation and perceptions and analyzing the gaps can further give direction for hospitals, viz. the management, in order to improve their services quality from the patients' perspectives, e.g., by evaluating hospitals' current services against the gaps.

A widely used scale for measuring service quality is proposed by Parasuraman, Zeithaml, and Berry (Pasuraman et al., 1985) namely SERVQUAL. SERVQUAL has 5 dimensions, viz., Tangible, Reliability, Assurance, Responsiveness, and Empathy. A previous study by Handayani et al. (2014a) adapts SERVQUAL and formulates a framework to identify and analyze strategic hospital service quality from the perspective of hospital management, government policy maker and academicians in Indonesia. It follows that in Handayani et al. (2014b) patient's expectation was being considered. However, Handayani's study did not address a more detailed and intensive review on the service quality from patient perspective in terms of perception-minus-expectation that is required in order to give directions for hospitals as previously mentioned especially in the case of a developing country. Therefore, this study's goal is to identify and analyse strategic service quality as perception-minus-expectation from patient perspective. Further, this study will adopt SERVQUAL dimensions of Handayani et al.'s framework (Handayani et al., 2014a; 2014b).

This paper is organized as follows: section 2 explains the literature review, while the research conceptual model is explained in section 3. The research methodology and result is discussed in section 4 and 5. Then, the discussion and implication of this research are discussed in section 6. The final sections discuss the conclusions and future works for limitations of this research.

LITERATURE REVIEW

Service Quality

SERVQUAL (Parasuraman et al., 1988) provides dimensions for measuring and managing service quality namely reliability, assurance, tangibles, empathy, and responsiveness as defined in Table 1. SERVQUAL has been widely used in various researches and some works such as of Al Bassam & Al Shawi (2011), Shahin & Samea (2010) and Buttle (1996) have been done to examine and evaluate the applicability of SERVQUAL and its dimensions. Modification as well as critics had been proposed towards SERVQUAL such as one of Cronin and Taylor (1994) which proposed SERVPERF instead of SERVQUAL. Nevertheless, Buttle (1996) states "despite these shortcomings, SERVQUAL seems to be moving rapidly toward institutionalized status". This is also supported by Rust and Zahorik (as cited in Buttle, 1996) who observe that "the general SERVQUAL dimensions … should probably be put on any first pass as a list of attributes of services". Thus, in a review of 20 years of SERVQUAL research, Ladhari (2009) concludes that SERVQUAL remains a useful instrument for service-quality research.

Hospital Service Quality from Patient's Perspective

Through a non-exhaustive literature search, a number of empirical studies concerning patient's perspective on hospital service quality have been found since the 90s such as of Tomes and Chee Peng (1995), Lam (1997), Sixma et al. (1998). Until recently some studies were performed in developing countries such as Bangladesh (Analeeb, 2001), Iran (Zarei et al., 2012; Aghamolaei et al., 2014), Qatar (Chaker

Table 1. SERVQUAL Dimensions (Parasuraman et al., 1988)

Dimension	Definition
Reliability	The ability to perform the promised service dependably and accurately
Assurance	The knowledge and courtesy of employees and their ability to convey trust and confidence
Tangibles	The appearance of physical facilities, equipment, personnel and communication materials
Empathy	The provision of caring, individualized attention to customers
Responsiveness	The willingness to help customers and to provide prompt service

Table 2. Previous Studies of Patients' Perspectives

Reference	Goal	Country	Conceptual Framework, Method	Result
Tomes & Peng, 1995	Assessing in-patient perceptions of service quality in an NHS or NHS Trust hospital	UK	A multi-item scale: Five intangible factors: empathy, relationship of mutual respect, dignity, understanding of illness and religious needs, and two tangible factors: food and physical environment	Patients' perceptions meet or exceed expectations in respect of four of the seven factors and 22 of the 49 individual variables.
Lam, 1997	Demonstrate the use of SERVQUAL for measuring patients' perceptions of health care quality in Hong Kong	Hong Kong	SERVQUAL	Perceived health care service performance generally falls short of expectations except in the physical elements of service quality. Timely, professional and competent services are what patients expect from health care providers.
Lim & Tang, 2000	Determine the expectations and perceptions of patients through the use of a generic, internationally used market research technique called SERVQUAL	Singapore	SERVQUAL	There was an overall service quality gap between patients' expectations and perceptions. Thus, improvements are required across all the six dimensions, namely, tangibility, reliability, responsiveness, assurance, empathy and accessibility and affordability.
Analeeb, 2001	Identifies the service quality factors that are important to patients; it also examines their links to patient satisfaction.	Bangladesh	Several dimensions of perceived service quality including responsiveness, assurance, communication, discipline, and baksheesh; Factor analysis and multiple regression	Associations were found between the five dimensions and patient satisfaction.
Kilbourne et al., 2004	Investigate the applicability of a modified SERVQUAL instrument as a means of measuring residents' perceptions of long-term health-care service quality in the USA and UK	UK & USA	Modified SERVQUAL instrument.	Confirm a stable, four-factor structure that is similar to previously defined service quality dimensions and is invariant across the countries studied.
Butt & de Run, 2010	Develop and test the SERVQUAL model scale for measuring Malaysian private health service quality.	Malaysia	Modified SERVQUAL scales. Means, correlations, principal component and confirmatory factor analysis.	A moderate negative quality gap for overall Malaysian private healthcare service quality. Results also indicate a moderate negative quality gap on each service quality scale dimension. However, scale development analysis yielded excellent results, which can be used in wider healthcare policy and practice.

Table 2. Continued

Reference	Goal	Country	Conceptual Framework, Method	Result
Padma et al., 2010	Conceptualize hospital service quality (SQ) into its component dimensions from the perspectives of patients and their attendants; and to analyse the relationship between SQ and customer satisfaction (CS) in government and private hospitals.	India	Hospital SQ is conceptualized as an eight-dimensional framework	Patients and attendants treat the interpersonal aspect of care as the most important one, as they cannot fully evaluate the technical quality of healthcare services. The study also revealed that the hospital service providers have to understand the needs of both patients and attendants in order to gather a holistic view of their services.
Chaker and Al-Azzab, 2011	Aims at determining the elements of the Inpatient Satisfaction.	Qatar	The main factors are: quality, access, and interpersonal issues.	The findings of the study suggest that respondents are satisfied with the services provided and they are getting during their visits to the hospital.
Zarei et al., 2012	Determine the different dimensions of the service quality in the private hospitals of Iran and evaluating the service quality from the patients' perspective.	Iran	SERVQUAL	The need for hospital staff to be responsive, credible, and empathetic when dealing with patients.
Yousapronpaiboon & Johnson, 2013	Determine the dimensions used in judging the hospital services quality; to develop a tool for measuring perceived service quality for hospitals; to test the validity and reliability of the new scale; and finally to use the results of the data collected to suggest improving service quality.	Thailand	SERVQUAL	SERVQUAL's five latent dimensions had a significant influence on overall service quality. Responsiveness had most influence; followed by empathy, tangibles, assurance; and finally reliability. Service quality can be assessed in diverse service settings such as hospital out-patient departments. SERVQUAL is robust enough to capture the critical elements used to assess overall service quality.
Aghamolaei et al., 2014	Determine the service quality gap of the main hospital of Hormozgan province	Iran	SERVQUAL; Wilcoxon and Kruskal-Wallis tests	Service quality gaps were seen in all five service quality dimensions and the overall quality of service. The highest perception was in assurance dimension and the highest expectation was in responsiveness and assurance dimensions. Also, the lowest perception was in responsiveness dimension and the lowest expectation was about empathy.

Table 2. Continued

Reference	Goal	Country	Conceptual Framework, Method	Result
Raheem et al., 2014	Determine the patient satisfaction at private hospital of Karachi for the in-patient departments.	Pakistan	Factos: Patient Satisfaction, Physical Appearance, Record-room Services, Reception staff Services, Pharmacy Services, Laboratory Services, Blood bank Services, X-ray Services, Ultrasound Services, Billing Services, OPD Services, Patient-ward Services, Emergency Services, Housekeeping Services, Food Services, Welfare Services	Majority of the patients are satisfied with the services provided by the in-patient departments.
Yeboah, 2014	With the outpatient services of a hospital as the empirical case, it aims to prioritize the use of various medical service technical items as an improvement directed towards hospitals' competitiveness.	Ghana	SERVQUAL and KANO model.	This paper identifies the main attributes in the healthcare as an empirical research subject for the purpose of patient satisfaction improvement.

and Al-Azzab, 2011), Pakistan (Raheem et al., 2014), Thailand (Johnson, 2013), India (Padma et al., 2010), Ghana (Yeboah, 2014), Malaysia (Butt and de Run, 2010) as well as in developed country such as Singapore (Cheng Lim & Tang, 2000) or UK and USA (Kilbourne et al., 2004). Those studies can be summarized in Table 2 as follows:

Some of the studies in Table 2 were using SERVQUAL or a modified SERVQUAL model. According to the literature study by Chakraborty and Majumdar (2011) SERVQUAL instruments remains popular and are still widely applied in measuring service quality or consumer satisfaction despite its drawbacks pointed by some researchers. Therefore, in assessing hospital service quality from patients' perceptions, SERVQUAL or using SERVQUAL as the basis for instrument is arguably reliable.

CONCEPTUAL MODEL

The literature study concluded that SERVQUAL is still a widely used approach in examining service quality. Therefore, this study, as previously mentioned, will adopt Handayani et al.'s framework which was heavily based on SERVQUAL and has been used to assess hospital service quality in Indonesia from management, government and academician perspectives, as shown in Figure 1. Level 1 Dimension, Level 2 Sub-dimension and Level 3 Subsub-dimension are adopted by this study and thus referred to as Dimension, Criteria and Sub-criteria respectively. There are 4 dimensions: people, process, infrastructure and policy. There are 5 of 6 criteria that are of SERVQUAL dimensions: empathy, responsiveness, reliability, tangibles and assurance. However, Handayani et. al. (2014a) adds professionalism as the second criterion for the people dimension besides empathy. Responsiveness and reliability criteria are in the process dimension while tangible criterion and assurance criterion belong to infrastructure and policy respectively.

Figure 1. The Evaluation Framework of the Healthcare Service Quality Model (Handayani et al., 2014a)

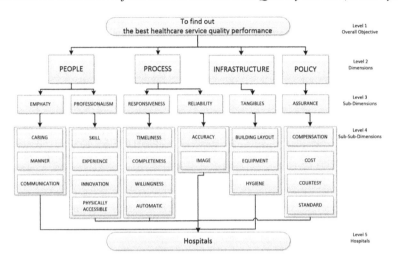

From the conceptual model in Figure 1, a measurement model was derived as in Handayani et al. (2014b) that will be adopted in this study to measure the hospitals service quality from patients' perspective based on SERVQUAL expectation-minus-perception score. The complete measurement model is shown in Table 3. The model consists of 6 criteria each of which is comprised of one or more sub-criteria: (1) empathy consists of caring, manner, communication; (2) professional consists of skill, experience, innovation, physically accessible; (3) responsiveness consists of timeliness, completeness, willingness, automatic; (4) reliability consists of accuracy, image; (5) tangible consists of building layout, equipment, hygiene; and (6) assurance consists of cost, courtesy, compensation and standard.

METHODOLOGY

Data Collecting Procedure

This research is a quantitative research using a survey technique. The survey instrument or questionnaire is developed based on the group criteria and the criteria to evaluate the quality of healthcare in general hospitals are shown in Figure 1. Before the questionnaire is being distributed, it is tested to identify errors and ambiguity for each statement. The questionnaire is assessed by four academicians involved in this research, i.e., three lecturers from the Faculty of Computer Science and one lecturer from the Faculty of Public Health Universitas Indonesia. Then, the questionnaire is being distributed directly to the patients. To gain more respondents, the survey also conducted online (accessible at http://healthcare. cs.ui.ac.id/kuesioner/).

Instruments

For each criterion in the measurement model, one or more indicators in the forms of statement items are defined. Eventually, we have a questionnaire which consists of 20 statements (as shown in Table 3 column 4) (Handayani et al., 2014b), each of which should be scored based on the expectation and

Table 3. The Measurement Model (adopted from Handayani et al., 2014b)

Dimension	Criteria	Sub Criteria	Definition
Human Resource	(1) Empathy	(1) Caring	Health workers provide individualized customer service based on patients' needs and preferences
		(2) Manner	Health workers listen carefully to patients' illness complaints and give solutions during consultation
		(3) Communication	Health workers always communicate medical information in the way that can be easily understood by patients and health workers willing to answer patients' questions so as to create a two-way interaction
	(2) Professionalism	(4) Skill	Health workers have appropriate competency in diagnosing and providing medical solution to patients' needs
		(5) Experience	Health workers are skillful in diagnosing and providing solution for patient's illness
		(6) Innovation	Health workers are able to use the latest technology devices properly and appropriately in treating patients.
		(7) Physically accessible	Health workers are easily encountered by patients in consultation or other medical treatment and can be contacted easily (e.g. by phone/SMS)
Process	(3) Responsiveness	(8) Timeliness	Health workers in the hospital serve patients perceptively (e.g., in waiting time, ease of appointment schedule changing) and emergency medical care procedures can be performed directly (without the need for appointment)
		(9) Completeness	Hospital provides all kind of services needed and available in order to handle patients' complaints
		(10) Willingness	Health workers willingly accept and serve all patients whenever needed regardless of their economic backgrounds.
		(11) Automatic	Hospital accommodates patients' needs in the administration process using online system (e.g. by phone, website, or SMS (short message service) and provides integrated patient medical information (e.g. complete medical resume for referral to another hospital including medical treatment, lab results, etc.)
	(4) Reliability	(12) Accuracy	Health workers provide information to patient before health services are provided, they explain about medical treatment to be performed and provide information about type of illness, the treatment and how to take medicine, completely.
		(13) Image	Health workers are able to assist every problem encountered by patients well
Infrastructure	(5) Tangible	(14) Building Layout	Hospital building is aesthetic, clean and comfortable, the signboards are easy to find and provide clear instructions in order to give guidance to patients.
		(15) Equipment	Hospital has waiting rooms, treatment rooms, beds, medical equipment, medicine, toilets and adequate sanitation
		(16) Hygiene	Health workers look clean and neat
Policy	(6) Assurance	(17) Cost	Hospital provides affordable services to patients
		(18) Courtesy	Courtesy of personnel and their ability to inspire trust and confidence, the health workers serve politely and convincing so that patients feel safe and comfortable, they show respect to patients
		(19) Compensation	Hospital gives guaranty in the event of problem arising from medical treatment performed
		(20) Standard	Comply with applicable standards for personnel, processes and infrastructure that are used (e.g. implementing ISO or perform hospital accreditation of the Ministry of Health

perception of the hospital health service by the respondents. The expectation will measure the extent to which level of quality is needed or desired by the respondents while the service perceived will measure the extent to which the level of quality is experienced by the respondents.

Thus, for each statement, a pair of Likert scale of 1 to 5 is provided to rate each sub-dimension of the services quality, one for expectation and one for perception. Scale 1 is used to express a very poor service, scale 2 is used to express a poor service, scale 3 is used to express a barely acceptable service, scale 4 is used to express a good service, and scale 5 is used to express an excellent service. The bigger the scale number chosen by the respondents indicates a higher expectation/perception for the selected sub-dimension of services quality in the hospital.

RESULTS

Respondents Profile

The questionnaires were distributed to more than 300 respondents. However, only 297 were filled in a complete order, thus deemed valid. The profiles are given as shown in Table 4. Our respondent's gender is quite in balance with 42% male and 58% female. As for age, they are fairly distributed although the age range of 26 – 35 is rather dominant with 32%. Most respondents are private employees (42%) and mostly (51%) earn 1-5 million rupiah per month. For education level, undergraduate degree seems to be predominant than others with 47% which is almost half of the respondents. Next, concerning hospitals, more than half of the respondents (65%) visited public (non-profit oriented) hospitals. The reason for picking hospital is mostly because of location factor, 61% respondents voted for this reason. The second reason backed by 32% of the respondents is whether the hospital is supported by their insurance or not. The remaining factors such as facility, recommendation, price and doctor are supported by 20-30% of the respondents. As for the unit, most respondents intend to visit polyclinic (67%) followed by inpatient unit (37%) and emergency unit 27%. Most respondents paid their visit to the hospital by insurance (47%). Nevertheless, the number of those who are paying in cash is still quite high (40%). The detailed respondents profile can be seen in Table 4.

Results

The reliability of the instruments was checked towards each criterion as well as sub-criterion. The internal reliability was measured using Cronbach's alpha via IBM SPSS Statistics Version 21. If Cronbach's alpha is greater than 0.7, the questionnaires was considered reliable.

The Cronbach's alpha of all criteria was found to be valid as can be seen in Table 5. The same holds for the sub-criteria as all Cronbach's alpha values of the sub-criteria were greater than 0.7.

Table 6 above shows a summary of the results of the paired t-test on the 6 criteria, i.e., empathy, professionalism, responsiveness, reliability, tangible and assurance.

From Table 7 column 1 and 2, it is exhibited that respondents perceive concerning service merit they experienced in downward order are: (1) tangible, (2) empathy, (3) reliability, (4) professionalism, (5) assurance and (6) responsiveness. Meanwhile, from Table 6 column 3 and 4, we can see that the respondents in this study expects, concerning service excellence in descending order are: (1) tangible, (2) assurance, (3) empathy, (4) reliability, (5) responsiveness and (6) professionalism.

Table 4. Respondents Profiles

Respondent Profile				
Sex			Type of Hospitals Visited	
Male	42%	Public (Non-profit oriented)		65%
Female	58%	owner: government		56%
Age		owner: non-gov org.		9%
< 17	2%	Private (Profit-oriented)		35%
17 - 25	25%	owner: private		32%
26 - 35	32%	owner: state owned company		3%
35 - 45	20%	Reason to Pick Hospital		
> 45	22%	Recommendation		22%
Occupation		Reputation		13%
Private employees	42%	Location		61%
Government employees	16%	Facility		27%
Enterpreneur	5%	Price		21%
Housewife	15%	Insurance		32%
Others	21%	Doctor		21%
Income		Others		8%
< 1 million	23%	Most Visited		
1- 3 million	27%	Inpatient unit		37%
3 - 5 million	24%	Polyclinic unit		67%
5 - 10 million	16%	Emergency unit		27%
> 10 million	10%	Others		14%
Education		Aim		
Elementary	5%	Check/control		14%
Junior	6%	Medical treatment		86%
Senior	27%	Lain-lain		14%
Undergraduate	47%	Payment Method		
Graduate	14%	Cash (own pocket)		40%
Doctoral	0%	Insurance		48%
		Jamkesmas (Government aid)		6%
		KJS (Healthy Jakarta Card)		5%
		Others		4%
		Total Respondents		297

Table 5. Reliability test result on the Criteria

Dimension	Criterion	Cronbach's Alpha	
		Perception	Expectation
Human Resources	Empathy	0.766	0.857
	Professionalism	0.764	0.867
Process	Responsiveness	0.746	0.876
	Reliability	0.788	0.831
Infrastructure	Tangible	0.799	0.872
Policy	Assurance	0.766	0.899

Table 6. Scores of Criteria

Dimension	Criterion		Mean	SD	Gap	T-Value	Result
Infrastructure	Tangible	P	3.883	0.811	-0.714	-26.303	Significant difference
			4.597	0.555			
Human Resource	Empathy	P	3.738	0.763	-0.800	-29.888	Significant difference
		E	4.539	0.608			
Process	Reliability	P	3.712	0.819	-0.815	-23.012	Significant difference
		E	4.527	0.623			
Human Resource	Professionalism	P	3.546	0.864	-0.948	-35.903	Significant difference
		E	4.494	0.664			
Policy	Assurance	P	3.516	0.936	-1.032	-35.754	Significant difference
		E	4.548	0.621			
Process	Responsiveness	P	3.443	0.884	-1.056	-36.766	Significant difference
		E	4.498	0.661			

* $p<0.05$

Table 7. Criteria orders based on Perception-mean and Expectation-mean

Criterion	Perception-mean	Criterion	Expectation-mean
Tangible	3.883	Tangible	4.597
Empathy	3.738	Assurance	4.548
Reliability	3.712	Empathy	4.539
Professionalism	3.546	Reliability	4.527
Assurance	3.516	Responsiveness	4.498
Responsiveness	3.443	Professionalism	4.494

Table 8. Scores of Sub-criteria

Sub-criterion		Paired Differences					t	df
		Mean-Gaps	Std. Deviation	Std. Error Mean	95% Confidence Interval of the Difference			
					Lower	Upper		
Pair 16	Hygiene	-0.5657	0.6852	0.0398	-0.6439	-0.4874	-14.2271	296
Pair 12	Accuracy	-0.7071	0.8127	0.0472	-0.7999	-0.6143	-14.9933	296
Pair 3	Communication	-0.7542	0.7992	0.0464	-0.8455	-0.6629	-16.2637	296
Pair 14	Building Layout	-0.7576	0.8787	0.0510	-0.8579	-0.6572	-14.8581	296
Pair 20	Standard	-0.7946	0.8311	0.0482	-0.8895	-0.6997	-16.4764	296
Pair 4	Skill	-0.8047	0.7899	0.0458	-0.8949	-0.7145	-17.5575	296
Pair 2	Manner	-0.8081	0.8262	0.0479	-0.9024	-0.7137	-16.8554	296
Pair 15	Equipment	-0.8182	0.8346	0.0484	-0.9135	-0.7229	-16.8946	296
Pair 6	Innovation	-0.8215	0.8086	0.0469	-0.9139	-0.7292	-17.5093	296
Pair 1	Caring	-0.8384	0.7716	0.0448	-0.9265	-0.7503	-18.7246	296
Pair 5	Experience	-0.8990	0.8402	0.0488	-0.9949	-0.8030	-18.4390	296
Pair 18	Courtesy	-0.9057	0.9288	0.0539	-1.0118	-0.7997	-16.8052	296
Pair 13	Image	-0.9226	0.8990	0.0522	-1.0252	-0.8199	-17.6856	296
Pair 9	Completeness	-0.9394	0.9059	0.0526	-1.0428	-0.8359	-17.8710	296
Pair 11	Automatic	-1.0101	1.0084	0.0585	-1.1253	-0.8950	-17.2634	296
Pair 17	Cost	-1.0101	0.9281	0.0539	-1.1161	-0.9041	-18.7562	296
Pair 10	Willingness	-1.0572	1.0101	0.0586	-1.1726	-0.9419	-18.0374	296
Pair 8	Timeliness	-1.2155	1.0138	0.0588	-1.3313	-1.0997	-20.6628	296
Pair 7	Physically Accessible	-1.2660	1.0936	0.0635	-1.3909	-1.1411	-19.9509	296
Pair 19	Compensation	-1.4175	1.1541	0.0670	-1.5493	-1.2857	-21.1678	296

$p<0.05$

Table 8 shows the gap for each sub-criterion.

Next, we analyse further by calculating the gap for each sub-criterion. The result is given in descending order for the perception-minus-expectation gap and shown in Table 8 above. The summary in Table 8 uncovers that all perception-minus-expectation gaps for sub-criteria were significantly different (see column t or 8). The negative value tells that each service was still delivered under the corresponding expectation (see column Mean or 3). We can pick the top 5 biggest sub-criteria gap with descending order, and thus we will have: compensation (of assurance criterion), physically accessible (of professionalism criterion), timeliness (of responsiveness), willingness (of responsiveness) and cost (of assurance criterion). On the other end, the 5 sub-criteria with the smallest gaps (starts from the smallest gap) are as follows: hygiene (of tangible criterion), accuracy (of reliability criterion), communication (of empathy criterion), building layout (of tangible criterion), standard (of assurance criterion).

Discussions and Implications

Apparently the gap, as shown in Table 5, for each criterion is shown to be significantly different which straightforwardly indicates the quality of the service delivered for each criterion is still below respondents' expectation. The order of the criteria gaps is given as follows (descending order): (1) responsiveness, (2) assurance, (3) professionalism, (4) reliability, (5) empathy and (6) tangible. If we look at the dimensions, i.e., Human Resources, Process, Infrastructure, and Policy, based on the gaps on the criteria, we can infer that the corresponding dimensions of the criteria can be ranked in descending order as follows: process, policy, human resource, process, human resource, and infrastructure. This means in Indonesia, from patients' perspective, the process dimension which is represented by responsiveness is shown as the biggest gap. Although responsiveness is seen from process point of view, if we elaborate further, there are several factors that might contribute for the lack of responsiveness. First that was identified is patients' overload which causes delay in giving service. As mentioned in the introduction section, the JKN program evidently surmounts patients especially in government-owned hospitals. To exacerbate, the lack of IT support in forms of automated systems in order to help scheduling, registering and dealing with bunch of administration details are not yet implemented in those hospitals. It is almost certain that utilizing hospital information system can improve and support the process dimension viz., to make the process become more effective and efficient. It can also help the hospitals to provide data/information in an accurate and integrated manner as well as to support the implementation of the Patient Safety Act in which patients are handled with adequate data. This can also help increase the professionalism degree as an element of human resource dimension, although professionalism in this context is only expected with the lowest quality relative to others by the respondents.

On the other hand, infrastructure aspect which is comprised of building layout, equipment and hygiene, is relatively closer to their quality perspective. This can also indicate that the improvement in the infrastructure aspect is going towards the right direction as to provide better service quality. However, this does not mean that this aspect does not need further improvement as the difference is still considered significant thus require effort to fill the gap.

When we compare both ranks, perception rank versus expectation rank, as shown in Table 6, we can directly see that tangible are both expected to be the highest and it turns out hospitals has been producing the highest service quality in tangible aspect as well. However, as shown by the t-value, the gap between perception and expectation for tangible is still significantly different. Interestingly, it is then revealed that assurance which is expected with the low quality relative to other criteria (5th rank) turns out to be provided in a quality second (2nd) only to tangible although from the t-value the gap between expectation and perception for empathy is still significantly different which means the quality delivered is still below expectation. Quite the contrary, professionalism, which is expected to be produced with moderate quality (4th rank relative to others), was delivered with the lowest quality compared to others (6th).

When we further scrutinize, 5 (out of 20 sub-criteria) biggest sub-criteria gaps are given as follows (descending order): compensation (of assurance criterion of policy dimension), physically accessible (of professionalism criterion of the human resource dimension), timeliness (of responsiveness of process dimension), willingness (of responsiveness of process dimension) and cost (of assurance criterion of policy dimension). This finding implies that assurance (compensation) seems to be crucial in these sub-criteria gaps. Our conjecture is that hospitals do not pass accreditation assessment or that people are not aware of this accreditation issues, therefore, they feel insecure as there is a lack of guarantee concerning the health services from the hospitals. A recommendation for hospitals is that they obviously must own good accreditation level and that both hospitals and the Ministry of Health familiarize this towards the community so that in turn the community could enforce hospitals for having good accreditation.

Based on the respondents' profiles which state that a significant number of respondents is paying in cash (40%) for the health service provided by hospitals we can conjecture that these people will most likely convert into JKN beneficiaries soon because 65% of those respondents were going to public (non-profit) hospitals. This means the JKN members are still continue expanding. The current state of the hospital capacity given the present member of JKN which is already overloaded should send alarms to hospitals as well as the Ministry of Health as this undesirable situation could worsen if there is no immediate action to overcome this lack of resources. In relation to the process dimension which has the biggest criterion gap, the Ministry of Health should take prompt action to accelerate the adoption of technological support in forms of IT support/automation in hospitals. In line with the suggestion of Handayani et al. (2014b), the Ministry of Health must form policy and its technical implementation for hospitals, especially those under the Ministry of Health, so that hospitals are supported by Hospital Information Systems which is expected to accelerate processes in hospitals and eliminate efficiencies. This could be a recommended solution that works in parallel with health personnel allocations or new health facility planning program of the Ministry of Health for a more evenly distributed health personnel and facilities in the entire regions.

CONCLUSION

Based on the results of the questionnaires, we can see that the criteria gaps is given as follows in descending order from the biggest gap: (1) responsiveness, (2) assurance, (3) professionalism, (4) reliability, (5) empathy and (6) tangible. Apparently the gap, for each criterion transpires to be significantly different which straightforwardly indicates the quality of the service delivered by hospitals for each criterion is still below respondents' expectations. Similar interpretation is also conveyed by the sub-criteria gaps which exhibits significant differences between perception and expectation. Recommendation towards hospitals is proposed from technological point of view in forms of IT support/automation in order to significantly improve the process as the dimension of the responsiveness criterion. Nonetheless, suggestion towards the Ministry of Health as the policy maker is also addressed that urges the establishment of policy and its implementation concerning IT support for accelerating hospitals automation.

LIMITATIONS

Given this research scope, the future works are expected to acquire a bigger number of respondents which are fairly distributed towards patients of hospitals of different type and class as in Indonesia there are several types and class of hospitals in order to give better accuracy on patients' perception towards hospital services. Furthermore, obtaining respondents which can sufficiently represent rural and urban areas would produce a better reflection on the expectation of patients as people's lifestyles which might influence expectation between urban and rural can be quite in contrast. Secondly, as this study presents a limited analysis concerning the respondent profiles, future research of this particular can employ technique such as cluster analysis for better analysis on the respondents.

ACKNOWLEDGMENT

We would like to express our gratitude towards the reviewers for their valuable feedbacks which substantially improve the quality of this article. We also want to express appreciation towards DIKTI for the financial support (PUPT research grant) for this research and also towards DRPM UI for managing the research grant.

REFERENCES

Aghamolaei, T., Eftekhaari, T. E., Rafati, S., Kahnouji, K., Ahangari, S., Shahrzad, M. E., & Hoseini, S. H. (2014). Service quality assessment of a referral hospital in Southern Iran with SERVQUAL technique: Patients' perspective. *BMC Health Services Research*, *14*(1), 322. doi:10.1186/1472-6963-14-322 PMID:25064475

Al Bassam, T., & Al Shawi, S. (2011). Analysing the Use of the SERVQUAL Model to Measure Service Quality in Specific-Industry Contexts. *Proceedings of 14th International Business Research Conference.*

Andaleeb, S. S. (2001). Service quality perceptions and patient satisfaction: A study of hospitals in a developing country. *Social Science & Medicine*, *52*(9), 1359–1370. doi:10.1016/S0277-9536(00)00235-5 PMID:11286361

BPJS (in Indonesian). (2001). Retrieved from http://www.jkn.kemkes.go.id/attachment/unduhan/UU%20No%2024%20Tahun%202011%20tentang%20BPJS.pdf

Butt, M. M., & de Run, E. C. (2010). Private Healthcare Quality: Applying A SERVQUAL Model. *International Journal of Health Care Quality Assurance*, *23*(7), 658–673. doi:10.1108/09526861011071580 PMID:21125961

Buttle, F. (1996). SERVQUAL: Review, critique, research agenda. *European Journal of Marketing*, *30*(1), 8–32. doi:10.1108/03090569610105762

Chaker, M., & Al-Azzab, N. (2011). Patient satisfaction in Qatar orthopedic and sports medicine hospital (ASPITAR). *International Journal of Business & Social Sciences*, *2*(7), 69–78.

Chakraborty, R., & Majumdar, A. (2011). Measuring consumer satisfaction in health care Sector: the applicability of servqual. *Journal of arts, science & commerce*, 2(4), 149-160.

Cheng Lim, P., & Tang, N. K. (2000). A study of patients' expectations and satisfaction in Singapore hospitals. *International Journal of Health Care Quality Assurance*, *13*(7), 290–299. doi:10.1108/09526860010378735 PMID:11484647

Cronin, J. J., & Taylor, S. A. (1994). SERVPERF versus SERVQUAL: Reconciling Performance -Based and Perceptions-Minus-Expectations Measurement of Service Quality. *Journal of Marketing*, *58*(1), 125–131. doi:10.2307/1252256

Handayani, P., Hidayanto, A. N., Sandhyaduhita, P., Junus, K., & Ayuningtyas, D. (2014a). Analysis on Strategic Hospital Service Quality based on the Perspective of Hospital Management, Government Policy Maker and Academicians in Indonesia. Proceedings of Technology Innovation and Industrial Management, Seoul, South Korea.

Handayani, P. W., Hidayanto, A. N., Sandhyaduhita, P. I., & Ayuningtyas, D. (2014b). Strategic hospital services quality analysis in Indonesia. *Expert Systems with Applications*, *42*(6), 3067–3078. doi:10.1016/j. eswa.2014.11.065

Hukor. (2014). Retrieved from http://www.hukor.depkes.go.id/up_prod_permenkes/PMK%20No.%20 001%20ttg%20Sistem%20Rujukan%20Pelayanan%20Kesehatan%20Perorangan.pdf

Kilbourne, W. E., Duffy, J. A., Duffy, M., & Giarchi, G. (2004). The applicability of SERVQUAL in cross-national measurements of health-care quality. *Journal of Services Marketing*, *18*(7), 524–533. doi:10.1108/08876040410561857

Ladhari, R. (2009). A Review of Twenty Years of SERVQUAL Research. *International Journal of Quality and Service Sciences*, *1*(2), 72–198. doi:10.1108/17566690910971445

Lam, S. S. (1997). SERVQUAL: A tool for measuring patients' opinions of hospital service quality in Hong Kong. *Total Quality Management*, *8*(4), 145–152. doi:10.1080/0954412979587

Padma, P., Rajendran, C., & Sai, L. P. (2010). Service quality and its impact on customer satisfaction in Indian hospitals: Perspectives of patients and their attendants. *Benchmarking: An International Journal*, *17*(6), 807–841. doi:10.1108/14635771011089746

Parasuraman, A., Zeithaml, V., & Berry, L. (1985). A conceptual model of service quality and its implications for future research. *Journal of Marketing*, *49*(4), 41–50. doi:10.2307/1251430

Parasuraman, A., Zeitmal, V., & Berry, L. (1988). SERVQUAL: A Multiple Item Scale for Measuring Consumer Perceptions of Service Quality. *Journal of Retailing*, *64*(1), 12–40.

Raheem, A. R., Nawaz, A., Nasir, F., & Khoso, I. (2014). Patients' Satisfaction and Quality Health Services: An Investigation from Private Hospitals of Karachi, Pakistan. *Research Journal of Recent Sciences*.

Shabila, N. P., Al-Tawil, N. G., Al-Hadithi, T. S., & Sondorp, E. (2014). Using Q-methodology to explore people's health seeking behavior and perception of the quality of primary care services. *BMC Public Health*, *14*(2). Retrieved from http://www.biomedcentral.com/1471-2458/14/2 PMID:24387106

Shahin, A., & Samea, M. (2010). Developing the models of service quality gaps: a critical discussion. *Business Management and Strategy*, 1(1), E2. Retrieved from http://www.macrothink.org/journal/index. php/bms/article/view/395/342

Sixma, H. J., Kerssens, J. J., Campen, C. V., & Peters, L. (1998). Quality of care from the patients' perspective: From theoretical concept to a new measuring instrument. *Health Expectations*, *1*(2), 82–95. doi:10.1046/j.1369-6513.1998.00004.x PMID:11281863

SJSN. (2004). Retrieved from http://www.jkn.kemkes.go.id/attachment/unduhan/UU%20No.%2040%20 Tahun%202004%20tentang%20SJSN.pdf

Sohail, M. S. (2003). Service Quality in Hospitals: More Favourable Than You Might Think. *Managing Service Quality*, *13*(3), 197–206. doi:10.1108/09604520310476463

Tomes, A. E., & Chee Peng Ng, S. (1995). Service quality in hospital care: The development of an in-patient questionnaire. *International Journal of Health Care Quality Assurance*, *8*(3), 25–33. doi:10.1108/09526869510089255 PMID:10143994

Yeboah, M. A., Ansong, M. O., Appau-Yeboah, F., Antwi, H. A., & Yiranbon, E. (2014). Empirical Validation of Patient's Expectation and Perception of Service Quality in Ghanaian Hospitals: An Integrated Model Approach. *American International Journal of Social Science*, *3*(3), 143–160.

Yousapronpaiboon, K., & Johnson, W. C. (2013). Out-patient Service Quality Perceptions in Private Thai Hospitals. *International Journal of Business and Social Science*, *4*(2).

Zarei, A., Arab, M., Froushani, A. R., Rashidian, A., & Tabatabaei, S. M. G. (2012). Service quality of private hospitals: The Iranian Patients' perspective. *BMC Health Services Research*, *12*(1), 31. doi:10.1186/1472-6963-12-31 PMID:22299830

ENDNOTES

[1]   http://www.bappenas.go.id/files/5413/9148/4109/Proyeksi_Penduduk_Indonesia_2010-2035.pdf

[2]   http://sirs.buk.depkes.go.id/rsonline/report/report_by_catrs.php

[3]   http://m.suaramerdeka.com/index.php/read/cetak/2013/04/10/221277

[4]   http://www.pdpersi.co.id/content/news.php?catid=2&mid=5&nid=1120

[5]   http://www.tribunnews.com/regional/2013/12/26/tempat-tidur-pasien-di-rs-masih-kurang

[6]   http://m.kabar24.com/health/read/20140424/54/217014/rsud-bekasi-kota-kekurangan-dokter

[7]   http://www.harianhaluan.com/index.php/berita/haluan-padang/32750-rsud-kekurangan-dokter-spesialis

Chapter 28
Applied Pervasive Patient Timeline in Intensive Care Units

André Braga
Universidade do Minho, Portugal

Filipe Portela
Universidade do Minho, Portugal

Manuel Filipe Santos
Universidade do Minho, Portugal

António da Silva Abelha
Universidade do Minho, Portugal

José Machado
Universidade do Minho, Portugal

Álvaro Silva
Centro Hospitalar do Porto, Portugal

Fernando Rua
Centro Hospitalar do Porto, Portugal

ABSTRACT

This study has the objective of introducing an innovative way of presenting and representing information concerning patients in Intensive Care Units. Therefore, the Pervasive Patient Timeline, which has the purpose of offering support to intensivists' decision-making process, by providing access to a real-time environment, was developed. The solution is patient-centred as it can be accessed from anywhere, at any time and it contains patients' clinical data since they are admitted to the ICU until their discharge. The environment holds data concerning vital signs, laboratory results, therapeutics, and data mining predictions, which can be analysed to have a better understanding of patients' present and future condition. Due to the nature of the critical care environment, the pervasive aspect is crucial because it allows intensivists make decisions when they have to be made. The Pervasive Patient Timeline is focused on improving the quality of care by helping the intensivists perform better in their daily activity.

DOI: 10.4018/978-1-7998-2451-0.ch028

Copyright © 2020, IGI Global. Copying or distributing in print or electronic forms without written permission of IGI Global is prohibited.

INTRODUCTION

Medicine is a field of study where many changes have occurred over the course of the years. Research projects allowed for discovering new vaccines, drugs, methods, techniques that resulted in the ability of healing diseases which previously could not be cured. Technological advancement is directly related to, not all, but many medical discoveries since it became possible to test and observe ideas that without the technology would not be possible. Technologies and information systems are not only used in medical discoveries but also support and improve existing methods and techniques involved in the decision process. Therefore, it is possible to infer that the introduction of e-health technologies intended to increase the effectiveness and efficiency of healthcare facilities (Direção Geral de Saúde, 2003; Haux, Ammenwerth, Winter, & Brigl, 2004).

Over the last century, a new approach to medicine emerged as a result of multidisciplinary effort in areas, such as physiopathology, therapeutics, and technology, called Intensive Medicine (IM) (Direção Geral de Saúde, 2003). This subfield of medicine saw many new technological devices being added over time. These devices drastically increased patients' chance of survival since they provide even more data and a constant feedback about the patients' condition (Silva, 2007). The growth of devices resulted in an increase of available data (Morris & Gardner, 1992). Even though this is a good thing, it can also represent a problem because the number of variables to consider in the decision process is bigger, and therefore it is harder to combine and analyse (Silva, 2007). The use of various and different technologies in Intensive Medicine (IM) represents another major problem. Each device or system presents data in its way, being it tables, text, graphs or any other. As a consequence of this fact, the intensivists have to make additional efforts to understand how each device works to interpret its content and retrieve information.

That is where Decision Support Systems (DSS) come to play. In the field of information systems, DSS are characterized as computer based interactive systems that help, those who need to make decisions, using data and models to solve non-structured problems (Sprague & Ralph, 1980). In medicine, they are called as Clinical DSS.

Therefore, exploiting computers high processing capacity, they seek to alleviate intensivists' difficulty in interpreting data and help them in making decisions. This study has the objective of filling this existent gap with the development of an interactive platform (pervasive timeline) that collects data from various devices and presents them into a single location with access in real-time and from anywhere. This platform standardizes the representation of data and sorts it chronologically, easing the interpretation of data and the observation of cause-effect relations.

The research project took place in the Intensive Care Unit (ICU) of the Hospital de Santo António, Centro Hospitalar do Porto, and ended with the development of the Pervasive Patient Timeline. The Pervasive Patient Timeline is an interactive web platform which seeks to address the difficulty felt by intensivists in having to deal with high amounts of data and the different ways the data is presented by each device or system. The platform developed solves this problem by collecting data from various devices / data sources and presents the information sorted chronologically in the interface. At the same time, the data representation is homogenized, as all the data collected follow the same pattern. The timeline possesses characteristics, such as adaptability, interactivity, flexibility, scalability, real-time access and pervasiveness. These aspects provide a faster, more intuitive, easier and efficient access to data so that intensivists can perform better when making decisions.

Concerning the structure of the article, it is composed of five sections. The first section is the Introduction; in the second section comes the Background which provides a problem context and it is divided into four sub-sections: Intensive Medicine and Intensive Care Units, INTCare, The Timeline and Pervasive Healthcare; the third section talks about the research methodology used during the study life-cycle; the fourth section is where the Pervasive Patient Timeline is presented along with its features; the fifth and last section is the Conclusion where the importance of the study and its results are discussed.

BACKGROUND

Intensive Medicine and Intensive Care Units

Intensive Medicine (IM) is described as a field of medicine that focuses on diagnosing and treating patients with severe health issues. These problems deteriorate the quality of life to a point that they start being a threat to the patients' life. Therefore, IM seeks to revert the patients' fragile condition to a state before hospital admission (Suter et al., 1994). The necessity to concentrate skills, knowledge and technology that can support these patients resulted in the creation of a specialized environment called Intensive Care Unit (ICU) (Direção Geral de Saúde, 2003). An ICU is a critical environment only for patients with life-threatening issues, and these patients usually are in a coma and under constant surveillance (Portela, Santos et al., 2014). In ICUs, there is a wider scope of resources that intensivists can use to try and revert the patients' condition (Silva, 2007). Technological devices allow for a constant monitoring and better assessment, which is combined with medication experiments and recovering tasks until the patient can live autonomously. For example, when a patient has a respiratory failure, he needs to be connected to a ventilation device (Ramon et al., 2007). These sets of devices collect data from the patient and give to intensivists more knowledge so that they can make decisions of higher quality.

INTCare

The INTCare is a research project conducted, in joint partnership, between the University of Minho and Centro Hospitalar do Porto (CHP). The project had the overall focus to modernize the Hospital de Santo António, Porto information system. Part of that modernization resulted in the development and implementation of the INTCare system in the Intensive Care Unit (ICU) (Portela, Santos, Silva, Machado, & Abelha, 2011).

The INTCare system is a Pervasive Decision Support System (PDSS) which has the objective of supporting the decision-making process of the intensivists. It works in real-time, autonomously and performs its tasks through intelligent agents, offering support to clinical decisions. In such a way, it makes predictions on organ failure and its consequences and suggests treatments based on that. The system is divided into four subsystems that interact between themselves through the previously mentioned intelligent agents: Data Acquisition, Knowledge Management, Inference and Interface (Portela, Santos et al., 2014; Santos, Portela, & Vilas-Boas, 2011). Six data sources provide the data used by the INTCare system: vital signs monitors, ventilation monitors, electronic health record, electronic nurse record, laboratory and drugs system (F. Portela, Santos et al., 2014). Since the system's purpose is to help and improve the decision-making process, it can monitor patient's condition, predict clinical events through data mining techniques and issue emergency messages when patients experience a critical event (Filipe Portela, Santos et al., 2014). These transformations applied to the hospital's information system allowed the creation of new and useful knowledge that end up making the decision processes inside UCIs more effective and efficient and reduce the level of uncertainty and stress associated with decision-making process

The study presented in this paper is part of the INTCare project, more specifically phase two.

Timeline

Chronology is the area that focuses on organizing dates or events by the order in which they happened. The ability of graphical representation is one of the most critical skills since it opened doors to the acquisition of new knowledge (Rosenberg & Grafton, 2010).

The timeline concept is one of many ways in which data can be represented. The fact that it represents data in chronological order is the main feature/reason that distinguishes it from other modes of representation.

The timeline allows observing things, such as, when events happened, for how long, overlaps between events, and possible cause-effect relations between events, among others. Granularity is also another main characteristic of timelines as it defines the level of detail presented in the contents of the timeline, such as hours, days and years.

Over the years, the way timelines are presented changed radically as it saw the rise and development of new digital technologies. Nowadays, due to the technology, it is possible to visualize timeline in computers, which allow the user to customize/change its characteristics and content much easier, without having to redo everything (Richardson, Reilly, & Kuntz, 2008).

It is very common to see timelines being used in representing historical milestones or events, such as social movements, wars, and natural catastrophes, discoveries, among others (Rosenberg & Grafton, 2010). Some fields of study, like mathematics, seismology, meteorology, the criminal investigation also use timelines in a way that fits their context. In medicine, they are often used to register events of diseases' outbreaks and clinical data representation. Specifically, in intensive medicine, timelines are used in monitoring heart rate, blood pressure, among others (McDonald & Gardner, 1987).

Overall, the use of timelines as a form of representation provides an easier understanding of relationships between data present in the timeline and how they possibly affect each other.

Pervasive HealthCare

Pervasive Healthcare can be seen as the application of an emerging approach called pervasive computing in clinical environments. This approach is deeply related with intelligent environments, in which technology applies artificial intelligence and machine learning techniques as a way to augment the capacity to control and adapt its surroundings (Lewis, 2004).

Therefore, pervasive computing can be defined as having the objective of creating intelligent environments where the devices that are connected and inserted into an environment offer a continuous, trustworthy and non-intrusive connection and services with added value to the users. In the end, the major focus of this approach on systems is to improve the quality of human life and experience, without a clear perception of the technical interactions between the technologies (Cook & Das, 2007).

These characteristics of pervasive computing allow for different types of implementations, such as body implanted devices, wearable devices in clothes and accessories, portable devices or even devices embedded in the environment (Varshney, 2009).

With this concept in mind, the idea of Pervasive Healthcare starts to become a reality, being defined as "healthcare to anyone, anytime, and anywhere by removing locational, time and other restraints while increasing both the coverage and the quality of healthcare" (Varshney, 2009).

The ever growing access to internet facilitates the evolution of technology towards these types of systems, which in turn results in the increase of the amount of wireless networks, communication systems (Portela, Santos, & Vilas-Boas, 2013), and mobile devices that are capable of retrieving, sharing and storing data (Cook & Das, 2012).

Concerning medicine, technologies have improved the quality of healthcare services provided, be it by reducing paperwork or more effective treatments. However, there are still many issues to solve, such as medical errors, healthcare professionals' stress, lack of access to healthcare in locations with less population, higher costs of healthcare services (Varshney, 2009).

In the case of Intensive Medicine (IM), the fact of having pervasive data available anywhere and at any time is a big step to increase the efficiency of Intensive Care Units (ICU). Many times in these environments the decisions need to be made under high pressure, and sometimes the information is not present at the moment that the intensivists need it, resulting in diagnosis with the lack of information and sometimes with incorrect data. With all of these challenges, pervasive technologies can be a case of doing more with less, reducing the impact of stated problems and many others, in favour of an improvement in the quality of care provided. For that, healthcare facilities have to adapt themselves to these new emerging paradigms of healthcare because they allow the creation of new knowledge and contribute to the improvement of human life.

RESEARCH METHODOLOGY

Design Science Research (DSR) methodology used during the research life-cycle. This method was selected as a tool to help the research process to achieve the project's goals successfully. (Peffers, Tuunanen, Rothenberger, & Chatterjee, 2007) presented a model of the DSR which is composed of six activities: Identify Problem and Motivation, Define Objectives of a Solution, Design and Development, Demonstration, Evaluation and Communication. Apart from these six activities the model also presents four possible research entry points: Problem-centred Initiation, Objective-centred Solution, Design and Development centred Initiation and Client/Context Initiated. That means it is not expected for researchers always to follow the same process, from the first activity to the last one. It also allows for the possibility to start any activity except Evaluation and Communication.

Concerning this study, the approach centred the problem. Therefore, it commenced in the first activity: Identify Problem and Motivate. This first activity objective was to understand in which ways the implementation of a Pervasive Patient Timeline would act as an improvement of the decision-making process in Intensive Care Units (ICU). The second activity, Define Objectives of a Solution, focused on defining the objective of research, being, in this case, the development of a Pervasive Patient Timeline, which would be capable of, without time and space restrictions, provide new knowledge to intensivists and therefore help in their decision-making process. In the third activity, Design and Development, the characteristics that the artefact would embody were defined, as well as the necessary requirements for the artefact development. After that, the development of the artefact started. The fourth activity, Demonstration, consists of adding clinical data from hospital's patients to distribute the information to the timeline's interface. In the fifth activity, Evaluation, which is a set of metrics for the purpose of evaluating the Pervasive Patient Timeline's performance in the clinical environment, was defined. The last activity is Communication. It consists of presenting the value of this study. That was done through the writing and publishing of scientific papers in journals and conferences, such as this one.

PERVASIVE PATIENT TIMELINE

The Pervasive Patient Timeline can be considered as a Clinical Decision Support System (CDSS) because it was developed to have an immediate impact on decisions taken by intensivists to treat patients in a clinical environment. Berner & La Lande (2007) define CDSS as a computer system designed to have an impact on clinical decisions, at the moment the decisions need to be made. It acts as a web platform that interoperates with the various hospitals' systems by collecting and presenting, in its interface, the necessary data for intensivists to make better-substantiated decisions. The centralization and standardization of data resulted in a better, faster, easier, concise way of understanding and reading data, since it obeys to the same pattern, discarding the need to learn how each system works. All the information that ends up being presented in the timeline is acquired by the INTCare system and passes through and Extract, Transform, and Load (ETL) process. This process corrects any found mistakes to ensure the quality of data.

This solution works in real-time as it is part of the INTCare system. It allows the intensivists see data concerning the moment that they are attending the patient's needs. As all recorded data are saved and presented, it is possible to consult it from the patient's hospital admission until his discharge.

The main characteristics are the real-time access by presenting data collected at the moment it was recorded, flexibility and adaptability which allow adding new and different events to the timeline and adapting it to the different environments. The other features are scalability since it is possible to increase the amount of data presented in the timeline, interactivity since the user can interact with the timeline and customize data's visualization, and pervasiveness.

The pervasive characteristic is an imperative aspect since it allows access to the timeline's content from any location. This feature helps the intensivists make a decision even if they are not near the patient, resulting in a more pro-active treatment since they can observe the situation from afar and act faster. Through the use of mobile or other wireless devices, the timeline is available anywhere and anytime with the features above mentioned.

Another important aspect of the timeline is the possibility to incorporate results provided by a data mining engine (Peixoto, Portela, & Santos, 2016). These models which were produced by the INTCare system are added to the timeline interface. That way, it is possible to observe future predictions, such as, critical events (Portela et al., 2015), organ failures (Santos, Portela, Vilas-Boas, Silva, & Rua, 2010), readmission (Braga, Portela, Santos, & Rua, 2014), vasopressors need (Braga et al., 2016. (accepted for publication)), length of stay (Veloso et al., 2014), patient outcome (Santos, Mathew, & Portela, 2011), patient discharge (Portela, Veloso, et al., 2014), among others. In the end, the Pervasive Patient Timeline provides intensivists new insights taking them to consider the relations between data: thus creating new knowledge that seeks to support the decision-making process.

Data Source

Regarding the data presented in the timeline's interface, they were taken from the information system presented in the Intensive Care Unit (ICU) of the Hospital de Santo António; Centro Hospitalar does Porto (CHP). The data were collected from six data sources. Before these data appear on the timeline, they go through an ETL process. This process ensures that only high-quality data are provided to intensivists. The data sources are:

- **Vital Signs Monitors:** Responsible for measuring and presentation of vital signs, such as blood pressure, heart rate, temperature
- **Ventilation Monitor:** Collect data concerning the patient's oxygen, positive end-expiratory pressure, and pulmonary compliance, among others
- **Drugs System:** Holds the medication prescribed which is used in the treatment
- **Laboratory:** This data source is where the result of medical exams is stored, such as haemoglobin, leukocytes, sodium, among others
- **Electronic Health Record:** Data concerning patient's admission and discharge from the hospital is saved in this system. Specifically, personal data and the patient's medical history
- **Electronic Nursing Record:** All the clinical data collected from the patient, after being validated, is registered manually into this system. That contains all hourly data collected near the patient bed

Development

The development of the Pervasive Patient Timeline was done following the Decision Making Process model for the development of decision support systems; It is composed of five phases: Intelligence, Design, Choice, Implementation (Sprague & Ralph, 1980) and Monitoring (Turban, Sharda, & Delen, 2014). In the Intelligence phase, the difficulty felt by intensivists in analysing data coming from various and different lines of evidence was identified. In this context, a set of the objectives for implementing a timeline model capable of helping intensivists make decisions was defined. After this, a search process was initiated to find timeline solutions that could be adapted to a clinical environment, and that would fit the minimum requirements.

In the Choice phase, the pros and cons of each solution found were weighed to access and have a better understanding of which would be optimal considering development constraints. The aspects evaluated were its features, interface, documentation, development time and extra functionalities. After that, the Implementation phase started.

Due to the fact of the Pervasive Patient Timeline is a web platform, the development resorted to using the XAMPP platform. In this work, the programming languages PHP and JavaScript, plus Oracle SQL for database management and data treatment were used. In this phase the following features in the timeline were implemented.

Data
- Display on the timeline's interface data belonging to databases of various data sources (ex: vital signs, clinical exams, etc.)

Granularity
- Maximum detail: 15 minutes to 15 minutes

- Minimum detail: Decade to Decade

Usability

- Choose a patient from a list to visualize his information in the timeline
- Choose the type of data to visualize: all data or only critical data
- Slide horizontally the timeline, to visualize the past and future events
- While visualizing the timeline, zoom in and zoom out the granularity
- Filter, through categories, the visible data in the timeline
- Adjust the events time according to the time zone
- Search bar to find events through title or description
- Click to go to the next or previous event
- Define a date and advance to the defined moment

Event Features

- Title, absolute values of the first hour and maximum, minimum and average hour values
- Event description, which can contain text, images, links
- Events can have start and end date
- Ability to add events to different categories
- Indicator importance level that defines the granularity the events can be seen (can be significant when there are too many events clutter the timeline)

These sets of features were deemed enough to make a difference on the daily job of an intensivist. More features can be added, and existing features can be improved to ensure the quality of the system. The system is already implemented in the hospital's information system, and the Monitoring phase has been initiated.

The purpose of this last phase was to evaluate the Pervasive Patient Timeline's performance while it is being used in the clinical environment by the intensivists. For this, a set of the main performance indicators was created. With this in mind, a questionnaire was elaborated to be answered by intensivists, in which the results would be used to achieve the performance indicators. By analysing the results, it would become possible to understand better the real appreciation of the users concerning the solution developed and if it fits their needs.

The timeline has a few requirements to make its implementation possible:

- There is the need of an internet connection
- Interoperability with the different systems of the hospital
- Securing the privacy of data being used in the timeline
- Restricting the data access
- Context awareness
- An existent database infrastructure that allows communication with the timeline to collect data
- Continuous availability of access to data

Timeline Interface

In Figure 1, it is possible to observe four examples of the Pervasive Patient Timeline's interface which represent different functionalities and capabilities.

The interface is first presented after selecting a patient's process number and the type of data (all data or just critical values using the critical event concept). Critical events occur when a patient has a higher or lower value than the predefined normal range, for a period of time. The range of values was determined after a literature review and counselling of specialized physicians to have the most reliable range possible (Portela et al., 2016). On the timeline, an event value is verified if it is between or outside the normal range, and then it is defined as critical or not. The patient admission's data are displayed in the toggleable black box on the timelines interface, being possible to toggle it on or off (top-left image). On the event, a description shows the name, the first value of the hour and the respective metric unit. However, it is also possible to display, if so desired, the maximum, minimum and average values registered at the time.

The granularity of the timeline is set to one hour, although it is possible to change the moment if the intensivist wants more or less detail.

In general, the timeline presents data of five categories, although more categories could be added: vital signs, medication, clinical exams, ventilation and data mining predictions. The vital signs are presented with a blue plus, medication with a yellow square, clinical exams with a green triangle, ventilation with a purple circle and predictions with a black infinity symbol. That allows for a faster tracking of the data on the timeline, being even possible to filter what is desired to see.

Some categories have different features which depend on the nature of the category itself. Medication, which usually has a different start and end date, has a grey bar which indicates where it started and where it ends (top and bottom left); vital signs, clinical exams, and ventilation may appear coloured in red in case critical values are registered (upper and lower left); concerning data mining predictions, the colours are attributed depending on the nature and result of the models, i.e., if it is predicting something right for the patient then high probability is coloured in green, and low probability is coloured in red; if it is something wrong then high probability is coloured in red and low probability in green. The addition of data mining models allows intensivists to take in consideration outcomes and make the necessary efforts to prevent them and in the end reduces stress on decisions, management and resources costs.

CONCLUSION

The life-cycle of this study ended with the development of the Pervasive Patient Timeline, which represents a continuous process of rethinking how the provided healthcare can be improved. The Pervasive Patient Timeline demonstrated the feasibility of presenting data in a new way. It can increase the efficiency and effectiveness of intensivists' job, through the ease of data readability and understanding, stress reduction, reduction of medical errors, the creation of new knowledge, among others.

Due to its adaptability and flexibility, this new approach has added value because it can be applied not only to different Intensive Care Units (ICU) but also to other completely different contexts and areas. Its pervasiveness is one of its most important features as it allows intensivists to access the timeline's content from any location and device; therefore, making decisions when they need to be made. The use of data mining models as a data type is a critical part of the timeline because they will help to reduce the uncertainty associated with making decisions, in favour of the patients.

The purpose of DSR was to guide the study, to make sure that it would be successful, instead of deviating from its objectives. Still, since it interoperates with many other systems and with people, there are barriers to implementation and development (financial, technical, human, etc.) that need to overcome

Figure 1. Pervasive patient timeline's interface

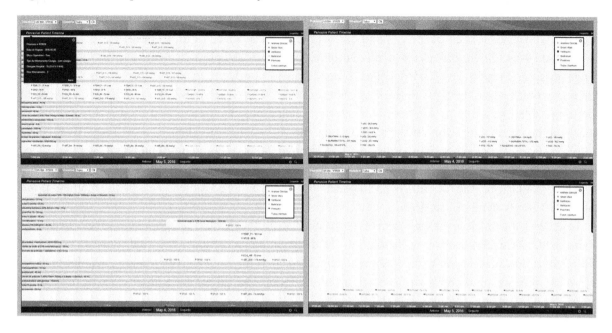

for the system to be successful. The Pervasive Patient Timeline has a major role in critical environments like ICU, where many devices work at the same time, and continuously collect and process significant amounts of data.

The conclusion of this study (by the feedback received by the intensivists) is that the use of timelines can be a viable solution to implement in critical environments like intensive care units; as it is a way to innovate the visualization of clinical data. It shows how important is to have an excellent presentation and chronological sorting of data when it is being displayed, how that can influence, in a right way, the decisions made by intensivists, and how the aggregation and homogenization of initially different data allow for a faster, easier and intuitive understanding. That way intensivists can acquire new knowledge which will make their decisions more reliable and accurate. On a side note, intensivists are motivated and interested in using the Pervasive Patient Timeline since it allows observing data as never before, with the plus of being able to access it in real-time and from anywhere.

Conclusively, the Pervasive Patient Timeline is people-centred, since it seeks to improve healthcare provided to patients, by upgrading the quality of the environment in which intensivists work.

ACKNOWLEDGMENT

This work has been supported by FCT - Fundação para a Ciência e Tecnologia within the Project Scope UID/CEC/00319/2013. The authors would like to thank FCT (Foundation of Science and Technology, Portugal) for the financial support through the contract PTDC/EEI-SII/1302/2012 (INTCare II).

REFERENCES

Berner, E. S., & La Lande, T. J. (2007). Overview of Clinical Decision Support Systems. In E.S. Berner (Eds.), Clinical Decision Support Systems. New York: Springer. doi:10.1007/978-0-387-38319-4_1

Braga, A., Portela, F., Filipe Santos, M., Machado, J., Abelha, A., Silva, Á., & Rua, F. (2016). Data Mining to predict the use of Vasopressors in Intensive Medicine Patients. Jurnal Teknolog.

Braga, P., Portela, F., Santos, M. F., & Rua, F. (2014). Data Mining Models to Predict Patient's Readmission in Intensive Care Units. *Paper presented at the ICAART - International Conference on Agents and Artificial Intelligence.*

Cook, D. J., & Das, S. K. (2007). How smart are our environments? An updated look at the state of the art. *Pervasive and Mobile Computing, 3*(2), 53–73. doi:10.1016/j.pmcj.2006.12.001

Cook, D. J., & Das, S. K. (2012). Pervasive computing at scale: Transforming the state of the art. *Pervasive and Mobile Computing, 8*(1), 22–35. doi:10.1016/j.pmcj.2011.10.004

Direção Geral de Saúde. (2003). *Cuidados Intensivos: Recomendações para o seu desenvolvimento.* Lisboa.

Haux, R., Ammenwerth, E., Winter, A., & Brigl, B. (2004). *Strategic information management in hospitals: an introduction to hospital information systems.* Springer. doi:10.1007/978-1-4757-4298-5

Lewis, F. (2004). *Smart Environments: Technologies, Protocols, and Applications.* New York: John Wiley.

McDonald, C., & Gardner, R. (1987). *Computerized Management of Intensive Care Patients Images, Signals and Devices* (pp. 31–45). New York: Springer.

Morris, A., & Gardner, A. (1992). Computer Applications. In J. Hall, G. Schmidt, & L. Wood (Eds.), *Principles of Critical Care* (pp. 500–514). New York: McGraw-Hill.

Peffers, K., Tuunanen, T., Rothenberger, M. A., & Chatterjee, S. (2007). A design science research methodology for information systems research. *Journal of Management Information Systems, 24*(3), 45–77. doi:10.2753/MIS0742-1222240302

Peixoto, R., Portela, F., & Santos, M. F. (2016). Towards a Pervasive Data Mining Engine—Architecture Overview. In Á. Rocha, M.A. Correia, H. Adeli, P.L. Reis, & M. Mendonça Teixeira (Eds.), New Advances in Information Systems and Technologies (WorldCist 2016 - Pervasive Information Systems Workshop) (Vol. 445, pp. 557-566). Cham: Springer International Publishing.

Portela, C. F., Santos, M. F., Silva, Á., Machado, J., & Abelha, A. (2011). Enabling a Pervasive Approach for Intelligent Decision Support in Critical Health Care. In M. Cruz-Cunha, J. Varajão, P. Powell, & R. Martinho (Eds.), *ENTERprise Information Systems* (Vol. 221, pp. 233–243). Springer Berlin Heidelberg. doi:10.1007/978-3-642-24352-3_25

Portela, F., Filipe Santos, M., Abelha, A., Machado, J., Rua Martins, F., & Silva, Á. (in press). Real-time Decision Support using Data Mining to predict Blood Pressure Critical Events in Intensive Medicine Patients.

Portela, F., Santos, M., Machado, J., Abelha, A., Silva, Á., & Rua, F. (2014). *Pervasive and Intelligent Decision Support in Intensive Medicine – The Complete Picture Information Technology in Bio- and Medical Informatics* (Vol. 8649, pp. 87–102). Springer International Publishing.

Portela, F., Santos, M. F., Machado, J., Abelha, A., Silva, A., & Rua, F. (2015). Preventing Patient Cardiac Arrhytmias by Using Data Mining Techniques. *Paper presented at the IEEE Conference on Biomedical Engineering and Sciences (IECBES)*, Kuala Lumpur.

Portela, F., Santos, M. F., Machado, J., Abelha, A., Silva, Á., & Rua, F. (2016). Critical Events in Mechanically Ventilated Patients. In Á. Rocha, M. A. Correia, H. Adeli, P. L. Reis, & M. Mendonça Teixeira (Eds.), *New Advances in Information Systems and Technologies* (Vol. 2, pp. 589–598). Cham: Springer International Publishing. doi:10.1007/978-3-319-31307-8_61

Portela, F., Santos, M. F., & Vilas-Boas, M. (2013, October 25-28). A Pervasive Approach to a Real-Time Intelligent Decision Support System in Intensive Medicine. In A. Fred, J.L.G. Dietz, K. Liu, & J. Filipe (Eds.), *Knowledge Discovery, Knowledge Engineering and Knowledge Management: Second International Joint Conference IC3K '10*, Valencia, Spain (pp. 368-381). Berlin, Heidelberg: Springer. 10.1007/978-3-642-29764-9_25

Portela, F., Veloso, R., Santos, M. F., Machado, J. M., Abelha, A., Silva, Á., & Oliveira, S. M. C. (2014). *Predict hourly patient discharge probability in Intensive Care Units using Data Mining*. ScienceAsia Journal. Doi: doi:10.17485/ijst/2015/v8i32/92043

Ramon, J., Fierens, D., Güiza, F., Meyfroidt, G., Blockeel, H., Bruynooghe, M., & Van Den Berghe, G. (2007). Mining data from intensive care patients. *Advanced Engineering Informatics*, *21*(3), 243–256. doi:10.1016/j.aei.2006.12.002

Richardson, M., Reilly, W., & Kuntz, J. (2008). How Timeglider Works. Retrieved from http://timeglider.com/how_it_works

Rosenberg, D., & Grafton, A. (2010). *Cartographies of time: A history of the timeline*. Princeton Architectural Press.

Santos, M.F., Mathew, W., & Portela, C.F. (2011). Grid Data Mining for Outcome Prediction in Intensive Care Medicine. In *ENTERprise Information Systems* (pp. 244-253).

Santos, M.F., Portela, F., & Vilas-Boas, M. (2011). Intcare: multi-agent approach for real-time intelligent decision support in intensive medicine.

Santos, M.F., Portela, F., Vilas-Boas, M., Silva, Á., & Rua, F. (2010). Hourly prediction of organ failure and outcome in intensive care based on data mining techniques.

Silva, Á.J.B.M.d. (2007). Modelos de intelegência artificial na análise da monitorização de eventos clínicos adversos, disfusão/falência de orgãos e prognóstico do doente crítico.

Sprague, J., & Ralph, H. (1980). A Framework for the Development of Decision Support Systems. *Management Information Systems Quarterly*, *4*(4), 1–26. doi:10.2307/248957

Suter, P., Armaganidis, A., Beaufils, F., Bonfill, X., Burchardi, H., Cook, D., ... Chang, R. (1994). Predicting outcome in ICU patients. *Intensive Care Medicine*, *20*(5), 390–397. doi:10.1007/BF01720917 PMID:7930037

Turban, E., Sharda, R., & Delen, D. (2014). *Business Intelligence and Analytics: Systems for Decision Support* (10th ed.). Prentice Hall.

Varshney, U. (2009). *Pervasive Computing*. Springer, US: Pervasive Healthcare Computing.

Veloso, R., Portela, F., Santos, M., Machado, J. M., Abelha, A., Silva, Á., & Rua, F. (2014). Real-time data mining models for predicting length of stay in intensive care units. *Paper presented at the KMIS 2014-International Conference on Knowledge Management and Information Sharing*. 10.5220/0005083302450254

This research was previously published in the International Journal of Reliable and Quality E-Healthcare (IJRQEH), 6(2); edited by Anastasius Moumtzoglou; pages 17-28, copyright year 2017 by IGI Publishing (an imprint of IGI Global).

Chapter 29
Estimating Key Performance Indicators of a New Emergency Department Model

Soraia Oueida
American University of Middle East, Kuwait

Seifedine Kadry
Beirut Arab University, Lebanon

Sorin Ionescu
Politehnica University of Bucharest, Romania

ABSTRACT

In this article, a real-life Emergency Department (ED) is studied and analyzed in order to propose areas for improvement in its operations and patient flow. EDs are in native very busy and complex systems where medical facility treatments are provided to arriving patients without any prior appointment. ED, a 24/7 open facility, interacts with the majority of other departments of the healthcare system. Due to this complexity and unplanned nature of patient surge, simulation modeling is proven to be very effective in order to study the necessary changes needed for better performance. As a consequence of these challenges, the patient LoS (Length of Stay) and the human-resource utilization rates are increased and thus leading to staff and customer dissatisfaction which need to be addressed for better performance. An emergency department of a hospital in Lebanon is chosen for simulation using Arena software where a model is designed to match the real system. This model is then verified, validated and enhanced by proposing some modifications in the resource allocation levels. These improvements are achieved by running different scenarios using Arena Process Analyzer and suggesting an optimal solution using Arena OptQuest tool without the need of interrupting the real system.

DOI: 10.4018/978-1-7998-2451-0.ch029

Copyright © 2020, IGI Global. Copying or distributing in print or electronic forms without written permission of IGI Global is prohibited.

INTRODUCTION

Healthcare, being a necessity for all nations, is considered as one of the effective and essential entity for all societies, where care treatment is given to needed patients (Mifflin, 2007). The media and politics are given much more attention to the challenges faced by healthcare since it threatens the health status of the nation. These challenges can be listed as staffing shortages ("Nurse Staffing", 2015; "Staffing Survey", 2001), aging population (Hellmich, 2008), rising costs (Bodenheimer, 2005), and inefficient hospital processes (Berwick & Hackbarth, 2012). Simulation Modeling is proved through the literature to be the most effective way to model the daily operations of a queuing, concurrent system such as the emergency department. The system chosen for study is the one of a hospital in Lebanon currently suffering from large waiting times caused by resource shortages (equipment and manpower), absence of computer technology and the heterogeneity of insurance types. These problems caused a loss of potential revenue where patients tend to leave the system before being treated and overcrowding/bottleneck because of the high length of stay; thus, leading to patient dissatisfaction and sometimes may affect patient's safety. The system is studied and analyzed using several methods in order to establish a comprehensive and solid view of the ED operation: collecting real data, conducting interviews with staff/patients and site visits' observations. Based on that, the model is designed, verified and validated leading to a reliable system. Patient flow is then improved using simulation experimentation and optimization techniques.

In order to ensure better process performance and provide efficient services to patients, always maintaining a high level of safety, improvements can be suggested by identifying new resource flow and allocation. Challenges arise here because of the various acuity levels of patients, the numerous ED processes and its different service time. Simulation modeling was proven to be efficient to combat such challenges and provide realistic results. Without interruption of the real system operations, a model can be designed to detect and imitate the flow of resources and patients through the system. Then, changes can be suggested to any process and effects can be easily analyzed before being applied. Using simulation, constraints, bottlenecks, and inefficiencies can be identified and combated thus guarantying patient and management satisfaction. The studied ED faces common issues in the healthcare industry: staffing shortage and inefficient operations. The ED is constituted of two different emergency rooms located in two different buildings and sharing some facilities, such as radiology and billing. This leads to patients' large waiting time and high staff utilization rates. Furthermore, this hospital suffers from the existence of various insurance coverage types which imposes on the billing department to deal with different insurance companies and indirectly affects the patient flow in the ED.

This journal is organized as follows: an introduction is presented in section 1 then a hospital background in section 2. Section 3, 4 and 5 represent the methodology followed in order to accomplish this project; including data collection and analysis, designing the Arena model and testing it in order to verify its functionality and validity, and output results. In section 6, experimentation is performed and different scenarios are suggested in order to explore the effects of changing specific metrics in the ED and areas for future improvement are suggested. In section 7, model optimization is performed using Arena OptQuest. Finally, the journal is concluded in section 8 and future work perspectives are suggested.

HOSPITAL BACKGROUND

The chosen ED is an emergency department for a hospital in Lebanon. It is a non- profit health institution recognized since 1952. Since this hospital was the only shelter for public services during the Lebanese Civil War (1975-1990) and because of the increasing number of patients, an extension became a must. Many achievements have been realized since then to expand the hospital and include new departments. In 2003, a new building was established in order to serve more beds and extend the hospital facilities. The two buildings were connected through an underground tunnel in order to safely transfer patients. The first building is a charitable suite building while the second one is a private suite building. Nevertheless, both buildings can serve all patients in need in case of overcrowding. The hospital includes almost 200 beds and covering most of the medical/surgical specialties. Its ED serves more than 40 000 patients yearly and open for 24/7. The main ED resources are classified as per the following:

- **Emergency Room Doctor (ER Dr.):** Responsible for high level decisions, final diagnosis, writing prescriptions, ordering extra facilities or special treatments.
- **Registered Nurse (RN):** Responsible for all triage activities once patient arrives to the ED. RN can make some decisions instead of the ER doctor in case of exceptional conditions like bottleneck or disaster conditions. RN is the chief of all nurses.
- **Nurse (N):** Responsible for collecting patients' data information once he enters the ED. The nurse is also responsible for preparing the patient until the doctor is available.
- **Transporter:** Responsible for transferring the patients to other units in case needed.
- **Specialist:** Responsible for extra diagnosis and assisting the ER doctor with final decisions if needed. Specialists are available in their clinics and are common for all the hospital.

METHODOLOGY

The main purpose of this study is to alleviate the patient flow delays and inefficiencies. This is achieved by defining the patient flow and operations inside the ED, designing a model that depicts the real system and testing this model to ensure it is reliable. After model validation, experimentation is approached in order to propose new scenarios for improving the system. As proven in previous related work (Centeno, 2003; Duguay & Chetouane, 2007), an efficient way for improving patient flow is related to performing some staff changes. In our methodology, these changes are performed to the designed model and assessed to check its effect on the key performance indicators: patient LoS and staff utilization rates. Resources are the main characteristics of the model and considered as the control variables while approaching experimentation. Because of the complexity of the system and the need for simulation modeling, Arena Rockwell Automation was selected as the DES (Discrete Event Simulation) tool for building the realistic ED model.

As first steps before designing the model, site visits and interviews with staff/patient were conducted in order to establish a clear overview of the ED operations and formulate the problems faced. Using these collected data, the model can then be designed, verified and validated. This model should depict the current status of the ED studied. These steps form the fundamentals of a simulation study in literature (Law & McComas, 2002; Baldwin et al., 2004). Finally, patient flow was improved by performing experimentation and analysis to the designed model taking into consideration also the cost analysis and hospital revenue.

Data Collection and Analysis

Data collection is the first important step before starting to build the model since the simulation quality depends on the ability of the model to imitate the behavior of the real system. Therefore, a deep and comprehensive understanding of the patient flow through the ED is necessary (Blake et al., 1996). Observations and interviews with staff/patients are performed during site visits to the ED. Data, such as, arrival time, routing probabilities and processes' service time are collected and analyzed in order to be fed to the simulation model. Patient arrivals vary from day to day and based on the time of the day. The routing probability is the percentage of patients moving from one stage to another in the process; they are mainly used after decisions. The service time is the average time needed in order to accomplish a process and it depends on both the resource type assigned along with the patient severity case.

As per previous related work, sources relied on for data collections were: records available in databases, interviews with resources/management, site visits and comparisons with other EDs (Paul et al., 2010). Once accurate data are collected and analyzed, Input Analyzer can be used in order to choose the best fitting distribution; which will be used later as inputs to the simulation model processes.

Patient Data

As mentioned before, patient data was collected and analyzed for the two ERs separately. From site visits and interviews it was concluded that they both follow the same process and flow of operation. The data recorded included patient arrival time, time spent for each activity and in each unit (such as registration, radiology, insurance, billing), acuity level (severe/non-severe), patient status (admitted or no), and patient departure time.

The data arrival rate is identified as the time the patient arrives to the ED and it is denoted in the model as Tnow. On the other hand, the time of departure is recorded as the time of discharge from ED. These records constitute the total length of stay (LoS) of a patient in the ED from the time he arrives until his discharge. Discharge from ED can be either to another unit for extra needed care or leaving home.

BUILDING A REALISTIC MODEL

In this section the services adopted by the ED, the flow of patients at each stage and the methodology followed in order to build the required model are presented along with the flowchart of the Arena simulation.

Emergency Department Overview

The studied ED is constituted of two emergency rooms (ERs). ER A offers public services and ER B offers private services. Each ER has its own operational flow and a fixed number of resources. Both ERs share the same radiology unit and billing center. The two ERs are split into six different zones:

1. A waiting room
2. A registration desk
3. A room dedicated for doctors/nurses
4. A triage zone

5.   Three examination rooms
6.   A dedicated room for small surgeries

Arrivals to the ED follow a random exponential process. Arrivals were modeled with an average arrival rate estimated based on a database of 48 weeks in our studied ED from August 2015 to August 2016.

The patient follows different stages during his journey in the ED and confronts several type of resources depending on the need. Therefore, all human resources are considered while designing the model processes. Each resource offers a certain type of service and generates a waiting time in order to accomplish this service; thus, affecting the overall process. These resources are presented in table 1 below.

Patient Journey in the ED

A patient must follow some essential steps during his journey at the ED: arrival, consultation, diagnosis, decision and finally either discharged or admitted to the hospital. Upon arrival, a nurse collects his data information and refers him to the initial consultation room where triage occurs. At this room, the RN responsible for triage will assign the severe cases immediately to an available doctor; whereas, the non-severe cases are transferred to a waiting room where they wait for a doctor to be available. This stage is very important since the ED has limited resources and needs to serve all arriving patients regardless of their case.

Next stage is the doctor examination. The high acuity patients are transferred immediately for examination using a transporter; While other patients wait for a free doctor. Once the patient is in the examination room and the doctor is available, examination starts. Based on the first examination, the doctor can diagnose the case and may request some additional tests (radiology/laboratory requests) in order to better assess the case and reach the optimal decision.

If the patient doesn't need any extra facility, he will be discharged with a prescription and some recommendations if necessary. Blood tests are taken in the ED and are transported to the laboratory unit using the medical transporter. For patients who need imaging services, they are transferred to the radiology unit (RU) by the medical transporter. It's worth to mention here that patients in ER B need to cross the tunnel in order to reach the RU while patients in ER A will be only moved to a different floor.

Table 1. Resources' Role and Capacity in the Model

Resource Type	Role	Capacity in the Model
Doctor	Diagnosis and final decision	1
Nurse: Triage, RN, N	Classifying patients based on severity	3
Transporter	Transporting patients to other units	1
Technician	Available for extra facilities such as in the radiology unit	3
Physician	Available in radiology unit to check the results and provide a report	1
Receptionist	Available for registration process and opening a file	1
Accountant	Responsible for billing	8
Specialist	A senior doctor to help ED doctor in critical decisions	On hospital duty (not included in the model)

Once arrived to the RU, patients should wait for an available technician. Waiting rooms are available. When the technician is available and the patient is served, he should wait again for the results that will be reported by a free physician. Only when the report is ready, the patient can leave the RU back to the corresponding ER. Here, he should wait again for an available doctor for final diagnosis. Before reaching the final examination, the patient is requested to go to the billing unit in order to open a file, provide insurance coverage type (if any) and finalize the payments.

At the final stage, the doctor will check the imaging/laboratory results and upon his diagnosis he may discharge the patient home with some prescriptions and necessary recommendations or may admit the patient to another unit in the hospital for extra necessary care. In case of admission, the patient should wait for an available bed before he is discharged from the ED. In some cases, the ER doctor may request the opinion of another specialist in order to finalize the diagnosis. Since, the specialist belongs to the whole hospital and may be shared by different units, a limitation for experimentation arises. Additional delays are added to the total time of the process and are considered in this designed model under the doctor examination process in order to avoid the limitation. As a final stage, the patient will be either transferred to another unit in the hospital to be admitted or totally discharged (exiting the system).

Flowchart of the Conceptual Model

The model, designed using Arena software, represents both ERs (ER A and ER B) and is presented in figure 1.

As mentioned before, the input data of the model are the data collected during site visits/databases. These data are fed to the Arena Input Analyzer and are fitted to the best corresponding distribution. Both ERs follow the same operational behavior and same flow except for when extra facilities are required. They share the radiology unit but the RU is located in the public building. Patient from private ED needs to be transferred across the tunnel in order to reach the RU and therefore resulting in extra process delays. We always refer to resource A corresponding to ER A and resource B corresponding to ER B.

Simulation

After building the model and fitting all data to the corresponding distributions, 10 replications were simulated in order to analyze the results and study the areas of interest. These replications will help getting the average of all performance measures and thus reaching a more realistic output. The base unit used is always minutes. The main performance measures recorded in order to verify and validate the model are: number of patients in and number of patients out, patient LoS, process service time and resource utilization. From the simulation results, the number of patients arriving to the ED is found to be on average 138 patients/day for both emergency rooms. While, the number of patients exiting the system is found to be on average 77 patients/day in total for both emergency rooms. The patient LoS is a user specified attribute that records the total time a patient spends in the system from the time he arrives to the ED until he exits. The average total time spent by patient A is found to be around 277 minutes and an average of 294 minutes for patient B. As per the resource utilization rates collected, we can conclude that the main problem exists with the transporters and the receptionist. These average utilization rates are 97% and 93% respectively.

Figure 1. ED Arena Model Flowchart

Public ER A

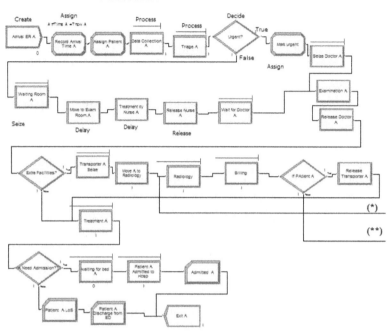

Private ER B

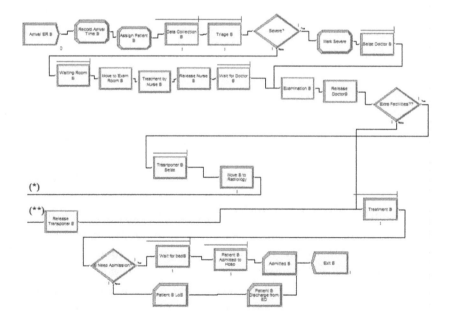

SIMULATION VALIDATION AND VERIFICATION

The results obtained from the simulation of the designed model should be verified and validated to match the behavior of the real system; otherwise any changes and suggestions for improvements will result in faulty decisions and unneeded costs.

Model Verification

As part of model verification, tests are applied in order to check desirable and undesirable situations. These tests are applied on the main perform measures that may highly affect the system: Patient flow, Arrivals/Departures, and Process service times. Processes are checked to be operating similarly for the different stages of the real system.

Model Validation

Since emergency departments are proven to be very complex systems, it is hard to take into consideration all its features while building the model. Studies showed that model accuracy is obtained from only 20% of the model's detail (Robinson, 1994). Therefore, we had to rely on some assumptions while designing the model which should be taken into account carefully.

In the validation stage, the behavior of four indicators are evaluated, compared to the real system and tested to ensure identical behavior: patient LoS, resources' workload, processes' service time, and the number of patients exiting the system (referred in the model by system number out). Any gaps or missing characteristics were identified and fixed until the designed model matched the real system. From the simulation output results, the number of patients exiting the system is 77 on average for both ERs while in the real system, the number of patients discharged from the ED per day is on average 40 to 45 patients per emergency room. As for the LoS, the simulation output shows a value of 277 and 294 minutes for ER A and ER B respectively. These numbers match the real system where patients' stay in the ED does not exceed 300 minutes. As for the resources' workload, the receptionist and transporters are super busy and face issues to serve all coming patients which match with the simulation output corresponding utilization rates of 97%. Other than the high utilization rate of resources, the billing department suffers from the heterogeneity of the insurance types which delays big time the process during acceptance. Therefore, the billing unit is a very busy one and it affects the daily operations of the ERs by increasing the average patient waiting time. The validation is said to be completed once the simulated model is compared, tested and found matching the behavior of the real system. We can say now that the designed model is reliable and experimentation can be approached for suggesting improvements on the system.

EXPERIMENTATION

The fact of experimentation falls under improving the system by suggesting some changes and analyze the effect of these changes on the system behavior. Different aspects can be relied on for experimentation as per the literature (Law & McComas, 2001): changing staffing schedules (Duguay & Chetouane, 2007), modifying a process behavior (Pallin & Kittell, 1992) or assessing the effect of external variables (Hannan et al., 1994). We started our experimentation by proposing different scenarios and comparing

Table 2. Resources' Salaries

Resource Type	Salary/Month
Doctor	$2000
RN	$1100
Nurse	$850
Specialist	$1200
Physician/Expert	$1200
Transporter	$650
Accountant	$1000
Receptionist	$500
Technician	$800

them to the original one using the Arena Process Analyzer tool. These scenarios focus on adding extra resources to the daily operation of the ED and assess the effect of this change to the overall performance. Since the major component here is the human resource, it is trustworthy to mention that resources get different salaries depending on their role, depicted in table 2 below.

Five different scenarios are proposed taking into consideration two performance measures while assessing the performance of the system: patient LoS, staff utilization and Cost; Thus, guarantying patient, staff and management satisfaction. Nevertheless, high utilization rates can also lead to medical errors in some cases which must be avoided.

Starting the experimentation, different controls and responses are added to the simulation. Controls represent the system resources. Responses are the outputs of theses simulations. The choice of these responses was based on the analysis of the model simulation output data. The five scenarios are as follows:

- **Scenario 1:** Addition of 2 doctors (one for ER A and one ER B), 2 transporters (one for ER A and one ER B), and one receptionist.
- **Scenario 2:** Addition of 2 nurses (one for ER A and one ER B), 2 transporters (one for ER A and one ER B), and one receptionist.
- **Scenario 3:** Addition of 2 RNs (one for ER A and one ER B), 2 transporters (one for ER A and one ER B), and one receptionist.
- **Scenario 4:** Addition of 4 transporters (two for ER A and two ER B), and two receptionists.
- **Scenario 5:** Addition of 2 doctors (one for ER A and one for ER B), 4 transporters (two for ER A and two ER B), and two receptionists.

After simulating these scenarios, the advantage of adding extra resources was obvious where patient LoS and transporters'/receptionist's utilization rates were noticeably reduced and the number of patient leaving the ED was increased. The best scenarios are 4 and 5. Another parameter should be highlighted as well while suggesting the optimal scenario: cost/revenue.

Average Waiting Time Analysis

The simulation outputs are presented in the figures below where the patient LoS is reduced and some staff workload is improved. Scenario 5 is found to be better compared to scenario 4 (for LoS and utilization rates measures), while scenario 4 better (for number of patient out measure). In figures 2 and 3, the average LoS of patients A and B is reduced from 277 min and 294 min (original scenario) to 82 min and 108 min (scenario 5) for ER A and ER B respectively.

In figure 4, the receptionist utilization is reduced from 93% in the original scenario to 69% and 67% in scenarios 4 and 5 respectively.

In figures 5 and 6, we can see that the transporters' utilization rates are reduced from 97% (original scenario) to 80% and 83% respectively in scenario 4 and 69% and 79% respectively in scenario 5.

In Figure 7, the number of patient out is highlighted to be highly increased in both scenarios 4 and 5 to be 134 and 124 respectively.

Figure 2. Reducing Patient A Los

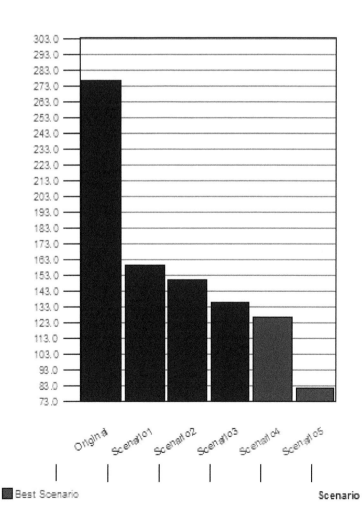

Figure 3. Reducing Patient B LoS

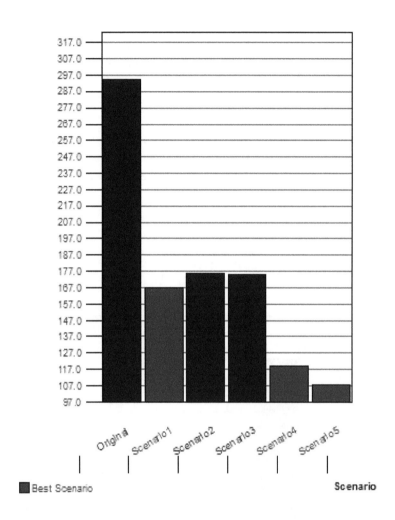

Cost Analysis

The suggestion of adding resources to the ED as part of improvement will result in additional costs. In order to guarantee management satisfaction and since the hospital suffers from some budget constraints, cost analysis is a very important step in order to convince the decision makers with the simulated scenarios. Calculating the additional costs and comparing this amount to the extra revenue resulted from the increased number of patient out, it is deducted that, for scenario 4 a net profit of $700,575 /year is reached while for scenario 5, only $563,150 /year net profit is reached. Therefore, scenario 4 seems more attracting for decision makers. The yearly cost/revenue proportion is depicted in table 3 below.

Figure 4. Reducing Receptionist Utilization

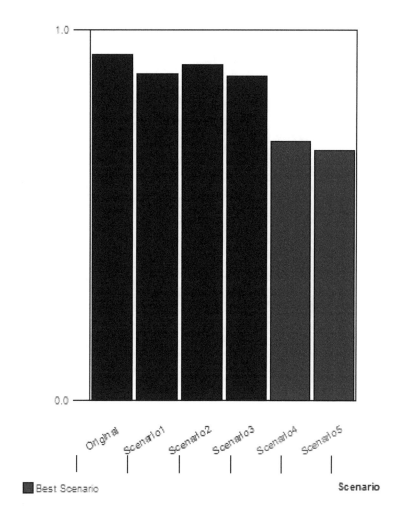

Decision

As per the simulation results of the five scenarios, scenario 4 is found better based on revenue measures whereas scenario 5 is found more reliable based on enhancing the performance measures studied. Noting that in both scenarios patient LoS is reduced and revenue is increased. Therefore, decision makers should compromise here and reach a decision to best fit the real system.

OPTIMIZATION

As mentioned in the previous section, many scenarios can be tested in order to alleviate the problems faced by the studied ED. Simulating different scenarios and comparing their performance in order to find the most efficient one is time consuming and may not lead to the optimal solution. Therefore,

Figure 5. Reducing Transporter A Utilization

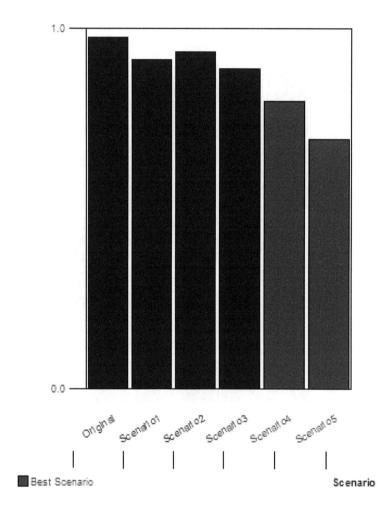

in order to find the optimal solution that best fits our case, simulation optimization is suggested and performed. This solution overcomes the problem of efficiency and accuracy and consists on searching automatically within the simulation model for optimal solutions. Simulation optimization is applied on the model using OptQuest. This tool is an application within Arena software that seeks a combination of defined variables in order to reach a minimum or a maximum set of objectives. This is the final phase of our experimentation.

The OptQuest for Arena includes three main elements:

1. **Controls:** Variables or resources that being changed can affect the performance of the system.
2. **Constraints:** Relationships among controls and responses.
3. **Objective:** One response that represents the model's objective; either minimizing or maximizing a certain parameter.

Figure 6. Reducing Transporter B Utilization

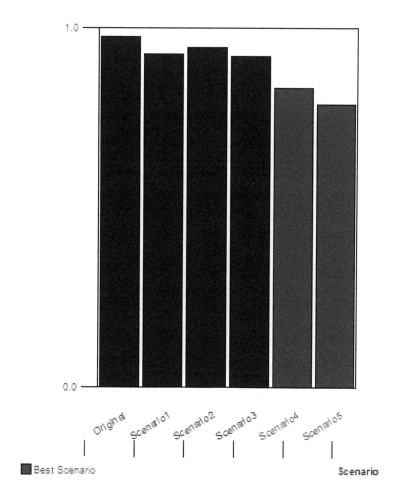

To begin with the OptQuest, a control list was defined and all human resources were chosen excluding the technicians, physician and accountants since the current number of these resources are enough for the operation of the ED (this conclusion was deducted from interviews and continuous visits to the ED). These controls were chosen in order to see the effect of resource changes on patient waiting time and system output (patients exiting the simulated system). Then, responses need to be chosen; which reflect the decisions for improvement. The chosen responses are: Transporter A and B Utilization, Receptionist Utilization, Patient A and B LoS, System Number Out, Transporter A and B Queues Waiting Time, Patient A and B Admitted to Hosp Queues Waiting Time, Billing Queue Waiting Time, Tnow A and Tnow B and finally Patient Number Out.

After defining our controls and responses, the replication number was set to 3 in order to get more accurate results and variation for each combination of controls. For each replication, a maximum of 300 simulations was chosen with an automatic stop option. The automatic stop option means that OptQuest would stop looking for solutions when it had not seen significant improvement for 100 different scenarios in a row.

Figure 7. Increasing the Number of Patient Out

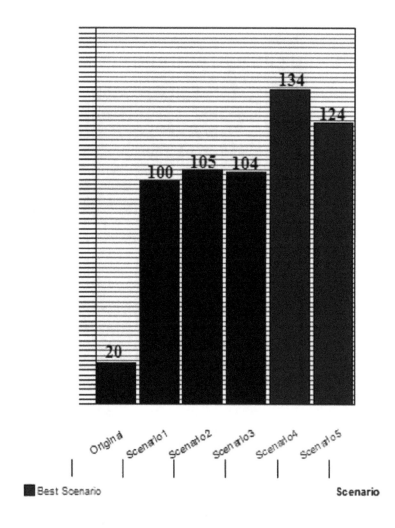

Table 3. Cost/Revenue Proportion for Scenarios 4 and 5

Scenario	Additional Cost	Revenue	Net Profit
4	$27,600	$728,175	$700,575
3	$75,600	$638,750	$563,150

Finally, before running the optimization, objectives were defined. The main goal for this optimization simulation is to minimize patients LoS and maximize the system number out at the same time. For this, the objective in OptQuest was set to be: "Maximizing the system number out". Running this simulation will both maximize this number and minimize the patient LoS in the system (further elaborated in the next section).

Simulation Objective

In this objective, the purpose is to reach the best or maximum number of patients exiting the system, taking into consideration all the responses defined earlier. The result from all simulations shows that the best solution is simulation 5 with an objective value of 138 (system number out). The best combination of resources is depicted in table 4 below.

Figure 8 shows the 10 best simulations resulted from the OptQuest run along with the corresponding best resource distribution. This new suggested solution helps the hospital management to improve its operations guarantying patient satisfaction by seeing more patients and increasing revenue in some cases (hospital satisfaction).

Scenario 5 suggests adding two nurses (one in each ER), adding two doctors (one in each ER), adding two receptionists, adding four transporters (two in each ER), and adding 2 RNs (one in each ER). The extra costs of adding these resources are $11,500 per month ($138,000 yearly) based on table 2 monthly

Table 4. Best Resource Distribution-Scenario 5

Resource Type	Best Capacity
Accountant	8
Doctor A	2
Doctor B	2
Nurse A	3
Nurse B	3
Physician	1
Receptionist	3
RN A	2
RN B	2
Technician	3
Transporter A	3
Transporter B	3

Figure 8. Best Scenarios for Maximizing System Out

Best Solutions   **Stopped due to the Auto Stop option.**

	Select	Simulation	Objective Value	Status	Doctor A	Doctor B	Nurse A	Nurse B	Receptionist	RN A	RN B	Transporter A	Transporter B
▶	✔	5	138.333333	Feasible	2	2	3	3	3	2	2	3	3
	✔	16	138.000000	Feasible	2	2	3	2	3	2	2	3	3
	✔	30	137.333333	Feasible	2	1	3	3	3	2	2	3	3
	✔	118	135.666667	Feasible	2	2	3	2	3	2	1	3	3
	✔	66	134.000000	Feasible	2	2	3	3	3	1	2	3	3
	✔	3	133.666667	Feasible	2	2	2	2	3	2	2	3	3
	✔	33	133.666667	Feasible	2	2	1	3	3	2	2	3	3
	✔	100	132.000000	Feasible	2	2	3	3	3	1	1	3	3
	✔	45	131.666667	Feasible	2	2	2	2	3	1	2	2	3
	✔	64	131.000000	Feasible	1	2	1	2	3	1	2	2	3

salary distributions. The system now is serving 138 patients which mean extra revenue of 61 consultation fees ($2,135 daily/779,275 yearly). The net profit will be $53,550 monthly. This is almost a $641,275 per year; which is huge yearly revenue that a hospital can add. Therefore, decision makers should take a look at this suggestion and think of considering and implementing it to the real running system.

Other parameters should be also highlighted as an efficient result from simulation 5 since a noticeable change occurs on these performance measures if we apply this suggested solution. These performance measures' improvements are depicted in table 5 below along with a comparison with the original scenario values.

Discussion

The comparison presented in table 5 shows that the output values are very efficient and the new distribution of resources suggested being the optimal solution are highly reliable; based on four measurement metrics:

1. Number of System Out
2. Patient LoS
3. Resource Utilization Rates
4. Hospital Revenue/Net profit

Where, Number of system out and revenue are increased and patient LoS is minimized.

Comparing the values obtained from OptQuest optimization tool with the results obtained using process analyzer, we found that these values are roughly similar to the results of best scenarios 4 and 5. Nevertheless, this optimal solution (scenario 5) using OptQuest optimization tool gave us a very efficient result by combining the 4 essential metrics mentioned above in one suggested solution only (system out, LoS, resource utilization and revenue); thus, the advantage of using OptQuest Arena Simulation.

Table 5. Comparison between original scenario and scenario 5

	Original scenario	Optimal scenario 5
Billing queue waiting time	9.7	0.74
Patient A admitted to hosp queue waiting time	28	7.79
Patient B admitted to hosp queue waiting time	29	14.22
Transporter A queue waiting time	410	19.7
Transporter B queue waiting time	426	52.9
Receptionist utilization	93%	72%
Transporter A utilization	97%	72%
Transporter B utilization	97%	72%
Patient A LoS	277	71
Patient B LoS	294	120

CONCLUSION AND FUTURE WORK

An emergency department of a hospital in North Lebanon was studied in order to build a simulation model using Arena software. The ED consists of two emergency rooms. The two ERs operate the same and have the same resource distribution but they share only the radiology and billing units. In order to establish a clear understanding of the ED services and operations, continuous visits and interviews with staff/patients were conducted. These records helped in designing a model that matches the real system and contributed in the verification and validation stages. By comparing the different performance measures' outputs from the Arena simulation to the ones of the real system, the model was found to be reliable and ready for experimentation. During the experimentation stage, five different scenarios were suggested in order to improve the system behavior and increase the performance of the system using Arena Process Analyzer tool. The scenarios consisted on adding extra resources to the system and assess the effect of these changes on the overall behavior. The performance measures taken into consideration are: patient LoS, resource utilization rates, number of patient out. Another very important parameter considered is the cost/revenue in order to guarantee management satisfaction and convince decision makers to adopt these changes regardless of budget constraints. Moreover, model optimization is performed using Arena OptQuest tool in order to achieve the optimal solution and best scenario for resource distribution; always taking into consideration patient satisfaction (decreasing LoS), staff satisfaction (decreasing the utilization rate) and management satisfaction (increasing revenue). To conclude, performing experimentation and/or optimization provides decision makers with better insights on how adding extra resources may improve the performance of the system without interrupting the operation of the real system.

As a future work, more performance measures will be studied while proposing new scenarios for experimentation and optimization. A new type of resource will be introduced in the model which consists of considering the use of equipment, medical devices, medical components, beds, etc. and study their effect on the flow of patients in the ED and how it affects the 4 already discussed metrics for system enhancement.

REFERENCES

Baldwin, L. P., Eldabi, T., & Paul, R. J. (2004). Simulation in healthcare management: A soft approach (MAPIU). *Simulation Modelling Practice and Theory, 12*(7), 541–557. doi:10.1016/j.simpat.2004.02.003

Berwick, D. M., & Hackbarth, A. D. (2012). Eliminating waste in US health care. *Journal of the American Medical Association, 307*(14), 1513–1516. doi:10.1001/jama.2012.362 PMID:22419800

Blake, J. T., Carter, M. W., & Richardson, S. (1996). An analysis of emergency room wait time issues via computer simulation. *INFOR, 34*(4), 263–273. doi:10.1080/03155986.1996.11732308

Bodenheimer, T. (2005). High and rising health care costs. Part 1: Seeking an explanation. *Annals of Internal Medicine, 142*(10), 847–854. doi:10.7326/0003-4819-142-10-200505170-00010 PMID:15897535

California Nurses Association. (2001, April 20). Staffing Survey. Mandatory Overtime Is Detrimental to Patient Care and the Health of Nurses.

Centeno, M. A., Giachetti, R., Linn, R., & Ismail, A. M. (2003, December). Emergency departments II: a simulation-ilp based tool for scheduling ER staff. In *Proceedings of the 35th conference on Winter simulation: driving innovation* (pp. 1930-1938).

Duguay, C., & Chetouane, F. (2007). Modeling and improving emergency department systems using discrete event simulation. *Simulation, 83*(4), 311–320. doi:10.1177/0037549707083111

Hannan, E. L., Giglio, R. J., & Sadowski, R. S. (1974). A simulation analysis of a hospital emergency department. In *Proceedings of the 7th conference on Winter simulation* (Vol. 1, pp. 379-388). ACM. 10.1145/800287.811199

Hellmich, N. (2008). Aging population making more visits to the doctor's. *USA today*. Retrieved from http://www.usatoday.com/news/health/2008-08-06-er_N.htm

Law, A. M., & McComas, M. G. (2001). How to Build Valid and Credible Simulation Models. In *Proceedings of the 2009 Winter Simulation Conference* (pp. 24–33). IEEE. 10.1109/WSC.2001.977242

Mifflin, H. (2007). The American Heritage Medical Directory.

Nursing World. (2015). State staffing plans. Retrieved from http://www.nursingworld.org/MainMenu-Categories/Policy-Advocacy/State/Legislative-Agenda-Reports/State-StaffingPlansRatios

Pallin, A., & Kittell, R. P. (1992). Mercy Hospital: "simulation techniques for ER processes. *Industrial Engineering (American Institute of Industrial Engineers), 24*(2), 35–37.

Paul, S. A., Reddy, M. C., & DeFlitch, C. J. (2010). A systematic review of simulation studies investigating emergency department overcrowding. *Simulation, 86*(8-9), 559–571. doi:10.1177/0037549709360912

Robinson, S. (1994). Simulation projects: building the right conceptual model. *Industrial Engineering-Norcross, 26*(9), 34–36.

This research was previously published in the International Journal of User-Driven Healthcare (IJUDH), 7(2); edited by Ashok Kumar Biswas; pages 1-16, copyright year 2017 by IGI Publishing (an imprint of IGI Global).

Chapter 30

A Review on the Contribution of Emergency Department Simulation Studies in Reducing Wait Time

Basmah Almoaber

University of Ottawa, Canada &King Khalid University, Saudi Arabia

Daniel Amyot

University of Ottawa, Canada

ABSTRACT

Background: Because of the important role of hospital emergency departments (EDs) in providing urgent care, EDs face a constantly large demand that often results in long wait times. Objective: To review and analyze the existing literature in ED simulation modeling and its contribution in reducing patient wait time. Methods: A literature review was conducted on simulation modeling in EDs. Results: A total of 41 articles have met the inclusion criteria. The papers were categorized based on their motivations, modeling techniques, data collection processes, patient classification, recommendations, and implementation statuses. Real impact is seldom measured; only four papers (~10%) have reported the implementation of their recommended changes in the real world. Conclusion: The reported implementations contributed significantly to wait time reduction, but the proportion of simulation studies that are implemented is too low to conclude causality. Researchers should budget resources to implement their simulation recommendations in order to measure their impact on patient wait time.

INTRODUCTION

An emergency department (ED) is considered the most important part of any hospital. It is responsible for providing care to patients who need immediate but unscheduled healthcare services, 24 hours a day, 7 days a week. However, because of an ED's important role in providing urgent care for ill or injured

DOI: 10.4018/978-1-7998-2451-0.ch030

Copyright © 2020, IGI Global. Copying or distributing in print or electronic forms without written permission of IGI Global is prohibited.

patients, EDs face a constantly large demand that often results in long wait time. Due to many factors, such as insufficient staffing, budget constraints, poor inpatient bed turnover, unscheduled arrivals, and growing and aging populations, ED services are seriously affected and patient wait time has reached a critical level in many hospitals, which in turn causes serious health consequences and adds an economic cost for both patients and societies. In this context, many healthcare organizations and research centers are wondering whether the analysis results of ED simulation models can help reduce patient wait time.

Background on Patient Wait Time

Wait time is usually known as the difference between the time of arrival in the ED and the time the patient has contact with a physician for the first time. Others define it as the time a patient has spent waiting for diagnostic tests (e.g., X-ray or blood test) or waiting after returning from external testing to get therapy (Chin & Fleisher, 1998). According to the Canadian Institute for Health Information (2012), four relevant measures can contribute to patient wait time in the ED:

- **ED Length of Stay:** Time from patient registration to discharge or admission;
- **Time Waiting for Initial Physician Assessment:** Time from patient registration to the moment a physician first assesses the patient;
- **Time to Disposition:** Time from patient registration to the moment the decision is taken to either discharge or admit the patient to a hospital bed; and
- **Time Waiting for Inpatient Bed:** Time from patient admission to the moment the patient leaves the ED to go to the inpatient unit (inside the hospital).

Different organizations have defined targets that give a maximum time a patient should spend in the ED. For instance, in Ontario (Canada), provincial targets for the ED length of stay are eight and four hours for the high acuity and low acuity patients, respectively (Ontario Ministry of Health and Long-Term Care, 2015). In Québec (Canada), the targeted provincial average wait time for ED length of stay is 12 hours (Ministère de la Santé et des Services Sociaux du Québec, 2011). In the UK, the target wait time is set to four hours from arrival to admission, transfer, or discharge (NHS Choices, 2015).

Unfortunately, in many cases, hospitals cannot meet their targets and patients wait longer than expected. Such long time causes negative effects on the patients and the service quality. Patients may experience delays in the treatment of pain or suffering, higher dissatisfaction, and higher risks of stronger or more permanent damage. Some patients even decide to leave without receiving treatment. On the other hand, the efficiency and stress level of physicians and nurses can also be affected negatively by such long waits (Waldrop, 2009).

Since long patient wait time is one of the most important issues in ED, and due to its direct impact on the quality of healthcare services and the satisfaction level of patients, it has attracted much attention lately. A variety of solutions have been considered toward shortening ED wait time, such as better resource allocation strategies (Day, Al-Roubaie, & Goldlust, 2013; Xu, Roger, Rohleder, & Cooke, 2008), improved staff working systems (Kuo, 2014; Kuo, Leung, & Graham, 2015; Wang, McKay, Jewer, & Sharma, 2013), and separate care programs for minor injuries (Khadem, Bashir, Al-Lawati, & Al-Azri, 2008; Maulla, Smarta, Harrisb, & Karasnehc, 2009; Rasheed, Lee, Kim, & Park, 2012). However, because ED is a dynamic system with complex interactions among different components and processes, the challenge with most of the suggested solutions is that, in addition to the possibility of failure, such solutions cost much money and time to be implemented. In this context, hospital decision makers need effective techniques to help them test proposed scenarios and predict results before the actual implementation. Simulation, which is used to imitate in an abstract way the operation of a real-world process or system over time, is a candidate technique that can likely help here.

ED Simulation Overview

Simulation is nowadays perceived as an effective technique for assessing organizations' efficiency, searching for more efficient processes, and testing recommended changes and improvements in a rapid, accurate, low cost, and low risk means. Simulation modeling approaches have been adapted to ED because of their ability to analyze patients flow, predict demand for services, address current problems in ED, and evaluate various interventions. They also help hospital administrators and practitioners examine many "what if" scenarios with an ED complex system by making changes in the system within a user-friendly graphical interface, without jeopardizing patient care (Friesen, McLeod, Strome, & Mukhi, 2011).

Simulation models are used in ED to either support strategic (long-term) decision making or to support operational (day-to-day) decision making. The former type includes improving the process by hiring additional physicians or nurses, or changing the ED layout or processes, whereas the latter type focuses on near real-time decisions such as calling for additional staff or diverting ambulances towards other hospitals (Bahrani, Tchemeube, Mouttham, & Amyot, 2013).

A number of simulation approaches have been used to model EDs such as system dynamics (SD), discrete event simulation (DES), or agent-based simulation (ABS).

The general simulation methodology, for every ED, contains five main steps:

1. Collecting the required data including arrival rates and different service times
2. Analyzing the data to develop statistical distributions and then feeding them to a simulation model of the ED
3. Running the model using the current state of the modeled ED
4. Verifying and validating the simulation model
5. Evaluating different alternatives/scenarios to mitigate patient wait time

The typical patient flow throughout an ED is presented in Figure 1. This flow starts with the patient's arrival to the ED entrance either by ambulance or by walking in and ends when the patient is either discharged from the ED or admitted into the hospital for further treatment. In between these endpoints, three stages are involved. First, in the triage station, patient acuity is decided by a nurse and higher

Figure 1. Typical patient flow in an ED

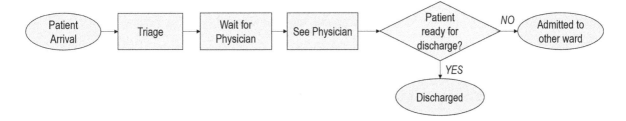

priority for treatment is given for patients with acute conditions. Second, the patient is moved to the waiting area or examination room until seen by a physician. Finally, the patient is seen by a physician, who decides whether to discharge or admit the patient.

Literature Review Objective

The objective of this review is to study and analyze the existing literature on ED simulation modeling and its contribution in reducing patient wait time to answer the following research question: How well has the simulation approach succeeded in achieving wait time reduction in emergency departments?

The review raises awareness about the gap that exists between the use of simulations for optimizing EDs and the implementation of the simulation recommendations in real environments to measure the concrete impact of these recommendations on wait time. This review is important as most hospitals around the globe that have an ED suffer from wait time issues and are continuously trying to minimize patient wait time. The review is also timely as there now exists a body of ED simulation work that can be analyzed. In addition, Scerbo (2016) reports on the increasing interest in the use of simulation in healthcare, be it for education, research, or operational optimization, as well as on major investments in specialized simulation centers.

The paper is organized as follows. The literature review section provides details on the methodology used to conduct the review and then reports on the findings. Next, the discussion section uses the findings to answer the research question and highlight important limitations of current studies. Threats to the validity of the review itself are then discussed. Finally, conclusions bring final thoughts and directions for future research.

LITERATURE REVIEW METHODOLOGY

To achieve the review objective and answer the research question, a systematized literature review, inspired by Kitchenham's systematic literature review approach (Kitchenham, 2004), is conducted. Kitchenham's popular approach has proven its value in guiding the rigorous collection, selection, and evaluation of research papers related to information technologies. Systematized reviews are done in three stages:

1. Searching as much relevant published (peer-reviewed) evidence as possible through a search query
2. Evaluating the retrieved publications against inclusion and exclusion criteria to only keep the most relevant studies
3. Synthesizing knowledge and conclusions by aggregating and interpreting the findings from individual studies

The specific details of our review protocol are presented next according to these three stages. These details are important for the readers to understand how the papers were selected and how knowledge was synthesized from them. Such details also enable the reproducibility of the review.

Searching Stage

In this first stage, three complementary databases were used to identify relevant papers:

- Scopus® in order to cover both the technology and health literature about simulations. Scopus also covers the journals from IEEE and those included in PubMed/Medline and Embase since 1996. Scopus claims to be the "world's largest abstract and citation database", with more than 60 million citations.
- IEEE Xplore® Digital Library to cover the technical literature related to ED simulation not already covered by Scopus (e.g., conference papers). Xplore includes over 4 million citations.
- PubMed to cover the biomedical/health literature about ED simulations not already covered by Scopus (e.g., conference papers). PubMed comprises over 26 million citations.

Groups of keywords were used to locate potentially relevant papers. In Scopus and IEEE Xplore, the following query was used *simulation AND model*ing AND "wait* time" AND "emergency department" AND healthcare*. In PubMed, Medical Subject Headings (MeSH) were used to search for *"computer simulation[MeSH Terms] AND emergency care[MeSH Terms] AND waiting list[MeSH Terms]"*.

Scopus was the main source for most of the retrieved papers. Then, IEEE Xplore came next (must of the returned papers were already founded by Scopus). Finally, PubMed was used but was not so effective in locating additional papers.

Evaluating Stage

In the second stage, the results were evaluated against inclusion criteria to only include papers with the following conditions:

- **Source Type**: Conference papers and scholarly journals
- **Language**: English

Additionally, the titles and abstracts of the retrieved papers were read to only include papers that satisfy the following selection criteria:

- The paper discusses an application of simulation models in emergency departments;
- The simulation model considers general ED and not only specific departments; and
- A reduction in the patient wait time is one of the simulation goals or results.

Synthesizing Stage

After evaluating the papers, the full text of each selected paper was retrieved and analyzed to extract the required data. The extracted data includes details about each study's reference, location (country and hospital), objectives, simulation tool, and implementation status.

RESULTS

The literature review, conducted in the spring of 2016, has resulted in 41 papers. They have been analyzed with respect to 1) project motivations, 2) modeling techniques, 3) data collection processes, 4) patients' classifications and flows, 5) recommendations, and 6) implementations. Table 3 in the Appendix presents a general summary of the selected papers. For each paper, Table 3 provides details on the target hospital and its country, the objectives of the ED simulation, the simulation tool used, and whether or not there was an actual implementation of the system following the simulation-based analysis.

Project Motivations

The motivations of reviewed papers can be broadly categorized as to 1) increase patient satisfaction, 2) increase service quality, 3) improve ED processes, or 4) improve resources management. Table 3 includes the objectives of every project.

To increase patient satisfaction and increase service quality, many projects worked towards reducing wait time as their main goal (Al-Ajeel et al., 2015; Day et al., 2013; Duguay & Chetouane, 2007; Eskandari, Riyahifard, Khosravi, & Geiger, 2011; Weng et al., 2011), and towards alleviating bottlenecks (Eskandari et al., 2011; MacDonald et al., 2005; Venugopal, Daniel Otero, Otero, & Centeno, 2013). A number of projects examined patient flows and introduced different tracks for different patients' acuity levels (Chonde, Parra, & Chang, 2013; Friesen et al., 2011; Konrad et al., 2013; Zeinali, Mahootchi, & Sepehri, 2015).

Different projects evaluated different procedural changes to improve ED processes. For instance, changes included introducing several discharging plans (Crawford, Parikh, Kong, & Thakar, 2014), reducing lab turn-around time (Storrow et al., 2008) and adding a separate track for pediatric and low acuity patients (Kim, Delbridge, & Kendrick, 2014; Chonde et al., 2013).

One of the primary motivations of some projects is to improve the management of resources such as staff. Several projects considered changing staff sizing (Al-Ajeel et al., 2015; Cabrera, Luque, Taboada, Epelde, & Iglesias, 2012; Cocke et al., 2016; Day et al., 2013; Eskandari et al., 2011; Komashie & Mousavi, 2005; Zeinali et al., 2015) and evaluating different staff schedules (Holm & Dahl, 2009; Kuo, 2014; Venugopal et al., 2013; Weng et al., 2011; Xu et al., 2008; Yeh & Lin, 2007). Other projects examined physician behaviors (Lim, Worster, Goeree, & Tarride, 2013; Wang et al., 2013) and heterogeneity (Y.H. Kuo et al., 2015). The effects of ED layout were also examined in (Khadem et al., 2008).

Modeling Techniques

Discrete event simulation (DES) is the main modeling approach that has been used in almost all reviewed papers, either alone or combined with other approaches, except for one paper that used an agent-based simulation (Cabrera et al., 2012). The high penetration level of DES in ED simulations is due to its ability to model complex non-linear systems while taking into account patient history, staff scheduling, and multiple resource constraints (Duguay & Chetouane, 2007). The DES approach has been used to explain patient flows through a series of queues and activities in discrete time intervals and to represent the relationships between different entities in the ED system.

Some papers integrated different techniques with DES to get a better representation of the actual ED system. For instance, Kuo (2014) introduced the use of simulated annealing (SA). Kuo proposed a simulation-optimization method, in which simulation is integrated as a subroutine to create realizations for evaluating system performances, and at the same time used a simulated annealing algorithm to search for a good solution to develop.

Ahmad et al. (2014) used hybrid simulation models that combine DES and system dynamics (SD) in order to get a better representation of the actual system than by using either modeling paradigm solely.

Another modeling possibility is the use of a Colored Petri Net model (Salimifard, Hosseini, & Moradi, 2013), which is first developed to analyze the performance of ED, and then employed in a DES model to capture patients flow and care processes.

In addition, Zeinali et al. (2015) combined both simulation and metamodels to design a decision support system. They used a metamodel-based optimization to obtain a configuration of resources to reduce the total average wait time of patients with consideration of budget and capacity constraints. Their main idea is to use DES to evaluate the ED performance, and then use a metamodel to allocate resources.

Weng et al. (2011) mixed DES and Data Envelopment Analysis (DEA) to evaluate potential bottlenecks, maximize throughput flows, and reduce wait time. The DEA model is developed to calculate the efficiency of different ED operation alternatives that have been generated by the DES model subject to the available budget.

In Yeh and Lin's work (2007), a genetic algorithm (GA) is utilized in combination with simulation to adjust nurses' schedules without hiring additional staff. They first developed a simulation model to simulate the patients flow through the ED. Then, they applied GA to find a near-optimal nurse schedule minimizes the patients' queue time.

Eskandari et al. (2011) proposed a new framework that integrates the simulation model of a patients' flow process with the group AHP (Analytic Hierarchy Process) and TOPSIS (Technique for Order Preference by Similarity to Ideal Solution) decision models to first identify bottlenecks of the ED and then to evaluate improving scenarios with the lowest possible expenditure developed for overcoming these bottlenecks. TOPSIS decision models take the weights of performance measures from the group AHP and the values of performance measures from the simulation model, and ranks the improvement scenarios.

As mentioned before, a large number of reviewed papers have used DES models in ED studies. In contrast, Cabrera et al. (2012) believed that using ABS to model EDs is more appropriate than DES because of the nature of healthcare systems, which are centered on human actions and interactions.

Table 1. Simulation tools references

Tool	Reference
Arena	Arena Simulation Software. https://www.arenasimulation.com/
AnyLogic	AnyLogic Multimethod Simulation Software. http://www.anylogic.com/
CPN Tools	Colored Petri Nets Tools. http://cpntools.org/
eM-Plant	Plant Simulation (formerly eM-Plant). https://www.simplan.de/en/software/tools/plant-simulation.html
Flexsim Healthcare	Flexsim HealthCare. https://healthcare.flexsim.com/
FORTRAN	Fortan Programming Language. http://fortranwiki.org/fortran/show/Fortran
MedModel	MedModel Patient Flow and Process Improvement. https://www.promodel.com/Products/MedModel
NetLogo	NetLogo. https://ccl.northwestern.edu/netlogo/
ProModel	ProModel Better Decision Faster. https://www.promodel.com/
Simio	Simio Forward Thinking. http://www.simio.com/index.php
SIMISCRIPT	SIMSCRIPT Modeling and Simulation Tools. http://www.simscript.com/partners/partners.html
SIMUL8	SIMUL8 Process Simulation Software. http://www.simul8.com/

A wide variety of commercial simulation tools have been used to build the models, including Arena (the most popular tool), AnyLogic, CPN Tools, eM-Plant, Flexsim Healthcare, FORTRAN, MedModel, NetLogo, ProModel, Simio, SIMISCRIPT, and SIMUL8. Table 1 gives a reference for each tool.

Data Collection Processes

Data collection is one of the most challenging issues in many simulation projects. The quality and availability of the data play an important role in providing accurate simulation results. To conduct a valid simulation for an emergency department, several datasets are required. For example, the required data includes but is not limited to i) patterns of patient arrivals, ii) time stamped events such as arrival, registration, discharge, and transfer location, iii) the capacity of each workstation, iv) the number of healthcare providers available at each workstation, v) staff work schedules, and vi) acuity levels. The number and type of collected data are different from one model to the other based on each ED' settings and the model goals. The nature of the required data also depends on the simulation goals. For example, if the model is built to evaluate different staff schedules, then the focus will be on collecting all the data related to the staff size, salaries, and schedules.

The reviewed papers used different sources to obtain the required data. Historic patient records are the most popular source (Cocke et al., 2016; Coughlan et al., 2011; Eskandari et al., 2011; Friesen et al., 2011; Holm & Dahl, 2009; Khadem et al., 2008; Konrad et al., 2013; Kuo, 2014; Kuo et al., 2015; Rasheed et al., 2012; Shim & Kumar, 2010; Wang et al., 2013; Weng, Cheng, et al., 2011; Xu et al., 2008). Open interviews with physicians, nurses, and other staff take the second place (Ahmad et al., 2014; Al-Ajeel et al., 2015; Duguay & Chetouane, 2007; Kang et al., 2014; Komashie & Mousavi, 2005; Konrad et al., 2013; Kuo, 2014; MacDonald et al., 2005; Salimifard et al., 2013; Shim & Kumar, 2010; Xu et al., 2008; Yeh & Lin, 2007). The third place is occupied by observation and monitoring data (Duguay & Chetouane, 2007; Khadem et al., 2008; Khurma et al., 2008; Komashie & Mousavi, 2005; Konrad et al., 2013; Maulla et al., 2009). Additionally, other sources were used such as surveys (Al-Ajeel et al., 2015; Holm & Dahl, 2009; Khadem et al., 2008), time-motion studies (Kang et al., 2014; MacDonald et al., 2005; Rasheed et al., 2012), and hospital administrative databases (Lim et al., 2013). In addition to hospital registers data, some papers collected and used data about special events to evaluate how to reduce wait time during those events. For instance, Malavisi et al. (2015) used data collected during the 1994 Northridge earthquake to simulate the seismic event in ED, and Al-Ajeel et al. (2015) collected data during both normal days and during sandstorm days to simulate the ED during a sandstorm.

Patients Classification

The reviewed papers stated that the patients' degree of acuity affects their wait time. For instance, patients who are classified as urgent but not critical, the largest group of patients, have the longest wait time in some ED (Day et al., 2013; Duguay & Chetouane, 2007; Friesen et al., 2011; Khurma et al., 2008; Konrad et al., 2013; Kuo, 2014; Kuo et al., 2015; Lim et al., 2013; MacDonald et al., 2005; Rasheed et al., 2012; Salimifard et al., 2013; Zeinali et al., 2015). The reason is that critical patients preempt all other patients whereas non-urgent patients are treated and discharged immediately. With this issue in mind, different projects categorized patients along different dimensions. The most popular dimension is based on the patients' level of acuity/urgency. In most cases, patients are classified into one of five categories: level 1 (critical), level 2 (emergency), level 3 (urgent), level 4 (less urgent) and level

5 (non-urgent) (Cocke et al., 2016; Day et al., 2013; Eskandari et al., 2011; Weng et al., 2011). Based on these categories, some papers reclassified the patients into other groups, for example, admitted and discharged patients (Chonde et al., 2013; Kang et al., 2014), or high (levels 1 and 2) and low (levels 3, 4 and 5) acuity (Komashie & Mousavi, 2005; Lim et al., 2013). Other projects put category 5 patients into category 4 because they have the same flow and priority in real practice, and there is only a small proportion of category 5 patients (Kuo, 2014; Kuo et al., 2015). In addition, other models consider different categories for the level of acuity: acute, sub-acute, and minor (Wang et al., 2013), or simply red, yellow, and green (Khadem et al., 2008).

Moreover, dimensions of categorization may include age (either adult or pediatric with a cutoff age of 18) (Ahmad et al., 2014; Coughlan et al., 2011), the mode of arrival (arriving by ambulance or arriving by walking in) (Ahmed & Alkhamis, 2009; Coughlan et al., 2011), or a combination of a mode of arrival with a level of acuity (Al-Ajeel et al., 2015; MacDonald et al., 2005).

Recommendations

Simulation models are built either to diagnose process issues or to test performance improvement ideas. The reviewed papers have tested different scenarios to improve the ED process and then presented their recommendations to reduce patient wait time. Most of the recommendations either suggest changing levels and allocation of resources (resources allocation) or suggest changing the ED processes themselves (process improvement). Not all recommendations are feasible; some of them are costly and cannot be implemented due to budget constraints in some EDs.

Processes Improvement

One of the most common recommendations is to introduce different queues for different patient classifications such as acuity level, or admitted or discharged statuses (see the typical patient flow in Figure 1).

Chonde et al. (2013) suggested using two patient flow models: Virtual Streaming (VS), which introduces two virtual queues for admitted and for discharged patients (see Figure 2), and Physician Directed Queuing (PDQ), which introduces a fast track PQD area for low acuity patients. Figure 3 summarizes the PDQ procedure.

Most of the patient redirections are recommended for low acuity patients to save time and resources for high acuity patients. A "fast-track" strategy (Figure 4) allows for the rapid assessment and treatment of less serious injuries and illnesses (Khadem et al., 2008; Maulla et al., 2009; Rasheed et al., 2012).

Kim et al. (2014), suggested dividing patients into two groups, adults and pediatric patients with a cutoff age of 18, and using a separate pediatric ED with its own patient flow management and medical resources in order to provide better quality emergency care to the target group.

Friesen et al. (2011) also recommended changing patient flows. They suggested redirecting the patients towards other EDs in order to balance ED loads using "crowdinforming", in which patients with non-urgent conditions consult a website or a smartphone-based service that provides insight into the "busyness" of an ED before deciding which one to attend.

The split-flow process of Konrad et al. (2013) is another example of patient redirection. Less sick patients are split off from the traditional ED process flow, which is then reserved for higher acuity patients, and redirected to a continuous care area.

Figure 2. Flowchart for virtual streaming (VS). Adapted from Chonde et al. (2013).

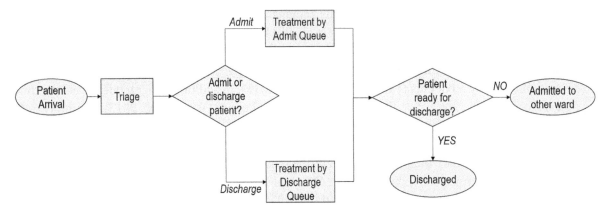

Figure 3. Flowchart for physician directed queuing (PDQ). Adapted from Chonde et al. (2013).

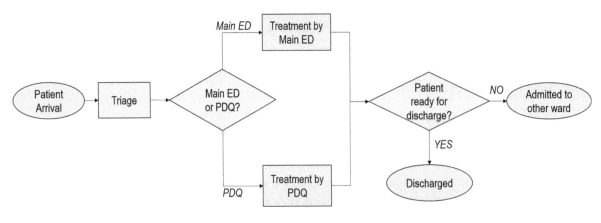

Figure 4. Example of "See and Treat" Model. Adapted from Maulla et al. (2009).

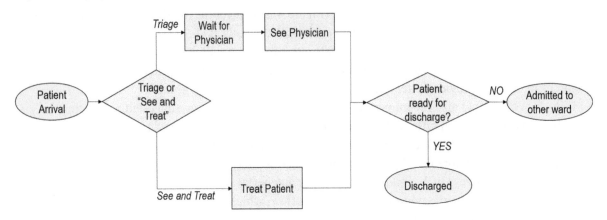

Another process-related recommendation is presented by Crawford et al. (2014). The authors suggested using two proactive inpatient discharge strategies to reduce ED waiting and boarding times. The two strategies differ in how they estimate the occurrence of ED crowding to start discharging inpatients based on their estimated readmission risk. The proactive strategy-waiting (PS-W) considers the number of patients waiting for an ED bed post triage, whereas proactive strategy-boarding (PS-B) considers the number of patients in an ED who are waiting for an inpatient unit bed after completion of treatment in the ED.

In addition, Storrow (2008) showed that decreasing lab turnaround time resulted in a reduction in the total number of diversion days, average diversion hours per day, percentage of days with diversion, and average ED LOS.

Giving priority to ED patients in need of limited/expensive medical equipment such as advanced scanners over non-ED patients was recommended by Eskandari et al. (2011) to reduce patient wait time.

Resources Allocation

Many papers suggested adding one or more physicians in order to reduce wait time and increase the number of treated patients (Duguay & Chetouane, 2007; Khadem et al., 2008; Konrad et al., 2013; Salimifard et al., 2013). Adding a physician to the split-flow area can reduce the length of stay for lower acuity patients (Konrad et al., 2013). The same result is obtained when adding a physician and mid-level provider in triage, absorbing fast-track patients into triage, and discharging low-acuity patients directly from triage whenever possible (Day et al., 2013). Doan et al. (2014) recommended the addition of physician assistants (PAs) to reduce time without increasing costs. Hung et al. (2007) recommended the addition of a hospital volunteer and a second triage nurse to reduce pre-triage wait time and the proportion of patients waiting longer than 30 to 60 minutes for pre-triage to manage the increase in patient arrival rates in the winter season. Cocke et al. (2016) found that increasing staff by 25% of the current schedule is the feasible solution to handle the upcoming yearly demand in their new ED facility. In contrast, Holm & Dahl (2009) found that no significant change in patient wait time results from replacing the nurse triage with a physician triage during busy hours.

Varying the layout of the ED by adding or removing rooms was also recommended in some papers. Examples include adding an additional triage room and combining reception with triage (Khadem et al., 2008), setting up a new short-stay ward for patients who need to be further observed and monitored for less than a day (Shim & Kumar, 2010), adding a separate load relief area for low acuity patients (Rasheed et al., 2012), adding five mobile beds in the inpatient ward (Eskandari et al., 2011), and establishing a Rapid Assessment and Treatment (RAT) area (MacDonald et al., 2005).

Other recommendations suggested considering physician behavior to reduce wait time, for example:

- Variation in physician service rates can help reducing wait time because employing more efficient physicians can speed up the overall consultation time (Kuo et al., 2015).
- Based on the idea that the speed of physician assessment varies considerably at the beginning and end of a shift, eight-hour shifts should start every four hours, so the shift beginning and shift ending periods overlap (Wang et al., 2013).

In addition, the simulation results of Kuo (2014) suggested that:

- The best staffing level has a similar profile to the patient arrival rate, but shifted 1.5 – 2 hours behind; and
- Staggered shifts are also helpful to match physicians with patient demand.

Other Recommendations

A few papers considered real-time decisions and near-future forecasting. For example, Hoot et al. (2008) developed a ForecastED simulation to predict near-future operating conditions in order to manage the problem of ED crowding proactively.

Furthermore, the work done by Tan et al. (2013) recommended the use of real-time information to manage demand surges or to release doctors to the backroom operations during low peak period. The authors proposed an intelligent model to adjust the number of doctors based on current and historical information about the patient arrival in the ED.

Implementations

Most of the papers' recommendations to improve ED processes and reduce wait time are only theoretically proposed by modelers and have not been implemented in the real world. To examine the impact of the changes recommended by the modeler, recommendations must be implemented and evaluated. From the 41 reviewed papers in Table 3, only four (i.e., less than 10%) have reported the implementation of their suggested changes Table 2.

To analyze the impact on the ED wait time of moving from a "triage and treat" strategy, where patients are treated in the triage area and discharged without reaching the main ED area, to a "see and treat" strategy, Maulla et al. (2009) constructed and implemented a DES model. The research was structured into three phases. Phase 1 was the model creation and validation based on ED data to represent the current processes. Phase 2 involved using the model to assess the impact of a "see and treat" strategy on wait time. Three scenarios have been tested in this phase. Lastly, Phase 3 compared pre- and post-implementation performances with the predicted results of the model. The comparison was conducted by analyzing three data sets: the actual pre-implementation performance, pre- and post-implementation predictions derived from the simulation model, and the actual results obtained from a post-implementation analysis. The results of the comparison show a significant reduction in patient wait time, from 13.2% of the population waiting longer than 4 h before the implementation to 1.4% after the implementation. The authors unfortunately have not mentioned the hospital's name.

Day et al. (2013) had a different objective when implementing their simulation model. Their aim was to assess the accuracy of the simulation in predicting the magnitude of the proposed changes. They suggested adding a physician and a mid-level provider in triage, and consolidating the Fast Track into triage to reduce the average length of stay (LOS) and the proportion of patients with over 6 hours of LOS. The assessment was done by comparing the two simulations (*before* and *after* models) with the real-world data before and after the implementation. The result showed no significant difference between the post-intervention states in the simulated and real-world ED.

Konrad et al. (2013) introduced the idea of using the split-flow concept to manage ED processes by splitting the flow of patients according to patient acuity. They compared seventeen scenarios, regarding Door-to-Doctor time and length-of-stay for different patient acuity levels, to estimate the likely impact of a split-flow process redesign, including staffing level changes and patient volume changes. Finally,

Table 2. Hospitals names and locations where simulation recommendations have been implemented

Reference	Country	Hospital Name
(Maulla et al., 2009)	UK	N/A
(Day et al., 2013)	USA	St. Louis Veterans Affairs Medical Center
(Konrad et al., 2013)	USA	Saint Vincent Hospital in Worcester
(Zeinali et al., 2015)	Iran	Modarres Hospital

they recommended adding a physician to the split-flow area. The hospital management added additional physician assistants based on this recommendation. The implementation resulted in significant improvements in Door-to-Doctor time, total length-of-stay, arrival to bed time, and the number of patients left without being seen. The success of the implementation was evaluated by comparing the performance metrics from three different sources: 1) Saint Vincent hospital data prior to split-flow implementation, 2) Saint Vincent hospital data after split-flow implementation, and 3) benchmark metrics.

A simulation-based metamodeling approach was used as a novel decision support system to improve the patients flow and minimize the average wait time in the Modarres Hospital, in Iran (Zeinali et al., 2015). The idea was to find the optimal number of ED resources within the ED's budget and capacity constraints and then implement the changes through three steps: first, develop a simulation of the ED in order to evaluate the measure (total average wait time of patients) for each configuration of resources; second, use different metamodel techniques and choose the one with the maximum efficiency through a cross-validation technique to replace the computationally expensive DES model, and finally, use the proposed model to minimize the total average wait time of patients. The paper declared that the proposed model has been implemented and has resulted in a 48% decrease in the total average wait time without any further details.

DISCUSSION AND LIMITATION

Discussion

Simulation models were introduced in the reviewed papers as a decision technique to help ED management explore options to improve patient wait time without the typical financial or physical risks that may result from implementing those options in a real ED. A few hospitals have implemented the proposed solutions and achieved not only a significant improvement in terms of reducing patient wait time, but also good predictability of the simulation models.

As explained in the introduction, many metrics are used in the different models to measure wait time. In many cases, the hospitals' historical records do not include data about the start and end of activities. Moreover, the rapid change in demands and the variety in acuity levels affect the accuracy of measured wait time. Almost all the papers consider the average wait time as a measure of ED capacity and quality of service provided except Chin & Fleischer (1998), who proposed the use of the maximum wait time because, in some cases, the maximum time can be much greater than the average.

The trend among the reviewed papers is to model the ED in isolation from other departments. They focus on internal factors that cause the long wait time while in reality there are other external contributing factors. For example, common factors include the delay in transferring admitted patients to other areas of the hospital, and labs turn-around time. On the other hand, the focus on the ED alone can affect other departments by pushing the bottleneck to other hospital units.

ED overcrowding, in which the number of patients in the waiting area exceeds the available resources, has been introduced as a main reason for long patient wait time (Friesen et al., 2011; Konrad et al., 2013; Kuo et al., 2015; Rasheed et al., 2012; Salimifard et al., 2013). Alleviating overcrowding in ED has a high impact on improving patient flow and reducing wait time. Several papers have produced solutions that improve wait time indirectly by solving the overcrowding problem. For example, Friesen et al. (2011) suggest the use of "crowedinforming" to divert incoming patients to an ED during busy periods. In a similar manner, Kuo et al. (2015) found that physician heterogeneity has a great impact in ED overcrowding. Variation in physician service rates can help relieve the ED overcrowding, which in turn reduces wait time.

The "see and treat" strategy provides a promising solution to long wait time. Many papers have evaluated the idea of "see and treat" and the results suggest the implementation of the strategy (Day et al., 2013; Duguay & Chetouane, 2007; Khadem et al., 2008; Konrad et al., 2013; MacDonald et al., 2005; Maulla et al., 2009; Rasheed et al., 2012; Salimifard et al., 2013). Since low acuity patients represent a large proportion of ED patients, the main goal is to discharge low acuity patients directly from triage whenever possible. Adding a physician to the triage succeeded in reducing wait time and in increasing the number of treated patients (Day et al., 2013; Duguay & Chetouane, 2007; MacDonald et al., 2005). One possible threat of using a "see and treat" strategy is that its focus on low-acuity patients may affect patients with higher acuity.

Some papers showed concerns about possible trade-offs when applying certain changes. The discharge strategy suggested by Crawford et al. (2014) may result in an increase in the number of patient readmissions because its main focus is on reducing the crowding by discharging inpatients early.

Papers Limitations

The reviewed simulation projects highlighted a number of useful solutions to reduce patient wait time. However, they have some limitations that could reduce their effectiveness.

First, ED settings vary from one hospital to the other. All the reviewed models were built to represent a specific ED with specific settings that may not be generalizable to other EDs.

Another limitation is that most of the simulation models have represented the ED in isolation from other departments. ED, in reality, is part of a wider system where different services are interacting together in order to achieve their goals. The simulation models need to represent the relationships between the ED and other units of the hospital to capture the big picture and include all the possible factors, internal or external, that may lead to long wait time.

The third limitation is related to the data collection. Acquiring the required data is costly and time consuming. Sometimes, it may be impossible to obtain certain data such as the service time or the data related to the patients or physicians' behavior variation. In that case, modelers tend to make assumptions to close the gap or use a small sample of patients to draw conclusions on system performance, which has an impact on the final results. Other concerns related to the data collection are that the data are collected during a short period. In this case, some useful data such as seasonal peak variations will be overlooked.

Other limitations are related to some common assumptions such as considering equal qualifications and efficiency for all healthcare providers and modeling EDs in stable situations without considering external factors such as different seasons and catastrophes. Also, few papers actually discussed the high cost of some solutions such as adding physicians or nurses.

THREATS TO VALIDITY

Validity refers to the degree of which correct conclusions can be interpreted accurately and confidently from the results of research. The validity of this review is subject to many external and internal threats. The following subsections address those threats and the extent to which they were mitigated.

Internal Validity

Internal validity reflects the extent to which a resulted conclusion is justified. In this review, not all papers that consider the wait time problem in ED may have been retrieved due to:

- Limiting the search to only English-language
- Limiting the search to only three databases
- Not considering referenced papers
- Including only papers that consider the general ED and excluded other papers that studied specific (sub-)departments within the ED

That being said, a sample of 41 relevant papers is large enough to make interesting observations and reach acceptable conclusions. The three databases selected are also quite general, complementary, and comprehensive (and actually Scopus itself also covers many other databases).

Internal validity also considers bias factors such as the number of reviewers. In this review, the retrieved papers were reviewed by a single researcher (the first author); this increases the risk of bias in selecting papers and extracting data. Having more than one reviewer for each paper would have helped but was impossible due to resource limitations. To mitigate this threat, previous related reviews have been considered to verify the research strategy.

External Validity

External validity reflects the ability to generalize the results confidently. From the conducted research, it is concluded that the proportion of implemented simulations is low. A possible reason is that the reviewed papers are limited to journals and conferences in which the focus is on the technical simulation design and not contributions to EDs. Considering the gray literature (magazines, government/hospital reports) may produce different results. Also, the conclusions here are limited to EDs; the ways simulations are used in other hospital departments might be different.

CONCLUSION

From the literature reviewed, a number of important conclusions can be drawn about simulation modeling in ED and its impact on wait time.

First, simulation models, especially DES, have attracted many researchers in ED because: 1) simulations enable researchers to model the uncertainties and variability that are involved in ED systems, 2) they facilitate the representation of the complexity of ED systems, and 3) they assist the communication between modelers and stakeholders.

Second, the use of separate flows for patients based on their acuity level has been proposed, evaluated and applied in real EDs. This recommendation has shown a significant contribution to reducing wait time for less critical patients. The addition of physicians to the triage area to treat and discharge patients has also shown a good result in reducing the waiting in most cases. However, it is still not clear if those approaches have had a negative impact on the wait time of critical patients.

Third, resource allocation has been examined extensively. In human resources, the interesting idea of employing other staff like hospital volunteers and physician assistance to help physicians in treating low acuity patients' needs more investigation to verify its validity and evaluate if this will affect patient readmission rates. Conversely, the expansion of the ED and the addition of more rooms did not lead to wait time reduction unless accompanied by additional staff.

Fourth, the number of reported implementations of the proposed recommendations is low. Without an implementation, some of the recommendations are just theories, and there is no evidence of their actual impact on real systems. It was expected that not all ED simulation papers would contain an implementation, but a mere 10% of implementations is somewhat disappointing. There are many factors that affect the decision to implement recommended changes to an ED. One obvious factor is that not all changes can be applied because of their cost; some changes require hiring an additional physician or adding a new room to the ED. Salimifard et al. (2013) have stated that although the results of the alternatives were promising, ED management may not implement them for unknown reasons: "Also ED staff reaction to our work was positive, and they helped us through the work but due to the reluctance of ED managers, we failed to implement the proposed changes in reality".

Back to the research question "How well has the simulation approach succeeded in achieving wait time reduction in emergency departments?", with the limited number of implemented simulation models, it may be difficult to assess the actual contribution of simulation in reducing patients wait time. One good news is that the implementations reported actually led to positive contributions on reducing patient wait time in EDs. However, as researchers and journals have a tendency to publish more positive results than negative ones, there might exist implemented recommendations that did not lead to positive impacts on wait time, but such results would not be published easily.

In the future, to improve the literature on simulations in EDs, researchers should budget appropriate resources (time, money, and access to data, EDs, and experts) in order to implement the recommendations resulting from the analysis of simulation models and to assess whether there is evidence of improvement. The time and effort spent on such research are huge and should not be wasted with incomplete validation. There is an opportunity to study what factors actually cause the gap between the number of modeled simulations and the number of implemented ones.

In terms of research directions, future ED simulation applications should focus on:

- Modeling ED as part of a larger view of a hospital system by incorporating the interactions between ED and other units. Although ED wait time can be affected by external factors such as labs wait time or inpatient admission processes, most current studies have modeled ED as an isolated unit.

- Modeling real-time decision making. Several studies have considered strategic decisions but only a few have considered real-time, operational decisions (at the patient level rather than at the process level). Forecasting the number of expected patients and dynamically adjusting the number of ED staff based on real-time (e.g., hourly) demand is a promising approach to improve wait time without much economic burden on hospitals.

ACKNOWLEDGMENT

Basmah Almoaber is sponsored by King Khalid University, Abha, Saudi Arabia.

REFERENCES

Ahmad, N., Ghani, N. A., Kamil, A. A., & Tahar, R. M. (2014). Managing resource capacity using hybrid simulation. *Proceedings of the 3rd International Conference on Quantitative Sciences and Its Applications: Fostering Innovation, Streamlining Development, ICOQSIA 2014 (Vol. 1635*, pp. 504–511). School of Quantitative Sciences, College of Arts and Sciences, Universiti Utara Malaysia, Sintok Kedah, Malaysia: American Institute of Physics Inc.

Ahmed, M. A., & Alkhamis, T. M. (2009). Simulation optimization for an emergency department healthcare unit in Kuwait. *European Journal of Operational Research, 198*(3), 936–942. doi:10.1016/j.ejor.2008.10.025

Al-Ajeel, F., Al-Thuwaini, L., Al-Qallaf, M., Al-Faraj, N., Al-Muzayan, S., & Joumaa, C. (2015). Deciding the minimum staffing level in an emergency medical center during sandstorms. *Proceedings of the 2015 IEEE International Conference on Industrial Engineering and Engineering Management (IEEM)* (pp. 711–716). 10.1109/IEEM.2015.7385740

Bahrani, S., Tchemeube, R. B., Mouttham, A., & Amyot, D. (2013). Real-time simulations to support operational decision making in healthcare. *Proceedings of the Summer Computer Simulation Conference, SCSC 2013 and Work in Progress, WIP 2013, Part of the 2013 Summer Simulation Multiconference, SummerSim 2013* (Vol. 45, pp. 374–380).

Cabrera, E., Luque, E., Taboada, M., Epelde, F., & Iglesias, M. L. (2012). ABMS optimization for emergency departments. *Proceedings of the 2012 Winter Simulation Conference (WSC)* (pp. 1–12). 10.1109/WSC.2012.6465116

Canadian Institute for Health Information. (2012). Health Care in Canada, 2012: A Focus on Wait Times. Retrieved from https://www.cihi.ca/en/hcic2012_ch2_en.pdf

Chin, L., & Fleisher, G. (1998). Planning model of resource utilization in an academic pediatric emergency department. *Pediatric Emergency Care, 14*(1), 4–9. doi:10.1097/00006565-199802000-00002 PMID:9516622

Chonde, S., Parra, C., & Chang, C.-J. (2013). Minimizing flow-time and time-to-first-treatment in an Emergency Department through simulation. *Proceedings of the 2013 43rd Winter Simulation Conference - Simulation: Making Decisions in a Complex World, WSC 2013* (pp. 2374–2385). 10.1109/WSC.2013.6721612

Cocke, S., Guinn, D., MacBlane, E., Walshak, S., Willenbrock, N., White, K. P., & Kang, H. (2016). UVA emergency department patient flow simulation and analysis. *Proceedings of the 2016 IEEE Systems and Information Engineering Design Symposium (SIEDS)* (pp. 118–123). 10.1109/SIEDS.2016.7489282

Coughlan, J., Eatock, J., & Patel, N. (2011). Simulating the use of re-prioritisation as a wait-reduction strategy in an emergency department. *Emergency Medicine Journal*, *28*(12), 1013–1018. doi:10.1136/emj.2010.100255 PMID:21068167

Crawford, E. A., Parikh, P. J., Kong, N., & Thakar, C. V. (2014). Analyzing discharge strategies during acute care: A discrete-event simulation study. *Medical Decision Making*, *34*(2), 231–241. doi:10.1177/0272989X13503500 PMID:24077016

Day, T. E., Al-Roubaie, A. R., & Goldlust, E. J. (2013). Decreased length of stay after addition of healthcare provider in emergency department triage: A comparison between computer-simulated and real-world interventions. *Emergency Medicine Journal*, *30*(2), 134–138. doi:10.1136/emermed-2012-201113 PMID:22398851

Doan, Q., Hall, W., Shechter, S., Kissoon, N., Sheps, S., Singer, J., ... Johnson, D. (2014). Forecasting the effect of physician assistants in a pediatric ED. *Journal of the American Academy of Physician Assistants*, *27*(8), 35–41. doi:10.1097/01.JAA.0000451860.95151.e1 PMID:25054792

Duguay, C., & Chetouane, F. (2007). Modeling and improving emergency department systems using discrete event simulation. *Simulation*, *83*(4), 311–320. doi:10.1177/0037549707083111

Eskandari, H., Riyahifard, M., Khosravi, S., & Geiger, C. D. (2011). Improving the emergency department performance using simulation and MCDM methods. *Proceedings of the 2011 Winter Simulation Conference (WSC)* (pp. 1211–1222). 10.1109/WSC.2011.6147843

Friesen, M. R., McLeod, R. D., Strome, T., & Mukhi, S. N. (2011). Load balancing at emergency departments using "crowdinforming." *Proceedings of the 2011 IEEE 13th International Conference on e-Health Networking, Applications and Services, HEALTHCOM 2011* (pp. 364–370). doi:10.1109/HEALTH.2011.6026780

Holm, L. B., & Dahl, F. A. (2009). Simulating the effect of physician triage in the emergency department of Akershus University Hospital. *Proceedings of the 2009 Winter Simulation Conference (WSC)* (pp. 1896–1905). 10.1109/WSC.2009.5429204

Hoot, N. R., LeBlanc, L. J., Jones, I., Levin, S. R., Zhou, C., Gadd, C. S., & Aronsky, D. (2008). Forecasting Emergency Department Crowding: A Discrete Event Simulation. *Annals of Emergency Medicine*, *52*(2), 116–125. doi:10.1016/j.annemergmed.2007.12.011 PMID:18387699

Hung, G. R., Whitehouse, S. R., ONeill, C., Gray, A. P., & Kissoon, N. (2007). Computer modeling of patient flow in a pediatric emergency department using discrete event simulation. *Pediatric Emergency Care*, *23*(1), 5–10. doi:10.1097/PEC.0b013e31802c611e PMID:17228213

Kang, H., Nembhard, H. B., Rafferty, C., & Deflitch, C. J. (2014). Patient flow in the emergency department: A classification and analysis of admission process policies. *Annals of Emergency Medicine, 64*(4), 335–342. doi:10.1016/j.annemergmed.2014.04.011 PMID:24875896

Khadem, M., Bashir, H. A., Al-Lawati, Y., & Al-Azri, F. (2008). Evaluating the layout of the emergency department of a public hospital using computer simulation modeling: A case study. *Proceedings of the 2008 IEEE International Conference on Industrial Engineering and Engineering Management, IEEM 2008* (pp. 1709–1713). 10.1109/IEEM.2008.4738164

Khurma, N., Bacioiu, G. M., & Pasek, Z. J. (2008). *Simulation-based verification of lean improvement for emergency room process. In 2008 Winter Simulation Conference* (pp. 1490–1499). WSC. doi:10.1109/WSC.2008.4736229

Kim, B. J. B., Delbridge, T. R., & Kendrick, D. B. (2014). Improving process quality for pediatric emergency department. *International Journal of Health Care Quality Assurance, 27*(4), 336–346. doi:10.1108/IJHCQA-11-2012-0117 PMID:25076607

Kitchenham, B. (2004). Procedures for performing systematic reviews. *Technical Report, Keele University and NICTA, Staffordshire, UK, 33*, 1–26.

Komashie, A., & Mousavi, A. (2005). Modeling emergency departments using discrete event simulation techniques. In 2005 Winter Simulation Conference (Vol. 2005, pp. 2681–2685). doi:10.1109/WSC.2005.1574570

Konrad, R., DeSotto, K., Grocela, A., McAuley, P., Wang, J., Lyons, J., & Bruin, M. (2013). Modeling the impact of changing patient flow processes in an emergency department: Insights from a computer simulation study. *Operations Research for Health Care, 2*(4), 66–74. doi:10.1016/j.orhc.2013.04.001

Kuo, Y. H. (2014). Integrating simulation with simulated annealing for scheduling physicians in an understaffed emergency department. *HKIE Transactions Hong Kong Institution of Engineers, 21*(4), 253–261. doi:10.1080/1023697X.2014.970748

Kuo, Y. H., Leung, J. M. Y., & Graham, C. A. (2015). Using Simulation to Examine the Effect of Physician Heterogeneity on the Operational Efficiency of an Overcrowded Hospital Emergency Department. *Journal of Physics: Conference Series 616*(1). 10.1088/1742-6596/616/1/012017

Lim, M. E., Worster, A., Goeree, R., & Tarride, J.-E. (2013). Simulating an emergency department: The importance of modeling the interactions between physicians and delegates in a discrete event simulation. *BMC Medical Informatics and Decision Making, 13*(1), 59. doi:10.1186/1472-6947-13-59 PMID:23692710

MacDonald, S. J., Karkam, I., Al-Shirrawi, N., Chowdhary, R. K., Escalante, E. M., & Afandi, A. (2005). Emergency department process improvement. *Proceedings of the 2005 IEEE Systems and Information Engineering Design Symposium* (Vol. 2005, pp. 253–261). 10.1109/SIEDS.2005.193266

Malavisi, M., Cimellaro, G. P., Terzic, V., & Mahin, S. (2015). Hospital emergency response network for mass casualty incidents. In I. N. & L. M. (Eds.), *Structures Congress 2015* (pp. 1573–1584). 10.1061/9780784479117.135

Maulla, R. S., Smarta, P. A., Harrisb, A., & Karasnehc, A. A.-F. (2009). An evaluation of fast track in A&E: A discrete event simulation approach. *Service Industries Journal, 29*(7), 923–941. doi:10.1080/02642060902749534

Ministère de la Santé et des Services Sociaux du Québec. (2011). *Rapport annuel de gestion 2010-2011.* Retrieved from http://publications.msss.gouv.qc.ca/ acrobat/f/documentation/2011/11-102-01F.pdf

N. H. S. Choices (2015). *Urgent and emergency care services in England.* Retrieved from http://www. nhs.uk/NHSEngland/AboutNHSservices/Emergencyandurgentcareservices/Pages/AE.aspx

Ontario Ministry of Health and Long-Term Care. (2015). *Ontario Wait Times. Emergency Room Wait Times - Emergency Room Targets.* Retrieved from http://www.health.gov.on.ca/en/pro/programs/wait-times/edrs/targets.aspx

Rasheed, F., Lee, Y. H., Kim, S. H., & Park, I. C. (2012). Development of emergency department load relief area-gauging benefits in empirical terms. *Simulation in Healthcare, 7*(6), 343–352. doi:10.1097/SIH.0b013e31825ded80 PMID:22960699

Salimifard, K., Hosseini, S. Y., & Moradi, M. S. (2013). Improving emergency department processes using Coloured Petri nets. M. D. in (Ed.), *Joint International Workshop on Petri Nets and Software Engineering, PNSE 2013 and the International Workshop on Modeling and Business Environments, ModBE 2013 - Co-located with the 34th International Conference on Application and Theory of Petri Nets and* (Vol. 989, pp. 335–349).

Scerbo, M. (2016). Simulation in Healthcare: Growin up*. *Simulation in Healthcare, 11*(4), 232–235. doi:10.1097/SIH.0000000000000190 PMID:27490084

Shim, S. J., & Kumar, A. (2010). Simulation for emergency care process reengineering in hospitals. *Business Process Management Journal, 16*(5), 795–805. doi:10.1108/14637151011076476

Storrow, A. B., Zhou, C., Gaddis, G., Han, J. H., Miller, K., Klubert, D., ... Aronsky, D. (2008). Decreasing lab turnaround time improves emergency department throughput and decreases emergency medical services diversion: A simulation model. *Academic Emergency Medicine, 15*(11), 1130–1135. doi:10.1111/j.1553-2712.2008.00181.x PMID:18638034

Tan, K. W., Tan, W. H., & Lau, H. C. (2013). Improving patient length-of-stay in emergency department through dynamic resource allocation policies. *Proceedings of the 2013 IEEE International Conference on Automation Science and Engineering, CASE 2013* (pp. 984–989). 10.1109/CoASE.2013.6653988

Venugopal, V., Daniel Otero, L., Otero, C. E., & Centeno, G. (2013). A simulation model for evaluating resource policies in a major emergency department. *Proceedings of IEEE Southeastcon* (pp. 1–5). 10.1109/SECON.2013.6567424

Waldrop, R. D. (2009). Don't be put out by throughput in the emergency department. *Physician Executive, 35*(3), 38–41. PMID:19534313

Wang, B., McKay, K., Jewer, J., & Sharma, A. (2013). Physician shift behavior and its impact on service performances in an emergency department. In *2013 Winter Simulations Conference WSC* (pp. 2350–2361). doi:10.1109/WSC.2013.6721610

Weng, S.-J., Cheng, B.-C., Kwong, S. T., Wang, L.-M., & Chang, C.-Y. (2011). Simulation Optimization for emergency department resources allocation. *Proceedings of the 2011 Winter Simulation Conference (WSC)* (pp. 1231–1238). 10.1109/WSC.2011.6147845

Weng, S.-J., Tsai, B.-S., Wang, L.-M., Chang, C.-Y., & Gotcher, D. (2011). Using simulation and Data Envelopment Analysis in optimal healthcare efficiency allocations. *Proceedings of the 2011 Winter Simulation Conference (WSC)* (pp. 1295–1305). 10.1109/WSC.2011.6147850

Xu, S., Roger, P., Rohleder, T. R., & Cooke, D. L. (2008). Improving emergency department physician management via computer simulation. *Proceedings of the IIE Annual Conference and Expo 2008* (pp. 834–839).

Yeh, J., & Lin, W. (2007). Using simulation technique and genetic algorithm to improve the quality care of a hospital emergency department. *Expert Systems with Applications*, *32*(4), 1073–1083. doi:10.1016/j.eswa.2006.02.017

Zeinali, F., Mahootchi, M., & Sepehri, M. M. (2015). Resource planning in the emergency departments: A simulation-based metamodeling approach. *Simulation Modelling Practice and Theory*, *53*, 123–138. doi:10.1016/j.simpat.2015.02.002

This research was previously published in the International Journal of E-Health and Medical Communications (IJEHMC), 8(3); edited by Joel J.P.C. Rodrigues; pages 1-21, copyright year 2017 by IGI Publishing (an imprint of IGI Global).

APPENDIX

Table 3. Summary of the 41 selected papers

Reference	Country	Hospital Name	Objectives	Simulation tool	Imple-mented?
(Chin & Fleisher, 1998)	USA	An urban, university affiliated pediatric teaching hospital	To quantify the effect of patient arrival time and physician practices on physician idle time and patient wait time	FORTRAN	NO
(Komashie & Mousavi, 2005)	UK	Hospital in London, no name.	(1) To model the system for better understanding of operations, (2) To determine the impact of critical resources on Key Performance Indicators (KPIs), and (3) To provide a cost-effective means of testing various scenarios for possible system improvement.	Arena	NO
(MacDonald et al., 2005)	USA	The University Medical Center in Tucson, Arizona	To propose recommendations that would alleviate bottlenecks in the patient flow process of the ED.	Arena	NO
(Duguay & Chetouane, 2007)	Canada	Dr. Georges-L. Dumont Hospital in Moncton	To reduce patient wait time and to improve overall service delivery and system throughput.	Arena	NO
(Hung, Whitehouse, O'Neill, Gray, & Kissoon, 2007)	Canada	British Columbia Children's Hospital (BCCH)	To determine what aspects of PED (Pediatric ED) activity could be modified to improve patient flow, reduce patient wait time, and increase staff efficiency and morale.	Arena	NO
(Yeh & Lin, 2007)	Taiwan	Show-Chwan Memorial Hospital	To appropriately adjust nurses' schedules without hiring additional staff.	eM-Plant	NO
(Hoot et al., 2008)	N/A	No name.	To forecast near-future operating conditions, and to validate the forecasts using several measures of ED crowding.	Standard C programming language	NO
(Khadem et al., 2008)	Oman	A public hospital, no name.	(1) Improving patient satisfaction through minimizing patient wait time, and (2) Expanding the capacity of the ED.	MedModel	NO
(Khurma, Bacioiu, & Pasek, 2008)	Canada	No name.	To increase the flow throughout the ED by introducing Lean and process improvement methodologies.	ProModel	NO
(Storrow et al., 2008)	USA	No name.	To determine the effect of decreasing turnaround times on emergency medical services (EMS) diversion, ED patient throughput, and total ED length of stay.	N/A	NO

continued on following page

Table 3. Continued

Reference	Country	Hospital Name	Objectives	Simulation tool	Imple-mented?
(Xu et al., 2008)	Canada	The Foothills Medical Centre in the Calgary	To test different ED physician management strategies, work practices, and alternative shift schedules to determine their impact on patient wait time in the ED.	Arena	NO
(Ahmed & Alkhamis, 2009)	Kuwait	A government hospital, no name.	To evaluate the impact of various staffing levels on service efficiency	SIMISCRIPT	NO
(Holm & Dahl, 2009)	Norway	Akershus University Hospital	To estimate the effect replacing nurse triage with a physician on patient wait time.	Flexsim Healthcare	NO
(Maulla et al., 2009)	UK	No name.	To evaluate the impact that a fast-track strategy in ED has on patient wait time.	N/A	YES
(Shim & Kumar, 2010)	Singapore	Tan Tock Seng Hospital	Reengineering emergency care process to improve patient wait time.	SIMUL8	NO
(Coughlan, Eatock, & Patel, 2011)	UK	A district general hospital in West London	To determine the impact a re-prioritization strategy has on the 4-hour target.	SIMUL8	NO
(Eskandari et al., 2011)	Iran	A government hospital, no name.	To identify and overcome bottlenecks that lead to long wait times of different patient types.	Arena	NO
(Friesen et al., 2011)	Canada	Different hospitals.	To investigate the application of existing available data and emerging data feeds towards developing an auxiliary ED process control strategy.	N/A	NO
(Weng, Tsai, et al., 2011)	Taiwan	Large teaching hospital center, no name.	To develop and deploy a mixed method incorporating DES and DEA to evaluate potential bottlenecks, maximize throughput flows, and identify solutions in reducing patient time in the ED while also increasing patient satisfaction.	Arena	NO
(Weng, Cheng, et al., 2011)	Taiwan	A medical center in Taiwan, no name.	To improve the flow of the ED by increasing the quality of treatment.	SIMUL8	NO
(Cabrera et al., 2012)	Spain	The Hospital of Sabadell	To identify the combination numbers of staff members of ED that optimize its performance.	NetLogo	NO
(Rasheed et al., 2012)	Korea	Hospital located in Seoul.	To assess the effects of an ED load relief area creation on ED effectiveness and service quality.	Arena	NO
(Chonde et al., 2013)	USA	No name.	To improve resource management strategies to combat the increasing costs of healthcare and overutilization of EDs.	Simio	NO

continued on following page

Table 3. Continued

Reference	Country	Hospital Name	Objectives	Simulation tool	Imple-mented?
(Day et al., 2013)	USA	St. Louis Veterans Affairs Medical Center	(1) To determine the effects of adding a provider in triage on the average length of stay (LOS) and proportion of patients with >6 h LOS, and (2) To assess the accuracy of computer simulation in predicting the magnitude of such effects on these metrics.	AnyLogic Professional	YES
(Konrad et al., 2013)	USA	Saint Vincent Hospital in Worcester	To evaluate the impact on patient throughput arising from different split-flow configurations.	Arena	YES
(Lim et al., 2013)	Canada	No name.	To present an alternative approach where physicians and their delegates in the ED are modeled as interacting pseudo-agents in a discrete event simulation and to compare it with the traditional approach ignoring such interactions.	Arena	NO
(Salimifard et al., 2013)	Iran	A general hospital in the city of Yazd, no name.	To improve ED processes, in order to solve the crowding problem.	Colored Petri Nets	NO
(Tan, Tan, & Lau, 2013)	Singapore	Local Hospital, no name.	To intelligently adjust the number of doctors based on current and historical information about the patient arrival.	N/A	NO
(Wang et al., 2013)	Canada	St. Mary's General Hospital	To study the impact of physician behaviors on the ED wait time performances.	Arena	NO
(Venugopal et al., 2013)	USA	A major emergency department in Melbourne, Florida.	To understand the ED system's behavior under different alternative staffing solutions.	Arena	NO
(Ahmad et al., 2014)	Malaysia	A government Hospital, no name.	To study patient flows and the complex interactions among hospital resources for ED operations	AnyLogic	NO
(Crawford et al., 2014)	USA	Generic model of an acute care hospital	To analyze the effect of discharge timing on several ED related measures and the number of readmissions.	Arena	NO
(Doan et al., 2014)	Canada	British Columbia Children's Hospital (BCCH)	To compare the effect on key pediatric ED efficiency indicators of extending physician coverage versus adding Physician Assistants with equivalent incremental costs.	Arena	NO
(Kang, Nembhard, Rafferty, & Deflitch, 2014)	USA	Hershey Medical Center.	To investigate the effect of admission process policies on patient flow in the ED.	Simio	NO

continued on following page

Table 3. Continued

Reference	Country	Hospital Name	Objectives	Simulation tool	Imple-mented?
(Kim et al., 2014)	USA	No name.	To explore different characteristics between ED pediatric and adult patient groups regarding process flow times and acuities, and to investigate developing pediatric EDs	Arena	NO
(Kuo, 2014)	Hong Kong	The Prince of Wales Hospital (PWH)	To explore different physician schedules iteratively to look for a good solution.	Arena	NO
(Al-Ajeel et al., 2015)	Kuwait	A government hospital, no name.	To determine the minimum number of staff needed to reduce the wait time during sandstorms without affecting the efficiency of the ED and its processes.	Arena	NO
(Kuo et al., 2015)	Hong Kong	The Prince of Wales Hospital (PWH)	To examine the effect of physician heterogeneity on the ED performance.	Arena	NO
(Malavisi, Cimellaro, Terzic, & Mahin, 2015)	Italy	Umberto I Mauriziano Hospital	To develop a simplified model in order to describe ED behavior during emergencies	ProModel	NO
(Zeinali et al., 2015)	Iran	Modarres Hospital	To improve the patient flow and relieve congestion by changing the number of ED resources (i.e., the number of receptionists, nurses, residents, and beds).	Arena	YES
(Cocke et al., 2016)	USA	University of Virginia (UVA) Medical Center	To examine whether the future ED facility would be able to handle the upcoming yearly demand and how different resource schedules would affect the average length of stay and average arrival to provider times.	Arena	NO

Index

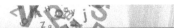

Purchase Print, E-Book, or Print + E-Book

IGI Global books are available in three unique pricing formats:
Print Only, E-Book Only, or Print + E-Book. Shipping fees apply.

www.igi-global.com

Recommended Reference Books

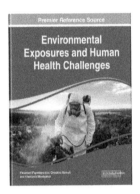

ISBN: 978-1-5225-7635-8
© 2019; 449 pp.
List Price: $255

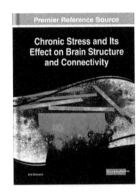

ISBN: 978-1-5225-7513-9
© 2019; 318 pp.
List Price: $225

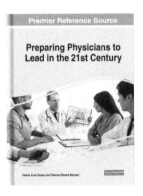

ISBN: 978-1-5225-7576-4
© 2019; 245 pp.
List Price: $245

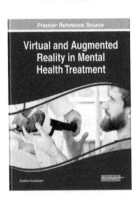

ISBN: 978-1-5225-7168-1
© 2019; 329 pp.
List Price: $265

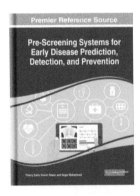

ISBN: 978-1-5225-7131-5
© 2019; 395 pp.
List Price: $245

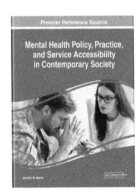

ISBN: 978-1-5225-7402-6
© 2019; 323 pp.
List Price: $245

Do you want to stay current on the latest research trends, product announcements, news and special offers?
Join IGI Global's mailing list today and start enjoying exclusive perks sent only to IGI Global members.
Add your name to the list at **www.igi-global.com/newsletters**.

Publisher of Peer-Reviewed, Timely, and Innovative Academic Research

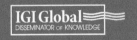

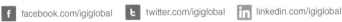

www.igi-global.com   Sign up at www.igi-global.com/newsletters   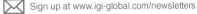 facebook.com/igiglobal   twitter.com/igiglobal   linkedin.com/igiglobal

Ensure Quality Research is Introduced to the Academic Community

Become an IGI Global Reviewer for Authored Book Projects

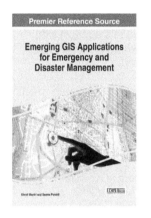

Premier Reference Source

Emerging GIS Applications for Emergency and Disaster Management

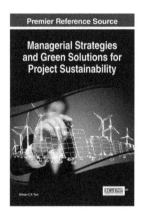

Premier Reference Source

Managerial Strategies and Green Solutions for Project Sustainability

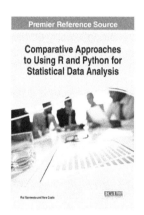

Premier Reference Source

Comparative Approaches to Using R and Python for Statistical Data Analysis

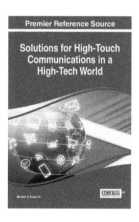

Premier Reference Source

Solutions for High-Touch Communications in a High-Tech World

The overall success of an authored book project is dependent on quality and timely reviews.

In this competitive age of scholarly publishing, constructive and timely feedback significantly expedites the turnaround time of manuscripts from submission to acceptance, allowing the publication and discovery of forward-thinking research at a much more expeditious rate. Several IGI Global authored book projects are currently seeking highly-qualified experts in the field to fill vacancies on their respective editorial review boards:

Applications and Inquiries may be sent to:
development@igi-global.com

Applicants must have a doctorate (or an equivalent degree) as well as publishing and reviewing experience. Reviewers are asked to complete the open-ended evaluation questions with as much detail as possible in a timely, collegial, and constructive manner. All reviewers' tenures run for one-year terms on the editorial review boards and are expected to complete at least three reviews per term. Upon successful completion of this term, reviewers can be considered for an additional term.

If you have a colleague that may be interested in this opportunity, we encourage you to share this information with them.

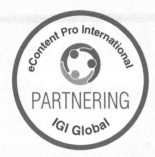

IGI Global Proudly Partners With eContent Pro International

Receive a 25% Discount on all Editorial Services

Editorial Services

IGI Global expects all final manuscripts submitted for publication to be in their final form. This means they must be reviewed, revised, and professionally copy edited prior to their final submission. Not only does this support with accelerating the publication process, but it also ensures that the highest quality scholarly work can be disseminated.

English Language Copy Editing

Let eContent Pro International's expert copy editors perform edits on your manuscript to resolve spelling, punctuaion, grammar, syntax, flow, formatting issues and more.

Scientific and Scholarly Editing

Allow colleagues in your research area to examine the content of your manuscript and provide you with valuable feedback and suggestions before submission.

Figure, Table, Chart & Equation Conversions

Do you have poor quality figures? Do you need visual elements in your manuscript created or converted? A design expert can help!

Translation

Need your documjent translated into English? eContent Pro International's expert translators are fluent in English and more than 40 different languages.

Hear What Your Colleagues are Saying About Editorial Services Supported by IGI Global

"The service was very fast, very thorough, and very helpful in ensuring our chapter meets the criteria and requirements of the book's editors. I was quite impressed and happy with your service."

– Prof. Tom Brinthaupt,
Middle Tennessee State University, USA

"I found the work actually spectacular. The editing, formatting, and other checks were very thorough. The turnaround time was great as well. I will definitely use eContent Pro in the future."

– Nickanor Amwata, Lecturer,
University of Kurdistan Hawler, Iraq

"I was impressed that it was done timely, and wherever the content was not clear for the reader, the paper was improved with better readability for the audience."

– Prof. James Chilembwe,
Mzuzu University, Malawi

Email: customerservice@econtentpro.com   www.igi-global.com/editorial-service-partners

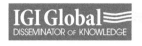

www.igi-global.com

Celebrating Over 30 Years of Scholarly
Knowledge Creation & Dissemination

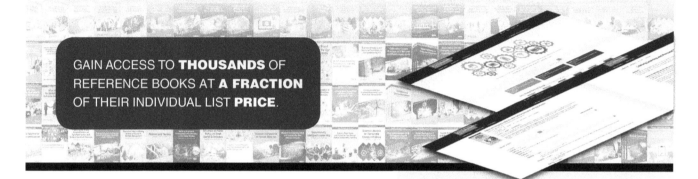

InfoSci®-Books

A Database of Over 5,300+ Reference Books Containing Over 100,000+ Chapters Focusing on Emerging Research

GAIN ACCESS TO **THOUSANDS** OF REFERENCE BOOKS AT **A FRACTION** OF THEIR INDIVIDUAL LIST **PRICE**.

InfoSci®-Books Database

The **InfoSci®-Books** database is a collection of over 5,300+ IGI Global single and multi-volume reference books, handbooks of research, and encyclopedias, encompassing groundbreaking research from prominent experts worldwide that span over 350+ topics in 11 core subject areas including business, computer science, education, science and engineering, social sciences and more.

Open Access Fee Waiver (Offset Model) Initiative

For any library that invests in IGI Global's InfoSci-Journals and/ or InfoSci-Books databases, IGI Global will match the library's investment with a fund of equal value to go toward **subsidizing the OA article processing charges (APCs) for their students, faculty, and staff** at that institution when their work is submitted and accepted under OA into an IGI Global journal.*

INFOSCI® PLATFORM FEATURES

- No DRM
- No Set-Up or Maintenance Fees
- A Guarantee of No More Than a 5% Annual Increase
- Full-Text HTML and PDF Viewing Options
- Downloadable MARC Records
- Unlimited Simultaneous Access
- COUNTER 5 Compliant Reports
- Formatted Citations With Ability to Export to RefWorks and EasyBib
- No Embargo of Content (Research is Available Months in Advance of the Print Release)

*The fund will be offered on an annual basis and expire at the end of the subscription period. The fund would renew as the subscription is renewed for each year thereafter. The open access fees will be waived after the student, faculty, or staff's paper has been vetted and accepted into an IGI Global journal and the fund can only be used toward publishing OA in an IGI Global journal. Libraries in developing countries will have the match on their investment doubled.

To Learn More or To Purchase This Database:
www.igi-global.com/infosci-books

eresources@igi-global.com • Toll Free: 1-866-342-6657 ext. 100 • Phone: 717-533-8845 x100

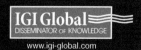

www.igi-global.com

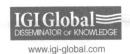

www.igi-global.com

Publisher of Peer-Reviewed, Timely, and
Innovative Academic Research Since 1988

IGI Global's Transformative Open Access (OA) Model:
How to Turn Your University Library's Database Acquisitions Into a Source of OA Funding

In response to the OA movement and well in advance of Plan S, IGI Global, early last year, unveiled their OA Fee Waiver (Offset Model) Initiative.

Under this initiative, librarians who invest in IGI Global's InfoSci-Books (5,300+ reference books) and/or InfoSci-Journals (185+ scholarly journals) databases will be able to subsidize their patron's OA article processing charges (APC) when their work is submitted and accepted (after the peer review process) into an IGI Global journal.*

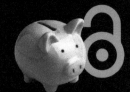

How Does it Work?

1. When a library subscribes or perpetually purchases IGI Global's InfoSci-Databases including InfoSci-Books (5,300+ e-books), InfoSci-Journals (185+ e-journals), and/or their discipline/subject-focused subsets, IGI Global will match the library's investment with a fund of equal value to go toward subsidizing the OA article processing charges (APCs) for their patrons.

   Researchers: Be sure to recommend the InfoSci-Books and InfoSci-Journals to take advantage of this initiative.

2. When a student, faculty, or staff member submits a paper and it is accepted (following the peer review) into one of IGI Global's 185+ scholarly journals, the author will have the option to have their paper published under a traditional publishing model or as OA.

3. When the author chooses to have their paper published under OA, IGI Global will notify them of the OA Fee Waiver (Offset Model) Initiative. If the author decides they would like to take advantage of this initiative, IGI Global will deduct the US$ 1,500 APC from the created fund.

4. This fund will be offered on an annual basis and will renew as the subscription is renewed for each year thereafter. IGI Global will manage the fund and award the APC waivers unless the librarian has a preference as to how the funds should be managed.

Hear From the Experts on This Initiative:

"I'm very happy to have been able to make one of my recent research contributions, 'Visualizing the Social Media Conversations of a National Information Technology Professional Association' featured in the *International Journal of Human Capital and Information Technology Professionals*, freely available along with having access to the valuable resources found within IGI Global's InfoSci-Journals database."

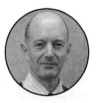

– Prof. Stuart Palmer,
Deakin University, Australia

For More Information, Visit: www.igi-global.com/publish/contributor-resources/open-access or contact IGI Global's Database Team at eresources@igi-global.com.

Are You Ready to Publish Your Research?

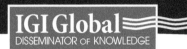

IGI Global offers book authorship and editorship opportunities across 11 subject areas, including business, computer science, education, science and engineering, social sciences, and more!

Benefits of Publishing with IGI Global:

- Free one-on-one editorial and promotional support.

- Expedited publishing timelines that can take your book from start to finish in less than one (1) year.

- Choose from a variety of formats including: Edited and Authored References, Handbooks of Research, Encyclopedias, and Research Insights.

- Utilize IGI Global's eEditorial Discovery® submission system in support of conducting the submission and blind review process.

- IGI Global maintains a strict adherence to ethical practices due in part to our full membership with the Committee on Publication Ethics (COPE).

- Indexing potential in prestigious indices such as Scopus®, Web of Science™, PsycINFO®, and ERIC – Education Resources Information Center.

- Ability to connect your ORCID iD to your IGI Global publications.

- Earn royalties on your publication as well as receive complimentary copies and exclusive discounts.

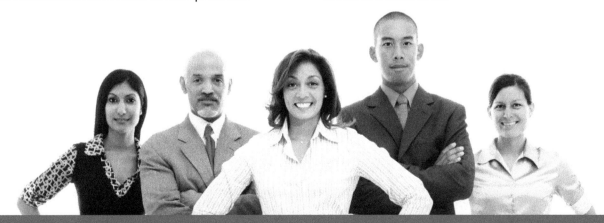

Get Started Today by Contacting the Acquisitions Department at:

acquisition@igi-global.com

Lightning Source UK Ltd.
Milton Keynes UK
UKHW051337121221
395490UK00002B/67